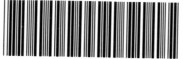

369 0246766

Handbook of Parkinson's Disease

Handbook of Parkinson's Disease

Fifth Edition

Edited by

Rajesh Pahwa, MD

Laverne and Joyce Rider Professor of Neurology
Director, Parkinson's Disease and Movement Disorder Center
University of Kansas Medical Center
Kansas City, Kansas, USA

Kelly E. Lyons, PhD

Research Professor of Neurology
Director of Research and Education
Parkinson's Disease and Movement Disorder Center
University of Kansas Medical Center
Kansas City, Kansas, USA

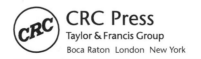

CRC Press
Taylor & Francis Group
Boca Raton London New York

CRC Press is an imprint of the
Taylor & Francis Group, an **informa** business

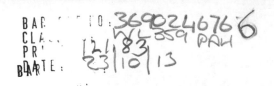

CRC Press
Taylor & Francis Group
6000 Broken Sound Parkway NW, Suite 300
Boca Raton, FL 33487-2742

© 2013 by Taylor & Francis Group, LLC
CRC Press is an imprint of Taylor & Francis Group, an Informa business

No claim to original U.S. Government works

Printed on acid-free paper
Version Date: 20130313

International Standard Book Number-13: 978-1-84184-908-9 (Hardback)

This book contains information obtained from authentic and highly regarded sources. While all reasonable efforts have been made to publish reliable data and information, neither the author[s] nor the publisher can accept any legal responsibility or liability for any errors or omissions that may be made. The publishers wish to make clear that any views or opinions expressed in this book by individual editors, authors or contributors are personal to them and do not necessarily reflect the views/opinions of the publishers. The information or guidance contained in this book is intended for use by medical, scientific or health-care professionals and is provided strictly as a supplement to the medical or other professional's own judgement, their knowledge of the patient's medical history, relevant manufacturer's instructions and the appropriate best practice guidelines. Because of the rapid advances in medical science, any information or advice on dosages, procedures or diagnoses should be independently verified. The reader is strongly urged to consult the drug companies' printed instructions, and their websites, before administering any of the drugs recommended in this book. This book does not indicate whether a particular treatment is appropriate or suitable for a particular individual. Ultimately it is the sole responsibility of the medical professional to make his or her own professional judgements, so as to advise and treat patients appropriately. The authors and publishers have also attempted to trace the copyright holders of all material reproduced in this publication and apologize to copyright holders if permission to publish in this form has not been obtained. If any copyright material has not been acknowledged please write and let us know so we may rectify in any future reprint.

Except as permitted under U.S. Copyright Law, no part of this book may be reprinted, reproduced, transmitted, or utilized in any form by any electronic, mechanical, or other means, now known or hereafter invented, including photocopying, microfilming, and recording, or in any information storage or retrieval system, without written permission from the publishers.

For permission to photocopy or use material electronically from this work, please access www.copyright.com (http://www.copyright.com/) or contact the Copyright Clearance Center, Inc. (CCC), 222 Rosewood Drive, Danvers, MA 01923, 978-750-8400. CCC is a not-for-profit organization that provides licenses and registration for a variety of users. For organizations that have been granted a photocopy license by the CCC, a separate system of payment has been arranged.

Trademark Notice: Product or corporate names may be trademarks or registered trademarks, and are used only for identification and explanation without intent to infringe.

Visit the Taylor & Francis Web site at
http://www.taylorandfrancis.com

and the CRC Press Web site at
http://www.crcpress.com

Contents

Contributors

Bastiaan R. Bloem   Donders Institute of Brain & Cognition, Department of Neurology, Radboud University Nijmegen Medical Centre, Nijmegen, the Netherlands

David J. Brooks   Hartnett Professor of Neurology, Hammersmith Hospital, Imperial College London, London, UK

K. Ray Chaudhuri   National Parkinson Foundation International Centre of Excellence, Centre Principal Investigator, MRC Centre of Neurodegeneration Research, King's College London, Kings College Hospital and University Hospital Lewisham, London, UK

Jack J. Chen   Movement Disorders Center, Schools of Medicine and Pharmacy, Loma Linda University, Loma Linda, California, USA

Shilpa Chitnis   Department of Neurology and Neurotherapeutics, UT Southwestern Medical Center, Dallas, Texas, USA

Kelvin L. Chou   Departments of Neurology and Neurosurgery, University of Michigan, Ann Arbor, Michigan, USA

Joseph S. Chung   Department of Neurology, Southern California Kaiser Permanente, Los Angeles, California, USA

Arif Dalvi   Department of Neurology, NorthShore University Health System, Glenview, Illinois, USA

Khashayar Dashtipour   Division of Movement Disorders, Department of Neurology, Loma Linda University School of Medicine, Loma Linda, California, USA

Richard B. Dewey Jr.   Department of Neurology and Neurotherapeutics, UT Southwestern Medical Center, Dallas, Texas, USA

Dennis W. Dickson   Robert E. Jacoby Professor of Alzheimer's Research, Department of Neuroscience, Mayo Clinic, Jacksonville, Florida, USA

Jill Giordano Farmer   Capital Institute for Neuroscience, Pennington, New Jersey, USA

Hubert H. Fernandez   Center of Neurological Restoration, Cleveland Clinic Foundation, Cleveland, Ohio, USA

Julie A. Fields   Department of Psychiatry and Psychology, Mayo Clinic College of Medicine, Rochester, Minnesota, USA

Cynthia Fox   National Center for Voice and Speech, Denver, Colorado, USA

Shinsuke Fujioka   Department of Neurology, Mayo Clinic, Jacksonville, Florida, USA

Christopher G. Goetz   Professor of Neurological Sciences, Rush University Medical Center, Chicago, Illinois, USA

Robert A. Hauser   Parkinson's Disease and Movement Disorders Center, National Parkinson Foundation Center of Excellence, Byrd Institute, University of South Florida, Tampa, Florida, USA

Neil M. Issar   School of Medicine, Vanderbilt University, Nashville, Tennessee, USA

Michael W. Jakowec   Department of Neurology, Keck School of Medicine, University of Southern California, Los Angeles, California, USA

Joseph Jankovic   Parkinson's Disease Center and Movement Disorders Clinic, Department of Neurology, Baylor College of Medicine, Houston, Texas, USA

Cherian Abraham Karunapuzha   Department of Neurology, The University of Oklahoma Health Sciences Center, Oklahoma City, Oklahoma, USA

Samyra H.J. Keus   Department of Neurology, Nijmegen Centre for Evidence Based Practice, Radboud University Nijmegen Medical Centre, Nijmegen, the Netherlands

Pravin Khemani   Department of Neurology and Neurotherapeutics, UT Southwestern Medical Center, Dallas, Texas, USA

Daniel E. Kremens   Department of Neurology, Jefferson Medical College of Thomas Jefferson University, Philadelphia, Pennsylvania, USA

Mark F. Lew   Division of Movement Disorders, Keck School of Medicine, University of Southern California, Los Angeles, California, USA

Thien Thien Lim   Center of Neurological Restoration, Cleveland Clinic Foundation, Cleveland, Ohio, USA

Raymond Y. Lo   Buddhist Tzu Chi General Hospital, Department of Neurology, Hualien, Taiwan

Kelly E. Lyons   Parkinson's Disease and Movement Disorder Center, Department of Neurology, University of Kansas Medical Center, Kansas City, Kansas, USA

Raja Mehanna   Parkinson's Disease Center and Movement Disorders Clinic, Department of Neurology, Baylor College of Medicine, Houston, Texas, USA

Shyamal H. Mehta   Movement Disorder Program, Department of Neurology, Georgia Health Sciences University, Augusta, Georgia, USA

Kulthida Methawasin   Department of Neurology, Parkinson's Disease and Movement Disorders Centre, National Neuroscience Institute, Singapore

M. Tanya Mitra   King's College Hospital and University Hospital, Lewisham, London, UK

Erwin B. Montgomery Jr.   Dr. Sigmund Rosen Scholar in Neurology, Division of Movement Disorders, Department of Neurology, University of Alabama at Birmingham School of Medicine, Birmigham, Alabama, USA

John C. Morgan   Movement Disorder Program, Department of Neurology, Georgia Health Sciences University, Augusta, Georgia, USA

Pouya Movahed   Division of Psychiatry, University Hospital, Lund, Sweden and National Parkinson Foundation International Centre of Excellence, King's College Hospital, London, UK

Marten Munneke   Department of Neurology, Nijmegen Centre for Evidence Based Practice, Radboud University Nijmegen Medical Centre, Nijmegen, the Netherlands

Jules M. Nazzaro   Departments of Neurology, Neurosurgery and Molecular and Integrative Physiology, University of Kansas Medical Center, Kansas City, Kansas, USA

Joseph S. Neimat   Department of Neurological Surgery, Vanderbilt University Medical Center, Nashville, Tennessee, USA

Gill Nelson   Division of Biostatistics and Epidemiology, School of Public Health, Faculty of Health Sciences, University of the Witwatersrand, Parktown, South Africa

Fernando L. Pagan   Department of Neurology, Georgetown University, Washington, DC, USA

Rajesh Pahwa   Parkinson's Disease and Movement Disorder Center, Department of Neurology, University of Kansas Medical Center, Kansas City, Kansas, USA

Giselle M. Petzinger   Section for Movement Disorders, Department of Neurology, Keck School of Medicine, University of Southern California, Los Angeles, California, USA

Ronald F. Pfeiffer   Department of Neurology, University of Tennessee Health Science Center, Memphis, Tennessee, USA

Brad A. Racette   Department of Neurology, Washington University School of Medicine, St. Louis, Missouri, USA

Alex Rajput   Division of Neurology, Royal University Hospital, University of Saskatchewan, Saskatoon, Saskatchewan, Canada

Lorraine Olson Ramig   Department of Speech, Language, Hearing Sciences, University of Colorado-Boulder, and National Center for Voice and Speech, Denver, Colorado, USA

Owen A. Ross   Department of Neuroscience, Mayo Clinic, Jacksonville, Florida, USA

David Salat   Universitat Autònoma de Barcelona, Barcelona, Spain

Shimon Sapir   Department of Communication Sciences and Disorders, Faculty of Social Welfare and Health Studies, University of Haifa, Haifa, Israel

Kapil D. Sethi   Movement Disorder Program, Department of Neurology, Georgia Health Sciences University, Augusta, Georgia, USA

Mark Stacy   Division of Neurology, Duke University Medical School, Durham, North Carolina, USA

Ingrid H.W.M. Sturkenboom   Department of Rehabilitation–Occupational Therapy, Nijmegen Centre for Evidence Based Practice, Radboud University Nijmegen Medical Centre, Nijmegen, the Netherlands

Christina Sundal   Department of Neurology, Mayo Clinic, Jacksonville, Florida, USA

Valerie Suski   Division of Neurology, University of Pittsburgh Medical Center, Pittsburgh, Pennsylvania, USA

Louis C.S. Tan   Department of Neurology, Parkinson's Disease and Movement Disorders Centre, National Neuroscience Institute, Singapore

Caroline M. Tanner   The Parkinson's Institute and Clinical Center, Department of Clinical Research, Sunnyvale, California, USA

Eduardo Tolosa   University of Barcelona, Barcelona, Spain

Alexander I. Tröster   Barrow Center for Neuromodulation and Muhammad Ali Parkinson Center, Barrow Neurological Institute, Phoenix, Arizona, USA

Zbigniew K. Wszolek   Department of Neurology, Mayo Clinic, Jacksonville, Florida, USA

Allan D. Wu   Division of Movement Disorders, Department of Neurology, David Geffen School of Medicine, University of California–Los Angeles, Los Angeles, California, USA

Theresa Zesiewicz   Frances J. Zesiewicz Foundation for Parkinson's Disease, Department of Neurology, University of South Florida, Tampa, Florida, USA

Foreword

The diagnosis and management of Parkinson's disease (PD) remains an ongoing challenge to clinicians of many specialties, particularly neurologists. The aging of our population and the wider recognition of the early symptoms of disease have put PD in the forefront of neurologic disorders. Furthermore, advancements in our understanding of disease mechanisms, the changing nosology of PD, and new additions to our therapeutic arsenal underscore the importance of an up-to-date comprehensive review of the state of the field.

The *Handbook of Parkinson's Disease* is now in its fifth edition. Previous editions have been comprehensive, current, and invaluable to both clinicians and basic scientists interested in PD. Yet even in the last several years, there has been a wealth of new information affecting our approach to PD. One example is our recognition of PD as a widespread disorder of the central and autonomic nervous system with extranigral pathology occurring early in the disease process. This has fueled the search for markers of PD that may be detected before neurologic symptoms emerge. A new chapter on pre-motor symptoms addresses this unique topic and lays the groundwork for an entirely new approach to disease modification. The neuroimaging of PD has also gone through a major evolution and new tools for imaging the dopamine system are now commercially available and will potentially alter our approach to early diagnosis. Similarly, advances in genetics have not only led to the recognition of new genetic causes of parkinsonism but have also expanded molecular biologic studies of the mechanisms of neurodegeneration in PD.

Although these advances will pave the way for novel therapeutic strategies to meaningfully impact the natural history of PD, the increasing number of treatments available now necessitates a more complex and comprehensive approach to patient care. The many nondopaminergic and dopaminergic drugs must be balanced in an individual patient to maximize improvement in symptoms and minimize long-term levodopa-related complications. Individual patients must be assessed for the myriad of nonmotor problems that affect disability and clinicians must be aware of the variable approaches now available to treat these common features, which can include a range of neurobehavioral problems, such as depression, personality changes, and dementia. The availability of surgical options has provided yet another dimension of care for many patients with motor complications.

The fifth edition of the *Handbook of Parkinson's Disease* addresses these many facets of PD. It is a comprehensive review of all aspects of PD, including diagnosis, early manifestations, genetics and epidemiology, motor and nonmotor management, surgical treatments, investigational treatments, and important basic science issues, including genetics and animal models. Finally, a more expansive view of nonpharmacologic approaches, including physical and occupational therapy, considerably enhances this version of the Handbook. It is an invaluable resource for anyone involved in PD care and research.

Matthew B. Stern, M.D.
Parker Family Professor of Neurology
Director, Parkinson's Disease and Movement Disorders Center
University of Pennsylvania

1 Early iconography of Parkinson's disease

Christopher G. Goetz

Parkinson's disease was first described in a medical context in 1817 by James Parkinson, a general practitioner in London. Numerous essays have been written about Parkinson himself and the early history of Parkinson's disease (*Paralysis agitans*), or the shaking palsy. Rather than repeat or resynthesize such prior studies, this introductory chapter focuses on a number of historical visual documents with descriptive legends. Some of these are available in prior publications, but the entire collection has not been previously presented. As a group, they present materials largely from the 19th century and very early 20th century and will serve as a base on which the subsequent chapters that cover progress of the 20th and budding 21st centuries are built. In 2005, as part of the Movement Disorder Society Annual International Congress, an extensive history exhibit was developed and this chapter's material is based in part on this exhibit.

HISTORICAL AND LITERARY PRECEDENTS

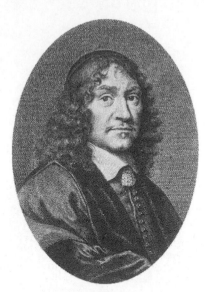

FIGURE 1.1   **Franciscus de le Boë (1614–1672).**   Also known as Sylvius de le Boë, and Franciscus Sylvius, this early physician was Professor of Leiden and a celebrated anatomist. In his medical writings, he also described tremor and he may be among the very earliest writers on involuntary movement disorders (1). (All figures are from the private collection of Christopher G. Goetz, MD, Chicago, IL, unless otherwise noted.)

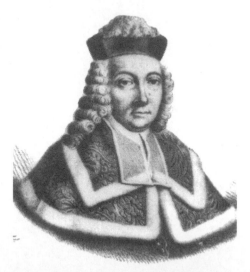

FIGURE 1.2   **François Boissier de Sauvages de la Croix (1706–1767).**   Sauvages was cited by Parkinson himself and described patients with "running disturbances of the limbs", *scelotyrbe festinans*. Such subjects had difficulty walking, moving with short and hasty steps. He considered the problem due to diminished flexibility of muscle fibers, possibly his manner of describing rigidity (1,2).

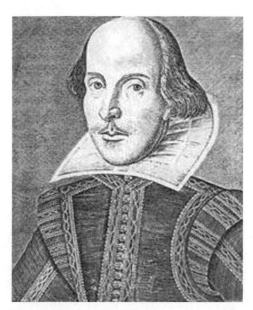

FIGURE 1.3 William Shakespeare. A brilliant medical observer and writer, Shakespeare described many neurologic conditions, including epilepsy, somnambulism, and dementia. In *Henry VI*, first produced in 1590, the character, Dick, notices that Say is trembling: "Why dost thou quiver, man," he asks, and Say responds, "The palsy and not fear provokes me" (1). Jean-Martin Charcot frequently cited Shakespeare in his medical lectures and classroom presentations and disputed the concept that tremor was a natural accompaniment of normal aging. He rejected "senile tremor" as a separate nosographic entity. After reviewing his data from the Salpêtrière service where 2000 elderly inpatients lived, he turned to Shakespeare's renditions of elderly figures: "Do not commit the error that many others do and misrepresent tremor as a natural accompaniment of old age. Remember that our venerated Dean, Dr. Chevreul, today 102 years old, has no tremor whatsoever. And you must remember in his marvelous descriptions of old age (*Henry IV* and *As You Like It*), the master observer, Shakespeare, never speaks of tremor" (3,4).

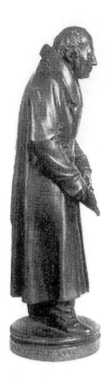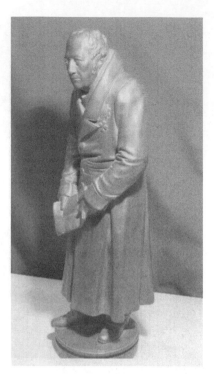

FIGURE 1.4 Wilhelm von Humboldt (1767–1835). The celebrated academic reformer and writer, von Humboldt, lived in the era of Parkinson and described his own neurologic condition in a series of letters, analyzed by Horowski (5). The statue by Friedrich Drake shown in the picture captures the hunched, flexed posture of Parkinson's disease, but von Humboldt's own words capture the tremor and bradykinesia of the disease:

> "Trembling of the hands…occurs only when both or one of them is inactive; at this very moment, for example, only the left one is trembling but not the right one that I am using to write…. If I am using my hands this strange clumsiness starts which is hard to describe. It is obviously weakness as I am unable to carry heavy objects as I did earlier on, but it appears with tasks that do not need strength but consist of quite fine movements, and especially with these. In addition to writing, I can mention rapid opening of books, dividing of fine pages, unbuttoning and buttoning up of clothes. All of these as well as writing proceed with intolerable slowness and clumsiness" (6).

JAMES PARKINSON

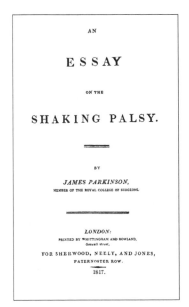

FIGURE 1.5   Front piece of James Parkinson's *an Essay on the Shaking Palsy.*   This short monograph is extremely difficult to find in its original 1817 version, but has been reproduced many times. In the essay, Parkinson describes a small series of subjects with a distinctive constellation of features. Although he had the opportunity to examine a few of the subjects, some of his reflections were based solely on observation (7).

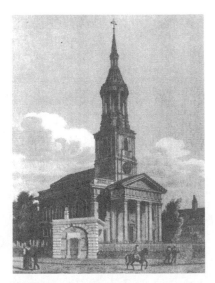

FIGURE 1.6   St. Leonard's Church.   The Shoreditch parish church was closely associated with James Parkinson's life as he was baptized, married and buried there (8).

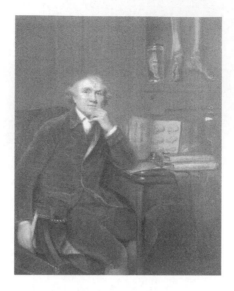

HUNTERIAN REMINISCENCES;

BEING THE SUBSTANCE OF A

COURSE OF LECTURES

ON THE

PRINCIPLES AND PRACTICE OF SURGERY,

DELIVERED BY THE LATE

MR. JOHN HUNTER,

IN THE YEAR 1785:

TAKEN IN SHORT-HAND, AND AFTERWARDS FAIRLY TRANSCRIBED, BY THE LATE

MR. JAMES PARKINSON,
AUTHOR OF "ORGANIC REMAINS OF A FORMER WORLD," &c.

EDITED BY HIS SON,

J. W. K. PARKINSON,
FELLOW OF THE ROYAL COLLEGE OF SURGEONS, IN LONDON:

BY WHOM ARE APPENDED

ILLUSTRATIVE NOTES.

LONDON:
SHERWOOD, GILBERT, AND PIPER, PATERNOSTER ROW.
1833.

FIGURE 1.7 John Hunter. The celebrated physician, Hunter [painted by J. Reynolds (9)] was admired by Parkinson, who transcribed the surgeon's lectures in his 1833 publication called *Hunterian Reminiscences* (10). In these lectures, Hunter offered observations on tremor. The last sentence of Parkinson's *Essay* reads:

> "...but how few can estimate the benefits bestowed on mankind by the labours of Morgagni, Hunter, or Baillie" (7).

Currier has posited that Parkinson's own interest in tremor was first developed under the direct influence of Hunter (11).

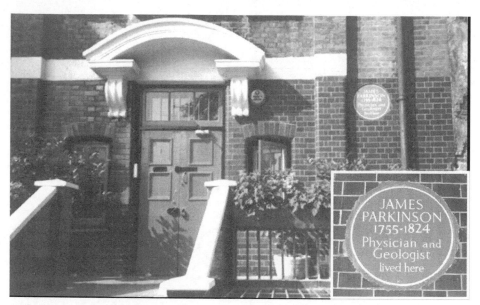

FIGURE 1.8 James Parkinson's home. No. 1 Hoxton Square, London, formerly Shoreditch, today carries a plaque honoring the birthplace of James Parkinson (12). The plaque that hangs by the entrance is shown close-up.

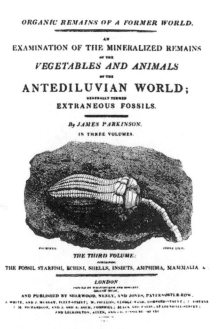

ORGANIC REMAINS OF A FORMER WORLD.

AN

EXAMINATION OF THE MINERALIZED REMAINS

OF THE

VEGETABLES AND ANIMALS

OF THE

ANTEDILUVIAN WORLD;

GENERALLY TERMED

EXTRANEOUS FOSSILS.

By JAMES PARKINSON.

IN THREE VOLUMES.

THE THIRD VOLUME;

CONTAINING

THE FOSSIL STARFISH, ECHINI, SHELLS, INSECTS, AMPHIBIA, MAMMALIA, &.

LONDON

FIGURE 1.9 James Parkinson as paleontologist. An avid geologist and paleontologist, Parkinson published numerous works on fossils, rocks, and minerals (13). He was an honorary member of the Wernerian Society of Natural History of Edinburgh and the Imperial Society of Naturalists of Moscow.

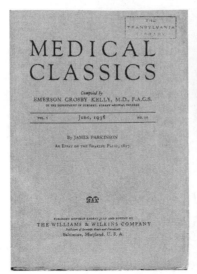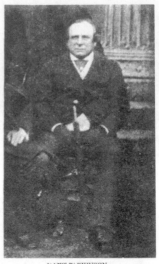

JAMES PARKINSON

FIGURE 1.10   Counterfeit portrait of James Parkinson.   To date, no portrait is known to exist
of James Parkinson. This photograph of a dentist by the same name was erroneously published and
widely circulated in 1938 as part of a *Medical Classics* edition of Parkinson's *Essay* (14). Because
Parkinson died prior to the first daguerreotypes, if a portrait is found, it will be a line drawing, paint-
ing or print. A written description does however exist. The paleontologist, Mantell wrote:

> "Mr. Parkinson was rather below middle stature, with an energetic intellect, and pleas-
> ing expression of countenance and of mild and courteous manners; readily imparting
> information, either on his favourite science or on professional subjects" (8).

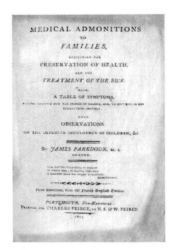

FIGURE 1.11   One of Parkinson's Medical Pamphlets.   As an avid writer, Parkinson compiled
many books and brochures that were widely circulated on basic hygiene and health. His *Medical
Admonitions to Families* and *The Villager's Friend and Physician* were among the most successful,
although he also wrote a children's book on safety entitled *Dangerous Sports* in which he traced the
mishaps of a careless child and lessons he learns through injury (12).

JEAN-MARTIN CHARCOT AND THE SALPÊTRIÈRE SCHOOL

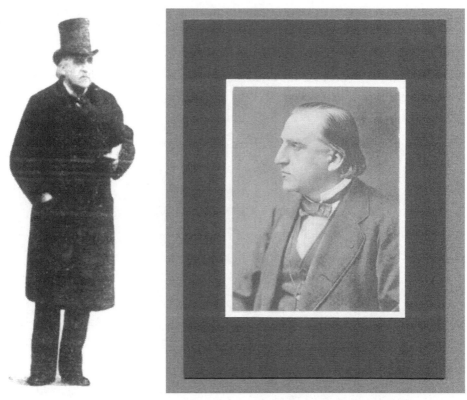

FIGURE 1.12 Jean-Martin Charcot. Working in Paris, in the second half of the 19th century, Charcot knew of Parkinson's description and studied the disorder in the large Salpêtrière hospital that housed elderly and destitute women. He identified the cardinal features of Parkinson's disease and specifically separated bradykinesia from rigidity (4,15):

"Long before rigidity actually develops, patients have significant difficulty performing ordinary activities: this problem relates to another cause. In some of the various patients I showed you, you can easily recognize how difficult it is for them to do things even though rigidity or tremor is not the limiting feature. Instead, even a cursory exam demonstrates that their problem relates more to slowness in execution of movement rather than to real weakness. In spite of tremor, a patient is still able to do most things, but he performs them with remarkable slowness. Between the thought and the action there is a considerable time lapse. One would think neural activity can only be affected after remarkable effort".

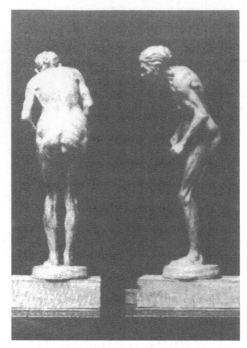

FIGURE 1.13   Statue of a parkinsonian woman by Paul Richer.   Richer worked with Charcot, and as an artist and sculptor produced several works that depicted the habitus, joint deformities, and postural abnormalities of patients with Parkinson's disease (13,16).

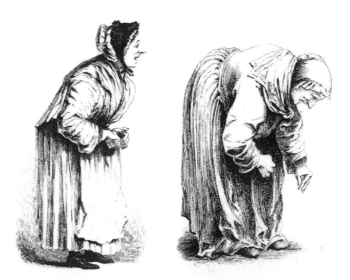

FIGURE 1.14   Evolution of parkinsonian disability.   These figures, drawn by Charcot's student, Paul Richer, capture the deforming posture and progression of untreated Parkinson's disease over a decade (14,17).

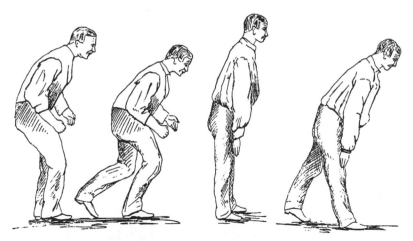

FIGURE 1.15 Parkinson's disease and its variants. Charcot's teaching method involved side-by-side comparisons of patients with various neurologic disorders. In one of his presentations on Parkinson's disease, he showed two subjects, one with the typical or archetypal form of the disorder with hunched posture and flexion (*left*) and another case with atypical parkinsonism, showing an extended posture. The latter habitus is more characteristic of the entity progressive supranuclear palsy, although this disorder was not specifically recognized or labeled by Charcot outside of the term "parkinsonism without tremor" (4).

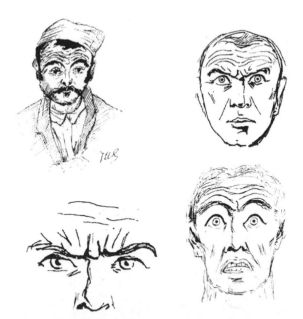

FIGURE 1.16 Atypical parkinsonism. These four drawings, from the same lesson, show the distinctive facial features of patients with atypical Parkinson's disease. (*upper left*) Portrait of Bachère, drawn by Charcot. (*upper right*) Forehead muscles and superior obicularis in simultaneous contraction. (*lower left*) Activation of the palpebral portion of the orbicularis. (*lower right*) Combined activation of frontalis superior portion of the orbicularis and platysma, giving a frightened expression in contrast to the placid, blank stare of typical Parkinson's disease patients (4).

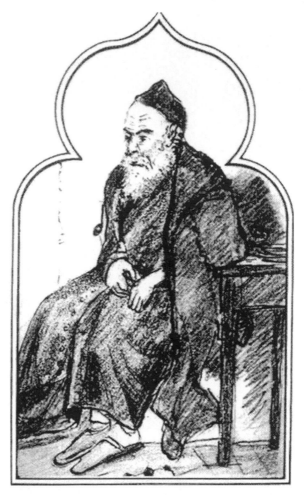

FIGURE 1.17 Charcot's sketch of a parkinsonian subject. Pencil sketch of a man with Parkinson's disease drawn by Charcot during a trip to Morocco in 1889 (18). Referring to the highly stereotyped clinical presentation of Parkinson's disease patients, Charcot told his students:

"I have seen such patients everywhere, in Rome, Amsterdam, Spain, always the same picture. They can be identified from afar. You do not need a medical history" (3,4).

Charcot's medical drawings form a large collection, which is housed at the Bibliothèque Charcot at the Hôpital de la Salpêtrière, Paris.

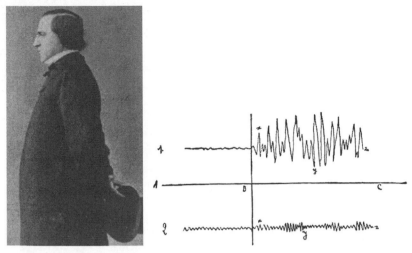

FIGURE 1.18 Charcot and "myographic curves." (*Left*) French neurologist Jean-Martin Charcot (1825–1893). (*Right*) Semi-diagrammatic "myographic curves" published by Charcot in 1887. The top tracing represents an intention tremor in multiple sclerosis. Segment AB indicates "at rest," and BC indicates increasing oscillations during voluntary movement. The lower tracing represents a Parkinsonian tremor. Segment AB indicates a tremor at rest, which persists in segment BC during voluntary movement. Charcot's graphical recording method upon which these drawings were based is not described, but in other circumstances he relied on various pneumatic tambour-like mechanisms (19).

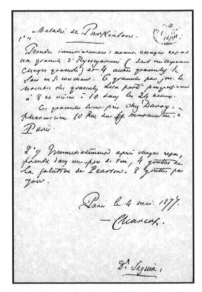

FIGURE 1.19 Treatment of Parkinson's disease. Prescription dated 1877 (20). In treating Parkinson's disease, Charcot used belladonna alkaloids (agents with potent anticholinergic properties) as well as rye-based products that had ergot activity, a feature of some currently available dopamine agonists (20). Charcot's advice was empiric and preceded the recognition of the well-known dopaminergic/cholinergic balance that is implicit to normal striatal neurochemical activity.

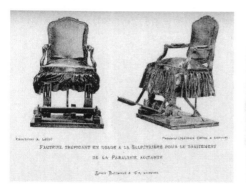 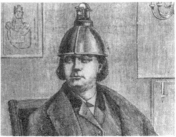

FIGURE 1.20 Vibratory therapy. Charcot observed that patients with Parkinson's disease experienced a reduction in their rest tremor after taking a carriage ride or after horseback riding. He developed a therapeutic vibratory chair that simulated the rhythmic shaking of a carriage (17). A vibratory helmet to shake the head and brain was later developed. Such therapies were not utilized widely, but have been studied with modern equipment in modern times (21).

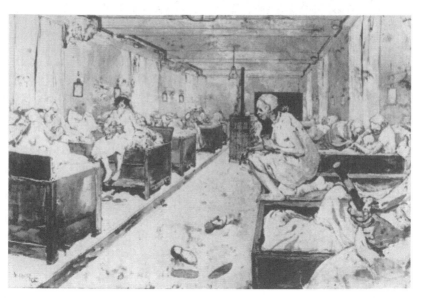

FIGURE 1.21 Dysautonomia in Parkinson's disease. This drawing by Daniel Vierge (1851–1904) shows the Salpêtrière inpatient wards with a single central furnace for heat (17). In this context, Charcot recognized the distinctive dysautonomia of Parkinson's disease, noting how patients experienced a sense of hyperthermia even in the drafty, cold wards of the French hospitals:

> "In the midst of winter (everyone on my service will substantiate this), you can see the parkinsonian patients with no blankets covering them and with only the lightest of clothes on…they feel hot especially around the epigastrium and back, although the face and extremities can also be the focus of their discomfort. When this heated sensation occurs, it is often accompanied by such severe sweating that the sheets and pajamas may need changing. I assure you that regardless of how hot these patients feel or how much they shake, their temperature remains normal" (17).

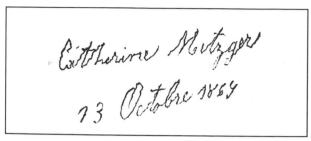

FIGURE 1.22 Micrographia and tremorous handwriting. Charcot recognized that one characteristic feature of Parkinson's disease was the handwriting impairment that included tremorous and tiny script. Charcot collected handwriting samples in his patient charts and used them as part of his diagnostic criteria, thereby separating the large and sloppy script of patients with action tremor from the micrographia of Parkinson's disease (15).

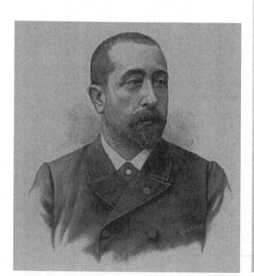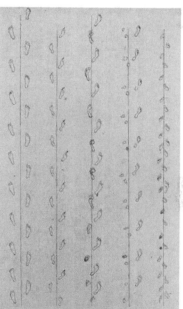

FIGURE 1.23 Gilles de la Tourette and footprint diagrams. (*Left*) French neurologist Georges Gilles de la Tourette (1857–1904). (*Right*) Footprint diagrams from the doctoral thesis of Gilles de la Tourette (1885) entitled *Etudes Cliniques et Physiologiques sur la Marche*. This student work analyzed normal gait as well as the walking patterns of patients with Parkinson's disease, locomotor ataxia, Friedreich's ataxia, and numerous neuropathies.

OTHER NINETEENTH CENTURY CONTRIBUTIONS

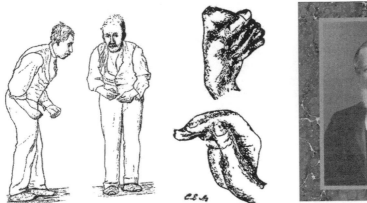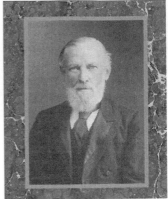

FIGURE 1.24 William Gowers' work. William Gowers' *A Manual of Diseases of the Nervous System* shows sketches of patients with Parkinson's disease (*left*) and diagrams of joint deformities (*right*) (22). More known for written descriptions than visual images, Gowers offered one of the most memorable similes regarding parkinsonian tremor:

> "the movement of the fingers at the metacarpal–phalangeal joints is similar to that by which Orientals beat their small drums" (22).

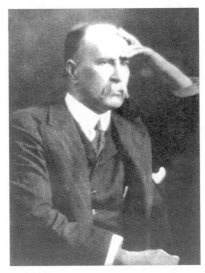

FIGURE 1.25 William Osler. Osler published his celebrated *Principles and Practice of Medicine* in 1892, one year before Charcot's death. As an internist always resistant to the concept of medical specialization, Osler was influential in propagating information to generalists on many neurologic conditions, including Parkinson's disease. Osler was less forthcoming than Charcot in appreciating the distinction between bradykinesia and weakness, and sided with Parkinson in maintaining that mental function was unaltered. Osler was particularly interested in pathologic studies and alluded to the concept of Parkinson's disease as a state of accelerated aging (23).

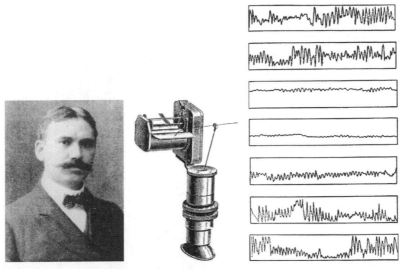

FIGURE 1.26 **Peterson and sphygmograph tracings of tremor.** (*Left*) New York neurologist
Fredrick Peterson (1859–1938). Photograph by courtesy of the National Library of Medicine. (*Middle*)
The Edward sphygmograph utilized by Peterson *c.* 1888. A wire stylus transfers perturbations onto
smoked paper, which moves forward at a fixed speed by clockwork-driven rollers (24). (*Right*) Nega-
tives of Peterson's sphygmographic recordings of tremors (each is 10 sec duration). Peterson's estimates of tremor frequency are generally consistent with modern estimates. These were the most
sophisticated tremor recordings made to this point (25).

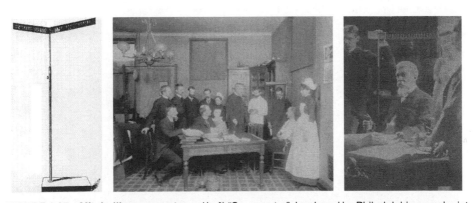

FIGURE 1.27 **Mitchell's sway meter.** (*Left*) "Sway meter" developed by Philadelphia neurologist
Silas Weir Mitchell (1829–1914). It consisted of a pair of graduated rulers oriented perpendicular to
each other and fixed on a stand (26). (*Middle*) Mitchell examining a patient at the Philadelphia
Orthopedic Hospital and Infirmary for Nervous Diseases *c.* 1890. In the background (*right*) is Mitchell's sway meter. In his right hand, Mitchell is holding a reflex hammer invented *c.* 1888 by his assis-
tant, John Madison Taylor (seated, recording Mitchell's observations). Photograph by courtesy of the
Library of the College of Physicians of Philadelphia. (*Right*) Another image of Mitchell at the Philadelphia Orthopedic Hospital and Infirmary for Nervous Diseases. In the background (on Mitchell's
right) a man is leaning on Mitchell's sway meter. Mitchell is holding his Taylor reflex hammer. Photograph by courtesy of the Library of the College of Physicians of Philadelphia.

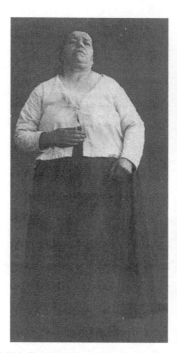 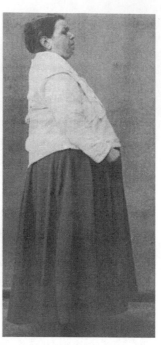

FIGURE 1.28   Progressive supranuclear palsy versus corticobasal degeneration.   Patient presented by A. Dutil as an atypical case of Parkinson's disease for two reasons; first she presented as a highly asymmetrical case of hemiplegic features, and second because of her extended posture. This case has been reviewed and published as a possible case of progressive supranuclear palsy, but the asymmetry of motor features and the flexed elbow and wrist suggest that corticobasal degeneration is another possibility. No autopsy information is available. The photos show a frontal view with asymmetry of arm posture, and profile view with truncal extension (27).

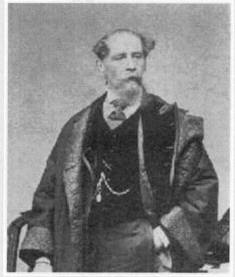

FIGURE 1.29 Progressive supranuclear palsy in the literature. Historical research on early medical diagnoses has occasionally benefited from nonmedical sources, especially literary descriptions. Because movement disorders are particularly visual in their character, it is reasonable to search the writings of celebrated authors known for their picturesque descriptive writings. In this context, Larner proposed that Charles Dickens captured the essential features of progressive supranuclear palsy in his description of a character in *The Lazy Tour of Two Idle Apprentices*. Dickens wrote:

"A chilled, slow, earthy, fixed old man. A cadaverous man of measured speech. An old man who seemed as unable to wink, as if his eyelids had been nailed to his forehead. An old man whose eyes (two spots of fire) had no more motion than if they had been connected with the back of his skull by screws driven through it and riveted and bolted outside, among his grey hair. He had come in and shut the door, and he now sat down. He did not bend himself to sit, as other people do, but seemed to sink bold upright, as if in water until the chair stopped him."

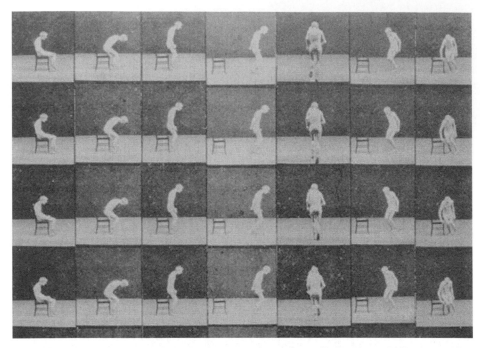

FIGURE 1.30 Early motion picture sequences of a patient with Parkinson's disease. From 1907 to 1912, with the assistance of photographer Sigmund Lubin, Philadelphia neurologist Theodore Weisenberg recorded approximately 10,000 feet of motion picture film of patients with nervous and mental diseases, including images of patients with Parkinson's disease. In 1911, Weisenberg was the first to include strips of motion picture images of various neurologic conditions in a medical textbook, *A Textbook of Medical Diagnosis* by James M. Anders and L. Napoleon Boston. The images shown were labeled "Moving picture of attitude and gait in Paralysis Agitans."

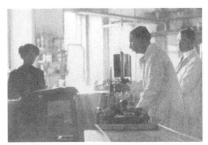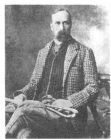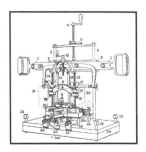

FIGURE 1.31 Early surgical interventions. (*Left*) Victor Horsley (1857–1916) was a celebrated British surgeon who attempted a surgical intervention on a patient having movement disorder with athetosis in 1909. He excised motor cortex with substantial improvement in involuntary movements. (*Middle*) Working in London with his physiologist colleague, Robert Henry Clarke (1850–1926), he developed early stereotaxic equipment, first for animal experiments and then for humans. (*Right*) This daunting surgical apparatus taken from their reports in Brain in 1908 guided them to deep brain centers, including the basal ganglia and the cerebellum.

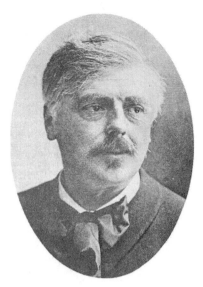

FIGURE 1.32 Eduard Brissaud. Brissaud was a close associate of Charcot and contributed several important clinical observations on Parkinson's disease in the late 19th century. Most importantly, however, he brought neuropathologic attention to the substantia nigra as the potential site of disease origin. In discussing a case of a tuberculoma that destroyed the substantia nigra and in association with contralateral hemiparkinsonism, he considered the currently vague knowledge of the nucleus and its putative involvement in volitional and reflex motor control. Extending his thoughts, he hypothesized that, "a lesion of the *locus niger* could reasonably be the anatomic basis of Parkinson's disease" (28).

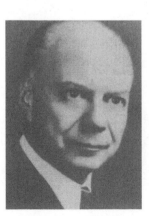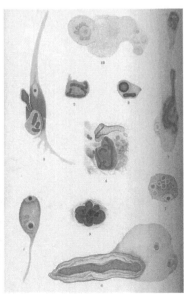

FIGURE 1.33   Lewy and Lewy bodies.   (*Left*) Friedrich Heinrich Lewy. (*Right*) Lewy's first illustration of microscopical changes (29).

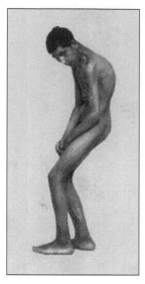

FIGURE 1.34 Postencephalitic parkinsonism of von Economo's disease. Among the late sequelae of von Economo's disease, parkinsonism was particularly common. Von Economo wrote:

> "the amyostatic–akinetic form…characterized by a rigidity, without a real palsy and without symptoms arising from the pyramidal tract…To look at these patients one would suppose them to be in a state of profound secondary dementia. Emotions are scarcely noticeable in the face, but they are mentally intact."

Photograph from Barcelona clinic of L. Barraquer Ferré (*c.* 1930) showing a patient with postencephalitic parkinsonism. Courtesy of L. Barraquer-Bordas, Barcelona.

REFERENCES

1. Finger S. Origins of Neuroscience. New York: Oxford University Press, 1994.
2. Sauvages de la Croix FB. Nosologia methodica. Amstelodami: Sumptibus Fratrum de Tournes, 1763.
3. Charcot J-M. Leçons du Mardi: Policlinique: 1887–1888. Paris: Bureaux du Progrès Médical, 1888.
4. Goetz CG. Charcot, the Clinician: The Tuesday Lessons. New York: Raven Press, 1987.
5. Horowski R, Horowski L, Vogel S, Poewe W, Kielhorn F-W. An essay on Wilhelm von Humboldt and the shaking palsy. Neurology 1995; 45: 565–8.
6. Leitzmann A. Briefe von Wilhelm von Humboldt an eine Freundin. Leipzig: Inselverlag, 1909.
7. Parkinson J. Essay on the Shaking Palsy. London: Whittingham and Rowland for Sherwood, Neeley and Jones, 1817.
8. Morris AD, Rose FC. James Parkinson: His Life and Times. Boston: Birkhauser, 1989.
9. Allen E, Turk JL, Murley R. The Case books of John Hunter FRS. London: Royal Society of Medicine, 1993.
10. Parkinson J. Hunterian Reminiscences. London: Sherwood, Gilbert and Piper, 1833.
11. Currier RD. Did John Hunter give James Parkinson an Idea? Arch Neurol 1996; 53: 377–8.
12. Robert D. Currier Parkinson Archives legged to Christopher G. Goetz.
13. Parkinson J. Organic Remains of a Former World (three volumes). London: Whittingham and Rowland for Sherwood, Neeley and Jones, 1804–1811.

14. Kelly EC. Annotated reprinting: essay on the shaking palsy by James Parkinson. Med Class 1938; 2: 957–98.
15. Charcot J-M. De la paralysie agitante (leçon 5). Oeuvres Complètes 1: 161–188. Paris: Bureaux du Progrès Médical, 1869: In English On paralysis agitans (Lecture 5). Lectures on the Diseases of the Nervous System. 105–7. Translated by G. Sigurson, Philadelphia: HC Lea and Company, 1879.
16. Historical art and document collection, Christopher G. Goetz.
17. Goetz CG, Bonduelle M, Gelfand T. Charcot: Constructing Neurology. New York: Oxford University Press, 1995.
18. Meige H. Charcot artiste. Nouvelle Iconographie de la Salpêtrière 1898; 11: 489–516.
19. Charcot JM. Tremors and choreiform movements. Rhythmical Chorea. In: Clinical Lectures on Diseases of the Nervous System: Delivered at the Infirmary of La Salpêtrière. Vol. 3 Translated by T. Savill London: New Sydenham Society, 1889: 183–97.
20. Philadelphia College of Physicians, Original manuscript and document collection, Philadelphia, PA.
21. Kapur SS, Stebbins GT, Goetz CG. Vibration therapy for Parkinson's disease: Charcot's studies revisited. J Parkinson's Dis 2012; 2: 23–7.
22. Gowers WRA. Manual of Diseases of the Nervous System. London: Churchill, 1886–1888.
23. Osler W. The Principles and Practice of Medicine. New York: Appleton and Company, 1892.
24. Peterson F. A Contribution to the study of Muscular Tremor. J Nerv Ment Dis 1889; 16: 99–112.
25. Peterson F. A clinical study of forty-seven cases of paralysis agitans. NY Med J 1890; 52: 93–398.
26. Mitchell SW, Dercum FX. Nervous diseases and their treatments: general considerations. In: Dercum FX, ed. A Textbook on Nervous Diseases by American Authors. Philadelphia: Lea Brothers & Co, 1895: 2–50.
27. Dutil A. Sur un cas de paralysis agitante a forme hemiplegique avec attitude anormale de la tete et du tronc (extension). Nouvelle Iconographie de la Salpetriere 1889; 2: 165–9.
28. Brissaud E. Nature et pathogénie de la maladie de Parkinson (leçon 23, 488-501). Leçons sur les maladies nerveuses: la Salpêtrière, 1893–1894. Paris: Masson, 1895.
29. Paralysis agitans I pathologische anatomie. In: Lewandowsky: Handbuch de Neurologie. Berlin: Springer, 1912.

2

Epidemiology

Raymond Y. Lo and Caroline M. Tanner

INTRODUCTION

Epidemiology is the study of the distribution and determinants of health-related states or events in specified populations, and the application of this study to control health problems (1). The ultimate goal of epidemiologic research of Parkinson's disease (PD) is to find the cause and prevent the occurrence of PD. This chapter focuses on describing the frequency, survival, and coexisting conditions of PD. We only briefly discuss the etiologic aspects of epidemiologic studies, because genetic and environmental risk factors are detailed in other chapters in this volume.

CASE DEFINITION IN EPIDEMIOLOGY: PARKINSONISM AND PARKINSON'S DISEASE

Case definition is the foundation of estimates of disease frequency and distribution. Like many neurologic disorders, PD has no diagnostic biomarker. Imaging using ligands with affinity for the dopamine transporter has been shown to distinguish PD from essential tremor, but to date these tests have been used in only a small number of cases (2). Dopamine transporter imaging cannot distinguish among parkinsonian syndromes. Studies seeking other biomarkers are now in progress, but at present, postmortem examination, combined with clinical information, remains the diagnostic gold standard. Pathology-based diagnosis is only feasible for PD patients after death. Thus, uncertain or inaccurate diagnosis is one potential source of error in most epidemiologic studies of PD.

Diagnostic criteria for PD have evolved over time, reflecting clinical and pathologic advances. Early studies often combined forms of parkinsonism, for example, postencephalitic, vascular, drug-induced, and idiopathic (3–5). The term "idiopathic PD" has been used to describe parkinsonism for which a single cause could not be identified. Because many cases in this category have disease risk factors that are now considered contributory to the cause of PD, in this chapter, we use the term "typical PD" rather than idiopathic; herein, "typical PD" refers to a progressive parkinsonian syndrome meeting modern clinical diagnostic criteria predictive of synuclein pathology, including nigral Lewy bodies at postmortem examination (5–8). The accuracy of a clinical diagnosis of PD was assessed in the early 1990s using postmortem brain pathologic findings as the gold standard. About 76% of clinically diagnosed PD cases fulfilled pathologic criteria for PD, and accuracy improved to 82% when the U.K. Brain Bank criteria were applied (9,10). Sensitivity and positive predictive value improved to more than 90% if diagnosis had been made by a movement disorder specialist (11). These findings suggest that the current clinical diagnosis of PD is not perfect but fairly satisfactory when a movement disorder expert applies uniform diagnostic criteria.

PREVALENCE AND INCIDENCE OF PARKINSON'S DISEASE

Prevalence is defined as the total number of existing cases in a given population at a certain period of time. More than 80 estimates of PD prevalence have been published; about 20 studies used intensive ascertainment methods, such as a door-to-door, two-stage approach (screening and clinical exam) (12–33). Most studies estimated the prevalence of PD to be 100–300 per 100,000 persons. In general, prevalence increased with older age and door-to-door surveys reported higher prevalence than registry- or record-based studies. However, the total number of cases identified in most of these studies was below 100, resulting in poor precision for age-specific estimates. Even among studies with rigorous ascertainment methods, prevalence estimates varied widely with a more than 10-fold difference worldwide. In a review of high-quality studies from the United States and European countries, the median prevalence of PD was 9.5 per 1000 persons of 65 years and above (34). Prevalence studies published after the year 2000 are shown in Table 2.1.

Differences in study design, population size and composition, and ascertainment methods, makes comparison of prevalence studies from various geographic regions challenging, even when estimates are adjusted to a standard population to minimize the effect of different population composition. An early review of worldwide occurrence of PD showed lower prevalence in many countries in Asia and Africa (35). Subsequent studies reported estimates similar to prevalence in European countries in some cases (27,29), but in other cases, despite intensive ascertainment methods, prevalence remained low (33). Whether these differences reflect true changes in prevalence or merely differences in methods is not known. Differences in population demographics, improved quality and accessibility of medical care with consequent improved survival, and changes in and environmental risk factors may all contribute to the apparent geographic variation of PD.

Systematic prospective determination of disease incidence using similar methods in all populations can provide important additional insights into the true distribution and determinants of PD worldwide. Incidence is the fundamental measure of disease distribution over time. Incidence is defined as the number of newly diagnosed cases divided by the amount of time-at-risk (e.g., person-years). PD is relatively rare and thus incidence estimates require surveys of many persons, particularly if the

TABLE 2.1 Parkinson's Disease Prevalence Reports After the Year 2000

Prevalence Study	Nation, Reference Year	Case Number	Prevalence Estimates; per 100,000 p (Age Group)
Chen et al. (2001) (21)	Taiwan, 1993	37	130.1 (for all age groups)
Kis et al. (2002) (22)	Italy, 1998	12	1500 (65+)
Benito-Leon et al. (2003) (23)	Spain, 1994	81	1500 (65+)
Nicoletti et al. (2003) (24)	Bolivia, 1994	5	286 (40+)
Bergareche et al. (2004) (25)	Spain, 1996	18	1500 (65+)
Tan et al. (2004) (26)	Singapore, 2001	46	290 (50+)
Zhang et al. (2005) (27)	China, 1997	277	1070 (55+)
Chan et al. (2005) (28)	Australia, 2002	36	780 (55+)
Barbosa et al. (2006) (29)	Brazil, 2001	39	3300 (64+)
Wirdefeldt et al. (2008) (31)	Sweden, 2002	132	496 (50+)
Morgante et al. (2008) (30)	Sicily, 2001	14	104.2 (for all age groups)
Das et al. (2010) (33)	India, 2007	41	52.85 (for all age groups)

TABLE 2.2   Parkinson's Disease Incidence Reports After the Year 2000

Incidence Study	Nation, Study Period	Case Number	Incidence Estimates; per 100,000 p-y (Age Group)
Baldereschi et al. (2000) (43)	Italy, 1992–1996	42	326 (65–85)
MacDonald et al. (2000) (44)	United Kingdom, 1995–1996	N/A	19 (for all age groups)
Chen et al. (2001) (21)	Taiwan, 1995–1997	15	10.4 (for all age groups)
Morioka et al. (2002) (45)	Japan, 1997	232	10.5 (for all age groups)
Van Den Eeden et al. (2003) (46)	United States, 1994–1995	588	13.4 (for all age groups)
Taba et al. (2003) (47)	Estonia, 1990–1998	264	16.8 (for all age groups)
Leentjens et al. (2003) (48)	Netherlands, 1990–2000	139	22.4 (for all age groups)
Benito-Leon et al. (2004) (49)	Spain, 1995–1998	30	186.8 (65–85)
de Lau et al. (2004) (50)	Netherlands, 1993–1999	67	49 (55–85)
Foltynie et al. (2004) (51)	United Kingdom, 2000–2003	201	10.8 (for all age groups)
Taylor et al. (2006) (52)	United Kingdom, 2002–2004	50	22.4 (for all age groups)
Tan et al. (2007) (53)	Singapore, 2002–2003	12	32 (50+)
Linder et al. (2010) (54)	Sweden, 2004–2007	112	22.5 (for all age groups)
Winter et al. (55)	Russia, 2006–2008	308	9.95 (for all age groups)
Hristova et al. (2010) (56)	Bulgaria, 2002–2004	244	11.7 (for all age groups)

Abbreviation: p-y, person-years.

time interval of observation is limited. For this reason, there are fewer incidence studies of PD than prevalence studies (21,36–56). Methods for case ascertainment vary. New PD cases have been identified via medical records, drug prescriptions, health insurance records, referral letters, self-report questionnaires, and direct exams. In most studies, the overall incidence rates of PD are estimated to be 10–20 per 100,000 person-years, with a median incidence of 14 per 100,000 person-years (34). In studies restricted to individuals of 65 years or above, the median incidence rate was 160 per 100,000 person-years. The incidence increased consistently with older age in all the studies. PD incidence reports after the year 2000 are shown in Table 2.2.

PD incidence may vary across racial or ethnic groups, but few studies have included diverse populations. In the United States, two reports suggest the highest incidence in Caucasians and those of Hispanic heritage and the lowest incidence in African Americans, but these estimates are based on few individuals and precision is limited (39,46). If PD incidence does vary by race or ethnicity, this could be due to genetic or environmental factors, or a combination of both. Dermal melanin is higher in races with putatively lower incidence and this led to the proposal that the free radical bonding properties of melanin could protect against environmental toxicants (57). More recently, persons homozygous for a variant of the gene encoding the melanocortin 1 receptor had increased PD risk, indicating an underlying genetic risk factor (58). However, this genotype is rare and does not explain all of the population variance.

SURVIVAL AND CAUSE OF DEATH IN PARKINSON'S DISEASE

The introduction of levodopa treatment in the late 1960s significantly changed the clinical care of PD patients. In 1967, Hoehn and Yahr reported that mortality in paralysis agitans was nearly three times greater than expected (5). Survival studies following the introduction of levodopa therapy have consistently reported an approximately twofold increase in mortality risk in PD patients compared with the general population (21,41,59–74). However, most of these studies were limited by the use of prevalent cases, which would overestimate the relative mortality risk because PD patients might become more fragile with increasing disease duration. For newly diagnosed PD patients, the risk of mortality may be no different from the general population during the first three to five years (60,63), although an analysis matching PD and controls with similar comorbidity found an excess risk of death in PD at all time points (71). The median survival length after diagnosis of PD was 10.3 years in one incidence study from Olmsted County, MN, U.S.A. (63), and 61% of PD cases had died 10 years after diagnosis in another large incident cohort from California (72). These incidence studies provide us a general picture of survival dynamics in PD.

Clinical features, such as postural instability, hallucinations, and cognitive impairment, when present early in the disease course, predict poor survival in PD (72,75). Among these, dementia is the most strongly associated with poor survival, almost doubling the mortality risk. In a 20-year follow-up study, dementia seemed nearly inevitable as PD progressed (76), and dementia is associated with shorter survival at any point in the disease course (77). Recent advances in PD therapeutics including new dopaminergic agents, agents with potential disease-modifying effects, deep brain stimulation, and treatments for dementia and depression and other nonmotor features may prolong survival, but to date there have been no systematic studies, and there is no solid evidence showing these novel therapies have prolonged survival in PD (78–82). Systematic population-based studies are warranted for evaluating the effects of these novel treatments on survival in PD.

Reporting of PD on death certificates is inconsistent, perhaps in part because PD per se is rarely the immediate cause of death. Numerous reports have shown that in nearly half of those diagnosed with PD, this diagnosis is not listed as a primary or contributing cause of death on the death certificate (83). For this reason, observations based on death certificates may not represent all persons with PD, and it may not be appropriate to generalize conclusions.

Death certificates have been investigated to determine cause of death in PD. Based on death certificates from the Michigan Department of Public Health during 1970–1990, PD patients were almost four times more likely to die of pneumonia (84). In community-based studies from Sweden and Norway, about twofold or more PD patients than the control group died of pneumonia, whereas PD patients had fewer deaths due to ischemic heart disease, cerebrovascular disease, or cancer (64,85). A 20-year follow-up study from Sydney also reported pneumonia as the major cause of death among PD patients (76). Although using death certificates for cause of death analysis is subject to various types of bias, including selection and reporting bias, the consistency of this finding across populations and time is compelling. The greater vulnerability to pneumonia among PD patients at advanced stages is likely multifactorial, reflecting the combined effects of dysphagia and ineffective cough with consequent aspiration risk, and recognition of these factors may improve care in vulnerable PD cases.

COMORBIDITY IN PARKINSON'S DISEASE

Comorbid illnesses are common in elderly populations. In persons with chronic diseases, such as PD, comorbid conditions can adversely affect quality of life, level of disability, response to therapy, and survival. Health services utilization and the costs of care are typically increased when comorbid illnesses are present in persons with PD (86). Etiologic clues may also be derived from patterns of comorbidity for conditions not thought to be part of the clinical spectrum of PD. For these reasons, investigating the effects of comorbid disease in PD is important, yet few systematic investigations of comorbidity in PD have been reported. Many comorbidity studies have focused on PD-associated nonmotor features, such as depression, anxiety, autonomic dysfunction, sleep disorders, and dementia, as comorbid conditions.

Cancer
Most cancers occur less often in patients with PD. Cancer incidence is lower in the period before as well as after the diagnosis of PD, and this is seen across many populations (87–92). Particularly low are those cancers associated with cigarette smoking. Since smoking is a behavior not commonly associated with PD, studies not able to incorporate information on smoking could have been confounded. One recent study using an incident cohort of PD with detailed smoking information reported that the overall cancer incidence in PD is not significantly different from the general population after controlling for smoking (93). In contrast to smoking-associated cancers, melanoma incidence is increased in persons with PD (94,95). The use of levodopa was once thought to be an etiologic factor for melanoma, because melanin is an oxidation product of dopamine. However, melanoma risk has been shown to be independent of levodopa therapy, and shared etiologic factors, either genetic or environmental, have been sought. A polymorphic variant in the gene encoding the melanocortin 1 receptor was associated with PD in one report, suggesting that PD and melanoma may have shared genetic risks, but this variant is not common and is not likely the only factor explaining this association (58).

Gout/Uric Acid
Uric acid has been proposed to protect against oxidative injury since the 1980s (96). In 1996, high normal serum urate levels in midlife were associated with a lower incidence of PD (97), a finding replicated in other prospective cohorts (98–100). Remarkably, higher levels of uric acid are related not only to lower incidence but also to slower clinical progression of PD (101). Gout would be expected to be an uncommon comorbid disorder in PD, and this has been observed (102). These data have been interpreted to support the key role of oxidative stress in the pathogenesis of PD and, suggest that antioxidant treatment may provide disease-modifying benefits (103).

Diabetes, Hypertension, Hypercholesterolemia, and Other Vascular Diseases
Cerebrovascular disease was considered a common cause of parkinsonism in early epidemiologic studies (104) as well as a commonly reported cause of death (84). This, combined with findings showing a vascular contribution in other neurodegenerative diseases, particularly Alzheimer's disease, prompted interest in investigating cardiovascular disease and risk factors for cardiovascular disease in PD. Stroke and cardiovascular diseases have more recently been proposed to be lower in PD, in keeping with the lower frequency of cigarette smoking, but neither decreased nor increased rates of these conditions have been consistently described (105–107). Risk factors for cardiovascular disease have not been associated with PD

either. For example, diabetes mellitus is not consistently increased in PD, and may even be inversely associated with PD, suggesting a lower risk of PD in diabetics (108–110). Similarly, hypertension was not associated with PD in several large cohort studies (111,112), and certain antihypertensive agents, such as L-type calcium channel blockers, are associated with a lower risk of PD (113) and may be useful as disease-modifying treatments (114). The relationship between cholesterol and PD remains inconclusive. High serum cholesterol was associated with lower PD risk in the Rotterdam study (115), but found to increase PD risk in a Finnish cohort (116) and reported no relationship with PD in the Nurses' Health Study and Health Professionals Study (112). Use of cholesterol-lowering agents has been associated with a modest reduction in PD risk, an association that is not easily separated from the indication for using these agents (117–119).

ETIOLOGY OF PARKINSON'S DISEASE: GENETICS, ENVIRONMENT, AND GENE–ENVIRONMENT INTERACTION
Genetics
The cause of PD can rarely be identified for a given individual. The exception is parkinsonism caused by genetic mutations inherited in a Mendelian pattern. A handful of specific genes causing parkinsonism have been identified (120,121), and these are described in detail in chapter 15. All of these are rare, but their investigation can provide important clues to the pathophysiologic mechanisms underlying PD. First identified was the *SNCA* gene on chromosome 4q21.3, which encodes α-synuclein, responsible for a rare, dominantly inherited disorder limited to a few families worldwide (122). The protein, α-synuclein, is a major component of Lewy bodies, the pathologic hallmark of PD. More common is the recessively inherited disorder caused by mutations in the *Parkin* gene on chromosome 6q25.2–27, accounting for most cases of parkinsonism beginning before the age of 30 years (123). However, parkinsonism with onset before the age of 50 years accounts for less than 10% of all disease worldwide, so this genetic form is also not a common cause of parkinsonism. Interestingly, the reported clinical features of *Parkin* mutation cases resembled typical PD, but postmortem findings often revealed nigral degeneration without Lewy bodies (124), leading to questions regarding the importance of Lewy pathology. Mutations in the *PINK1* and *DJ-1* genes are also limited to very few families worldwide. Most common are mutations in the leucine-rich repeat kinase 2 or *LRRK2* gene on chromosome 12q12 (125). The G2019S mutation is the most common mutation of the *LRRK2* gene in North African and Jewish populations, and is associated with an autosomal dominant inheritance pattern with incomplete penetrance and typical late-onset PD features. In North America, *LRRK2* mutations account for 1–2% of PD cases. In Asian populations, several variants in the *LRRK2* gene confer susceptibility but are not considered causative (126,127). The glucocerebrosidase or *GBA* gene mutation, known to cause Gaucher's disease, has recently been identified as a cause of PD (128).

Familial aggregation studies have facilitated the identification of genetic causes of PD, but PD cases with multiple afflicted family members or cases of PD caused by known mutations are not common. In a meta-analysis of genetic associations with PD, only specific mutations in the *LRRK2* and *GBA* genes yielded odds ratios above 2 in the PD gene database. In a study of twins, a strong genetic contribution is evident only when PD begins before the age of 50 years (129). Recent genome-wide association studies suggest that small increases in risk of 10–20% may be associated with a number of common polymorphic variants, such as variation in the tau gene (130–133).

Environment

The idea that environmental exposure might cause PD was triggered by the observation of a cluster of parkinsonism in narcotics addicts. The causative agent was identified as 1-methyl-4-phenyl-1,2,4,6-tetrahydropyridine (MPTP) (134). MPTP caused irreversible, levodopa responsive parkinsonism without other symptoms or signs, compellingly similar to PD. In postmortem studies of animals and a few humans, the distribution of nerve cell injury within the brain also paralleled that seen in PD, although whether Lewy bodies occurred was uncertain. These findings sparked a search for environmental factors that might increase or decrease the risk of PD. In this sense, "environmental" refers to all exposures not intrinsic to the organism. Among these are exposures due to occupation, place of residence, lifestyle, diet, and infectious agents. In this section, only a few environmental factors are considered and a more detailed review can be found in chapter 16.

The most frequently observed association between an exposure and PD is the inverse association between cigarette smoking and PD risk (111,135,136). This pattern has been seen in nearly every population in which it has been investigated, independent of race, nationality, or time. Many of the Bradford–Hill criteria for causation are met, including strength of association, consistency, temporality and dose–response. Although nicotine, a key component of cigarette smoke, appears to stimulate dopaminergic neurons and inhibit the formation of α-synuclein fibrils, a biologically plausible model of the protective effect of smoking against PD has not yet been established. Cigarette smoke contains hundreds of compounds, and identification of a causative agent is challenging. The causal relationship between smoking and PD cannot be verified directly, because conducting a trial to test smoking on PD is not ethically feasible. However, experimental evidence suggests a potentially neuroprotective role for nicotine (137).

Coffee intake is also associated with decreased risk of PD in many large cohort studies (138–140). Most believe that pharmacologic properties of caffeine, an adenosine receptor antagonist, may have a neuroprotective effect on dopaminergic neurons. As has been observed for many PD-associated risk factors, the inverse relationship is less significant in postmenopausal women and particularly in those who used estrogen (141). Experimental evidence also suggests that the use of estrogen might block the neuroprotective effect of coffee on PD (142). An inverse association between tea consumption and PD has also been reported. In one study from Singapore, intake of black tea rather than green tea was inversely associated with PD, even after taking caffeine intake into account, suggesting that compounds other than caffeine in black tea may be neuroprotective (143).

PD risk is increased in association with farming or pesticide exposure in several large cohort studies (144–146). Increasing cumulative time of pesticide exposure is associated with increasing risk of incident PD. Most studies have investigated only broad categories, but specific agents associated with mitochondrial complex I inhibition or oxidative stress, such as paraquat, rotenone and certain organochlorines, have been associated with a two- to threefold increased risk of PD in populations with good exposure information (147–149). *In vitro,* rotenone, dieldrin, and paraquat cause aggregation of the protein α-synuclein, and cause experimental parkinsonism *in vivo*, supporting the strength, consistency, and biologic plausibility of pesticide exposure as one environmental cause of PD. In a prospective cohort, the prevalence of pesticide exposure in PD cases was less than 10% in a large nutrition cohort (144), more common than the genes associated with PD. Measuring occupational pesticide exposure is challenging, and studies measuring only broad categories of exposure likely miss associations of individual chemicals, underestimating the true association (150). Moreover pesticide exposure is not limited to the workplace, but even more difficult is measurement of nonoccupational exposure to pesticides, such as residential exposure, home use, and exposure through food or water. Nonetheless, investigation using geographic mapping of pesticide use has found paraquat, maneb, and ziram exposure and well water use to be associated with PD risk, suggesting that pesticide exposure may contribute to the development of PD in many more cases (151–153).

In addition to pesticides, metal and solvent exposures also appear to increase the risk of PD. Occupational manganese has long been known to produce parkinsonism, but the cases described do not resemble typical PD, and whether PD can be caused by chronic low-level manganese exposure remains controversial, and in the United States scientific investigation is impeded by litigation (154–157). The concentration of lead in tibial bone, a measure of chronic exposure to lead, was also associated with a higher risk of PD (158), although the underlying mechanism remains to be determined. A cluster of PD patients among industrial coworkers was reported in association with extensive trichloroethylene (TCE) exposure, a widely used solvent additive in many household products (159). Exposure to TCE and two other chlorinated solvents, perchlorothylene and carbon tetrachloride, was also observed to increase PD risk two- to threefold in a study of occupational exposure in twin pairs discordant for PD (160). TCE also causes experimental parkinsonism and mitochondrial dysfunction. Solvent exposure, similar to pesticide exposure, is common but not easily measured, suggesting that solvent exposure may be another under-recognized risk factor for PD.

Recent experimental work has shown that even mild head injury can cause chronic physiologic changes, such as disruption of the blood–brain barrier, increased inflammatory cytokines, and increased production of α-synuclein, providing biologic plausibility for an association of head injury and PD. In support of this, case–control studies have reported an association between head trauma and PD, although results are inconsistent, leading some to argue that this association is due to recall bias or reverse causation (161). Evidence against the former is provided by studies in which head injury was verified by medical record evidence (162,163). Evidence against reverse causation is provided by studies finding the association between head injuries occurring 10 years or more before PD onset, when disease-associated balance problems would not be manifest (162).

Gene–Environment Interaction

Typical PD cases are often called "idiopathic" because neither a clear hereditary pattern or single gene mutation nor a single environmental exposure is thought to be the cause of disease. Penetrance of most of the genes associated with PD is low, and the effects of most environmental factors identified are not universal. These observations suggest that PD in most cases results from the combined effects of environmental exposures and genetic make-up (164). Examples include gene–environment interaction but the interaction of multiple genes, multiple environmental exposures and even more complex combinations are likely. Investigating such effects in humans requires very large populations with well-characterized exposures as well as extensive genetic information, and few such population studies have been possible. Examples of gene–environment interaction include the recent report of a more than 350% increased risk of PD in those with a promoter region variant of the α-synuclein gene and head injury, but not in those with head injury without the variant (165). Pesticide exposure was associated with PD in those with the poor metabolizer genotype for cytochrome P450 2D6, responsible for metabolizing many xenobiotics, but not in those with other geneotypes (166). The multidrug resistance protein 1 gene (*MDR1* or *ABCB1*), which encodes xenobiotic metabolizing enzymes, is not associated with PD; but the G2677 (A, T) polymorphism modified the risk of PD in the presence of organochlorine insecticide exposure (167). A genome-wide association study found the rs4998386_T allelic variant in the glutamate receptor gene *GRIN2A* to be associated with lower PD risk in coffee drinkers but not in others (168). Pesticide exposure was associated with greater risk of PD only in nonsmokers and those not habitually consuming coffee in one prospective cohort study (169).

These observations are among those providing support for a complex etiology for most PD cases, and suggest that studies of PD etiology should routinely include environmental as well as genetic risk factor assessment. "Hypothesis-free" genome-wide association studies and investigations of epigenetic changes will be most informative when combined with well-characterized information on environmental exposures. Investigations incorporating both genetic and environmental information can provide key insights into the causes of PD, and, ultimately, means for disease prevention.

REFERENCES
1. Last J. A Dictionary of Epidemiology, 4th edn. New York: Oxford University Press, 2001.
2. Tolosa E, Borght TV, Moreno E. Accuracy of DaTSCAN (123I-Ioflupane) SPECT in diagnosis of patients with clinically uncertain parkinsonism: 2-year follow-up of an open-label study. Mov Disord 2007; 22: 2346–51.
3. Kurland LT. Epidemiology: incidence, geographic distribution and genetic considerations. In: Fields WS, ed. Pathogenesis and Treatment of Parkinsonism. Thomas, Springfield, 1958: 5–49.
4. Pollock M, Hornabrook RW. The prevalence, natural history and dementia of Parkinson's disease. Brain 1966; 89: 429–48.
5. Hoehn MM, Yahr MD. Parkinsonism: onset, progression and mortality. Neurology 1967; 17: 427–42.
6. Gibb WR, Lees AJ. The relevance of the Lewy body to the pathogenesis of idiopathic Parkinson's disease. J Neurol Neurosurg Psychiatry 1988; 51: 745–52.
7. Calne DB, Snow BJ, Lee C. Criteria for diagnosing Parkinson's disease. Ann Neurol 1992; 32(Suppl): S125–7.
8. Gelb DJ, Oliver E, Gilman S. Diagnostic criteria for Parkinson disease. Arch Neurol 1999; 56: 33–9.
9. Hughes AJ, Daniel SE, Kilford L, et al. Accuracy of clinical diagnosis of idiopathic Parkinson's disease: a clinico-pathological study of 100 cases. J Neurol Neurosurg Psychiatry 1992; 55: 181–4.
10. Hughes AJ, Ben-Shlomo Y, Daniel SE, et al. What features improve the accuracy of clinical diagnosis in Parkinson's disease: a clinicopathologic study. Neurology 1992; 42: 1142–6.

11. Hughes AJ, Daniel SE, Ben-Shlomo Y, et al. The accuracy of diagnosis of parkinsonian syndromes in a specialist movement disorder service. Brain 2002; 125: 861–70.
12. Schoenberg BS, Anderson DW, Haerer AF. Prevalence of Parkinson's disease in the biracial population of Copiah county, Mississippi. Neurology 1985; 35: 841–5.
13. Li SC, Schoenberg BS, Wang CC, et al. A prevalence survey of Parkinson's disease and other movement disorders in the People's Republic of China. Arch Neurol 1985; 42: 655–7.
14. Okada K, Kobayashi S, Tsunematsu T. Prevalence of Parkinson's disease in Izumo City, Japan. Gerontology 1990; 36: 340–4.
15. Wang YS, Shi YM, Wu ZY, et al. Parkinson's disease in China. Coordinational Group of Neuroepidemiology, PLA. Chin Med J (Engl) 1991; 104: 960–4.
16. Morgante L, Rocca WA, Di Rosa AE, et al. Prevalence of Parkinson's disease and other types of parkinsonism: a door-to-door survey in three Sicilian municipalities. The Sicilian Neuro-Epidemiologic Study (SNES) Group. Neurology 1992; 42: 1901–7.
17. Tison F, Dartigues JF, Dubes L, et al. Prevalence of Parkinson's disease in the elderly: a population study in Gironde, France. Acta Neurol Scand 1994; 90: 111–15.
18. de Rijk MC, Breteler MM, Graveland GA, et al. Prevalence of Parkinson's disease in the elderly: the Rotterdam Study. Neurology 1995; 45: 2143–6.
19. Wang SJ, Fuh JL, Teng EL, et al. A door-to-door survey of Parkinson's disease in a Chinese population in Kinmen. Arch Neurol 1996; 53: 66–71.
20. Melcon MO, Anderson DW, Vergara RH, et al. Prevalence of Parkinson's disease in Junin, Buenos Aires Province, Argentina. Mov Disord 1997; 12: 197–205.
21. Chen RC, Chang SF, Su CL, et al. Prevalence, incidence, and mortality of PD: a door-to-door survey in Ilan county, Taiwan. Neurology 2001; 57: 1679–86.
22. Kis B, Schrag A, Ben-Shlomo Y, et al. Novel three-stage ascertainment method: prevalence of PD and parkinsonism in South Tyrol, Italy. Neurology 2002; 58: 1820–5.
23. Benito-Leon J, Bermejo-Pareja F, Rodriguez J, et al. Prevalence of PD and other types of parkinsonism in three elderly populations of central Spain. Mov Disord 2003; 18: 267–74.
24. Nicoletti A, Sofia V, Bartoloni A, et al. Prevalence of Parkinson's disease: a door-to-door survey in rural Bolivia. Parkinsonism Relat Disord 2003; 10: 19–21.
25. Bergareche A, De La Puente E, Lopez de Munain A, et al. Prevalence of Parkinson's disease and other types of Parkinsonism. A door-to-door survey in Bidasoa, Spain. J Neurol 2004; 251: 340–5.
26. Tan LC, Venketasubramanian N, Hong CY, et al. Prevalence of Parkinson disease in Singapore: Chinese vs Malays vs Indians. Neurology 2004; 62: 1999–2004.
27. Zhang ZX, Roman GC, Hong Z, et al. Parkinson's disease in China: prevalence in Beijing, Xian, and Shanghai. Lancet 2005; 365: 595–7.
28. Chan DK, Cordato D, Karr M, et al. Prevalence of Parkinson's disease in Sydney. Acta Neurol Scand 2005; 111: 7–11.
29. Barbosa MT, Caramelli P, Maia DP, et al. Parkinsonism and Parkinson's disease in the elderly: a community-based survey in Brazil (the Bambui study). Mov Disord 2006; 21: 800–8.
30. Morgante L, Nicoletti A, Epifanio A, et al. Prevalence of Parkinson's disease and other types of parkinsonism in the Aeolian Archipelago, Sicily. Parkinsonism Relat Disord 2008; 14: 572–5.
31. Wirdefeldt K, Gatz M, Bakaysa SL, et al. Complete ascertainment of Parkinson disease in the Swedish Twin Registry. Neurobiol Aging 2008; 29: 1765–73.
32. Racette BA, Good LM, Kissel AM, et al. A population-based study of parkinsonism in an Amish community. Neuroepidemiology 2009; 33: 225–30.
33. Das SK, Misra AK, Ray BK, et al. Epidemiology of Parkinson disease in the city of Kolkata, India: a communiNeurologyty-based study. Neurology 2010; 75: 1362–9.
34. Hirtz D, Thurman DJ, Gwinn-Hardy K, et al. How common are the "common" neurologic disorders? Neurology 2007; 68: 326–37.
35. Zhang ZX, Roman GC. Worldwide occurrence of Parkinson's disease: an updated review. Neuroepidemiology 1993; 12: 195–208.

36. Brewis M, Poskanzer DC, Rolland C, Miller H. Neurological disease in an English city. Acta Neurol Scand 1966: 42: 1–89.
37. Marttila RJ, Rinne UK. Epidemiology of Parkinson's disease in Finland. Acta Neurol Scand 1976; 53: 81–102.
38. Granieri E, Carreras M, Casetta I, et al. Parkinson's disease in Ferrara, Italy, 1967 through 1987. Arch Neurol 1991; 48: 854–7.
39. Mayeux R, Marder K, Cote LJ, et al. The frequency of idiopathic Parkinson's disease by age, ethnic group, and sex in northern Manhattan, 1988–1993. Am J Epidemiol 1995; 142: 820–7.
40. Fall PA, Axelson O, Fredriksson M, et al. Age-standardized incidence and prevalence of Parkinson's disease in a Swedish community. J Clin Epidemiol 1996; 49: 637–41.
41. Morens DM, Davis JW, Grandinetti A, et al. Epidemiologic observations on Parkinson's disease: incidence and mortality in a prospective study of middle-aged men. Neurology 1996; 46: 1044–50.
42. Bower JH, Maraganore DM, McDonnell SK, et al. Incidence and distribution of parkinsonism in Olmsted county, Minnesota, 1976-1990. Neurology 1999; 52: 1214–20.
43. Baldereschi M, Di Carlo A, Rocca WA, et al. Parkinson's disease and parkinsonism in a longitudinal study: two-fold higher incidence in men. ILSA Working Group. Italian Longitudinal Study on Aging. Neurology 2000; 55: 1358–63.
44. MacDonald BK, Cockerell OC, Sander WAS, Shorvon SD. The incidence and lifetime prevalence of neurological disorders in a prospective community-based study in the UK. Brain 2000; 123: 665–76.
45. Morioka S, Sakata K, Yoshida S, et al. Incidence of Parkinson disease in Wakayama, Japan. J Epidemiol 2002; 12: 403–7.
46. Van Den Eeden SK, Tanner CM, Bernstein AL, et al. Incidence of Parkinson's disease: variation by age, gender, and race/ethnicity. Am J Epidemiol 2003; 157: 1015–22.
47. Taba P, Asser T. Incidence of Parkinson's disease in Estonia. Neuroepidemiology 2003; 22: 41–5.
48. Leentjens AF, Van den Akker M, Metsemakers JF, et al. The incidence of Parkinson's disease in the Netherlands: results from a longitudinal general practice-based registration. Neuroepidemiology 2003; 22: 311–12.
49. Benito-Leon J, Bermejo-Pareja F, Morales-Gonzalez JM, et al. Incidence of Parkinson disease and parkinsonism in three elderly populations of central Spain. Neurology 2004; 62: 734–41.
50. de Lau LM, Giesbergen PC, de Rijk MC, et al. Incidence of parkinsonism and Parkinson disease in a general population: the Rotterdam Study. Neurology 2004; 63: 1240–4.
51. Foltynie T, Brayne CEG, Robbins TW, Barker RA. The cognitive ability of an incident cohort of Parkinson's patients in the UK. The CamPaIGN study. Brain 2004; 127: 550–60.
52. Taylor KS, Counsell CE, Harris CE, et al. Pilot study of the incidence and prognosis of degenerative Parkinsonian disorders in Aberdeen, United Kingdom: methods and preliminary results. Mov Disord 2006; 21: 976–82.
53. Tan LC, Venketasubramanian N, Jamora RD, et al. Incidence of Parkinson's disease in Singapore. Parkinsonism Relat Disord 2007; 13: 40–3.
54. Linder J, Stenlund H, Forsgren L. Incidence of Parkinson's disease and parkinsonism in northern Sweden: a population-based study. Mov Disord 2010; 25: 341–8.
55. Winter Y, Bezdolnyy Y, Katunina E, et al. Incidence of Parkinson's disease and atypical parkinsonism: Russian population-based study. Mov Disord 2010; 25: 349–56.
56. Hristova D, Zachariev Z, Mateva N, et al. Incidence of Parkinson's disease in Bulgaria. Neuroepidemiology 2010; 34: 76–82.
57. Marsden CD. Neuromelanin and Parkinson's disease. J Neural Transm Suppl 1983; 19: 121–41.
58. Gao X, Simon KC, Han J, et al. Genetic determinants of hair color and Parkinson's disease risk. Ann Neurol 2009; 65: 76–82.
59. Louis ED, Marder K, Cote L, et al. Mortality from Parkinson disease. Arch Neurol 1997; 54: 260–4.

60. Hely MA, Morris JG, Traficante R, et al. The Sydney multicentre study of Parkinson's disease: progression and mortality at 10 years. J Neurol Neurosurg Psychiatry 1999; 67: 300–7.
61. Berger K, Breteler MM, Helmer C, et al. Prognosis with Parkinson's disease in Europe: a collaborative study of population-based cohorts. Neurologic Diseases in the Elderly Research Group. Neurology 2000; 54: S24–7.
62. Morgante L, Salemi G, Meneghini F, et al. Parkinson disease survival: a population-based study. Arch Neurol 2000; 57: 507–12.
63. Elbaz A, Bower JH, Peterson BJ, et al. Survival study of Parkinson disease in Olmsted County, Minnesota. Arch Neurol 2003; 60: 91–6.
64. Fall PA, Saleh A, Fredrickson M, et al. Survival time, mortality, and cause of death in elderly patients with Parkinson's disease: a 9-year follow-up. Mov Disord 2003; 18: 1312–16.
65. Herlofson K, Lie SA, Arsland D, et al. Mortality and Parkinson disease: A community based study. Neurology 2004; 62: 937–42.
66. Hughes TA, Ross HF, Mindham RH, et al. Mortality in Parkinson's disease and its association with dementia and depression. Acta Neurol Scand 2004; 110: 118–23.
67. de Lau LM, Schipper CM, Hofman A, et al. Prognosis of Parkinson disease: risk of dementia and mortality: the Rotterdam Study. Arch Neurol 2005; 62: 1265–9.
68. Marras C, McDermott MP, Rochon PA, et al. Survival in Parkinson disease: thirteen-year follow-up of the DATATOP cohort. Neurology 2005; 64: 87–93.
69. D'Amelio M, Ragonese P, Morgante L, et al. Long-term survival of Parkinson's disease: a population-based study. J Neurol 2006; 253: 33–7.
70. Chen H, Zhang SM, Schwarzschild MA, et al. Survival of Parkinson's disease patients in a large prospective cohort of male health professionals. Mov Disord 2006; 21: 1002–7.
71. Driver JA, Kurth T, Buring JE, Gaziano JM, Logroscino G. Parkinson disease and risk of mortality: a prospective comorbidity-matched cohort study. Neurology 2008; 70: 1423–30.
72. Lo RY, Tanner CM, Albers KB, et al. Clinical features in early Parkinson's disease and survival. Arch Neurol 2009; 66: 1353–8.
73. Diem-Zangerl A, Seppi K, Wenning GK, et al. Mortality in Parkinson's disease: a 20-year follow-up study. Mov Disord 2009; 24: 819–25.
74. Posada IJ, Benito-León J, Louis ED, et al. Mortality from Parkinson's disease: a population-based prospective study (NEDICES). Mov Disord 2011; 26: 2522–9.
75. Goetz CG, Leurgans S, Pappert EJ, et al. Prospective longitudinal assessment of hallucinations in Parkinson's disease. Neurology 2001; 57: 2078–82.
76. Hely MA, Reid WG, Adena MA, et al. The Sydney multicenter study of Parkinson's disease: the inevitability of dementia at 20 years. Mov Disord 2008; 23: 837–44.
77. Buter TC, van den Hout A, Matthews FE, et al. Dementia and survival in Parkinson disease: a 12-year population study. Neurology 2008; 70: 1017–22.
78. Merola A, Zibetti M, Angrisano S, et al. Parkinson's disease progression at 30 years: a study of subthalamic deep brain-stimulated patients. Brain 2011; 134: 2074–84.
79. Emre M. Treatment of dementia associated with Parkinson's disease. Parkinsonism Relat Disord 2007; 13: S457–61.
80. Richard IH. Depression and apathy in Parkinson's disease. Curr Neurol Neurosci Rep 2007; 7: 295–301.
81. Rascol O, Fitzer-Attas CJ, Hauser R, et al. A double-blind, delayed-start trial of rasagiline in Parkinson's disease (the ADAGIO study): prespecified and post-hoc analyses of the need for additional therapies, changes in UPDRS scores, and non-motor outcomes. Lancet Neurol 2011; 10: 415–23.
82. Schupbach MW, Welter ML, Bonnet AM, et al. Mortality in patients with Parkinson's disease treated by stimulation of the subthalamic nucleus. Mov Disord 2007; 22: 257–61.
83. Pressley JC, Tang MX, Marder K, et al. Disparities in the recording of Parkinson's disease on death certificates. Mov Disord 2005; 20: 315–21.
84. Gorell JM, Johnson CC, Rybicki BA. Parkinson's disease and its comorbid disorders: an analysis of Michigan mortality data, 1970 to 1990. Neurology 1994; 44: 1865–8.

85. Beyer MK, Herlofson K, Arsland D, et al. Causes of death in a community-based study of Parkinson's disease. Acta Neurol Scand 2001; 103: 7–11.
86. Pressley JC, Louis ED, Tang MX, et al. The impact of comorbid disease and injuries on resource use and expenditures in parkinsonism. Neurology 2003; 60: 87–93.
87. Elbaz A, Peterson BJ, Yang P, et al. Nonfatal cancer preceding Parkinson's disease: a case-control study. Epidemiology 2002; 13: 157–64.
88. Elbaz A, Peterson BJ, Bower JH, et al. Risk of cancer after the diagnosis of Parkinson's disease: a historical cohort study. Mov Disord 2005; 20: 719–25.
89. Olsen JH, Friis S, Frederiksen K. Malignant melanoma and other types of cancer preceding Parkinson disease. Epidemiology 2006; 17: 582–7.
90. Driver JA, Kurth T, Buring JE, et al. Prospective case-control study of nonfatal cancer preceding the diagnosis of Parkinson's disease. Cancer Causes Control 2007; 18: 705–11.
91. Driver JA, Logroscino G, Buring JE, et al. A prospective cohort study of cancer incidence following the diagnosis of Parkinson's disease. Cancer Epidemiol Biomarkers Prev 2007; 16: 1260–5.
92. Olsen JH, Friis S, Frederiksen K, et al. Atypical cancer pattern in patients with Parkinson's disease. Br J Cancer 2005; 92: 201–5.
93. Lo RY, Tanner CM, Van Den Eeden SK, et al. Comorbid cancer in Parkinson's disease. Mov Disord 2010; 25: 1809–17.
94. Olsen JH, Tangerud K, Wermuth L, et al. Treatment with levodopa and risk for malignant melanoma. Mov Disord 2007; 22: 1252–7.
95. Bajaj A, Driver JA, Schernhammer ES. Parkinson's disease and cancer risk: a systematic review and meta-analysis. Cancer Causes Control 2010; 21: 697–707.
96. Ames BN, Cathcart R, Schwiers E, et al. Uric acid provides an antioxidant defense in humans against oxidant- and radical-caused aging and cancer: a hypothesis. Proc Natl Acad Sci USA 1981; 78: 6858–62.
97. Davis JW, Grandinetti A, Waslien CI, et al. Observations on serum uric acid levels and the risk of idiopathic Parkinson's disease. Am J Epidemiol 1996; 144: 480–4.
98. Weisskopf MG, O'Reilly E, Chen H, et al. Plasma urate and risk of Parkinson's disease. Am J Epidemiol 2007; 166: 561–7.
99. de Lau LM, Koudstaal PJ, Hofman A, et al. Serum uric acid levels and the risk of Parkinson disease. Ann Neurol 2005; 58: 797–800.
100. Chen H, Mosley TH, Alonso A, et al. Plasma urate and Parkinson's disease in the Atherosclerosis Risk in Communities (ARIC) study. Am J Epidemiol 2009; 169: 1064–9.
101. Ascherio A, LeWitt PA, Xu K, et al. Urate as a predictor of the rate of clinical decline in Parkinson disease. Arch Neurol 2009; 66: 1460–8.
102. Alonso A, Rodriguez LA, Logroscino G, et al. Gout and risk of Parkinson disease: a prospective study. Neurology 2007; 69: 1696–700.
103. Schwarzschild MA, Marek K, Eberly S, et al. Serum urate and probability of dopaminergic deficit in early "Parkinson's disease". Mov Disord 2011; 26: 1864–8.
104. Kurland LT, Darrell PH, Darrell RW. Epidemiologic and genetic characteristics of parkinsonism: a review. Int J Neurol 1961; 2: 11–24.
105. Herishanu YO, Medvedovski M, Goldsmith JR, et al. A case-control study of Parkinson's disease in urban population of southern Israel. Can J Neurol Sci 2001; 28: 144–7.
106. McCann SJ, LeCouteur DG, Green AC, et al. The epidemiology of Parkinson's disease in an Australian population. Neuroepidemiology 1998; 17: 310–17.
107. Becker C, Jick SS, Meier CR. Risk of stroke in patients with diopathic Parkinson disease. Parkinsonism Relat Disord 2010; 16: 31–5.
108. Hu G, Jousilahti P, Bidel S, et al. Type 2 diabetes and the risk of Parkinson's disease. Diabetes Care 2007; 30: 842–7.
109. Driver JA, Smith A, Buring JE, et al. Prospective cohort study of type 2 diabetes and the risk of Parkinson's disease. Diabetes Care 2008; 31: 2003–5.
110. Becker C, Brobert GP, Johansson S, et al. Diabetes in patients with idiopathic Parkinson's disease. Diabetes Care 2008; 31: 1808–12.
111. Grandinetti A, Morens DM, Reed D, et al. Prospective study of cigarette smoking and the risk of developing idiopathic Parkinson's disease. Am J Epidemiol 1994; 139: 1129–38.

112. Simon KC, Chen H, Schwarzschild M, et al. Hypertension, hypercholesterolemia, diabetes, and risk of Parkinson disease. Neurology 2007; 69: 1688–95.
113. Ritz B, Rhodes SL, Qian L, et al. L-type calcium channel blockers and Parkinson disease in Denmark. Ann Neurol 2010; 67: 600–6.
114. Simuni T, Borushko E, Avram MJ, et al. Tolerability of isradipine in early Parkinson's disease: a pilot dose escalation study. Mov Disord 2010; 25: 2863–6.
115. de Lau LM, Koudstaal PJ, Hofman A, et al. Serum cholesterol levels and the risk of Parkinson's disease. Am J Epidemiol 2006; 164: 998–1002.
116. Hu G, Antikainen R, Jousilahti P, et al. Total cholesterol and the risk of Parkinson disease. Neurology 2008; 70: 1972–9.
117. Gao X, Simon KC, Schwarzschild MA, et al. Prospective study of statin use and risk of Parkinson disease. Arch Neurol 2012; 69: 380–4.
118. Tanner CM. Advances in environmental epidemiology. Mov Disord 2010; 25 Suppl 1: S58–62.
119. Huang X, Abbott RD, Petrovitch H, et al. Low LDL cholesterol and increased risk of Parkinson's disease: prospective results from Honolulu-Asia Aging Study. Mov Disord 2008; 23: 1013–18.
120. Klein C, Schlossmacher MG. Parkinson disease, 10 years after its genetic revolution: multiple clues to a complex disorder. Neurology 2007; 69: 2093–104.
121. Lill CM, Roehr JT, McQueen MB, et al. Comprehensive research synopsis and systematic meta-analyses in Parkinson's disease genetics: the PDGene database. PLoS Genet 2012; 8: e1002548.
122. Polymeropoulos MH, Lavedan C, Leroy E, et al. Mutation in the alpha-synuclein gene identified in families with Parkinson's disease. Science 1997; 276: 2045–7.
123. Kitada T, Asakawa S, Hattori N, et al. Mutations in the parkin gene cause autosomal recessive juvenile parkinsonism. Nature 1998; 392: 605–8.
124. Takahashi H, Ohama E, Suzuki S, et al. Familial juvenile parkinsonism: clinical and pathologic study in a family. Neurology 1994; 44: 437–41.
125. Zimprich A, Biskup S, Leitner P, et al. Mutations in LRRK2 cause autosomal-dominant parkinsonism with pleomorphic pathology. Neuron 2004; 44: 601–7.
126. Tan EK, Shen H, Tan LC, et al. The G2019S LRRK2 mutation is uncommon in an Asian cohort of Parkinson's disease patients. Neurosci Lett 2005; 384: 327–9.
127. Tan EK. Identification of a common genetic risk variant (LRRK2 Gly2385Arg) in Parkinson's disease. Ann Acad Med Singapore 2006; 35: 840–2.
128. Sidransky E, Nalls MA, Aasly JO, et al. Multicenter analysis of glucocerebrosidase mutations in Parkinson's disease. N Engl J Med 2009; 361: 1651–61.
129. Tanner CM, Ottman R, Goldman SM, et al. Parkinson disease in twins: an etiologic study. JAMA 1999; 281: 341–6.
130. Satake W, Nakabayashi Y, Mizuta I, et al. Genome-wide association study identifies common variants at four loci as genetic risk factors for Parkinson's disease. Nat Genet 2009; 41: 1303–7.
131. Fung HC, Xiromerisiou G, Gibbs JR, et al. Association of tau haplotype-tagging polymorphisms with Parkinson's disease in diverse ethnic Parkinson's disease cohorts. Neurodegener Dis 2006; 3: 327–33.
132. Do CB, Tung JY, Dorfman E, et al. Web-based genome-wide association study identifies two novel loci and a substantial genetic component for Parkinson's disease. PLoS Genet 2011; 7: e1002141.
133. Nalls MA, Plagnol V, Hernandez DG, et al. Imputation of sequence variants for identification of genetic risks for Parkinson's disease: a meta-analysis of genome-wide association studies. Lancet 2011; 377: 641–9.
134. Langston JW, Ballard P, Tetrud JW, et al. Chronic Parkinsonism in humans due to a product of meperidine-analog synthesis. Science 1983; 219: 979–80.
135. Ritz B, Ascherio A, Checkoway H, et al. Pooled analysis of tobacco use and risk of Parkinson disease. Arch Neurol 2007; 64: 990–7.
136. Hernan MA, Takkouche B, Caamano-Isorna F, et al. A meta-analysis of coffee drinking, cigarette smoking, and the risk of Parkinson's disease. Ann Neurol 2002; 52: 276–84.

137. Quik M, O'Leary K, Tanner CM. Nicotine and Parkinson's disease: implications for therapy. Mov Disord 2008; 23: 1641–52.
138. Ross GW, Abbott RD, Petrovitch H, et al. Association of coffee and caffeine intake with the risk of Parkinson disease. JAMA 2000; 283: 2674–9.
139. Ascherio A, Zhang SM, Hernan MA, et al. Prospective study of caffeine consumption and risk of Parkinson's disease in men and women. Ann Neurol 2001; 50: 56–63.
140. Hu G, Bidel S, Jousilahti P, et al. Coffee and tea consumption and the risk of Parkinson's disease. Mov Disord 2007; 22: 2242–8.
141. Ascherio A, Weisskopf MG, O'Reilly EJ, et al. Coffee consumption, gender, and Parkinson's disease mortality in the cancer prevention study II cohort: the modifying effects of estrogen. Am J Epidemiol 2004; 160: 977–84.
142. Xu K, Xu Y, Brown-Jermyn D, et al. Estrogen prevents neuroprotection by caffeine in the mouse 1-methyl-4-phenyl-1,2,3,6-tetrahydropyridine model of Parkinson's disease. J Neurosci 2006; 26: 535–41.
143. Tan EK, Tan C, Fook-Chong SM, et al. Dose-dependent protective effect of coffee, tea, and smoking in Parkinson's disease: a study in ethnic Chinese. J Neurol Sci 2003; 216: 163–7.
144. Ascherio A, Chen H, Weisskopf MG, et al. Pesticide exposure and risk for Parkinson's disease. Ann Neurol 2006; 60: 197–203.
145. Kamel F, Tanner C, Umbach D, et al. Pesticide exposure and self-reported Parkinson's disease in the agricultural health study. Am J Epidemiol 2007; 165: 364–74.
146. Petrovitch H, Ross GW, Abbott RD, et al. Plantation work and risk of Parkinson disease in a population-based longitudinal study. Arch Neurol 2002; 59: 1787–92.
147. Tanner CM, Kamel F, Ross GW, et al. Rotenone, paraquat, and Parkinson's disease. Environ Health Perspect 2011; 119: 866–72.
148. Tanner CM, Ross GW, Jewell SA, et al. Occupation and risk of parkinsonism: a multicenter case-control study. Arch Neurol 2009; 66: 1106–13.
149. Elbaz A, Clavel J, Rathouz PJ, et al. Professional exposure to pesticides and Parkinson disease. Ann Neurol 2009; 66: 494–504.
150. Dick FD. Parkinson's disease and pesticide exposures. Br Med Bull 2006; 79-80: 219–31.
151. Gatto NM, Cockburn M, Bronstein J, et al. Well-water consumption and Parkinson's disease in rural California. Environ Health Perspect 2009; 117: 1912–18.
152. Costello S, Cockburn M, Bronstein J, et al. Parkinson's disease and residential exposure to maneb and paraquat from agricultural applications in the central valley of California. Am J Epidemiol 2009; 169: 919–26.
153. Wang A, Costello S, Cockburn M, et al. Parkinson's disease risk from ambient exposure to pesticides. Eur J Epidemiol 2011; 26: 547–55.
154. Racette BA, Tabbal SD, Jennings D, et al. Prevalence of parkinsonism and relationship to exposure in a large sample of Alabama welders. Neurology 2005; 64: 230–5.
155. Jankovic J. Searching for a relationship between manganese and welding and Parkinson's disease. Neurology 2005; 64: 2021–8.
156. Martin WR. Fuming over Parkinson disease: are welders at risk? Neurology 2011; 76: 1286–7.
157. Santamaria AB, Cushing CA, Antonini JM, et al. State-of-the-science review: Does manganese exposure during welding pose a neurological risk? J Toxicol Environ Health B Crit Rev 2007; 10: 417–65.
158. Weisskopf MG, Weuve J, Nie H, et al. Association of cumulative lead exposure with Parkinson's disease. Environ Health Perspect 2010; 118: 1609–13.
159. Gash DM, Rutland K, Hudson NL, et al. Trichloroethylene: Parkinsonism and complex 1 mitochondrial neurotoxicity. Ann Neurol 2008; 63: 184–92.
160. Goldman SM, Quinlan PJ, Ross GW, et al. Solvent exposures and Parkinson disease risk in twins. Ann Neurol 2011.
161. Rugbjerg K, Ritz B, Korbo L, et al. Risk of Parkinson's disease after hospital contact for head injury: population based case-control study. BMJ 2008; 337: a2494.
162. Goldman SM, Tanner CM, Oakes D, et al. Head injury and Parkinson's disease risk in twins. Ann Neurol 2006; 60: 65–72.

163. Bower JH, Maraganore DM, Peterson BJ, et al. Head trauma preceding PD: a case-control study. Neurology 2003; 60: 1610–15.
164. Tanner CM, Langston JW. Do environmental toxins cause Parkinson's disease? A critical review. Neurology 1990; 40: 17–30; discussion 30–1.
165. Goldman SM, Kamel F, Ross GW, et al. Head injury, alpha-synuclein Rep1, and Parkinson's disease. Ann Neurol 2012; 71: 40–8.
166. Elbaz A, Levecque C, Clavel J, et al. CYP2D6 polymorphism, pesticide exposure, and Parkinson's disease. Ann Neurol 2004; 55: 430–4.
167. Dutheil F, Beaune P, Tzourio C, et al. Interaction between ABCB1 and professional exposure to organochlorine insecticides in Parkinson disease. Arch Neurol 2010; 67: 739–45.
168. Hamza TH, Chen H, Hill-Burns EM, et al. Genome-Wide Gene-Environment Study Identifies Glutamate Receptor Gene GRIN2A as a Parkinson's Disease Modifier Gene via Interaction with Coffee. PLoS Genet 2011; 7: e1002237.
169. Abbott RD, Ross GW, White LR, et al. Environmental, life-style, and physical precursors of clinical Parkinson's disease: recent findings from the Honolulu-Asia Aging Study. J Neurol 2003; 250(Suppl 3): 30–9.

3

Differential diagnosis

John C. Morgan, Shyamal H. Mehta, and Kapil D. Sethi

Parkinsonism refers to a clinical syndrome characterized by a variable combination of rest tremor, bradykinesia or akinesia, cogwheel rigidity, and postural instability. In general, two of these four features must be present to make a diagnosis of parkinsonism. However, the situation is complicated by rare cases of pure akinesia in the absence of tremor and rigidity that have the classic pathology of Parkinson's disease (PD) (1). Within the rubric of parkinsonism there are a myriad of disorders, some yet unclassified (Table 3.1).

The most common cause of parkinsonism is PD. Pathologically, PD is characterized by cell loss in the substantia nigra (SN) and other pigmented nuclei of the brainstem. Characteristic inclusions called Lewy bodies are found in the remaining neurons and the term "Lewy body parkinsonism" is sometimes used synonymously with PD. Some researchers consider it most appropriate to refer to even the clinical picture of PD as "Parkinson's syndrome" on the premise that PD may not be one disease. Whereas the purists demand the presence of Lewy bodies at autopsy to diagnose PD, these inclusions may not be present in some inherited forms of otherwise classic PD. Currently, one such condition, the *parkin* mutation, has been mapped to chromosome 6 (2). This autosomal recessive young-onset parkinsonism differs pathologically from sporadic disease as Lewy bodies are usually absent. The clinical picture can be similar to idiopathic PD, including the presence of tremor (3). There are other forms of inherited parkinsonism, including the *LRRK2* mutation, where typical Lewy body pathology is found (4,5).

In the absence of a known biologic marker, the challenge facing the clinician is to make an accurate diagnosis of PD and differentiate it from other similar conditions. This review will give a practical approach to the differential diagnosis of parkinsonism and examine the diagnostic accuracy of a clinical diagnosis of PD.

IDIOPATHIC PARKINSON'S DISEASE

The onset of PD is gradual and the course slowly progressive albeit at different rates in different individuals. In most series, 65–70% of the patients present with an asymmetric tremor, especially of the upper extremity (6). After a variable delay, the disorder progresses to the other side with bilateral bradykinesia and gait difficulty that takes the form of festination and in advanced cases freezing. Postural instability and falls tend to be a late feature. Eye movements may show saccadic pursuit and upgaze may be limited in the elderly. Downgaze is normal. Autonomic disturbances may occur, but are not severe in early disease. Depression may occur early in the disease but dementia, as a presenting manifestation is not a feature of PD. Several signs should ring alarm bells when considering a diagnosis of PD. These include early dementia, early autonomic dysfunction, gaze difficulty (especially

TABLE 3.1 Classification of Parkinsonism

Primary Parkinson's Disease	Other Degenerative Disorders
Sporadic	Corticobasal degeneration
Familial	Dementia with Lewy bodies
Secondary Parkinsonism	Multiple system atrophy
Drug-induced parkinsonism	Progressive supranuclear palsy (Steele Richardson
Toxin-induced parkinsonism	Olszewski Syndrome)
Infectious	Spinocerebellar ataxias
Creutzfeld–Jakob disease	Neurodegeneration with brian iron accumulation 1
Metabolic	Huntington's disease
Structural	Neuroacanthocytosis
Tumor	Wilson's disease
Subdural hematoma	X-linked dystonia parkinsonism (Lubag)
Vascular	

TABLE 3.2 Features Indicating an Alternative Diagnosis to Parkinson's Disease

Early or Predominant Feature	Disease
Young onset	Drug- or toxin-induced parkinsonism, Wilson's disease, NBIA1
Minimal or absent tremor	PSP, vascular parkinsonism
Atypical tremor	CBD, MSA
Postural instability	PSP, MSA
Ataxia	MSA
Pyramidal signs	MSA, vascular parkinsonism
Amyotrophy	MSA, parkinsonism dementia of Guam
Symmetric onset	PSP, SND
Myoclonus	CBD, CJD, MSA
Dementia	DLB
Apraxia, Cortical sensory loss	CBD
Alien limb sign	CBD
Gaze palsies	PSP, OPCA, CBD, DLB, and PSG
Dysautonomia	MSA
Hallucinations (non-drug related)	DLB
Acute onset	Vascular parkinsonism, toxin-induced, psychogenic
Step-wise deterioration	Vascular parkinsonism

Abbreviations: PSP, progressive supranulear palsy; CBD, cortiobasal degeneration; MSA, multiple system atrophy; CJD, Creutzfeld–Jakob disease; DLB, dementia with Lewy bodies; NBIA1, neurodegeneration with brain iron accumulation type 1; OPCA, olivopontocerebellar atrophy; PSG, progressive subcortical gliosis; SND, striatonigral degeneration.

looking down), signs of upper motor neuron lesion or cerebellar signs in addition to parkinsonism, step-wise deterioration, and apraxia (Table 3.2).

Conditions Mimicking Parkinsonism

Essential tremor (ET) is more common than PD and results in tremor that affects primarily the upper extremities, head, and voice (7). The tremor is absent at rest except in the most severe cases and is increased by maintained posture and voluntary movement. Mild cogwheeling may be present but bradykinesia is not a feature (Table 3.3). The confusion occurs when a patient with a long history of ET begins to develop signs of parkinsonism. Patients with PD may have a prominent action tremor adding to the diagnostic uncertainty. In addition there are elderly patients with ET who exhibit mild bradykinesia on detailed testing (8). It is debatable if patients with ET are at an increased risk to develop PD (9). Psychomotor slowing in a severely depressed individual may resemble PD but there is no tremor and patients improve with antidepressant therapy.

OTHER CAUSES OF PARKINSONISM
Drug-Induced Parkinsonism

Drug-induced parkinsonism is a common complication of antipsychotic drug use with a reported prevalence of 15–60% (10). In one study, 51% of 95 patients referred for evaluation to a geriatric medicine service had neuroleptic-induced parkinsonism (11). Frequently these patients are misdiagnosed as PD and treated with dopaminergic drugs without any benefit. In a community study, 18% of all cases initially thought to be PD were subsequently diagnosed as drug-induced parkinsonism (12).

The symptoms of drug-induced parkinsonism may be indistinguishable from PD. Drug-induced parkinsonism is often described as symmetrical, whereas PD is often asymmetrical. However, one series found asymmetry of signs and symptoms in 30% of drug-induced patients (13). Patients with drug-induced parkinsonism are as varied in their clinical manifestations as patients with PD. Some patients have predominant bradykinesia, whereas others are tremor predominant. Postural reflexes may be impaired, festination is uncommon, and freezing is rare (13,14).

When the patient is on a dopamine blocking agent it is difficult to distinguish underlying PD from drug-induced parkinsonism. If possible, the typical dopamine blocking agents should be stopped or substituted with atypical antipsychotics and the symptoms and signs of parkinsonism should resolve within a few weeks to a few months, but it could take up to six months or more for signs and symptoms to resolve completely (15). Cerebrospinal fluid (CSF) dopamine

TABLE 3.3 Differentiating Essential Tremor from Parkinson's Disease

Body Parts	Essential Tremor Arms > Head > Voice > Legs	Parkinson's Disease Arms > Jaw > Legs
Rest tremor	−	+++
Postural tremor	+++	+
Kinetic tremor	+++	+
Frequency	7–12 Hz	4–6 Hz
Bradykinesia	−	++
Rigidity	+	++
Family history	++	+
Response to beta blockers	+	−
Response to levodopa	−	++
Postural instability	−	+

metabolites have been studied in drug-induced parkinsonism. These may be low in untreated PD but are relatively normal or increased in drug-induced parkinsonism. However, the DATATOP cohort CSF study showed that there is a significant overlap between PD and normal controls making this test of doubtful clinical value (16). One study utilizing 6-fluorodopa positron emission tomography (PET) scanning showed that a normal PET scan predicted good recovery from drug-induced parkinsonism upon cessation of the dopamine blocking agent and an abnormal PET scan was associated with persistence of signs in some but not all patients (17).

Drug-induced parkinsonism should be considered and inquiry should be made about intake of antipsychotic drugs and other dopamine blocking agents, such as metoclopramide (Table 3.4). Once drug-induced parkinsonism has been considered and ruled out, the most common conditions confused with PD include progressive supranuclear palsy (PSP), multiple system atrophy (MSA), dementia with Lewy bodies (DLB), corticobasal degeneration (CBD), and frontotemporal dementia (FTD) with parkinsonism. Together these entities are referred to as atypical forms of parkinsonism.

TABLE 3.4   Drugs Known to Cause Parkinsonism

Generic Name	Trademark
Chlorpromazine	Thorazine
Thiordazine	Mellaril
Mesoridazine	Serentil
Chlorprothixine	Taractan
Triflupromazine hydrochloride	Vesprin
Carphenazine maleate	Proketazine
Acetophenazine maleate	Tindal
Prochlorperazine	Compazine
Piperacetazine	Quide
Butaperazine maleate	Repoise maleate
Perphenazine	Tilafon
Molindone hydrochloride	Moban
Thiothixene	Navane
Trifluoperazine hydrochloride	Stelazine
Haloperidol	Haldol
Fluphenazine hydrochloride	Prolixin, 5 mg
Amoxapine	Asendin
Loxapine	Loxitane, Daxolin
Metoclopramide	Reglan
Promazine	Sparine
Promethazine	Phenergan
Thiethylperazine	Torecan
Trimeprazine	Temaril
Risperidone	Risperdal[a]
Olanzapine	Zyprexa[a]
Ziprasidone	Zeodon[a]
Combination drugs	Etrafon, Triavil

[a]In high dosages.

Progressive Supranuclear Palsy

PSP also known as Steele–Richardson–Olszewski syndrome is easy to diagnose in advanced stages (18). However, diagnostic confusion may occur early in the disease and in cases that have atypical features. Typically, the disorder presents with a gait disturbance with resultant falls in over half the cases (19). Measurable bradykinesia in the upper extremity may not be present at the initial presentation. The clinical features of PSP consist of supranuclear gaze palsy, especially involving the down-gaze with nuchal extension and predominant truncal extensor rigidity. Varying degrees of bradykinesia, dysphagia, personality changes, and other behavioral disturbances coexist. Patients often exhibit a motor recklessness and get up abruptly out of a chair (Rocket sign) even if this results in a fall. Another sign is the "applause sign" where the patient is unable to stop clapping after given directions to clap the hands three times (20).

Extraocular movement abnormalities are characteristic but may not be present at the onset of the illness or for several years (21). These abnormalities consist of square wave jerks, instability of fixation, slow or hypometric saccades, and predominantly a downgaze abnormality (22,23). Asking the patient to generate a saccade in the direction opposite to a stimulus (antisaccade test) is frequently abnormal in PSP (23). The oculocephalic responses are present in early disease but may be lost with advancing disease suggesting a nuclear element to the gaze palsy. Bell's phenomenon may be lost in advanced cases. Some patients with PSP have a limb dystonia that can be asymmetric (24), which can cause confusion with CBD. Rest tremor is rare but has been reported in pathologically confirmed PSP (25).

Radiologically PSP differs from PD in that in advanced cases there is atrophy of the mid-brain tectum and tegmentum with resultant diminution of the anteroposterior diameter of the midbrain (26,27). There may be dilatation of the third ventricle and sometimes a signal alteration may be seen in the tegmentum of the midbrain (28). PET scanning utilizing 6-fluorodopa may distinguish PSP from PD in that the uptake is diminished equally in both the caudate and putamen in PSP, whereas in PD the abnormalities are largely confined to the putamen (29). PET scans using raclopride binding show that the D2 receptor sites are diminished in PSP, whereas in PD these are normal (30).

Clinically, CBD, DLB, MSA, progressive subcortical gliosis (PSG), and even prion diseases have been misdiagnosed as PSP because of the presence of supranuclear gaze palsies (31–34). PSP also needs to be distinguished from other causes of supranuclear gaze palsy, including cerebral Whipple's disease, adult-onset Niemann–Pick type C, and multiple cerebral infarcts (35–37). The presence of prominent early cerebellar symptoms or early, unexplained dysautonomia would favor MSA over PSP (38) and the presence of alien limb syndrome, cortical sensory deficits, and focal cortical atrophy on magnetic resonance imaging (MRI) would favor CBD (39). The clinical diagnostic criteria proposed by Litvan et al. may be helpful (40,41).

Multiple System Atrophy

MSA, originally coined by Graham and Oppenheimer (42), refers to a variable combination of parkinsonism, autonomic, pyramidal, or cerebellar symptoms and signs. MSA can be subdivided into three types: striatonigral degeneration (SND), olivopontocerebellar atrophy (OPCA), and Shy–Drager syndrome (SDS) (43). All subtypes of MSA may have parkinsonian features. It is especially difficult to differentiate SND and PD. SND was originally described by Van Eecken et al. (44).

The parkinsonian features of MSA consist of progressive bradykinesia, rigidity, and postural instability (43). However, in a clinicopathologic report one of four patients had a rest tremor characteristic of PD (45). Although symptoms are usually bilateral, unilateral presentations have been described (46). The autonomic failure is more severe than seen in idiopathic PD and occurs early in MSA. Other useful clinical clues for the diagnosis of MSA include disproportionate anterocollis and the presence of cold blue hands.

The response to levodopa is usually incomplete in MSA (47). However, patients with MSA may initially respond to levodopa but the benefit usually declines within one or two years of treatment (48). Levodopa-induced dyskinesia may occur in MSA. Dyskinesia typically involves the face and neck but may also involve the extremities (49). Therefore, the presence of levodopa-induced dyskinesia cannot be used to make a definite diagnosis of PD. The situation is further complicated by the fact that PD patients may develop autonomic dysfunction including postural hypotension, urinary problems, constipation, impotence, and sweating disturbances. The autonomic dysfunction in PD may be worsened by dopaminergic therapy. Autonomic dysfunction tends to be severe in MSA and occurs early (50). Stridor can also occur early in MSA but not in PD (51). Urinary symptoms are very common in MSA. On urodynamic testing, there is a combination of detrusor hyperreflexia and urethral sphincter weakness (52). In addition neurogenic anal and urethral sphincter abnormalities are very common in MSA (53). However, this finding is not diagnostic and may occur in other conditions, such as PSP (54). Neuroimaging may show nonspecific abnormalities, such as diffuse hypointensity involving the putamen but more specific findings include a strip of lateral putaminal hyperintensity or pontine atrophy with an abnormal "hot cross bun" sign in the pons (55). Cardiac autonomic innervation may be tested using [123I] meta-iodobenzylguanidine (MIBG) scintigraphy. There is growing evidence that the MIBG scintigraphy is abnormal in PD and DLB due to postsynaptic sympathetic denervation (56). In contrast, in MSA the uptake in the heart is normal due to the presynaptic nature of the pathology. There is some overlap between normal individuals and patients with parkinsonism that decreases the sensitivity and specificity of this technique.

Dementia with Lewy Bodies

DLB, Lewy bodies are found in the neocortex as well as brain stem and diencephalic neurons (57). Some of these patients may have associated neurofibrillary tangles. The parkinsonian syndrome of DLB may be indistinguishable from PD. However, these patients have early-onset dementia and may have hallucinations, delusions, and even psychosis in the absence of dopaminergic therapy (58,59). Another characteristic feature is wide fluctuations in cognitive status. It may be difficult to distinguish PD dementia (PDD) from DLB. Resting tremor is typically less of a feature of DLB relative to PD. As a rule, if the dementia precedes or appears within one year of motor symptoms, the diagnosis of DLB is made (57). Rarely, patients with DLB may develop supranuclear gaze palsy resulting in confusion with PSP (31,32). Some patients respond partially and temporarily to dopaminergic therapy; however, occasionally the response to levodopa is robust.

Corticobasal Degeneration

Rabeiz et al. initially described this disorder as corticodentatonigral degeneration with neuronal achromasia (60). CBD typically presents in the 6th or 7th decade with slowly progressive unilateral, tremulous, apraxic, and rigid upper limb (61). The disorder tends to be gradually progressive with progressive gait disturbances, cortical sensory loss, and stimulus sensitive myoclonus resulting in a "jerky useless hand" (62–64). Jerky useless lower extremity is uncommon but may occur. Rarely these patients may develop Babinski signs and supranuclear gaze palsy.

When typical, the clinical picture is distinct and easily recognizable. However, atypical cases may be confused with PSP and the myoclonic jerking may be confused with the rest tremor of PD. The gait disturbance typically consists of slightly wide-based apraxic gait rather than the typical festinating gait of PD. Fixed limb dystonia may be prominent and strongly suggests CBD; however, some patients with PSP may also have asymmetric limb dystonia (24). Patients with CBD do not benefit from levodopa and the course is relentlessly progressive.

Rare cases of a parietal form of Pick's disease may be confused with CBD (65). The clinical spectrum of CBD has been expanded to include early-onset dementia and aphasia (66); however, in general these patients have a conspicuous absence of cognitive deficits. MRI in CBD shows focal atrophy especially in the parietal areas (67) and PET scans show asymmetric decrease of regional cerebral metabolic rates for glucose utilization (68). Tables 3.5 and 3.6 summarize some of the differential diagnostic features.

TABLE 3.5   Differential Diagnosis of Parkinson's Disease

	PD	PSP	MSA	CBD	DLB
Symmetry of deficit	+	+++	+++	−	+
Axial rigidity	+	+++	++	+	+
Limb dystonia	+	+	+	+++	+
Postural instability	++	+++	++	+	++
Vertical gaze palsy	+	+++	+	++	+
Dysautonomia	+	−	++	−	+
L-dopa response	+++	−	+	−	++
Asymmetric cortical atrophy	−	−	−	++	−
Hallucinations	+	−	−	−	++

Abbreviations: PD, Parkinson's disease; PSP, progressive supranuclear palsy; MSA, multiple system atrophy; CBD, corticobasal degeneration; DLB, dementia with Lewy bodies.

TABLE 3.6   MRI Features of Some Cases of Parkinsonism

	PSP	PD	MSA (OPCA)	MSA (SND)	CBD
Cortical atrophy	+	+	±	+	++
Putaminal atrophy	−	−	−	++	−
Pontine atrophy	+	−		+++	−
Midbrain atrophy	++	−	+	−	−
Cerebellar atrophy	−	−	++	−	−
High putaminal iron	−	−	+	+	−

Abbreviations: PSP, progressive supranuclear palsy; PD, Parkinson's disease; MSA, multiple system atrophy; OPCA, olivopontocerebellar atrophy; SND, striatonigral degeneration; CBD, corticobasal degeneration.

Frontotemporal Dementia with Parkinsonism

FTD is characterized by profound behavioral changes and an alteration in personality and social conduct with relative preservation of memory (69,70). Extrapyramidal symptoms are common and parkinsonism occurs in 40% of patients (71). Akinesia, rigidity, and a shuffling gait are the most common with typical tremor being rare (72). The PET scan reveals an equal decrease in the beta CFT uptake in the caudate and the putamen as opposed to PD where putamen is preferentially involved (72). This disorder is generally easy to distinguish from PD but may be confused with DLB and other disorders causing dementia and parkinsonism.

Toxin-Induced Parkinsonism

In general, these disorders are uncommon and may pose less of a differential diagnostic problem. 1-methyl-4-phenyl-1,2,3,6-tetrahydropyridine (MPTP)-induced parkinsonism is distinct from dopamine blocking agent–induced parkinsonism in that it is irreversible and is due to the destruction of the SN neurons (73). The clinical features have some similarities to PD except that the onset is abrupt and the affected individuals are younger than typical PD (74,75). These patients respond to levodopa with early levodopa-induced fluctuations (76). The patients may worsen gradually even in the absence of continued exposure to the toxin (77). In manganese poisoning, patients may superficially resemble PD, including soft speech, clumsiness, and impaired dexterity; however, they have a peculiar cock-walk gait in which they swagger on their toes (78,79). Typical resting tremor is absent. They may also have limb and truncal dystonia that is very unusual in untreated PD. Dementia and psychosis may occur and these patients do not respond well to dopaminergic drugs. Manganese is a component of welding rods and welders have been said to develop typical PD at an earlier age of onset compared with controls (80). However, many studies fail to show a relationship between welding and PD (81).

Parkinsonism as a result of carbon monoxide intoxication has been well described earlier (82). The parkinsonism may be delayed after the acute episode. These patients often show a slow shuffling gait, loss of arm swing, retropulsion, bradykinesia, rigidity, and occasionally, a rest tremor. The pull test tends to be markedly abnormal. A computed tomography (CT) scan or MRI may show necrotic lesions of the globus pallidus (83,84). There may also be associated white matter lesions that may progress without further exposure to carbon monoxide (85). Other toxins that have been reported to cause parkinsonism include carbon disulfide (86), cyanide (87,88), and methanol (89,90). These patients often have an acute onset and in some cases show basal ganglia lesions on neuroimaging. Posthypoxic parkinsonism has an acute evolution following a bout of severe prolonged hypoxia. Variable degrees of intellectual deterioration often accompany posthypoxic parkinsonism and the patients usually do not have rest tremor.

Posttraumatic Parkinsonism

Isolated head trauma is rarely a cause of parkinsonism (91). Parkinsonism may be seen in the setting of diffuse severe cerebral damage after severe brain injury (92). However, repeated minor trauma to the head as in boxers (dementia pugilistica) may be complicated by the late onset of dementia, parkinsonism, and other clinical features (93,94). Boxers are not immune to developing typical PD; however, the onset of parkinsonism and dementia in a boxer would be suggestive of dementia pugilistica. Imaging studies may show a cavum septum pellucidum and cerebral atrophy. A PET study using 6-fluorodopa showed damage to the caudate and the putamen in posttraumatic parkinsonism, whereas in PD the putamen is more severely involved.

Multi-Infarct Parkinsonism

Arteriosclerotic or multi-infarct parkinsonism is a debatable entity (95). However, patients are seen who have predominant gait disturbance with slightly wide-based gait with some features of gait apraxia and frequent freezing (96). These patients are labeled lower-half parkinsonism and they usually lack the typical rest tremor or other signs in the upper extremities (97). The gait disorder may not be distinct from senile gait and a similar gait disorder may also be seen in patients with Binswanger's disease (98,99). Levodopa responsiveness is uncommon but has been demonstrated occasionally in patients with pathologically confirmed multi-infarct parkinsonism.

The proposed criteria for the diagnosis of vascular parkinsonism include acute or subacute onset with a step-wise evolution of akinesia and rigidity along with vascular risk factors (100). This should be supplemented by at least two or more infarcts in the basal ganglia on neuroimaging. In some cases there may be more widespread MRI white matter abnormalities. Spontaneous improvement in symptoms and signs without dopaminergic therapy is suggestive of vascular parkinsonism.

Some patients with multiple cerebral infarction have a clinical picture characterized by gaze palsies, akinesia, and balance difficulties consistent with PSP. In fact, one study found that 19 out of 58 patients with a clinical diagnosis of PSP had radiographic evidence of multiple small infarcts in the deep white matter and the brainstem (35).

Parkinsonism with Hydrocephalus

Varying degrees of hypomimia, bradykinesia, and rigidity in the absence of tremor may occur in high pressure as well as in normal pressure hydrocephalus (NPH) (101). High pressure hydrocephalus rarely poses any diagnostic difficulties because of the relatively acute onset in the presence of signs of raised intracranial pressure. However, NPH may be more difficult to distinguish from PD. The classic triad of NPH includes a subacute onset of dementia, gait difficulty and urinary incontinence (102). The gait is slightly wide based with features of gait apraxia or slight ataxia. Rarely levodopa responsiveness has been demonstrated (103). In some patients the gait might improve for a few hours to days by the removal of CSF (104).

Parkinsonism Due to Structural Lesions of the Brain

Blocq and Marinesco were the first to report a clinicopathologic correlation of midbrain tuberculoma involving the nigra and contralateral parkinsonism (105,106). In most cases the responsible lesions have been tumors, chiefly gliomas and meningiomas. Interestingly these are uncommon in the striatum and have usually involved the frontal or parietal lobes. Subdural hematoma may present with subacute onset of parkinsonism with some pyramidal signs (107). Other rare causes of parkinsonism and structural lesions have included striatal abscesses (108) and vascular malformations. However, the structural lesions are easily confirmed by neuroimaging. Occasionally parkinsonism has been reported in patients with basal ganglia calcifications that usually occur in the setting of primary hypoparathyroidism. The calcification should be obvious on neuroimaging (109).

Infectious and Postinfectious Causes of Parkinsonism

The classic postencephalitic parkinsonism is not seen currently. It was characterized by a combination of parkinsonism and other movement disorders. Particularly characteristic were "oculogyric crises," which resulted in forceful and painful ocular deviation lasting minutes to hours. Other causes of oculogyric crises are Tourette's syndrome, neuroleptic induced acute dystonia, paroxysmal attacks in multiple sclerosis, and possibly conversion reaction. The parkinsonism may improve with levodopa but response deteriorates quickly. Parkinsonism rarely occurs as a sequelae of other sporadic encephalitides. Human immunodeficiency virus dementia has also been reported with parkinsonian features. Other infectious causes include striatal abscesses and neurosyphilis.

Psychogenic Parkinsonism

As compared with other psychogenic movement disorders, such as tremor, psychogenic parkinsonism is uncommon (110). A tremor of varying rates with marked distractibility along with inconsistent slowness and the presence of feigned weakness and numbness might lead to the correct diagnosis.

PARKINSONISM IN YOUNG ADULTS

The onset of parkinsonism under the age of 40 years is called young-onset parkinsonism. When symptoms begin under the age of 20 years, the term "juvenile parkinsonism" is sometimes used (111). Under the age of 20 years, parkinsonism typically occurs as a component of a more widespread degenerative disorder. However, *parkin* mutations have been described in some young patients (2).

Dopa-Responsive Dystonia

There is a significant overlap in young patients with dystonia and parkinsonism. Patients with young-onset parkinsonism manifest dystonia that may be responsive to dopaminergic drugs (112). However, the response may deteriorate upon long-term follow-up. Patients with hereditary dopa-responsive dystonia have an excellent and sustained response to low doses of levodopa (113). In addition, PET scans show markedly reduced 6-fluorodopa uptake in patients with young-onset PD, whereas the fluorodopa uptake is normal in patients with dopa-responsive dystonia (114). Patients with dopa-responsive dystonia have a guanosine triphosphate-cyclohydrolase deficiency that is not a feature of PD in young adults.

Wilson's Disease

Wilson's disease usually presents primarily with neuropsychiatric impairment. It should be considered in every case of young-onset parkinsonism because it is eminently treatable and the consequences of nonrecognition can be grievous. The most common neurologic manifestations are tremor, dystonia, rigidity, dysarthria, drooling, and ataxia. A combination of parkinsonism and ataxia is particularly indicative of neurologic Wilson's disease (115). Parkinsonism is the most prevalent motor dysfunction, whereas about 25% of patients present with disabling cerebellar ataxia, tremor, or dysarthria (116). Typically, the tremor involves the upper limbs and the head and rarely the lower limbs. It can be present at rest, with postural maintenance and may persist with voluntary movements. The classic tremor is coarse and irregular and present during action. Holding the arms forward and flexed horizontally can emphasize that the proximal muscles are active (wing-beating tremor). Less commonly, tremor may affect just the tongue and the orofacial area (117). Dystonia is also quite common in Wilson's disease. The characteristic feature is an empty smile due to facial dystonia. Dysarthria is very common and may take the form of a dystonic or scanning dysarthria. Approximately 30% of patients present with behavioral and mental status changes (118). The psychiatric disorder may take the form of paranoid symptoms sometimes accompanied by delusional thinking and hallucinations. Early presentation may be a decline in memory and school performance. Patients may develop anxiety, moodiness, disinhibited behavior, and loss of insight. A characteristic feature is inappropriate laughter. Although eye movements are typically normal, some cases of Wilson's disease may show a saccadic pursuit, gaze distractibility, or difficulty in fixation (119).

Kayser–Fleischer rings (KF rings) due to copper deposition in the cornea may be easy to recognize in patients with a light-colored iris; however, in patients with brown irises these rings may be very difficult to see. Usually the ring is golden-brown in color and involves the whole circumference of the cornea. However, in the early stages the ring may be more apparent in the upper than the lower pole. Rarely these rings can be unilateral. KF rings are best appreciated by a slit-lamp examination done by a neuro-ophthalmologist. Typically the absence of KF rings on the slit-lamp examination rules out neurologic Wilson's disease. However, there are reports of patients with typical neurologic Wilson's disease without any KF rings (120,121).

Radiologically, advanced cases of Wilson's disease may have cavitation of the putamen (122). However, putaminal lesions are not specific to Wilson's disease. Other causes of putaminal cavitation or lesions include hypoxic ischemic damage, methanol poisoning, mitochondrial encephalomyopathy, and wasp-sting encephalopathy. Nearly half the patients of established neurologic Wilson's disease have hypodensities of the putamina on CT scans in contrast to patients with hepatic disease who frequently have normal CT scans (123). MRI is more sensitive and almost all patients with neurologic features have some disturbance on T2-weighted images in the basal ganglia with a pattern of symmetric, bilateral, concentric-laminar T2 hyperintensity and the involvement of the pars compacta of the SN, periaqueductal gray matter, pontine tegmentum, and thalamus (124). The hepatic component of Wilson's disease may cause increased T1 signal intensity in the globus pallidus (125). In the adult age group, the basal ganglia lesions may be different from those in the pediatric group. The putaminal lesions may not be present and the globus pallidus and SN may show increased hypointensity on T2-weighted images. Cortical and subcortical lesions may also be present with a predilection to the frontal lobe. However, rare cases of neurologic Wilson's disease may have a normal MRI (126). PET scans of Wilson's disease may show a reduction of 6-fluorodopa uptake (127).

The most useful diagnostic test is serum ceruloplasmin and a 24-hour urinary copper excretion supplemented by a slit-lamp examination for KF rings. Unfortunately, not all patients with Wilson's disease have a low ceruloplasmin level (128). The measurement of copper concentration in the liver makes a definitive diagnosis. In heterozygotes it is between 50 and 100 µg/g of tissue and in patients with Wilson's disease it may be over 200 µg/g (129).

Neurodegeneration with Brain Iron Accumulation 1
Previously known as Hallervorden–Spatz disease or pantothenate kinase–associated neurodegeneration (PKAN), this is usually a disease found in children but young

adults may also be affected. Typically, the disease occurs before the age of 20 years. Facial dystonia tends to be prominent, coupled with gait difficulty and postural instability. Patients may have night blindness progressing to visual loss secondary to retinitis pigmentosa. Other extrapyramidal signs include choreoathetosis and a tremor that has been poorly characterized. Cognitive problems include impairment of frontal tasks and memory disturbances and psychiatric manifestations have been reported. CT scans are often normal; however, low-density lesions have been described in the globus pallidus. MRI, especially using a high field strength magnet, shows decreased signal intensity in the globus pallidus with a central hyperintensity. This has been called the "eye of the tiger sign" (130). Genetic testing for PANK 2 mutation is now commercially available and may be performed in doubtful cases (131).

Juvenile Huntington's Disease

This autosomal dominant neurodegenerative disorder typically presents with chorea, difficulty with gait, and cognitive problems. However, the "Westphal variant" of the disease affecting the young may manifest bradykinesia, tremulousness, myoclonic jerks, and occasionally seizures and cognitive disturbances (132). Eye movement abnormalities, including apraxia, can be remarkable. When coupled with a lack of family history these young patients may be confused with young-onset PD; however, neuroimaging and genetic testing should easily distinguish the two.

Hemiparkinsonism–Hemiatrophy Syndrome

These patients have a long-standing hemiatrophy of the body and develop progressive bradykinesia and dystonic movements around the age of 40 years (133). Ipsilateral corticospinal tract signs may be found, which are not a feature of PD. Neuroimaging reveals brain asymmetry with atrophy of the contralateral hemisphere with compensatory ventricular dilatation. Regional cerebral metabolic rates are diminished in the hemisphere contralateral to the clinical hemiatrophy in the putamen and the medial frontal cortex, whereas in PD the regional cerebral metabolic rates are normal or increased contralateral to the clinically affected side (134).

X-linked Dystonia Parkinsonism (Lubag)

This inherited disorder usually occurs in the Philippines. However, rare cases are seen in other parts of the world (135). Typical age of presentation is around the age of 30–40 years. Focal dystonia or tremor is the initial finding followed by other parkinsonian features. Rarely parkinsonian features may precede dystonia. Clinically this disorder is differentiated from idiopathic PD by the presence of marked dystonia and the pattern of inheritance.

Neuroacanthocytosis

This is a rare cause of parkinsonism and typically presents with a hyperkinetic movement disorder, including chorea, tic-like features, and polyneuropathy. MRI shows a characteristic atrophy of the caudate and a hyperintensity in the putamen on T2-weighted images and acanthocytes are revealed on a fresh blood smear (136).

DIAGNOSTIC CRITERIA FOR PARKINSON'S DISEASE

From the preceding discussion it is obvious that there are a large number of disorders that can be confused with PD. In an effort to improve diagnostic accuracy several sets of clinical diagnostic criteria for PD have been proposed (137–141). Table 3.7 lists the UK Parkinson's Disease Society Brain Bank clinical diagnostic criteria (138).

The first clinicopathologic study found that only 69–75% of the patients with an autopsy-confirmed diagnosis of PD had at least two of the three cardinal manifestations of PD: tremor, rigidity, and bradykinesia (141). Furthermore, 20–25% of patients who showed two of these cardinal features had a pathologic diagnosis other than PD. Even more concerning, 13–19% of patients who demonstrated all three cardinal features typically associated with a clinical diagnosis of PD had another pathologic diagnosis. Rajput et al. reported autopsy results in 59 patients with parkinsonian syndromes (142). After a long-term follow-up period, the clinical diagnosis of PD was retained in 41 of 59 patients. However, only 31 of 41 (75%) patients with clinically determined PD showed histopathologic signs of PD at autopsy examination.

A third series comprised 100 patients with a clinical diagnosis of PD, who had been examined during their life by different neurologists using poorly defined

TABLE 3.7 UK Parkinson's Disease Society Brain Bank Clinical Diagnostic Criteria (138)

Inclusion Criteria	Exclusion Criteria	Supportive Criteria
Bradykinesia (slowness of initiation of voluntary movement with progressive reduction in speed and amplitude of repetitive actions) And at least one of the following: • muscular rigidity • 4–6 Hz rest tremor • postural instability not caused by primary visual, vestibular, cerebellar, or proprioceptive dysfunction	• History of repeated strokes with stepwise progression of parkinsonian features • History of repeated head injury • History of definite encephalitis • Oculogyric crises • Neuroleptic treatment at onset of symptoms • More than one affected relative • Sustained remission • Strictly unilateral features after 3 years • Supranuclear gaze palsy • Cerebellar signs • Early severe autonomic involvement • Early severe dementia with disturbances of memory, language, and praxis • Babinski sign • Presence of cerebral tumour or communicating hydrocephalus on CT scan • Negative response to large doses of levodopa (if malabsorption excluded) • MPTP exposure	(Three or more required for diagnosis of definite PD) • Unilateral onset • Rest tremor present • Progressive disorder • Persistent asymmetry affecting side of onset most • Excellent response (70–100%) to levodopa • Severe levodopa-induced chorea • Levodopa response for 5 years or more • Clinical course of 10 years or more

Abbreviations: CT, computed tomography; MPTP, 1-methyl-4-phenyl-1,2,3,6-tetrahydropyridine; PD, Parkinson's disease.

diagnostic criteria. When autopsies were performed (mean interval between symptom-onset and autopsy 11.9 years), PD was found in 76 patients. The authors reviewed the charts of these patients and applied the UK Parkinson's Disease Society Brain Bank clinical criteria for PD requiring bradykinesia and at least one other feature, including rigidity, resting tremor, or postural instability and focusing on clinical progression, asymmetry of onset, and levodopa response. Sixteen additional exclusion criteria were also applied (Table 3.7). With the application of these diagnostic criteria, 89 of the original 100 patients were considered to have PD, but, again, only 73 (82%) were confirmed to have PD at autopsy. When the authors re-examined the patients with all three cardinal features (excluding the postural instability), only 65% of patients with an autopsy diagnosis of PD fit this clinical category.

These authors studied another 100 patients with a clinical diagnosis of PD that came to neuropathologic examination (144). Ninety fulfilled pathologic criteria for PD. Ten were misdiagnosed: MSA (six), PSP (two), post–encephalitic parkinsonism (one), and vascular parkinsonism (one). They next examined the accuracy of diagnosis of parkinsonian disorders in a specialist movement disorders service (145). They reviewed the clinical and pathologic features of 143 cases of parkinsonism, likely including many of the patients previously reported (144). They found a surprisingly high positive predictive value (98.6%) of clinical diagnosis of PD among the specialists. In fact, only 1 of 73 patients diagnosed with PD during life was found to have an alternate diagnosis. This study demonstrated that the clinical diagnostic accuracy of PD may be improved by utilizing stringent criteria and a prolonged follow-up. A retrospective study showed that the hallucinations are very predictive of Lewy body pathology, either PD or DLB (146).

The Emerging Role of Neuroimaging in the Differential Diagnosis of Parkinson's Disease

Brain MRI has revealed potential biomarkers in the differential diagnosis of parkinsonism. Radiotracer neuroimaging is currently one of the most used imaging techniques in the differential diagnosis of PD. ^{123}I-ioflupane (DaTscan) single photon emission computed tomography was approved for use in Europe in 2000 and in the United States in 2011. Approximately 300,000 patients have undergone DaTscan in Europe and this ligand of the dopamine transporter has been routinely used in practice to aid in the differential diagnosis of PD (147). DaTscan is helpful in the differential diagnosis of PD, but patients with multiple forms of parkinsonism (PD, DLB, PSP, and MSA) demonstrate striatal binding deficits with this scan. DaTscan does appear quite useful for differentiating between Parkinsonian syndromes and ET, psychogenic parkinsonism, many cases of vascular parkinsonism, and drug-induced parkinsonism. Although a recent study calls into question whether DaTscan is any better than a clinical diagnosis of PD in neurologic practice (147), it can be quite helpful for both the patient and the clinician in numerous select cases.

Another neuroimaging technique used for the diagnosis of parkinsonism is 6-fluorodopa PET, which has been available for many years at numerous research institutions and has been helpful in identifying presynaptic versus postsynaptic parkinsonism in the small number of patients who have been scanned. The combination of imaging the nigrostriatal pathway with 6-fluorodopa PET and brain metabolism using fluorodeoxyglucose PET may provide better diagnostic accuracy of PD and Parkinson's plus syndromes (148).

In 2009, Vaillancourt et al. reported that diffusion tensor imaging reveals reduced fractional anisotropy (a measure of the directional diffusivity of water) in the SN of subjects with PD relative to healthy controls with a sensitivity and specificity of 100% (149). The sample size was small (28 subjects total) and this research needs further study, but these results hold some promise. Quantitative MRI may also help differentiate between PD and other Parkinsonian syndromes, but these specialized measurement techniques are not currently a part of routine radiologic practice (150). Most recently, 7.0 Tesla MRI of the SN revealed clear-cut alterations in the dorsomedial portion of the nigra in PD subjects relative to controls, but the availability of 7.0 Tesla MRI is currently limited (151). Further refinements in MRI are likely to improve the clinical accuracy of early PD diagnosis in the future.

Transcranial ultrasound (TCUS) has also emerged as a potential tool in the diagnosis and differential diagnosis of PD. Hyperechogenicity of the SN is characteristic of PD on TCUS and it is unfortunately present in perhaps 9% or more of healthy controls (152). However, SN hyperechogenicity may be a risk factor for future development of PD in elderly subjects without neurodegenerative disease at baseline, with a three-year relative risk of incident PD of 17.4 in one published study (153). In Parkinson's plus syndromes, there is some evidence that third ventricle dilatation and hyperechogenicity of the lenticular nuclei on TCUS is associated with PSP and MSA, respectively (154). Although TCUS appears promising in the differential diagnosis of PD, it remains somewhat controversial to date.

Further refinements in neuroimaging are likely to improve accuracy in the differential diagnosis of PD in the future.

REFERENCES

1. Quinn NP, Luthert P, Hanover M, Marsden CD. Pure akinesia due to Lewy body. Parkinson's disease: a case with pathology. Mov Disord 1989; 4: 885–92.
2. Rajput AH. Pathologic and biochemical studies of juvenile parkinsonism linked to chromosome 6q. Neurology 1999; 53: 1375.
3. Klein C, Pramstaller PP, Kis B, et al. Parkin deletions in a family with adult-onset, tremor-dominant parkinsonism: expanding the phenotype. Ann Neurol 2000; 48: 65–71.
4. Polymeropoulos MH. Autosomal dominant Parkinson's disease and alpha-synuclein. Ann Neurol 1998; 44: S63–4.
5. Ross OA, Toft M, Whittle AJ, et al. LRRK2 and Lewy body disease. Ann Neurol 2006; 59: 388–93.
6. Paulson HL, Stern MB. Clinical manifestations of Parkinson's disease. In: Watts RL, Koller WC, eds. Movement Disorders: Neurological Principles and Practice. New York: McGraw-Hill, 1997: 183–99.
7. Findley LJ, Koller WC. Essential tremor. Clin Neuropharm 1989; 12: 453–82.
8. Montgomery EB, Baker KB, Lyons K, Koller WC. Motor initiation and execution in essential tremor and Parkinson's disease. Mov Disord 2000; 15: 511–15.
9. Pahwa R, Koller WC. Is there a relationship between Parkinson's disease and essential tremor? Clin Neuropharm 1993; 16: 30–5.
10. Hardie RJ, Lees AJ. Neuroleptic induced Parkinson's syndrome: clinical features and results of treatment with levodopa. Neurology 1987; 37: 850–4.
11. Stephen PJ, Williams J. Drug-induced Parkinsonism in the elderly. Lancet 1987; 2: 1082.
12. Mutch WJ, Dingwall-Fordyce I, Downie AW, et al. Parkinson's disease in a Scottish city. Br Med J 1986; 292: 534–6.
13. Sethi KD, Zamrini EY. Asymmetry in clinical features of drug-induced parkinsonism. J Neuropsychiatry Clin Neurosci 1990; 2: 64–6.
14. Giladi N, Kao R, Fahn S. Freezing phenomenon in patients with Parkinsonian syndromes. Mov Disord 1997; 12: 302–5.

15. Klawans HL, Bergan D, Bruyn GW. Prolonged drug induced parkinsonism. Confin Neurol 1973; 35: 368–77.
16. LeWitt PA, Galloway MP, Matson W, et al. Markers of dopamine metabolism in Parkinson's disease. Neurology 1992; 42: 2111–17.
17. Burn DJ, Brooks DJ. Nigral dysfunction in drug-induced parkinsonism: an [18]flurodopa PET study. Neurology 1993; 43: 552–6.
18. Steele JC, Richardson JC, Olszewski J. Progressive supranuclear palsy. Arch Neurol 1964; 10: 333–59.
19. Golbe LI, Davis PH, Schoenberg BS, Duvoisin RC. Prevalence and natural history of progressive supranuclear palsy. Neurology 1988; 38: 1031–4.
20. Dubois B, Slachevsky A, Pillon B, et al. "Applause sign" helps to discriminate PSP from FTD and PD. Neurology 2005; 64: 2132–3.
21. Nuwer MR. Progressive supranuclear palsy despite normal eye movements. Arch Neurol 1981; 38: 784.
22. Troost B, Daroff R. The ocular motor defects in progressive supranuclear palsy. Ann Neurol 1977; 2: 397–403.
23. Vidailhet M, Rivaud S, Gouider-Khouja N, et al. Eye movements in Parkinsonian syndromes. Ann Neurol 1994; 35: 420–6.
24. Barclay CL, Lang AE. Dystonia in progressive supranuclear palsy. J Neurol Neurosurg Psychiatry 1997; 62: 352–6.
25. Masucci EF, Kurtzke JF. Tremor in progressive supranuclear palsy. Acta Neurol Scand 1989; 80: 296–300.
26. Schonfeld SM, Golbe LI, Sage JI, Safer JN, Duvoisin RC. Computed tomographic findings in progressive supranuclear palsy: correlation with clinical grade. Mov Disord 1987; 2: 263–78.
27. Savoiardo M, Girotti F, Strada L, Cieri E. Magnetic resonance imaging in progressive supranuclear palsy and other Parkinsonian disorders. J Neural Transm Suppl 1994; 42: 93–110.
28. Yagishita A, Oda M. Progressive supranuclear palsy: MRI and pathological findings. Neuroradiology 1996; 38: S60–6.
29. Brooks DJ, Ibanez V, Sawle GV, et al. Differing patterns of striatal F-dopa uptake in Parkinson's disease, multiple system atrophy, and progressive suprauclear palsy. Ann Neurol 1990; 28: 547–55.
30. Brooks DJ, Ibanez V, Sawle GV, et al. Striatal D2 receptor status in patients with Parkinson's disease, striatonigral degeneration, and progressive supranuclear palsy, measures with C-raclopride and positron emission tomography. Ann Neurol 1992; 31: 184–92.
31. Fearnley JM, Revesz T, Brooks DJ, Frackowiak RS, Lees AJ. Diffuse Lewy body disease presenting with a supranuclear gaze palsy. J Neurol Neurosurg Psychiatry 1991; 54: 159–61.
32. De Bruin VM, Lees AJ, Daniel SE. Diffuse Lewy body disease presenting with supranuclear gaze palsy, parkinsonism, and dementia: a case report. Mov Disord 1992; 7: 355–8.
33. Foster NL, Gilman S, Berent S, et al. Progressive subcortical gliosis and progressive supranuclear palsy can have similiar clinical and PET abnormalities. J Neurol Neurosurg Psychiatry 1992; 55: 707–13.
34. Lees AJ, Gibb W, Barnard RO. A case of progressive subcortical gliosis presenting clinically as Steele-Richardson Olszewski syndrome. J Neurol Neurosurg Psychiatry 1988; 51: 1224–7.
35. Dubinsky RM, Jankovic J. Progressive supranuclear palsy and a multi-infarct state. Neurology 1987; 37: 570–6.
36. Winikates J, Jankovic J. Vascular progressive supranuclear palsy. J Neural Transm Suppl 1994; 42: 189–201.
37. Fink JK, Filling- Katz MR, Sokol J, et al. Clinical spectrum of Niemann- Pick disease type C. Neurology 1989; 39: 1040–9.
38. Quinn N. Multiple system atrophy. In: Marsden C, Fahn S, eds. Movement Disorders 3 Newton. Massachusetts: Butterworth-Heinemann, 1994: 262–81.

39. Gibb WR, Luthert PJ, Marsden CD. Corticobasal degeneration. Brain 1989; 112: 1171–92.
40. Litvan I, Agid Y, Jankovic J, et al. Accuracy of clinical criteria for the diagnosis of progressive supranuclear palsy (Steele-Richardson-Olszewski syndrome). Neurology 1996; 46: 922–30.
41. Litvan I, Agid Y, Calne D, et al. Clinical research criteria for the diagnosis of progressive supranuclear palsy (Steele-Richardson-Olszewski syndrome) report of the NINDS-SPSP international workshop. Neurology 1996; 47: 1–9.
42. Graham JG, Oppenheimer DR. Orthostatic hypotension and nicotine sensitivity in a case of multiple system atrophy. J Neurol Neurosurg Psychiatry 1969; 32: 28–34.
43. Wenning GK, Ben Shlomo Y, Magalhaes M, Daniel SE, Quinn NP. Clinical features and natural history of multiple system atrophy; an analysis of 100 cases. Brain 1994; 117: 835–45.
44. Van Eecken H, Adams RD, Van Bogaert, L. Striatopallidal-nigral degeneration. J Neuropath Exp Neurol 1960; 19: 159–66.
45. Adams RA, Van Bogaert L, Van der Eecken H. Striato-nigral degeneration. J Neuropathol Exp Neurol 1964; 23: 584–608.
46. Wenning GK, Tison F, Ben-Shlomo Y, Daniel SE, Quinn NP. Multiple system atrophy: a review of 203 pathologically proven cases. Mov Disord 1997; 12: 133–47.
47. Rajput AH, Kazi KH, Rozdilsky B. Striatonigral degeneration, response to levodopa therapy. J Neuro Sci 1972; 16: 331–41.
48. Hughes AJ, Colosimo C, Kleedorfer B, Daniel SE, Lees AJ. The dopaminergic response in multiple system atrophy. J Neurol Neurosurg Psychiatry 1992; 55: 1009–13.
49. Lang AE, Birnbaum A, Blair RDG, Kierans C. Levodopa related response fluctuations in presumed olivopontocerebellar atrophy. Mov Disord 1986; 1: 93–102.
50. Shy GM, Drager GA. A neurologic syndrome associated with orthostatic hypotension. Arch Neurol 1960; 2: 511–27.
51. Wu YR, Chen CM, Ro LS, Chen ST, Tang LM. Vocal cord paralysis as an initial sign of multiple system atrophy in the central nervous system. J Formos Med Assoc 1996; 95: 804–6.
52. Bonnet AM, Pichon J, Vidailhet M, et al. Urinary disturbances in striatonigral degeneration and Parkinson's disease: clinical and urodynamic aspects. Mov Disord 1997; 12: 509–13.
53. Kirby R, Fowler C, Gosling J, Bannister R. Urethro-vesical dysfunction in progressive autonomic failure with multiple system atrophy. J Neurol Neurosurg Psychiatry 1986; 49: 554–62.
54. Valldeoriola F, Valls-Sole E, Tolosa S, Marti MJ. Striated anal sphincter denervation in patients with progressive supranuclear palsy. Mov Disord 1995; 10: 550–5.
55. Schrag A, Good CD, Miszkiel K, et al. Differentiation of atypical parkinsonian syndromes with routine MRI. Neurology 2000; 54: 697–702.
56. Nagayama H, Hamamoto M, Ueda M, Nagashima J, Katayama Y. Reliability of MIBG myocardial scintigraphy in the diagnosis of Parkinson's disease. J Neurol Neurosurg Psychiatry 2005; 76: 249–51.
57. McKeith IG, Dickson DW, Lowe J, et al. Diagnosis and management of dementia with Lewy bodies: third report of the DLB Consortium. Neurology 2005; 65: 1863–72.
58. Mega MS, Masterman DL, Benson DF, et al. Dementia with Lewy bodies: reliability and validity of clinical and pathologic criteria. Neurology 1996; 47: 1403–9.
59. Ala TA, Yang KH, Sung JH, Frey WH. Hallucinations and signs of parkinsonism help distinguish patients with dementia and cortical Lewy bodies from patients with Alzheimer's disease at presentation: a clinicopathological study. J Neurol Neurosurg Psychiatry 1997; 62: 16–21.
60. Rebeiz JJ, Kolodny EH, Richardson EP. Corticodentatonigral degeneration with neuronal achromasia. Arch Neurol 1968; 18: 220–3.
61. Riley De, Lang AE, Lewis A, et al. Cortical-basal ganglionic degeneration. Neurology 1990; 40: 1203–12.
62. Rinne Jo, Lee MS, Thompson PD, Marsden CD. Corticobasal degeneration: a clinical study of 36 cases. Brain 1994; 117: 1183–96.

63. Chen R, Ashby P, Lang AE. Stimulus-sensitive myoclonus in akinetic-rigid syndromes. Brain 1992; 115: 1875–88.
64. Litvan I, Agid Y, Gostz C, et al. Accuracy of the clinical diagnosis of corticobasal degeneration: a clinicopathological study. Neurology 1997; 48: 119–25.
65. Lang AE, Bergeron C, Pollanen MS, Ashby P. Parietal Pick's disease mimicking cortical-basal ganglionic degeneration. Neurology 1994; 44: 1436–40.
66. Katai S, Maruyama T, Nakamura A, et al. A case of corticobasal degeneration presenting with primary progressive aphasia Rinsho Shinkeigaku. Clin Neurol 1997; 37: 249–52.
67. Grisoli M, Fetoni V, Savoiardo M, Girotti F, Bruzzone MG. MRI in corticobasal degeneration. Eur J Neurol 1995; 2: 547–52.
68. Nagasawa H, Tanji H, Nomura H, et al. PET study of cerebral glucose metabolism and fluorodopa uptake in patients with corticobasal degeneration. J Neurol Sci 1996; 139: 210–17.
69. Neary D, Snowden J, Gustafsson L, et al. Frontotemporal lobar degeneration: a consensus on clinical diagnostic criteria. Neurology 1998; 51: 1546–54.
70. Gustaffson L. The clinical picture of frontal lobe degeneration of non-Alzheimer type. Dementia 1993; 4: 143–8.
71. Pasquier F, Lebert F, Lavenu I, Guillaume B. The clinical picture of frontotemporal dementia: diagnosis and follow-up. Geriatr Cogn Disord 1999; 109: 10–14.
72. Rinne JO, Laine M, Kaasinen V, et al. Striatal dopamine transporter and extrapyramidal symptoms in frontotemporal dementia. Neurology 2002; 58: 1489–93.
73. Davis GC, Williams AC, Markey SP, et al. Chronic parkinsonism secondary intravenous injection of meperidine analogues. Psychiatry Res 1979; 1: 249–54.
74. Langston JW, Ballard P, Tetrud J, Irwin I. Chronic Parkinsonism in humans due to a product of meperidine-analog synthesis. Science 1983; 219: 979–80.
75. Tetrud JW, Langston JW, Garbe PL, Ruttenber JA. Early Parkinsonism in persons exposed to 1-methyl-4-phenyl-1, 2,3,6-tetrahydropyridine (MPTP). Neurology 1989; 39: 1482–7.
76. Langston JW, Ballard PA. Parkinsonism induced by 1-methyl-4-phenyl 1,2,3,6-tetrahydropyridine (MPTP): implications for treatment and the pathogenesis of Parkinson's disease. Can J Neurol Sci 1984; 11: 160–5.
77. Langston JW. MPTP-induced Parkinsonism: how good a model is it? In: Fahn S, Marsden CD, Teychenne P, Jenner P, eds. Recent Advances in Parkinson's Disease. New York: Raven Press, 1986: 119–26.
78. Huang CC, Chu NS, Song C, Wang JD. Chronic manganese intoxication. Arch Neurol 1989; 46: 1104–12.
79. Barbeau A. Manganese and extrapyramidal disorders. Neurotoxicology 1984; 5: 113–36.
80. Racette BA, McGee-Minnich L, Moerlein SM, et al. Welding-related parkinsonism: clinical features, treatment, and pathophysiology. Neurology 2001; 56: 8–13.
81. Fored CM, Fryzek JP, Brandt L, et al. Parkinson's disease and other basal ganglia or movement disorders in a large nationwide cohort of Swedish welders. Occup Environ Med 2006; 63: 135–40.
82. Lee MS, Marsden CD. Neurological sequelae following carbon monoxide poisoning: clinical course and outcome according to the clinical types and brain computed tomography scan findings. Mov Disord 1994; 9: 550–8.
83. Miura T, Mitomo M, Kawai R, Harada K. CT of the brain in acute carbon monoxide intoxication. Characteristic features and prognosis. AJNR 1985; 6: 739–42.
84. Kobayashi K, Isaki K, Fukutani Y, et al. CT findings of the interval form of carbon monoxide poisoning compared with neuropathological findings. Eur Neurol 1984; 23: 34–43.
85. Vieregge P, Klostermann W, Blumm RG, Borgis KJ. Carbon monoxide poisoning. Clinical, neurophysiological and brain imaging observations in acute phase and follow up. J Neurol 1989; 239: 478–81.
86. Peters HA, Levine RL, Matthews CG, Chapman LJ. Extrapyramidal and other neurological manifestations associated with carbon disulfide fumigant exposure. Arch Neurol 1988; 45: 537–40.

87. Uitti RJ, Rajput AH, Aashenhurst EM, Rozkilsky B. Cyanide-induced Parkinsonism: a clinicopathologic report. Neurology 1985; 35: 921–5.
88. Rosenberg NL, Myers JA, Wayne WR. Cyanide-induced Parkinsonism: clinical, MRI, and 6-fluorodopa PET studies. Neurology 1989; 39: 142–4.
89. Guggenheim MA, Couch JR, Weinberg W. Motor dysfunction as a permanent complication of methanol ingestion. Arch Neurol 1971; 24: 550–4.
90. Mclean DR, Jacobs H, Mielki BW. Methanol poisoning a clinical and pathological study. Ann Neurol 1980; 8: 161–7.
91. Factor SA, Sanchez-Ramos J, Weiner WJ. Trauma as an etiology of Parkinsonism: a historical review of the concept. Mov Disord 1988; 3: 30–6.
92. Factor SA. Posttraumatic parkinsonism. In: Stern MB, Koller WC, eds. Parkinsonian Syndromes. New York: Marcel Dekker, 1993: 95–110.
93. Critchley M. Medical aspects of boxing, particularly from a neurological standpoint. Br Med J 1957; 1: 357–62.
94. Martland HS. Punch drink. J Am Med Assoc 1928; 91: 1103–7.
95. Critchley M. Arteriosclerotic parkinsonism. Brain 1929; 52: 23–83.
96. Fitzgerald PM, Jankovic J. Lower body Parkinsonism: evidence for a vascular etiology. Mov Disord 1989; 4: 249–60.
97. Parkes JD, Marsden CD, Rees JE, et al. Parkinson's disease: cerebral arteriosclerosis and senile dementia. Q J Med 1974; 43: 49–61.
98. Thompson PD, Marsden CD. Gait disorder of subcortical arteriosclerotic encephalopathy: Binswanger's disease. Mov Disord 1987; 2: 8.
99. Mark MH, Sage JI, Walters AS, et al. Binswanger's disease presenting as L-dopa-responsive Parkinsonism: clinicopathologic study of three cases. Mov Disord 1995; 10: 450–4.
100. Hurtig HI. Vascular parkinsonism. In: Stern MB, Koller WC, eds. Parkinsonian Syndromes. New York: Marcel Dekker, 1993: 81–93.
101. Krauss JK, Regel JP, Droste DW, et al. Movement disorders in adult hydrocephalus. Mov Disord 1997; 12: 53–60.
102. Hakim S, Adams RD. The special clinical problem of symptomatic hydrocephalus with normal cerebrospinal fluid hydrodynamics. J Neurol Sci 1965; 2: 307–27.
103. Jacobs L, Conti D, Kinkel WR, Manning EJ. Normal pressure hydrocephalus: relationship of clinical and radiographic findings to improvement following shunt surgery. JAMA 1976; 235: 510–12.
104. Ahlberg J, Norlen L, Blomstrand C, Wikkelso C. Outcome of shunt operation on urinary incontinence in normal pressure hydrocephalus predicted by lumbar puncture. J Neurol Neurosurg Psychiatry 1988; 51: 105–8.
105. Waters CH. Structural lesions and parkinsonism. In: Stern MB, Koller WC, eds. Parkinsonian Syndromes. New York: Marcel Dekker, 1993: 137–44.
106. Blocq P, Marinesco G. Sur un cas tremblement parkinsonien hemiplegique symptomatique d'une tumeur de pedoncule cerebral. C R Soc Biol 1893; 45: 105–11.
107. Samiy E. Chronic subdural hematoma presenting a parkinsonian syndrome. J Neurosurg 1963; 20: 903.
108. Adler CH, Stern MB, Brooks ML. Parkinsonism secondary to bilateral striatal fungal abscesses. Mov Disord 1989; 4: 333–7.
109. Murphy MJ. Clinical correlations of CT scan-detected calcification of the basal ganglia. Ann Neurol 1979; 6: 507–11.
110. Lang AE, Koller WC, Fahn S. Psychogenic Parkinsonism. Arch Neurol 1995; 52: 802–10.
111. Quinn N, Critchley P, Marsden CD. Young onset Parkinson's disease. Mov Disord 1987; 73–91.
112. Gershanik OS. Early-onset parkinsonism. In: Jankovic J, Tolosa E, eds. Parkinson's Disease and Movement Disorders. Baltimore: Williams & Wilkins, 1993: 235–52.
113. Nygaard TG, Marsden CD, Fahn S. Dopa-responsive dystonia: long-term treatment response and prognosis. Neurology 1991; 41: 174–81.
114. Snow BJ, Nygaard TG, Takahashi H, Calne DB. Positron emission tomographic studies of dopa-responsive dystonia and early-onset idiopathic Parkinsonism. Ann Neurol 1993; 34: 733–8.

115. Dobyns WB, Goldstein NNP, Gordon H. Clinical spectrum of Wilson's disease (hepato-lenticular degeneration). Mayo Clin Proc 1979; 54: 35–42.
116. Walshe JM, Yealland M. Wilson's disease: the problem of delayed diagnosis. J Neurol Neurosurg Psychiatry 1992; 55: 692–6.
117. Topaloglu H, Gucuyener K, Orkun C, Renda Y. Tremor of tongue and dysarthria as the sole manifestation of Wilson's disease. Clin Neurol Neurosurg 1990; 92: 295–6.
118. Sheinberg IH, Sternlieb I, Richman J. Psychiatric manifestations of Wilson's disease. Birth Defects 1968; 4: 85–6.
119. Wilson SAK. Progressive lenticular degeneration: a familial nervous disease associated with cirrhosis of the liver. Brain 1912; 34: 295–509.
120. Weilleit J, Kiechl SG. Wilson's disease with neurological impairment but no Kayser-Fleischer rings. Lancet 1991; 337: 1426.
121. Demirkiran M, Jankovic J, Lewis RA, Cox DW. Neurologic presentation of Wilson disease without Kayser-Fleischer rings. Neurology 1996; 46: 1040–3.
122. Nelson RF, Guzman DA, Grahovaac Z, Howse DCN. Computerized tomography in Wilson's disease. Neurology 1979; 29: 866–8.
123. Dettori P, Rochelle MB, Demalia L, et al. Computerized cranial tomography in pres-ymptomatic and hepatic form of Wilson's disease. Eur Neurol 1984; 23: 56–63.
124. King AD, Walshe JM, Kendall BE, et al. Cranial MR imaging in Wilson's disease. Am J Roentgenol 1996; 167: 1579–84.
125. Steindl P, Ferenci P, Dienes HP, et al. Wilson's disease in patients presenting with liver disease: a diagnostic challenge. Gastroenterology 1997; 113: 212–18.
126. Saatci I, Topcu M, Baltaoglu FF, et al. Cranial MR findings in Wilson's disease. Acta Radiol 1997; 38: 250–8.
127. Snow BJ, Bhatt M, Martin WR, et al. The nigrostriatal dopaminergic pathway in Wilson's disease studied with positron emission tomography. J Neurol Neurosurg Psychiatry 1991; 54: 12–17.
128. Scheinberg IH, Sternlieb I. Wilson's Disease: Major Problems in Internal Medicine. Vol. 3 Philadelphia, PA: WB Saunders, 1984.
129. Brewer GJ, Yuzbasiyan-Gurkan V. Wilson's disease. Medicine 1992; 71: 139–64.
130. Sethi KD, Adams RJ, Loring DW, EL Gammal T. Hallervorden-Spatz syndrome: clinical and magnetic resonance imaging correlations. Ann Neurol 1988; 24: 692–4.
131. Hayflick SJ, Westaway SK, Levinson B, et al. Genetic, clinical, and radiographic delineation of Hallervorden-Spatz syndrome. N Engl J Med 2003; 348: 33–40.
132. Adams P, Falek A, Arnold J. Huntington's disease in Georgia: Age at onset. Am J Hum Genet 1988; 43: 695–704.
133. Klawans HL. Hemiparkinsonism as a late complication of hemiatrophy: a new syndrome. Neurology 1981; 31: 625–8.
134. Przedborski S, Giladi N, Takikawa S, et al. Metabolic topography of the hemiparkinsonism-hemiatrophy syndrome. Neurology 1994; 44: 1622–8.
135. Waters CH, Faust PL, Powers J, et al. Neuropathology of lubag (X-linked dystonia-Parkinsonism). Mov Disord 1993; 8: 387–90.
136. Spitz MC, Jankovic J, Killian JM. Familial tic disorder, Parkinsonism, motor neuron disease and acanthocytosis: a new syndrome. Neurology 1985; 35: 366–70.
137. Litvan I, Bhatia KP, Burn DJ, et al. Movement Disorder Society Scientific Issues Committee report: SIC Task Force appraisal of clinical diagnostic criteria for Parkinsonian disorders. Mov Disord 2003; 18: 467–8.
138. Hughes AJ, Ben-Shlomo Y, Daniel SE, Lees AJ. What features improve the accuracy of clinical diagnosis in Parkinson's disease: a clinicopathologic study. Neurology 1992; 42: 1142–6.
139. Gelb DJ, Oliver E, Gilman S. Diagnostic criteria for Parkinson disease. Arch Neurol 1999; 56: 33–9.
140. Gibb WR, Lees AJ. The relevance of the Lewy body to the pathogenesis of idiopathic Parkinson's disease. J Neurol Neurosurg Psychiatry 1988; 51: 745–52.
141. Ward CD, Gibb WR. Research diagnostic criteria for Parkinson's disease. Adv Neurol 1990; 53: 245–9.

142. Rajput AH, Rozdilsky B, Rajput A. Accuracy of clinical diagnosis in parkinsonism prospective study. Can J Neurol Sci 1991; 18: 275–8.
143. Hughes AJ, Daniel SE, Kilford L, Lees AJ. Accuracy of clinical diagnosis of idiopathic Parkinson's disease: a clinico-pathological study of 100 cases. J Neurol Neurosurg Psychiatry 1992; 55: 181–4.
144. Hughes AJ, Daniel SE, Lees AJ. Improved accuracy of clinical diagnosis of Lewy body Parkinson's disease. Neurology 2001; 57: 1497–9.
145. Hughes AJ, Daniel SE, Ben-Shlomo Y, Lees AJ. The accuracy of diagnosis of parkinsonian syndromes in a specialist movement disorder service. Brain 2002; 125: 861–70.
146. Williams DR, Lees AJ. Visual hallucinations in the diagnosis of idiopathic Parkinson's disease: a retrospective autopsy study. Lancet Neurol 2005; 4: 605–10.
147. de la Fuente-Fernández R. Role of DaTSCAN and clinical diagnosis in Parkinson disease. Neurology 2012; 78: 696–701.
148. Tang CC, Eidelberg D. Abnormal metabolic brain networks in Parkinson's disease from blackboard to bedside. Prog Brain Res 2010; 184: 161–76.
149. Vaillancourt DE, Spraker MB, Prodoehl J, et al. High-resolution diffusion tensor imaging in the substantia nigra of denovo Parkinson disease. Neurology 2009; 72: 1378–84.
150. Focke NK, Helms G, Pantel PM, et al. Differentiation of typical and atypical Parkinson syndromes by quantitative MR imaging. AJNR Am J Neuroradiol 2012; 32: 2087–92.
151. Kwon DH, Kim JM, Oh SH, et al. Seven-Tesla magnetic resonance images of the substantia nigra in Parkinson disease. Ann Neurol 2012; 71: 267–77.
152. Berg D, Becker G, Zeiler B, et al. Vulnerability of the nigrostriatal system as detected by transcranial ultrasound. Neurology 1999; 53: 1026–31.
153. Berg D, Seppi K, Behnke S, et al. Enlarged substantia nigra hyperechogenicity and risk for Parkinson disease: a 37-month 3-center study of 1847 older persons. Arch Neurol 2011; 68: 932–7.
154. Walter U, Dressler D, Probst T, et al. Transcranial brain sonography findings in discriminating between parkinsonism and idiopathic Parkinson disease. Arch Neurol 2007; 64: 1635–40.

4

Pathophysiology and clinical assessment

Joseph Jankovic and Raja Mehanna

INTRODUCTION

In his 1817 *An Essay on the Shaking Palsy,* Parkinson (1) recorded many features of the condition that now bears his name. Parkinson emphasized tremor at rest, flexed posture, festinating gait (Fig. 4.1), dysarthria, dysphagia, and constipation. Charcot and others later pointed out that the term paralysis agitans used by Parkinson was inappropriate, because in Parkinson's disease (PD), strength was usually well preserved and many patients did not shake.

Although traditionally regarded as a motor system disorder, PD is now considered to be a much more complex syndrome involving motor as well as nonmotor systems (2–6). For example, oily skin, seborrhea, pedal edema, fatigability, and weight loss are recognized as nonspecific but typical parkinsonian features. The autonomic involvement is responsible for orthostatic hypotension, paroxysmal flushing, diaphoresis, problems with thermal regulation, constipation, and bladder, sphincter, and sexual disturbances. The involvement of the thalamus and the spinal dopaminergic pathway may explain some of the sensory complaints such as pains, aches and burning–tingling paresthesias (7). The special sensory organs may also be involved in PD and cause visual, olfactory and vestibular dysfunction (8). A number of studies have drawn attention to the protean neurobehavioral abnormalities in PD, such as apathy, fearfulness, anxiety, emotional lability, social withdrawal, increasing dependency, depression, dementia, bradyphrenia, a type of anomia termed the "tip-of-the-tongue phenomenon," visual–spatial impairment, sleep disturbance, psychosis, and other psychiatric problems (9). To take into account these nonmotor features the original Unified Parkinson's Disease Rating Scale (UPDRS) has been modified and the new scale, developed by the Movement Disorders Society (MDS), designated as the MDS-UPDRS now includes an expanded section on nonmotor experiences of daily living (10,11).

The rich and variable expression of PD often causes diagnostic confusion and a delay in treatment (12). In the early stages, parkinsonian symptoms are often mistaken for simple arthritis or bursitis, depression, normal aging, Alzheimer's disease, or stroke (Fig. 4.2). PD often begins on one side of the body, but usually becomes bilateral. However, parkinsonism may remain unilateral, particularly when it is a late sequelae of posttraumatic hemiatrophy, perinatal and early childhood cerebral injury or when it is due to a structural lesion in the basal ganglia (13). In a survey of 181 treated PD patients, Bulpitt et al. (14) found at least 45 different symptoms attributable to PD. However, only nine of these symptoms were reported by the patients in more than fivefold excess when compared with those of a control population of patients randomly selected from a general practice. These common symptoms included being frozen or rooted to a spot, grimacing, jerking of the arms and legs, shaking hands, clumsy hands, salivation, poor

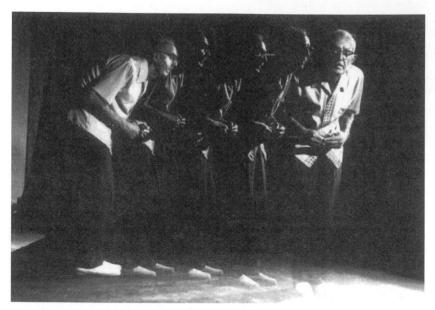

FIGURE 4.1 A 74-year-old man with nine years of bilateral parkinsonism demonstrated by hypo-mimia, hand tremor and posturing, stooped posture, and a shuffling gait.

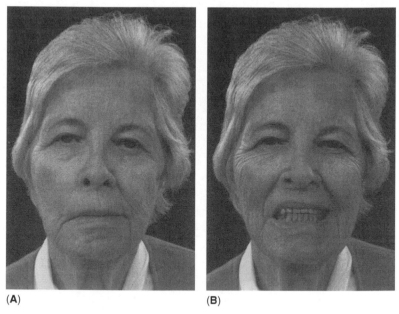

(A)   (B)

FIGURE 4.2 **(A)** A 74-year-old woman with facial asymmetry and right hemiatrophy for five years associated with right hemiparkinsonism. **(B)** Voluntary facial contraction reveals no evidence of right facial weakness.

concentration, severe apprehension, and hallucinations. However, even these frequent symptoms are relatively nonspecific and do not clearly differentiate PD patients from diseased controls. In many cases, a follow-up for several years is needed before the diagnosis becomes apparent. Gonera et al. (15) found that, four to six years prior to the onset of classic PD symptoms, patients experience a prodromal phase characterized by more frequent visits to general practitioners and specialists compared with normal controls. During this period, PD patients, compared with normal controls, had a higher frequency of mood disorder, "fibromyalgia," and shoulder pain.

Different diagnostic criteria for PD, based on clinical and pathologic findings, have been proposed but their reliability has not been vigorously tested. In one study of 800 patients diagnosed with PD and prospectively followed by trained parkinsonologists from early, untreated stages, the final diagnosis after a mean of 7.6 years of follow-up was considered to be other than PD in 8.1% of cases (16). In a study of 143 cases of parkinsonism who came to autopsy and had a clinical diagnosis made by neurologists specializing in movement disorders, the positive predictive value of the clinical diagnosis of PD was 98.6% and for the other parkinsonian syndromes, it was 71.4% (17). Although the emphasis in PD research has been on dopaminergic deficiency underlying motor dysfunction, there is growing body of evidence that the caudal brainstem nuclei (e.g., dorsal motor nucleus of the glossopharyngeal and vagal nerves), anterior olfactory nucleus, and other nondopaminergic neurons may be affected long before the classic loss of dopaminergic neurons in the substantia nigra (18). In a positron emission tomography (PET) study with [11C] methyl-4-piperidinyl propionate acetylcholinesterase in 58 PD patients, cholinergic denervation of the limbic archicortex was found to be a more robust determinant of hyposmia than nigrostriatal dopaminergic denervation in subjects with moderately severe PD (19). Furthermore, greater deficits in odor identification correlated with increased risk for clinically significant cognitive impairment.

According to the Braak staging (18), during the presymptomatic stages 1 and 2, the PD-related inclusion body pathology remains confined to the medulla oblongata and olfactory bulb. In stages 3 and 4, the substantia nigra and other nuclear grays of the midbrain and basal forebrain are the focus of initially subtle and then severe changes, and the illness reaches its symptomatic phase. In the end-stages 5 and 6, the pathologic process encroaches upon the telencephalic cortex. This staging proposal has been challenged, as there have been no cell counts to correlate with the described synuclein pathology and there was no observed asymmetry in the pathologic findings that would correlate with the asymmetry of clinical findings. In addition, there is controversy as to the classification of dementia with Lewy bodies, viewed by Braak as part of stage 6, but others suggest that it is a separate entity since these patients often have behavioral and psychiatric problems before or at the same time as the onset of motor or other signs of PD.

Although systemic, mental, sensory, and other nonmotor symptoms of PD are often quite disabling, PD patients are usually most concerned about the motor symptoms (2–6,20). Several studies have demonstrated that patients who predominantly manifest "axial" symptoms such as dysarthria, dysphagia, loss of equilibrium, and freezing are particularly disabled by their disease compared with those who have predominantly limb manifestations (21). The poor prognosis of patients in whom axial symptoms predominate is partly due to a lack of response of these symptoms to dopaminergic drugs.

The specific mechanisms underlying PD symptoms are poorly understood. An accurate assessment of the disorder's motor signs should help to differentiate them from the motor changes associated with normal aging. Normal elderly subjects may have mild extrapyramidal impairment, including slow movement and a shuffling gait as well as disinhibition of the nuchocephalic reflex, glabellar blink reflex, snout reflex, head-retraction reflex, and the presence of paratonia, impaired vertical glaze, and cogwheel visual pursuit (22,23). Although these signs occur more frequently in parkinsonian patients than other aged individuals, they are not specific to PD. They may indicate an age-dependent loss of striatal dopamine and dopamine receptors (24). Receptor loss may explain why these age-related motor signs do not improve with levodopa treatment (25).

This chapter focuses on the pathophysiology and clinical assessment of the cardinal signs of PD: bradykinesia, tremor, rigidity, and postural instability (Table 4.1).

TABLE 4.1   Motor Features of Parkinsonism

Tremor at rest[a]
Rigidity[a]
Bradykinesia[a]
Loss of postural reflexes[a]
Hypomimia (masked facies)
Speech disturbance (hypokinetic dysarthria)
Hypophonia
Dysphagia
Sialorrhea
Respiratory difficulties
Loss of associated movements
Shuffling, short-step gait
Festination
Freezing
Micrographia
Difficulty turning in bed
Slowness in activities of daily living
Stooped posture, kyphosis, and scoliosis,
Dystonia, myoclonus, and orofacial dyskinesia
Neuro-ophthalmologic findings
Impaired visual contrast sensitivity
Visuospatial impairment
Impaired upward gaze, convergence, and smooth pursuit
Impaired vestibuloocular reflex
Hypometric saccades
Decreased blink rate
Spontaneous and reflex blepharospasm (glabellar or Myerson's sign)
Lid apraxia (opening or closure)
Motor findings related to dopaminergic therapy
Levodopa-induced dyskinesia (chorea, dystonia, myoclonus, tic)

[a]Cardinal signs.

BRADYKINESIA

Bradykinesia, or slowness of movement, is the most characteristic symptom of basal ganglia dysfunction in PD (26). It may be manifested by a delay in the initiation and slowness of execution of a movement as well as a reduced frequency and amplitude of spontaneous movement, particularly noticeable in automatic movements (27). There is some evidence that amplitude is disproportionately more affected than speed in patients with PD and may be due to different motor mechanisms and might have to be assessed separately (28). Other aspects of bradykinesia include a delay in arresting movement, decrementing amplitude and speed of repetitive movement, and an inability to execute simultaneous or sequential actions. In addition to whole body slowness and impairment of fine motor movement, other manifestations of bradykinesia include drooling due to impaired swallowing of saliva (29), monotonous (hypokinetic) dysarthria, loss of facial expression (hypomimia), and reduced arm swing when walking (loss of automatic movement). Micrographia has been postulated to result from an abnormal response due to reduced motor output or weakness of agonist force coupled with distortions in visual feedback (30). Although affecting all types of movements in PD, there is some evidence that bradykinesia affects more self-initiated movement than externally triggered movements, as exemplified by gait improvement when external cues are provided (31). Bradyphrenia is slowness of thought and does not always correlate with bradykinesia. Therefore, different biochemical mechanisms may underlie these two parkinsonian disturbances (32).

Bradykinesia can be understood as the inability to "energize" the appropriate neurons and thus muscles (33,34). The movement patterns are adequately selected, but parameters such as speed and amplitude of movement are inadequately set (28,34) despite the preserved capacity to choose the appropriate parameters (35). Moreover, electromyography (EMG) bursts are normally timed but the amount of EMG activity is under-scaled relative to the desired movement parameters (36) and PD patients therefore need a series of multiple agonist bursts to accomplish a larger movement. Micrographia, a typical PD symptom, is an example of a muscle energizing defect (33). The impaired generation and velocity of ballistic movement can be ameliorated with levodopa (37,38). Demirci (39) also demonstrated a problem in sensory scaling of kinesthesia, which is the perception of the amplitude of passive angular displacement of the joints. When kinesthesia is used to match a visual target, distances are perceived to be shorter by the PD patients. Assuming that visual perception is normal, this reduced kinesthesia implies that the sensorimotor apparatus is "set" smaller in PD patients than in normal subjects.

Bradykinesia, more than any other cardinal sign of PD, correlates well with striatal dopamine deficiency. Measuring brain dopamine metabolism of rats running on straight and circular treadmills, Freed and Yamamoto (40) found that dopamine metabolism in the caudate nucleus was more affected by posture and direction of movement. Dopamine metabolism in the nucleus accumbens was more linked to the speed and direction of the antagonists, appears to be normal in PD, and is probably more under cerebellar than basal ganglia control (33). In other words, in PD, the simple motor program to execute a fast ballistic movement is intact, but it fails because the initial agonist burst is insufficient. The degree of bradykinesia correlates with a reduction in the striatal fluorodopa uptake measured by PET scans and with nigral damage (41).

Studies performed in monkeys made parkinsonian with the toxin 1-methyl-4-phenyl-1,2,3,6-tetrahydropyridine (MPTP) (42), in rats made parkinsonian with the toxin 6- hydroxydopamine (6-OHDA) (43) and in patients with PD provide evidence that bradykinesia results from excessive activity in the subthalamic nucleus (STN) and the internal segment of the globus pallidus (GPi) (44). This has been further demonstrated by increased blood oxygenation level-dependent (BOLD) activation in the basal ganglia and thalamus on functional magnetic resonance imaging (fMRI) (45), without increased activation in the motor cortex (46). In rats made parkinsonian with 6-OHDA-induced nigrostriatal lesions, almost half the substantia nigra pars reticulata (SNpr) units had abnormal slow oscillations of discharge that were cortically driven and on which motor cortex stimulation induced abnormal augmented excitations. D1 or D2 dopamine agonists reduced the abnormal excitations but had no effect on the pathologic oscillations. In this case, if a motor cortex input to the basal ganglia during movement could elicit a transient overactivity of the basal ganglia output, this could contribute to impeding movement initiation or execution in PD (47). Thus, there is both functional and biochemical evidence of increased activity in the outflow nuclei, particularly STN and GPi, in patients with PD.

The motor circuit of the basal ganglia has two entry points receiving cortical input, the striatum and the STN, and an output, the GPi, which connects to the cortex via the motor thalamus. Neuronal afferents coding for a given movement or task project to the basal ganglia by two different systems: the direct disynaptic projections to the GPi via the STN and the striatum; and the indirect trisynaptic projections to the GPi via the globus pallidus pars externa (GPe). Corticostriatal afferent's primary actions on the medium spiny neurons are inhibition via the indirect pathway and facilitation via the direct pathway. Dopaminergic depletion in PD disrupts this corticostriatal balance and leads to reduced activity in the direct circuit and increased activity the indirect circuit, thus decreasing movement. However, the precise chain of events leading to increased STN activity is not completely understood (48). As a result of the abnormal neuronal activity at the level of the GPi, the muscle discharge in patients with PD changes from the normal high (40 Hz) to pulsatile (10 Hz) contractions. These muscle discharges can be auscultated with a stethoscope (49). This exaggerated beta synchronization within and between structures in the basal ganglia circuitry is largely suppressed by treatment with dopamine replacement therapies that promote faster oscillations (about 70 Hz), similar to the high frequency stimulation associated with deep brain stimulation (50,51), in tandem with clinical improvement (52,53). Further studies showed that the beta band oscillations are reduced prior to and during self- and externally paced voluntary movements (54,55) and after a "go" signal (56,57), yet increase after a "no go" signal (56). This suggests that increased beta activity is involved in movement inhibition. Furthermore, beta suppression does not seem to be related to peripheral feedback, but to feed forward organization of movements (57) as the power suppression prior to movement is longer in duration when more motor processing following the "go" cue is required.

Beta oscillatory activity and suppression are not unique to the parkinsonian state as they are also manifest in the striatum of the healthy monkey (58) and in the healthy human putamen (59) and cortex (60). Since the baseline level of synchrony within and between basal ganglia structures is elevated in PD, it might be relatively resistant to suppression and thus lead to difficulty in movement initiation (61). This is supported by studies in PD patients in whom 10- or 20-Hz stimulation of the STN resulted in decreased motor performance, mainly seen as bradykinesia (62,63).

However, it is still unclear if there is a single frequency having a critical negative influence on PD symptoms and what this frequency might be. Chen et al. (64) demonstrated a 15% slowing in the grip force task during a 20 Hz stimulation of the STN, but not during stimulation with other frequencies. In other studies measuring finger tapping, a frequency between 5 and 10 Hz had the largest influence. It thus seems that there is no single pathologic oscillation frequency that is responsible for all parkinsonian symptoms, but specific frequencies lead to changes in specific performance parameters evaluated in particular tasks (65). It thus seems that excessive neuronal synchronization in the STN and GPi might contribute to bradykinesia in PD, and that bradykinesia can be seen as a failure of the motor circuit to generate a phasic and time-locked inhibition of GPi neurons and to achieve a significant desynchronization in the beta band to facilitate recruitment of cortical motor neurons appropriately adjusted for the intended movement (66,67).

The incidence of oscillatory neurons does not correlate with the severity of symptoms before treatment, suggesting that the degree of beta oscillatory activity does not fully account for the motor impairments. Instead, it appears to be related more to the amplitude of the response of the STN to dopaminergic agents (61). Moreover, these abnormally amplified beta oscillations seem to be a delayed consequence of chronic dopamine depletion rather than the result of an acute absence of dopamine receptor stimulation (68,69). Nevertheless, the exaggerated beta synchronization in PD may contribute to rigidity and akinesia by limiting the ability of neurons to code information in time and space, as both adjacent and spatially distributed neurons are preferentially locked to the beta rhythm (70,71). Indeed, bradykinesia worsens when more than one body part is activated simultaneously (27). It should be noted however that the synchrony of the oscillation is more important than the exact frequency in the beta range in the genesis of bradykinesia (72).

Bradykinesia, similar to other parkinsonian symptoms, is dependent on the emotional state of the patient. With a sudden surge of emotional energy, the immobile patient may catch a ball or make other fast movements. This curious phenomenon, called "kinesia paradoxica," demonstrates that the motor programs are intact in PD, but that patients have difficulty in utilizing or accessing the programs without the help of an external trigger (73). Bradykinesia thus results from a failure of the basal ganglia output to reinforce the cortical mechanisms preparing and executing the commands to move. This is more apparent in the midline cortical motor areas and leads to difficulty with self-paced movements and prolonged reaction times. Movement can be quickened by sensory cues, maybe because of the over activity observed in the lateral premotor areas during task performance (36). Therefore, parkinsonian patients are able to make use of prior information to perform an automatic or a preprogrammed movement, but they cannot use this information to initiate or select a movement.

Another fundamental defect in PD is the inability to execute learned sequential motor plans automatically (74). This impairment of normal sequencing of motor programs probably results from a disconnection between the basal ganglia and the supplementary motor cortex, an area that subserves planning function for movement. The supplementary motor cortex receives projections from the motor basal ganglia (via the GPi and ventrolateral thalamus) and, in turn, projects to the motor cortex. In PD, the early component of the premovement potential (Bereitschaftspotential) is reduced, probably reflecting inadequate basal ganglia activation of the supplementary motor area (75) and seems to normalize with levodopa (76). Recording from the motor cortex of MPTP monkeys, Tatton et al. (77) showed markedly increased gain of the long latency (M2) segments of the mechanoreceptor-evoked responses. This and other findings indicate that PD patients have an abnormal processing of sensory input necessary for the generation and execution of movement.

Most neurophysiologic and neurobehavioral studies in PD have concluded that the basal ganglia and possibly the supplementary motor cortex play a critical role in planning and sequencing voluntary movements (78). For example, when a patient rises from a chair, he/she may "forget" any one of the sequential steps involved in such a seemingly simple task: to flex forward, place hands on the arm rests, place feet under the chair, and then push out of the chair into an erect posture. Similar difficulties may be encountered when sitting down, squatting, kneeling, turning in bed, and walking. Lakke (73) suggests that since the patient can readily perform these activities under certain circumstances, such as when emotionally stressed, the intrinsic program is not disturbed, and, therefore, these axial motor abnormalities are a result of apraxia. Thus, the PD patient has an ability to "call up" the axial motor program on command.

The inability to combine motor programs into complex sequences seems to be a fundamental motor deficit in PD.

The study of reaction time and velocity of movement provides some insight into the mechanisms of the motor deficits at an elementary level. Evarts et al. (79) showed that both reaction and movement times are independently impaired in PD. In patients with asymmetrical findings, reaction time is slower on the more affected side (80). Reaction time is influenced not only by the degree of motor impairment but also by the interaction between cognitive processing and motor response. This is particularly evident when choice reaction time is used and compared with simple reaction time (32). Bradykinetic patients with PD have more specific impairment in choice reaction time, which involves a stimulus categorization and a response selection, and reflects disturbance at more complex levels of cognitive processing (81). However, Teräväinen and Calne supported that reaction time was only of limited value in the measure of hypokinesia in PD, by contrast to movement time (82).

Reduced dopaminergic function has been hypothesized to disrupt normal motor cortex activity leading to bradykinesia. While recording from single cortical neurons in free-moving rats, a decrease in firing rate correlated with haloperidol-induced bradykinesia, demonstrating that reduced dopamine action impairs the ability to generate movement and causes bradykinesia (83). The movement time, particularly when measured for proximal muscles, is less variable than the reaction time and more consistent with the clinical assessment of bradykinesia. Both movement and reaction times are better indicators of bradykinesia than the speed of rapid alternating movements.

Ward et al. (84) attempted to correlate the median movement and reaction times with tremor, rigidity, and manual dexterity in 10 patients. The only positive correlations were found between movement time and rigidity and between reaction time and manual dexterity. Of the various objective assessments of bradykinesia, movement time correlated best with the total clinical score, but it was not as sensitive an indicator of the overall motor deficit as the clinical rating. Ward et al. (84) concluded that although movement time was a useful measurement, it alone did not justify the use of elaborate and expensive technology. Other studies suggested that computer-assisted Motor Performance Test Series (MPS) (85), computer-connected sensors (tremor pen, touch recording plate, reaction time handle, and force plate for balance recording) (86) or a gyrosensor could be used to quantitatively measure bradykinesia (87). However, all these expensive and time-consuming techniques had to be compared with the UPDRS for validation, confirming the latter as the most accurate tool to accurately reflect the patient's disability, because it includes more relevant observations.

Although many patients with PD complain of "weakness," this subjective symptom is probably due to a large number of factors, including bradykinesia, rigidity, fatigue, and also reduced power due to muscle weakness, particularly when lifting heavy objects (88).

TREMOR

Tremor, although less specific than bradykinesia, is one of the most recognizable symptoms of PD. However, only half of all patients present with tremor as the initial manifestation of PD, and 15% never have tremor (89). Although tremor at rest (4–6 Hz) is the typical parkinsonian tremor, most patients also have tremor during activity, and this postural tremor (5–8 Hz) may be more disabling than the resting tremor. Postural tremor without parkinsonian features and without any other known etiology is often diagnosed as essential tremor (ET) (Table 4.2). However, isolated postural tremor clinically identical to ET may be the initial presentation of PD and may be found with higher-than-expected frequency in relatives of patients with PD (90,91). The two forms of postural tremor can be differentiated by a delay in the onset of tremor when arms assume an outstretched position. While most patients with PD have a latency of a few seconds (up to a minute) before the tremor re-emerges during postural holding, hence called re-emergent tremor, postural

TABLE 4.2 Differential Diagnosis of Parkinsonian and Essential Tremor

	Parkinsonian Tremor	Essential Tremor
Age at onset (years)	55–75	10–80
Gender	M > F	M < F
Family history	–	+
Site of involvement	Hands, legs, jaw, chin, tongue	Hands, head, voice
Characteristics	Supination-pronation	Flexion-extension
Influencing factors		
Rest	↑	↓
Action	↓	↑
Mental concentration, walking	↑	↓
Frequency (Hz)	4–7	8–12
Electromyography	Alternating contractions	Simultaneous contractions
Associated features	Cogwheel rigidity (±)	Dystonia, Charcot–Marie–Tooth disease
Neuropathology	Nigrostriatal degeneration, alpha-synucluin accumulation, Lewy bodies	No discernible pathology
Treatment	Anticholinergics, amantadine, dopaminergic drugs,	Alcohol, beta-blockers, primidone, topiramate, botulinum toxin

tremor of ET usually appears immediately after arms assume a horizontal posture (92). Since the re-emergent tremor has similar frequency to that of rest tremor and both tremors generally respond to dopaminergic drugs, it is postulated that the re-emergent tremor represents a variant of the more typical rest tremor. Some patients with long-standing, even childhood-onset, ET evolve into tremor-dominant PD, which usually has a slower progression than the "postural instability gait difficulty" (PIGD) form of PD (93).

While bradykinesia and rigidity are most likely associated with nigrostriatal dopaminergic deficit, the pathophysiology of PD rest tremor is probably more complicated and most likely results from dysfunction of both the striato-pallidal-thalamo-cortical and the cerebello-dentato-thalamocortical circuits (94). It has been postulated that the typical tremor at rest results from nigrostriatal degeneration and consequent disinhibition of the pacemaker cells in the thalamus (95). These thalamic neurons discharge rhythmically at 5–6 Hz, a frequency similar to the typical parkinsonian tremor at rest (96,97). Some support for the thalamic pacemaker theory of PD tremor also comes from the studies of Lee and Stein (98), which show that the resting 5 Hz tremor is remarkably constant and relatively resistant to resetting by mechanical perturbations. Furthermore, during stereotactic thalamotomy, 5 Hz discharges are usually recorded in the nucleus ventralis intermedius of the thalamus in parkinsonian subjects, even in the absence of visible tremor (99). This rhythmic bursting is not abolished by deafferentation or paralysis. However, in an attempt to determine if parkinsonian tremor might be produced by the activity of an intrinsic thalamic pacemaker or by the oscillation of an unstable long loop reflex arc, Zirh et al. examined 42 thalamic cells and found that 11 had a sensory feedback pattern, one had a pacemaker pattern, 21 had a completely random pattern, and nine did not have any pattern (100). Another study (101) did show some thalamic cells with a pacemaker pattern, but these did not participate in the rhythmic activity correlating with tremor. These results suggest the thalamic cells are not the pacemaker.

Another theory would be that rest tremor originates from the basal ganglia rather than the thalamus. Indeed, rhythmic and synchronous neuronal firing recorded in the STN and the GPi correlates with tremor in the limbs in both monkeys treated with MPTP and in patients with PD (102,103). The pallidum, in particular, seems to play a fundamental role in generating tremor as suggested by a 4–8 Hz GPi neuronal firing in primate models of parkinsonism, correlation of tremor severity with pallidal (but not striatal) dopamine depletion, and complete abolition or a marked improvement of tremor with GPi ablation or DBS (104). Furthermore, BOLD activation in the contralateral GPi is related to tremor (45). As a result of the abnormal neuronal activity at the level of the GPi, the muscle discharge in patients with PD changes from the normal high (40 Hz) to pulsatile (10 Hz) contractions. These muscle discharges, which may be viewed as another form of PD-associated tremor, can be auscultated with a stethoscope (105).

On the other hand, a 5 Hz stimulation of the GPi of MPTP-treated monkeys is unable to recruit and drive motor cortex activity, revealing a low frequency activity filtering in the motor circuit (106). This means that rhythmic activity in the basal ganglia is unlikely to generate the tremor on its own. However, the increased basal ganglia output can increase the excitability of the primary motor cortex neurons (107,108) and the sensitivity to muscle stretching and synchronous basal ganglia firing. Muscle stretching thus evokes neuronal responses in the STN of PD patients, which show a pronounced tendency to oscillate at the tremor frequency (27).

Whether the pacemaker is in the thalamus or basal ganglia, some affirm that increased activity as well as increased synchronization of these central oscillators are equally important and need to coexist simultaneously for the tremor to be clinically evident (109). Wherever the pacemaker might be, transcranial magnetic stimulation can reset the tremor, indicating a role of the motor cortex in the genesis of the tremor (110,111). It is also important to note that, although the tremor is synchronous within a limb, it is not synchronous between limbs (112), suggesting that a single pacemaker does not influence the whole body. It thus seems that oscillations in both the ventral intermediate nucleus (VIM) of the thalamus and the basal ganglia play an efferent role in tremor generation, but also that the tremor itself feeds back to these same structures to influence the oscillation (113). This does suggest that in some sense the whole loop is responsible for the tremor (114). The basal ganglia loop may well trigger the cerebellar loop to produce the tremor (104).

Contrary to bradykinesia, rest tremor does not seem to be dependent on beta oscillatory synchronization (115,116). Furthermore, tremulous PD patients have a lower proportion of beta oscillatory neurons in the STN and a decrease in the ratio of beta (11–30 Hz) to low-gamma (35–55 HZ) oscillation during stronger tremor (117). Some authors also consider tremor and rigidity as downstream compensatory mechanisms for bradykinesia (118). Because the frequency (6 Hz) of the postural (action) tremor is the same as the frequency of the cogwheel phenomenon elicited during passive movement, some authors have suggested that the postural tremor and cogwheel phenomenon have similar pathophysiologies (Fig. 4.3) (119).

The biochemical defect underlying either resting or postural parkinsonian tremor is uncertain. Dopamine deficiency as measured by F-fluorodopa PET striatal uptake does not correlate with tremor severity (120) and resting tremor is not

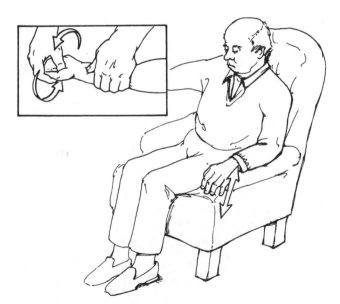

FIGURE 4.3 Parkinsonian cogwheel rigidity elicited by passive rotation of the wrist is enhanced by voluntary repetitive movement of the contralateral hand.

associated with striatal lesions (27). However, the tremor seems associated with a serotoninergic deficiency as suggested by a PET study (121) and the fact that a stereotactic lesion or deep brain stimulation of the VIM nucleus of the thalamus, a cerebellar relay nucleus, may successfully treat it (122,123). Bernheimer et al. (124) showed that the severity of tremor paralleled the degree of homovanillic acid reduction in the pallidum. In contrast, bradykinesia correlated with dopamine depletion in the caudate nucleus. In an experimental monkey model of parkinsonian tremor, a pure lesion in the ascending dopaminergic nigrostriatal pathway is not sufficient to produce the alternating rest tremor (125). Experimental parkinsonian tremor requires nigrostriatal disconnection combined with a lesion involving the rubrotegmentospinal and the dentatorubrothalamic pathways. Atypical PD tremor is observed in humans and animals exposed to MPTP, which presumably affects, rather selectively, the nigrostriatal dopaminergic system (126). However, the cerebellorubrothalamic system has not been examined in detail in this MPTP model. Furthermore, in MPTP subjects, a prominent action tremor was more typically seen than a tremor at rest.

In early studies, mechanical and optic devices were used to record tremor (127). EMG recordings and accelerometers, assisted by computer analysis, have been utilized to measure the characteristics of tremor. However, most accelerometers record tremor in a single plane. By using computed triaxial accelerometry, the distortion of the normal motion characteristics in patients with PD and ET during voluntary arm abduction–adduction movement was recorded (37). There was a good correlation between the reduction in the distortion and the clinical improvement in response to medications. More recent tools have been used to measure tremor, such as a software for automatic detection of tremor and measurement of its frequency from video recordings (128), continuous ambulatory multichannel accelerometry (CAMCA) which simultaneously measures hypo- and bradykinesia and body position in addition to tremor (129), gyroscopes fixed to forearms (130), 3D electromagnetic position sensors fixed to a finger (131), combined use of a laser system, surface EMG of the extensor digitorum and an accelerometer (132), and the Kinesia portable wireless system (133). However, the quantitative recordings of tremor, although accurate, are time consuming, costly, and influenced by the emotional state of the patient. Moreover, it is questionable whether such recordings provide a reliable index of a meaningful therapeutic response.

RIGIDITY AND POSTURAL ABNORMALITIES

Rigidity is less variable than tremor, and it probably better reflects the patient's functional disability. Rigidity may contribute to subjective stiffness and tightness, a common complaint in patients with PD. However, there is relatively poor correlation between the sensory complaints experienced by most patients and the degree of rigidity (134,135). In mild cases, cogwheel rigidity can be brought out by a passive rotation of the wrist or flexion–extension of the forearm while the patient performs a repetitive voluntary movement in the contralateral arm (Fig. 4.3) (136). Rigidity may occur proximally (e.g., neck, shoulders, and hips) and distally (e.g., wrists and ankles). At times, it can cause discomfort and actual pain. Painful shoulder, probably due to rigidity but frequently misdiagnosed as arthritis, bursitis, or rotator cuff, is one of the most frequent initial manifestations of PD (137,138).

In a prospective, longitudinal study of 6038 individuals, subjective complaints of stiffness, tremor, and imbalance were associated with increased risk of PD with hazard ratios of 2.11, 2.09, and 3.47, respectively (139). During the mean 5.8 years of follow-up, 56 new cases of PD were identified. Rigidity is often associated with postural deformity, resulting in flexed neck and trunk posture and flexed elbows and knees. Some patients develop ulnar deviation of the hands (striatal hand), and there may be extension of the big toe ("striatal toe") or flexion of the other toes, which can be confused with arthritis (140–142). Other skeletal abnormalities include neck flexion (dropped head or bent spine) (142–147) and truncal flexion (campto-cormia) (Figs. 4.4 and 4.5) (148–152).

Duvoisin and Marsden (153) studied 20 PD patients with scoliosis and found that 16 of the patients tilted away from the side with predominant parkinsonian symptoms but subsequent studies could not confirm this observation (154). Tilting of the trunk, referred to as the Pisa syndrome can also be seen in PD patients (155). In some cases, dystonia may be the presenting symptom of PD; particularly the early-onset PD variety such as is seen in patients with the *parkin* mutation (140,156). Another form of dystonia associated with PD is paroxysmal exercise-induced foot dystonia, which may be the presenting feature of young-onset PD (157).

The neurophysiologic mechanisms of rigidity are poorly understood. Spinal monosynaptic reflexes involving spinal motor neuron response to afferents from muscle spindles (type Ia fibers) are normal in PD. However, there is a reduction in the inhibition normally evoked from tendon organs (type Ib fibers) (158), whereas interneurons activated by secondary muscle afferents (type II fibers) are hyperactive. Furthermore, rigidity is abolished by dorsal root sectioning, local dural injection of anesthetics or procaine infiltration of the muscle, supporting a reflexive origin (159). All this suggests an increased activity of spinal cord motor neurons in response to

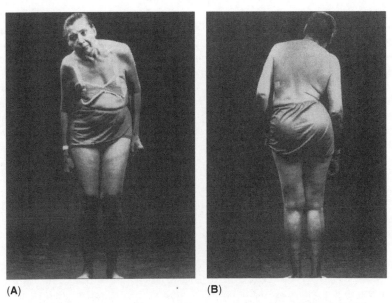

(A)   (B)

FIGURE 4.4 A 63-year-old woman with progressive scoliosis to the right side for 20 years and left hemiparkinsonism manifested by hand and leg tremor, rigidity, and bradykinesia. (**A**) Front view. (**B**) Back view.

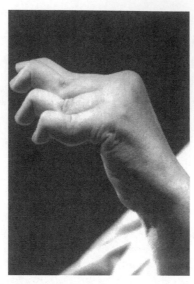

FIGURE 4.5 A 44-year-old woman with Parkinson's disease showing typical dystonic ("striatal") hand with flexion at the metacarpophalengeal joints, extension at the proximal interphalangeal joints, and flexion of the distal interphalangeal joints. The dystonia completely resolved with levodopa. *Source*: From Ref. 140.

peripheral stimulation (27), but there is no convincing evidence of a primary defect of fusimotor function in parkinsonian rigidity (160).

Passive shortening of a rigid muscle, due to PD or seen in tense subjects, produces an involuntary contraction called the Westphal phenomenon. Although the mechanism of this sign is unknown, it probably is the result of excessive supraspinal drive on normal spinal mechanism as demonstrated by the increased primary motor cortex excitability detected by magnetic cortical stimulation (161) and the correlation of the motor cortex BOLD activation on fMRI with upper limb rigidity (46). Similarly, the primary motor cortex of MPTP-treated monkeys responds more vigorously and less specifically to passive limb movements, without change in the firing rate at rest (162). If the motor circuit seems to play a direct role in the genesis of rigidity, as demonstrated by the clear beneficial effect of basal ganglia surgery on rigidity, it is still unclear how dopamine deficiency and increased basal ganglia output activity are associated with rigidity (27). Rigidity is not explained by the classic model of basal ganglia pathophysiology as discussed above. For some, rigidity probably involves disinhibition of brainstem mechanisms such as the reticulospinal projections (163) mediating muscle tone and posture. For others, rigidity, similar to tremor, is a downstream compensatory mechanism for bradykinesia (118).

The measurement of torque or resistance during passive flexion–extension movement has been used most extensively as an index of rigidity. It has been demonstrated that rigidity correlated with increased amplitude of the long-latency (transcerebral) responses to sudden stretch. These long-latency stretch reflexes represent a positive (release) phenomenon, mediated by motor pathways that do not traverse the basal ganglia. The earlier techniques of passively flexing and extending the limbs were later refined by Mortimer and Webster (159), who designed a servo-controlled electronic device to move the limb at a constant angular velocity. They and others (164–166) demonstrated a close relationship between the enhanced long-latency stretch reflexes and the degree of activated rigidity. Using measurements of the tonic stretch reflex as an index of rigidity, Meyer and Adorjani (167) found an inverse correlation between the "dynamic sensitivity" (ratio between the increase in reflex EMG at a high vs. low angular velocity) and the severity of parkinsonian rigidity. In contrast, the "static" component of the tonic stretch reflex (the maximum reflex activity at greatest stretch or at sustained stretch) positively correlated with the severity of rigidity. Both the dynamic and the static components of the tonic stretch reflex may be reduced by antiparkinson drugs (167). Although Lee and Tatton (165) showed diminution of the amplitude of the reflex after treatment, correlating it with improvement in rigidity, the measurement of long-latency responses is quite cumbersome, time-consuming, and possibly unreliable (168). Moreover, a marked overlap in the long-latency response between PD and normal subjects has been noted (169).

More recent devices suggested to measure rigidity include a computerized method for measuring rigidity with an elbow device (170), the measure of angular impulse scores (which reflect the relationship between change in total resistive torque and time) (171), an isokinetic dynamometer to assess trunk rigidity (172), myotonometry to measure the passive stiffness of the relaxed biceps brachii muscle (173) and a more complex system composed of two compact force sensors, a gyroscope and EMG surface electrodes measuring passive extension and flexion of the elbow joint (174). However, these techniques are time consuming and have been studied only on a small number of patients.

POSTURAL INSTABILITY

The loss of balance associated with propulsion and retropulsion is probably the least specific, but most disabling, of all parkinsonian symptoms. Purdon-Martin (175), after studying nine brains of patients with postencephalitic parkinsonism, concluded that globus pallidum degeneration was most responsible for the loss of righting reflexes and postural instability in parkinsonian patients. More recently, however, cellular loss in nondopaminergic structures, including the locus coeruleus with the consequent central norepinephrine deficit (176) as well as the pedunculopontine nucleus (PPN) with the consequent decrease in cortical and subcortical acetylcholine have been involved in the pathophysiology of postural instability in PD (177,178). Postural instability in PD patients has been correlated with reduced or absent vestibular responses (8).

Traub et al. (179) studied postural reflexes in 29 PD patients by recording anticipatory postural responses in the legs (triceps surae) in response to perturbations of one of the arms. In normal subjects, a burst of activity can be recorded from the calf muscles at a latency of 80 msec after the perturbation. This postural adjustment occurs even before any movement can be recorded in the legs (with a latency of 150 msec). Therefore, this reflex adjustment is anticipatory and centrally generated. In PD, the anticipatory postural reflexes are absent or markedly diminished. Such abnormalities were present in 10 of the 18 patients with moderately severe PD and in two of 11 PD patients without obvious postural instability. Since some patients with normal anticipatory reflexes can still fall, it is likely that other mechanisms contribute to the falls of parkinsonian patients (20,180). One of these would be an excessive response to vibratory stimulation of the neck or calves, as measured by static posturography. In comparing PD patients with healthy controls, Valkovic et al. (181,182) showed no intergroup difference in the pattern or latencies of the responses, but significantly larger amplitudes in advanced PD patients, whereas controls did not differ from early-stage PD patients. Furthermore, patients with progressive supranuclear palsy (PSP), who are much more prone to falling than PD patients, have normal anticipatory postural responses (179). Weiner et al. (183) found moderate or severe loss of balance in response to a standing postural perturbation in 68% of 34 patients in a geriatric care facility. They suggested that a postural reflex dysfunction was largely responsible for the unexplained falls in the elderly.

One of the distinguishing features of PD fallers is their tendency to overestimate balance performance on functional reach testing compared with controls. This overestimation worsens with worsening disease severity and when concurrently performing complex motor (e.g., carrying a tray) and cognitive tasks (e.g., performing mental arithmetic). In contrast to controls, PD patients are willing to sacrifice motor performance to complete competing tasks and make significantly more motor errors when performing a complex motor-cognitive task, whereas controls were more likely to preserve motor performance while sacrificing cognitive accuracy (184).

Loss of postural reflexes usually occurs in more advanced stages of PD and, along with freezing, is the most common cause of falls, often resulting in hip fractures. The loss of protective reactions further contributes to fall-related injuries. Many patients with postural instability, particularly when associated with flexed truncal posture, have festination, manifested by faster and faster walking in order to prevent falling. When combined with axial rigidity and bradykinesia, loss of postural reflexes causes the patient to collapse into the chair when attempting to sit down. The "pull test" (pulling the patient by the shoulders) is commonly used to determine the degree of retropulsion or propulsion (185).

FREEZING AND OTHER GAIT ABNORMALITIES

A slow, shuffling, narrow-based gait is one of the most characteristic features of PD (186). The gait and postural problems associated with PD probably result from a combination of bradykinesia, rigidity, loss of protective reaction to a fall, gait and axial apraxia (187), ataxia, loss of anticipatory proprioceptive reflexes (188), vestibular dysfunction, and orthostatic hypotension.

There is a decrease in gait speed, step length, and swing phase duration associated with a partial increase in cadence in an effort to compensate for these disorders in the early stages of the disease (189). This appears to be directly related to dopamine deficiency as it responds very well to dopamine replacement therapy (187). Freezing, festination and postural instability develop later (189) and are less dopamine responsive. These may be linked to propagation of neurodegeneration to structures directly involved in gait control and to nondopaminergic neurotransmitter systems, such as the noradrenergic locus coeruleus, the acetylcholinergic pedunculopontine nucleus and lateral pontine tegmentum, the serotoninergic raphe nuclei (although less affected) and the dopamine-depletion induced glutamatergic hyperactivity of the efferent pathways from the STN to the pedunculopontine nucleus (187). On the other hand, the use of an artificial neural network model, which simulates the behavior of the basal ganglia and produces stride time intervals, showed that the main cause of freezing of gait is probably severe decreased dopamine as well as increased resistance to dopaminergic drugs and that using gabapentin with a glutamate antagonist may be a relevant management for decreasing freezing of gait episodes (190). Other authors describe freezing of gait as the consequence of a transient period of increased synchronization within the basal ganglia oscillations leading to "cross-talk" between competing inputs and consequent paroxysmal excessive inhibition of the thalamus and pedunculopontine nucleus (191).

When gait disorder, with or without freezing and postural instability, is the dominant motor dysfunction, "lower body" parkinsonism should be considered in the differential diagnosis (192). This syndrome is thought to represent a form of "vascular" parkinsonism associated with a multi-infarct state (193). Furthermore, gait disorder and postural instability are typically associated with PSP (194,195).

One of the most disabling symptoms of PD is freezing or motor blocks, a form of akinesia (196,197). Although it most often affects the legs when walking, it can also involve upper limbs and the eyelids (apraxia of eyelid opening or eyelid closure) (198). The observation that some patients even with severe bradykinesia have no freezing and other patients have a great deal of freezing, but minimal or no bradykinesia, suggests that the two signs have different pathophysiologies. Furthermore, that bradykinesia usually responds well to levodopa and freezing does not indicates that freezing may be a manifestation of a nondopaminergic disturbance. Freezing, thought to be related to noradrenergic deficiency as a result of degeneration of the locus coeruleus (199), consists of a sudden, transient (a few seconds) inability to move. It typically causes "start hesitation" when initiating walking and the sudden inability to move the feet (as if "glued to the ground") when turning or walking through narrow passages (such as the door or the elevator) (200), when crossing streets with heavy traffic, or when approaching a destination (target hesitation). Patients often learn a variety of tricks to overcome freezing, such as marching to command ("left, right, left, right"); visual cues, such as stepping over objects (end of a walking stick, pavement stone, cracks in the floor, and so on); walking to music or metronome; shifting body weight; rocking movements; and others (201,202). "Off" gait freezing was found to correlate with dopa-responsive abnormal discriminatory processing as determined by abnormally increased temporal discrimination threshold (203). Freezing may be a manifestation of the "off" phenomenon in PD patients who fluctuate, but may also occur during "on" time ("on freezing"), independent of bradykinesia and tremor (204).

Neurophysiologic studies in monkeys treated with MPTP found that dopamine depletion is associated with impaired selection of proprioceptive inputs in the supplementary motor area, which could interfere with motor planning and may be related to motor freezing (205). Integrating EMG signals over real time while recording EMG activity from lower extremities before and during movement has shown freezing. Nieuwboer and colleagues (206) found significantly abnormal timing in the tibialis anterior and gastrocnemius muscles, although reciprocity is preserved. Thus, before freezing, the tibialis anterior and gastrocnemius contract prematurely, and the duration of contraction is shortened in the tibialis anterior, but the amplitude of the EMG burst is increased (probably a compensatory strategy pulling the leg into swing), whereas the contraction is prolonged in the gastrocnemius during the actual swing phase (207).

When freezing occurs early in the course of the disease or is the predominant symptom, a diagnosis other than PD should be considered. Disorders associated with prominent freezing include PSP, multiple system atrophy (MSA), and vascular parkinsonism (192,208).

OTHER MOTOR MANIFESTATIONS

There are many other motor findings in PD (Table 4.1), most of which are directly related to one of the cardinal signs. For example, the loss of facial expression (hypomimia, masked facies) and the bulbar symptoms (dysarthria, hypophonia, dysphagia, and sialorrhea) result from orofaciallaryngeal bradykinesia and rigidity (209). Respiratory difficulties result from a variety of mechanisms, including a restrictive component due to rigid respiratory muscles and levodopa-induced respiratory dyskinesia (210).

Of the various oculomotor problems characteristically seen in PD, the following are most common: impaired saccadic and smooth pursuit, limitation of upward gaze and convergence, oculogyric crises, spontaneous and reflex blepharospasm, apraxia of lid opening (involuntary levator inhibition), and apraxia of eyelid closure (211). Although supranuclear ophthalmoplegia is often used to differentiate PSP from PD, this oculomotor abnormality has also been described in two patients with otherwise typical parkinsonism (212). Abnormal spontaneous blinking, particularly the longer pauses between the closing and opening phase in PD patients reflects underlying bradykinesia (213).

Some patients exhibit the re-emergence of primitive reflexes attributed to a breakdown of the frontal lobe inhibitory mechanisms normally present in infancy and early childhood, hence the term "release signs." The glabellar tap reflex, also known as Meyerson's sign, has often been associated with PD. Its diagnostic accuracy, however, has not been subjected to rigorous studies. The glabellar reflex and the palmomental reflex were examined in 100 subjects, which included patients with PD ($n = 41$), PSP ($n = 12$), MSA ($n = 7$), and healthy, age-matched, controls ($n = 40$). Although relatively sensitive signs of parkinsonian disorders, particularly PD, these primitive reflexes lack specificity, as they do not differentiate between the three most common parkinsonian disorders (214). In one study, 24 of 27 patients with asymmetric PD exhibited mirror movements on the less affected side, the mechanism of which is unknown (215). In addition to these primitive reflexes, there are other "frontal" and "cortical disinhibition" signs, such as the applause sign (216), but none of them is specific for PD.

Besides the classic cardinal signs, there are many other motor abnormalities that may be equally or even more disabling. One of the most prominent features of motor impairment in PD is the inability to perform multiple tasks simultaneously possibly associated with limited attentiveness and defective central executive function (217).

ASSESSMENT OF DISABILITY

The assessment of PD is difficult, because it is expressed variably in an individual patient at different times and it is influenced by emotional state, response to medication, and other variables. Moreover, there is a marked intersubject variability of symptoms and signs. To study this heterogeneity and to determine possible patterns of clinical associations, the clinical findings in 334 patients with PD were analyzed and identified at least two distinct clinical populations of parkinsonian patients (218). One subtype was characterized by a prominent tremor, an early age at onset, and a greater familial tendency. Another subtype was dominated by PIGD and was associated with a greater degree of dementia, bradykinesia, functional disability, and a less favorable long-term prognosis.

These findings are supported by the results of an analysis of 800 patients with untreated PD included in the multicenter trial Deprenyl and Tocopherol Antioxidative Therapy of Parkinson's Disease (DATATOP). The PIGD group had greater occupational disability and more intellectual impairment, depression, lack of motivation, and impairment in activities of daily living than a corresponding group of patients with tremor-dominant PD (21). The investigators concluded that patients with older age of onset, a presentation with PIGD and bradykinesia are more likely to have a more aggressive course than those with early symptoms dominated by tremor (219). In order to determine the overall rate of functional decline and to assess the progression of different signs of PD, 297 PD patients were prospectively followed for at least three years (219). Data from 1731 visits, over a period of an average of 6.36 years (range = 3–17 years), were analyzed. The annual rate of decline in the total UPDRS scores was 1.34 units in the on state and 1.58 units in the off state. Patients with older age at onset had a more rapid progression of disease than those with younger age at onset. Furthermore, the older onset group had significantly more progression in mentation, freezing, and UPDRS activities of daily living subscores. Handwriting was the only component of the UPDRS that did not significantly deteriorate during the observation period. Regression analysis of 108 patients, whose symptoms were rated during the off state, showed a faster rate of cognitive decline as age at onset increased. The slopes of progression in UPDRS scores, when adjusted for age at initial visit, were steeper for the PIGD group of patients as compared to the tremor-dominant group. These findings, based on longitudinal follow-up data, provide evidence for a variable course of progression of the different PD symptoms, thus implying different biochemical or degenerative mechanisms for the various clinical features associated with PD.

PD should be considered a syndrome with characteristic patterns of symptoms, course, response to therapy, and different etiologies. The different subsets of PD may have a different pathogenesis and even a different genetic predisposition (207). Using cluster analysis, a systematic review identified four subtypes of PD: (i) Young age-at-onset and slow disease progression, (ii) old age-at-onset and rapid disease progression, (iii) Tremor-dominant (benign tremulous PD), and (iv) PIGD dominated by bradykinesia and rigidity (220).

Longitudinal studies of PD progression utilizing imaging ligands targeting both dopamine metabolism ([^{18}F]DOPA) and dopamine transporter density (β-CIT) using both PET and single photon emission computed tomography (SPECT), respectively, have demonstrated an annualized rate of reduction in striatal [^{18}F] DOPA or [^{123}I]β-CIT uptake of about 6–13% in PD patients compared with a 0–2.5% change in healthy controls (221). With improved methodology of β-CIT SPECT scans, the annualized rate of decline is now estimated to be 4–8% (222). These functional imaging studies are consistent with pathologic studies, showing that the rate of nigral degeneration in PD is 8- to 10-fold higher than that of healthy age-matched controls. Several studies have suggested that the rate of progression of PD may not be linear and that the disease progresses more rapidly initially and the rate of deterioration slows with more advanced disease, arguing against the "long-latency" hypothesis for a presymptomatic period in PD (223–226). In a study of 227 patients, 82 of whom were followed for up to eight years, Forsaa et al. (227) found that the steepest progression was in physical mobility, followed by social isolation and emotional reactions.

The United States Food and Drug Administration (FDA) approved the [^{123}I] FP-CIT SPECT imaging, DaTscan, to help in distinguishing parkinsonism from essential tremor. It was approved in Europe in 2000 to distinguish parkinsonism from essential tremor and Lewy body disease (LBD) from Alzheimer's disease. It may also be useful in distinguishing PD and "parkinson plus" syndromes from normal pressure hydrocephalus, psychogenic parkinsonism, vascular parkinsonism, and drug-induced parkinsonism (228–230). However, it does not help in distinguishing between PD and other "parkinson plus" syndromes such as MSA, PSP, or LBD. There is no good correlation between clinical and radiologic worsening, and this technique is not currently used to monitor disease progression (231,232). One must be aware that neurostimulants such as methylphenidate, cocaine, amphetamines, and modafinil, as well as the antidepressant wellbutrin, and, to a lesser degree, selective serotonin reuptake inhibitors, estrogen, fentanyl, and anticholinergic drugs can interfere with DaTscan sensitivity and specificity and should be held prior to the test being performed (233,234). DaTscan can be used as a diagnostic aid, but an accurate and reliable evaluation of patient history and motor dysfunction is essential for and accurate diagnosis of PD and determination of an appropriate treatment plan.

In assessing the motor symptoms and signs of PD, two approaches have been used, both of which strive to quantify the motor findings (168). One method utilizes neurologic history and an examination with subjective rating of symptoms, signs, and functional disability, and the other method utilizes timing of specific tasks or neurophysiologic tests of particular motor disturbances. Although the latter method is considered to be more objective and scientific, it is not necessarily more accurate, reliable, or relevant than the clinical rating. However, both approaches have certain advantages and disadvantages and, when combined, may provide a useful method of assessing the severity of the disability and the response to therapy.

Most of the subjective methods of assessment of parkinsonian disability utilize rating scales of various symptoms and disabilities. The most widely used method of staging PD is the Hoehn and Yahr scale (235). Although this staging scale is useful in comparing populations of PD patients, it is relatively insensitive to changes in the clinical state. Therefore, the Hoehn and Yahr scale is not useful in monitoring the response of individual patients to therapy. Thus, it is important that the severity of the disease is objectively assessed in the context of the individual's goals and needs.

Although a variety of neurophysiologic- and computer-based methods have been proposed to quantify the severity of the various parkinsonian symptoms and signs, most studies rely on clinical rating scales, particularly the UPDRS (11,236–238). Despite having a number of limitations (239), such as ambiguities in the written text, inadequate instructions for raters, some metric flaws, and inadequate screening questions for nonmotor symptoms, the UPDRS is the most frequently used instrument in clinical trials. In order to address some of the limitations of the original UPDRS, a revised scale, the MDS-UPDRS, was developed (11,240). The MDS-UPDRS includes an expanded section on non-motor experiences of daily living, has been refined to be more sensitive to small changes, and the section on motor fluctuations and dyskinesia related to levodopa therapy has been revised (10,11).

In some studies, the UPDRS is supplemented by more objective timed tests such as the Purdue Pegboard or movement and reaction times (12). There are also many scales such as the Parkinson's Disease Questionnaire-39 (PDQ-39), the PDQ-8 which is a briefer version of PDQ-39 and the Parkinson's Disease Quality of Life Scale (241–243), all of which assess quality of life and the impact of the disease on the performance of activities of daily living. The Non-Motor Symptom Questionnaire (NMS-Quest) was developed to assess the impact of the various non-motor symptoms and is a self-report assessment. It is a 30-item questionnaire containing nine dimensions: cardiovascular, sleep/fatigue, mood/cognition, perceptual problems, attention/memory, gastrointestinal, urinary, sexual function, and a variety of miscellaneous other symptoms (244). The Non-Motor Scale (NMS Scale) is a physician-completed assessment of non-motor symptoms in PD (245). An important factor contributing to quality of life is the ability to drive and patients with PD are significantly less safe than controls. In addition, the driver's perception of his or her ability to drive correlates poorly with the examiner's assessment (246). Formal assessments should be completed if safety is in question.

When a particular aspect of parkinsonism requires more detailed study, separate scales should be employed, such as tremor scales or the Gait and Balance Scale (247). Also, it is important that when performing the UPDRS, the instructions are followed exactly. For example, one study of 66 pull tests, part of the UPDRS used to assess postural instability (248), performed by 25 examiners showed marked variability in the technique among the examiners and only 9% of the examinations were rated as error-free (249). Another study showed that the "push and release test" predicts which PD patients will be fallers better than the pull test (185). The standard pull test consists of a sudden, firm, and quick shoulder pull without prior warning, but with prior explanation, and executed only once (250). If the patient takes more than two steps backward, this is considered abnormal. When performing the push and release test, patients are instructed to stand in a comfortable stance with their eyes open while the examiner stands behind them. The patient is then instructed to push backward against the palms of the examiner's hands placed on the patient's scapulae while the examiner flexes his elbows to allow slight backward movement of the trunk. The examiner then suddenly removes his hands, requiring the patient to take a backward step to regain balance. Other scales include the Schwab–England activities of daily living (251), the Short (0–3) Parkinson's Evaluation Scale (SPES)/Scale for Outcomes in Parkinson's Disease (SCOPA) (252).

The search for biomarkers for presymptomatic detection of PD and for progression of PD is becoming increasingly important because pathogenesis-targeted neuroprotective strategies are being developed for future use in at-risk populations, even before clinical onset of disease. Symptoms and signs suggested as possible premonitory features of PD include olfactory dysfunction, sleep disturbances, depression, anxiety, apathy, low impulsiveness, constipation, and other dysautonomic features. However, these are not specific for PD. Functional imaging such as DaTscan and [^{18}F] DOPA can be used to detect preclinical evidence of dopamine deficiency in people deemed to be at increased risk of PD, and may be also used to differentiate PD from ET, dystonic tremor, depression, and psychogenic parkinsonism (253). In some cases patients may present as PD, but are found to have scans without evidence of dopaminergic deficit (SWEDD). SWEDDs have been found in up to 20% of patients enrolled in PD trials (254,255). Functional MRI, transcranial sonography which measures hyperechogenicity, and cardiac metaiodobenzylguanidine scintigraphy are also being studied as potential imaging biomarkers for PD. Some neurochemical biomarkers have been suggested, such as alpha-synuclein in the blood or CSF, but with limited sensitivity and specificity (256). The future goal is to find a reliable biomarker of neurodegenerative diseases in peripheral blood, CSF, or other readily accessible tissues. The Parkinson Progression Marker Initiative (PPMI) is an ongoing comprehensive observational, international, multicenter study designed to identify PD progression biomarkers (257).

REFERENCES

1. Parkinson J. An Essay on the Shaking Palsy. London: Sherwood, Neely, and Jones, 1817.
2. Barone P, Antonini A, Colosimo C, et al. PRIAMO Study Group. The PRIAMO study: a multicenter assessment of nonmotor symptoms and their impact on quality of life in Parkinson's disease. Mov Disord 2009; 24: 1641–9.
3. Gallagher DA, Lees AJ, Schrag A. What are the most important nonmotor symptoms in patients with Parkinson's disease and are we missing them? Mov Disord 2010; 25: 2493–500.
4. Mostile G, Jankovic J. Treatment of dysautonomia associated with Parkinson's disease. Parkinsonism Relat Disord 2009; 15S3: S224–32.
5. Ha AD, Jankovic J. Pain in Parkinson's disease. Mov Disord 2012; 27: 485–91.
6. Lim SY, Fox SH, Lang AE. Overview of the extranigral aspects of Parkinson disease. Arch Neurol 2009; 66: 167–72.
7. Ford B, Louis ED, Greene P, Fahn S. Oral and genital pain syndromes in Parkinson's disease. Mov Disord 1996; 11: 421–6.
8. Pollak L, Prohorov T, Kushnir M, Rabey M. Vestibulocervical reflexes in idiopathic Parkinson disease. Neurophysiol Clin 2009; 39: 235–40.
9. Aarsland D, Andersen K, Larsen JP, et al. Risk of dementia in Parkinson's disease. A community-based, prospective study. Neurology 2001; 56: 730–6.
10. Jankovic J. Parkinson's disease: clinical features and diagnosis. J Neurol Neurosurg Psychiatry 2008; 79: 368–76.
11. Goetz CG, Fahn S, Martinez-Martin P, et al. Movement Disorder Society-sponsored revision of the Unified Parkinson's Disease Rating Scale (MDS-UPDRS): process, format, and clinimetric testing plan. Mov Disord 2007; 22: 41–7.
12. Jankovic J, Lang AE. Movement disorders: diagnosis and assessment. In: Bradley WG, Daroff RB, Fenichel GM, Jankovic J, eds. Neurology in Clinical Practice, 6th edn. Philadelphia, PA: Butterworth-Heinemann (Elsevier), 2012: 230–59.
13. Wijemanne S, Jankovic J. Hemiparkinsonism-hemiatrophy syndrome. Neurology 2007; 69: 1585–94.
14. Bulpitt CJ, Shaw K, Clifton P, et al. The symptoms of patients treated for Parkinson's disease. Clin Neuropharmacol 1985; 8: 175–83.
15. Gonera EG, van't Hof M, Berger HJC, et al. Symptoms and duration of the prodromal phase in Parkinson's disease. Mov Disord 1997; 12: 871–6.
16. Jankovic J, Rajput AH, McDermott MP, Perl DP. The evolution of diagnosis in early Parkinson disease. Arch Neurol 2000; 57: 369–72.
17. Hughes AJ, Daniel SE, Ben-Shlomo Y, Lees AJ. The accuracy of diagnosis of parkinsonian syndromes in a specialist movement disorder service. Brain 2002; 125: 861–70.
18. Braak H, Ghebremedhin E, Rub U, et al. Stages in the development of Parkinson's disease-related pathology. Cell Tissue Res 2004; 318: 121–34.
19. Bohnen NI, Müller ML, Kotagal V, et al. Olfactory dysfunction, central cholinergic integrity and cognitive impairment in Parkinson's disease. Brain 2010; 133: 1747–54.
20. Jankovic J. Movement disorders. In: Daroff RB, Fenichel GM, Jankovic J, Maziotta J, eds. Bradley's Neurology in Clinical Practice, 6th Edition, Butterworth-Heinemann (Elsevier), Philadelphia, PA, 2012: 1762–1801.

21. Jankovic J, McDermott M, Carter J, et al. Variable expression of Parkinson's disease: A base-line analysis of the DATATOP cohort. Neurology 1990; 40: 1529–34.
22. Clark D, Eggenberger E. Neuro-ophthalmology of movement disorders. Curr Opin Ophthalmol 2012; 23: 491–6.
23. Jenkyn LR, Reeves AG, Warren T, et al. Neurologic signs in senescence. Arch Neurol 1985; 42: 1154–7.
24. Seidler RD, Bernard JA, Burutolu TB, et al. Motor control and aging: links to age-related brain structural, functional, and biochemical effects. Neurosci Biobehav Rev 2010; 34: 721–33.
25. Newman RP, LeWitt PA, Jaffe M, et al. Motor function in the normal aging population: treatment with levodopa. Neurology 1985; 35: 571–3.
26. Jankovic J, Ben-Arie L, Schwartz K, et al. Movement and reaction times and fine coordination tasks following pallidotomy. Mov Disord 1999; 14: 57–62.
27. Rodriguez-Oroz MC, Jahanshahi M, Krack P, et al. Initial clinical manifestations of Parkinson's disease: features and pathophysiological mechanisms. Lancet Neurol 2009; 8: 1128–39.
28. Espay AJ, Beaton DE, Morgante F, et al. Impairments of speed and amplitude of movement in Parkinson's disease: a pilot study. Mov Disord 2009; 24: 1001–8.
29. Bagheri H, Damase-Michel C, Lapeyre-Mestre M, et al. A study of salivary secretion in Parkinson's disease. Clin Neuropharmacol 1999; 22: 213–15.
30. Teulings HL, Contreras-Vidal JL, Stelmach GE, Adler CH. Adaptation of handwriting size under distorted visual feedback in patients with Parkinson's disease and elderly and young controls. J Neurol Neurosurg Psychiatry 2002; 72: 315–24.
31. Morris ME, Iansek R, Matyas TA, Summers JJ. Stride length regulation in Parkinson's disease. Normalization strategies and underlying mechanisms. Brain 1996; 119: 551–68.
32. Press DZ, Mechanic DJ, Tarsy D, Manoach DS. Cognitive slowing in Parkinson's disease resolves after practice. J Neurol Neurosurg Psychiatry 2002; 73: 524–8.
33. Hallett M, Khoshbin S. A physiological mechanism of bradykinesia. Brain 1980; 103: 301–14.
34. Berardelli A, Dick JP, Rothwell JC, et al. Scaling of the size of the first agonist EMG burst during rapid wrist movements in patients with Parkinson's disease. J Neurol Neurosurg Psychiatry 1986; 49: 1273–9.
35. Mazzoni P, Hristova A, Krakauer JW. Why don't we move faster? Parkinson's disease, movement vigor, and implicit motivation. J Neurosci 2007; 27: 7105–16.
36. Berardelli A, Rothwell JC, Thompson PD, Hallett M. Pathophysiology of bradykinesia in Parkinson's disease. Brain 2001; 124: 2131–46.
37. Jankovic J, Frost JD. Quantitative assessment of parkinsonian and essential tremor: clinical application of triaxial accelerometry. Neurology 1981; 31: 1235–40.
38. Baroni A, Benvenuti F, Fantini L, et al. Human ballistic arm abduction movements: effects of L-dopa treatment in Parkinson's disease. Neurology 1984; 34: 868–76.
39. Demirci M, Grill S, McShane L, Hallett M. A mismatch between kinesthetic and visual perception in Parkinson's disease. Ann Neurol 1997; 41: 781–8.
40. Freed CR, Yamamoto BK. Regional brain dopamine metabolism: a marker for the speed, direction, and posture of moving animals. Science 1985; 229: 62–5.
41. Vingerhoets FJ, Schulzer M, Calne DB, Snow BJ. Which clinical sign of Parkinson's disease best reflects the nigrostriatal lesion? Ann Neurol 1997; 41: 58–64.
42. Bergman H, Wichmann T, DeLong MR. Reversal of experimental parkinsonism by lesions of the subthalamic nucleus. Science 1990; 249: 1436–8.
43. Lintas A, Silkis IG, Albéri L, Villa AE. Dopamine deficiency increases synchronized activity in the rat subthalamic nucleus. Brain Res 2012; 1434: 142–51.
44. Dostrovsky JO, Hutchinson WD, Lozano AM. The globus pallidus, deep brain stimulation and Parkinson's disease. Neuroscientist 2002; 8: 284–90.
45. Prodoehl J, Spraker M, Corcos D, et al. Blood oxygenation level-dependent activation in basal ganglia nuclei relates to specific symptoms in de novo Parkinson's disease. Mov Disord 2010; 25: 2035–43.
46. Yu H, Sternad D, Corcos DM, Vaillancourt DE. Role of hyperactive cerebellum and motor cortex in Parkinson's disease. Neuroimage 2007; 35: 222–33.

47. Belluscio MA, Riquelme LA, Murer MG. Striatal dysfunction increases basal ganglia output during motor cortex activation in parkinsonian rats. Eur J Neurosci 2007; 25: 2791–804.
48. Obeso JA, Rodríguez-Oroz MC, Benitez-Temino B, et al. Functional organization of the basal ganglia: therapeutic implications for Parkinson's disease. Mov Disord 2008; 23:S548–59.
49. Brown P. Muscle sounds in Parkinson's disease. Lancet 1997; 349: 533–5.
50. Farmer S. Neural rhythms in Parkinson's disease. Brain 2002; 125: 1175–6.
51. Levy R, Ashby P, Hutchison WD, et al. Dependence of subthalamic nucleus oscillations on movement and dopamine in Parkinson's disease. Brain 2002; 125: 1196–209.
52. Priori A, Foffani G, Pesenti A, et al. Rhythm-specific pharmacological modulation of subthalamic activity in Parkinson's disease. Exp Neurol 2004; 189: 369–79.
53. Silberstein P, Pogosyan A, Kuhn AA, et al. Cortico-cortical coupling in Parkinson's disease and its modulation by therapy. Brain 2005; 128: 1277–91.
54. Doyle LM, Kuhn AA, Hariz M, et al. Levodopa-induced modulation of subthalamic beta oscillations during self-paced movements in patients with Parkinson's disease. Eur J Neurosci 2005; 21: 1403–12.
55. Kempf F, Kuhn AA, Kupsch A, et al. Premovement activities in the subthalamic area of patients with Parkinson's disease and their dependence on task. Eur J Neurosci 2007; 25: 3137–45.
56. Kuhn AA, Williams D, Kupsch A, et al. Event-related beta desynchronization in human subthalamic nucleus correlates with motor performance. Brain 2004; 127: 735–46.
57. Williams D, Kuhn A, Kupsch A, et al. The relationship between oscillatory activity and motor reaction time in the parkinsonian subthalamic nucleus. Eur J Neurosci 2005; 21: 249–58.
58. Courtemanche R, Fujii N, Graybiel AM. Synchronous, focally modulated betaband oscillations characterize local field potential activity in the striatum of awake behaving monkeys. J Neurosci 2003; 23: 11741–52.
59. Sochurkova D, Rektor I. Event-related desynchronization/synchronization in the putamen. An SEEG case study. Exp Brain Res 2003; 149: 401–4.
60. Doyle LM, Yarrow K, Brown P. Lateralization of event-related beta desynchronization in the EEG during pre-cued reaction time tasks. Clin Neurophysiol 2005; 116: 1879–88.
61. Weinberger M, Hutchison WD, Dostrovsky JO. Pathological subthalamic nucleus oscillations in PD: can they be the cause of bradykinesia and akinesia? Exp Neurol 2009; 219: 58–61.
62. Chen CC, Litvak V, Gilbertson T, et al. Excessive synchronization of basal ganglia neurons at 20 Hz slows movement in Parkinson's disease. Exp Neurol 2007; 205: 214–21.
63. Eusebio A, Chen CC, Lu CS, et al. Effects of low-frequency stimulation of the subthalamic nucleus on movement in Parkinson's disease. Exp Neurol 2009; 209: 125–30.
64. Chen CC, Lin WY, Chan HL YT, et al. Stimulation of the subthalamic region at 20 Hz slows the development of grip force in Parkinson's disease. Exp Neurol 2011; 231: 91–6.
65. Timmermann L, Florin E. Parkinson's disease and pathological oscillatory activity: is the beta band the bad guy? New lessons learned from low-frequency deep brain stimulation. Exp Neurol 2012; 233: 123–5.
66. Boraud T, Bezard E, Bioulac B, Gross CE. Ratio of inhibited-to-activated pallidal neurons decreases dramatically during passive limb movement in the MPTP-treated monkey. J Neurophysiol 2000; 83: 1760–3.
67. Escola L, Michelet T, Macia F, et al. Disruption of information processing in the supplementary motor area of the MPTP-treated monkey: a clue to the pathophysiology of akinesia? Brain 2003; 126: 95–114.
68. Mallet N, Pogosyan A, Sharott A, et al. Disrupted dopamine transmission and the emergence of exaggerated beta oscillations in subthalamic nucleus and cerebral cortex. J Neurosci 2008; 28: 4795–806.
69. Degos B, Deniau JM, Chavez M, Maurice N. Chronic but not acute dopaminergic transmission interruption promotes a progressive increase in cortical beta frequency synchronization: relationships to vigilance state and akinesia. Cereb Cortex 2009; 19: 1616–30.

70. Brown P. Abnormal oscillatory synchronisation in the motor system leads to impaired movement. Curr Opin Neurobiol 2007; 17: 656–64.
71. Hammond C, Bergman H, Brown P. Pathological synchronization in Parkinson's disease: networks, models and treatments. Trends Neurosci 2007; 30: 357–64.
72. Kühn AA, Tsui A, Aziz T, et al. Pathological synchronisation in the subthalamic nucleus of patients with Parkinson's disease relates to both bradykinesia and rigidity. Exp Neurol 2009; 215: 380–7.
73. Lakke JP. Axial apraxia in Parkinson's disease. J Neurol Sci 1985; 69: 37–46.
74. Marsden CD. The mysterious motor function of the basal ganglia. Neurology 1982; 32: 514–39.
75. Colebatch JG. Bereitschaftspotential and movement-related potentials: origin, significance, and application in disorders of human movement. Mov Disord 2007; 22: 601–10.
76. Dick PJR, Cantello R, Buruma O, et al. The Bereitschaftspotential, L-dopa and Parkinson's disease. Electroencephalogr Clin Neurophysiol 1987; 66: 263–74.
77. Tatton WG, Eastovan MJ, Bedingham W, et al. Defective utilization of sensory input as the basis for bradykinesia, rigidity and decreased movement repertoire in Parkinson's disease: a hypothesis. Can J Neurol Sci 1984; 11: 136–47.
78. Tanji J. Sequential organization of multiple movements: involvement of cortical motor areas. Annu Rev Neurosci 2001; 24: 631–51.
79. Evarts EV, Teravainen M, Calne DB. Reaction time in Parkinson's disease. Brain 1981; 104: 167–1861.
80. Yokochi F, Nakamura R, Narabayashi H. Reaction time of patients with Parkinson's disease with reference to asymmetry of neurological signs. J Neurol Neurosurg Psychiatry 1985; 48: 702–5.
81. Pirozzolo FJ, Jankovic J, Mahurin RK. Differentiation of choice reaction time performance in Parkinson's disease on the basis of motor symptoms. Neurology 1985; 35: 222.
82. Terävänen H, Calne DB. Assessment of hypokinesia in Parkinsonism. J Neural Transm 1981; 51: 149–59.
83. Parr-Brownlie LC, Hyland BI. Bradykinesia induced by dopamine D2 receptor blockade is associated with reduced motor cortex activity in the rat. J Neurosci 2005; 25: 5700–9.
84. Ward CD, Sanes JN, Dambrosia JM, Calne DB. Methods for evaluating treatment in Parkinson's disease. In: Fahn S, CaIne DB, Shoulson I, eds. Experimental Therapeutics of Movement Disorders. New York: Raven Press, 1983: 1–7.
85. Pinter MM, Helscher RJ, Nasel CO, et al. Quantification of motor deficit in Parkinson's disease with a motor performance test series. J Neural Transm Park Dis Dement Sect 1992; 4: 131–41.
86. Papapetropoulos S, Katzen HL, Scanlon BK, et al. Objective quantification of neuromotor symptoms in Parkinson's disease: implementation of a portable, computerized measurement tool. Parkinsons Dis 2010; 2010: 760196.
87. Kim JW, Lee JH, Kwon Y, et al. Quantification of bradykinesia during clinical finger taps using a gyrosensor in patients with Parkinson's disease. Med Biol Eng Comput 2011; 49: 365–71.
88. Allen NE, Canning CG, Sherrington C, Fung VS. Bradykinesia, muscle weakness and reduced muscle power in Parkinson's disease. Mov Disord 2009; 24: 1344–51.
89. Louis ED, Klatka LA, Liu Y, Fahn S. Comparison of extrapyramidal features in 31 pathologically confirmed cases of diffuse Lewy body disease and 34 pathologically confirmed cases of Parkinson's disease. Neurology 1997; 48: 376.
90. Jankovic J. Essential tremor: a heterogenous disorder. Mov Disord 2002; 17: 638–44.
91. Shahed J, Jankovic J. Exploring the relationship between essential tremor and Parkinson's disease. Parkinsonism Relat Disord 2007; 13: 67–76.
92. Jankovic J, Schwartz KS, Ondo W. Re-emergent tremor of Parkinson's disease. J Neurol Neurosurg Psychiatry 1999; 67: 646–50.
93. Fekete R, Jankovic J. Revisiting the relationship between essential tremor and Parkinson's disease. Mov Disord 2011; 26: 391–8.
94. Boecker H, Brooks DJ. Resting tremor in Parkinson disease: is the pallidum to blame? Ann Neurol 2011; 69: 229–31.

95. Trost M, Su S, Su P, et al. Network modulation by the subthalamicnucleus in the treatment of Parkinson's disease. Neuroimage 2006; 31: 301–7.
96. Llinas R, Jahnsen H. Electrophysiology of mammalian thalamic neurons in vitro. Nature 1982; 297: 406–8.
97. Lamarre Y. Animal models of physiological, essential and parkinsonian-like tremors. In: Findley LJ, Capildeo R, eds. Movement Disorders: Tremor. New York: Oxford University Press, 1984: 183–94.
98. Lee RG, Stein RB. Resetting of tremor by mechanical perturbations: a comparison of essential tremor and parkinsonian tremor. Ann Neurol 1981; 10: 523–31.
99. Kelly PJ, Ahlskog JE, Goerss SJ, et al. Computer-assisted stereotactic ventralis lateralis thalamotomy with microelectrode recording control in patients with Parkinson's disease. Mayo Clin Proc 1987; 62: 655–64.
100. Zirh TA, Lenz FA, Reich SG, Dougherty PM. Patterns of bursting occurring in thalamic cells during parkinsonian tremor. Neuroscience 1998; 83: 107–21.
101. Magnin M, Morel A, Jeanmonod D. Single-unit analysis of the pallidum, thalamus and subthalamic nucleus in parkinsonian patients. Neuroscience 2000; 96: 549–64.
102. Rodriguez MC, Guridi OJ, Alvarez L, et al. The subthalamic nucleus and tremor in Parkinson's disease. Mov Disord 1998; 13: 111–18.
103. Rivlin-Etzion M, Elias S, Heimer G, Bergman H. Computational physiology of the basal ganglia in Parkinson's disease. Prog Brain Res 2010; 183: 259–73.
104. Helmich RC, Janssen MJ, Oyen WJ, et al. Pallidal dysfunction drives a cerebellothalamic circuit into Parkinson tremor. Ann Neurol 2011; 69: 269–81.
105. Brown P. Muscle sounds in Parkinson's disease. Lancet 1997; 349: 533–5.
106. Rivlin-Etzion M, Marmor O, Saban G, et al. Low-pass filter properties of basal ganglia cortical muscle loops in the normal and MPTP primate model of parkinsonism. J Neurosci 2008; 28: 633–49.
107. Pogosyan A, Kühn AA, Trottenberg T, et al. Elevations in local gamma activity are accompanied by changes in the firing rate and information coding capacity of neurons in the region of the subthalamic nucleus in Parkinson's disease. Exp Neurol 2006; 202: 271–9.
108. Foffani G, Priori A. Information theory, single neurons and gamma oscillations in the human subthalamic nucleus. Exp Neurol 2007; 205: 292–3.
109. Bartolić A, Pirtosek Z, Rozman J, Ribaric S. Tremor amplitude and tremor frequency variability in Parkinson's disease is dependent on activity and synchronisation of central oscillators in basal ganglia. Med Hypotheses 2010; 74: 362–5.
110. Britton TC, Thompson PD, Day BL, et al. Modulation of postural wrist tremors by magnetic stimulation of the motor cortex in patients with Parkinson's disease or essential tremor and in normal subjects mimicking tremor. Ann Neurol 1993; 33: 473–9.
111. Pascual-Leone A, Valls-Solé J, Toro C, et al. Resetting of essential tremor and postural tremor in Parkinson's disease with transcranial magnetic stimulation. Muscle Nerve 1994; 17: 800–7.
112. Hurtado JM, Lachaux JP, Beckley DJ, et al. Inter- and intralimb oscillator coupling in parkinsonian tremor. Mov Disord 2000; 15: 683–91.
113. Tass P, Smirnov D, Karavaev A, et al. The causal relationship between subcortical local field potential oscillations and Parkinsonian resting tremor. J Neural Eng 2010; 7: 16009.
114. Fahn S, Jankovic J, Hallet M. Motor control: physiology of voluntary and involuntary movement. In: Fahn S, Jankovic J, Hallett M, eds. Principles and Practice of Movement Disorders, 2nd edn. Philadelphia, PA: Elsevier, 2011: 38–42.
115. Kühn AA, Kupsch A, Schneider GH, Brown P. Reduction in subthalamic 8-35 Hz oscillatory activity correlates with clinical improvement in Parkinson's disease. Eur J Neurosci 2006; 23: 1956–60.
116. Ray NJ, Jenkinson N, Wang S, et al. Local field potential beta activity in the subthalamic nucleus of patients with Parkinson's disease is associated with improvements in bradykinesia after dopamine and deep brain stimulation. Exp Neurol 2008; 213: 108–13.
117. Weinberger M, Hutchison WD, Lozano AM, et al. Increased gamma oscillatory activity in the subthalamic nucleus during tremor in Parkinson's disease patients. J Neurophysiol 2009; 101: 789–802.

118. Rosin B, Nevet A, Elias S, et al. Physiology and pathophysiology of the basal ganglia-thalamo-cortical networks. Parkinsonism Relat Disord 2007; 13: S437–9.
119. Findley LJ, Gresty MA, Halmagyi GM. Tremor, the cogwheel phenomenon and clonus in Parkinson's disease. J Neurol Neurosurg Psychiatry 1981; 44: 534–46.
120. Otsuka M, Ichiya Y, Kuwabara Y, et al. Differences in the reduced 18F-Dopa uptakes of the caudate and the putamen in Parkinson's disease: correlations with the three main symptoms. J Neurol Sci 1996; 136: 169–73.
121. Doder M, Rabiner EA, Turjanski N, et al. Tremor in Parkinson's disease and serotoner-gic dysfunction: an 11C-WAY 100635 PET study. Neurology 2003; 60: 601–5.
122. Jankovic J, Cardoso F, Grossman RG, Hamilton WJ. Outcome after stereotactic thala-motomy for parkinsonian, essential, and other types of tremor. Neurosurgery 1995; 37: 680–6.
123. Benabid AL, Pollak P, Gao D, et al. Chronic electrical stimulation of the ventralis inter-medius nucleus of the thalamus as a treatment of movement disorders. J Neurosurg 1996; 84: 203–14.
124. Bernheimer H, Birkmayer W, Hornykiewicz O, et al. Brain dopamine and the syn-dromes of Parkinson and Huntington: clinical morphological and neurochemical cor-relations. J Neurol Sci 1973; 20: 415–55.
125. Pechadre JC, Larochelle L, Poirier LJ. Parkinsonian akinesia, rigidity and tremor in the monkey. Histopathological and neuropharmacological study. J Neurol Sci 1976; 28: 147–157.
126. Fox SH, Brotchie JM. The MPTP-lesioned non-human primate models of Parkinson's disease. Past, present, and future. Prog Brain Res 2010; 184: 133–57.
127. Holmes G. Clinical symptoms of cerebellar disease and their interpretation. Lancet 1922; 1: 1231–7.
128. Uhríková Z, Sprdlík O, Hoskovcová M, et al. Validation of a new tool for automatic assessment of tremor frequency from video recordings. J Neurosci Methods 2011; 198: 110–13.
129. Hoff JI, Wagemans EA, van Hilten BJ. Ambulatory objective assessment of tremor in Parkinson's disease. Clin Neuropharmacol 2001; 24: 280–3.
130. Salarian A, Russmann H, Wider C, et al. Quantification of tremor and bradykinesia in Parkinson's disease using a novel ambulatory monitoring system. EEE Trans Biomed Eng 2007; 54: 313–22.
131. Rajaraman V, Jack D, Adamovich SV, et al. A novel quantitative method for 3D mea-surement of Parkinsonian tremor. Clin Neurophysiol 2000; 111: 338–43.
132. Norman KE, Edwards R, Beuter A. The measurement of tremor using a velocity trans-ducer: comparison to simultaneous recordings using transducers of displacement, acceleration and muscle activity. J Neurosci Methods 1999; 92: 41–54.
133. Mostile G, Giuffrida JP, Adam OR, et al. Correlation between Kinesia system assessments and clinical tremor scores in patients with essential tremor. Mov Disord 2010; 25: 1938–43.
134. Snider SR, Fahn S, Isgreen WP, et al. Primary sensory symptoms in parkinsonism. Neu-rology 1979; 26: 423–9.
135. Koller WC. Sensory symptoms in Parkinson's disease. Neurology 1984; 34: 957–9.
136. Matsumoto K, Rossomann F, Lin TH, Cooper IS. Studies on induced exacerbation of parkinsonian rigidity. The effect of contralateral voluntary activity. J Neurol Neurosurg Psychiatry 1963; 26: 27–32.
137. Riley D, Lang AE, Blair RDG, et al. Frozen shoulder and other disturbances in Parkin-son's disease. J Neurol Neurosurg Psychiatry 1989; 52: 63–6.
138. Stamey W, Davidson A, Jankovic J. Shoulder pain: a presenting symptom of Parkinson disease. J Clin Rheumatol 2008; 14: 253–4.
139. de Lau LM, Koudstaal PJ, Hofman A, Breteler MM. Subjective complaints precede Par-kinson disease: The Rotterdam study. Arch Neurol 2006; 63: 362–5.
140. Jankovic J, Tintner R. Dystonia and parkinsonism. Parkinsonism Relat Disord 2001; 8: 109–21.
141. Ashour R, Tintner R, Jankovic J. "Striatal" hand and foot deformities in Parkinson's disease. Lancet Neurol 2005; 4: 423–31.

142. Ashour R, Jankovic J. Joint and skeletal deformities in Parkinson's disease, multiple system atrophy, and progressive supranuclear palsy. Mov Disord 2006; 21: 1856–63.
143. Kashihara K, Ohno M, Tomita S. Dropped head syndrome in Parkinson's disease. Mov Disord 2006; 21: 1213–16.
144. Gdynia HJ, Sperfeld AD, Unrath A, et al. Histopathological analysis of skeletal muscle in patients with Parkinson's disease and 'dropped head'/'bent spine' syndrome. Parkinsonism Relat Disord 2009; 15: 633–9.
145. Oyama G, Hayashi A, Mizuno Y, Hattori N. Mechanism and treatment of dropped head syndrome associated with parkinsonism. Parkinsonism Relat Disord 2009; 15: 181–6.
146. Doherty KM, van de Warrenburg BP, Peralta MC, et al. Postural deformities in Parkinson's disease. Lancet Neurol 2011; 10: 538–49.
147. Askmark H, Edebol Eeg-Olofsson K, Johnsson A, et al. Parkinsonism and neck extensor myopathy. A new syndrome or coincidental findings. Arch Neurol 2001; 58: 232–7.
148. Azher SN, Jankovic J. Camptocormia: pathogenesis, classification, and response to therapy. Neurology 2005; 65: 355–9.
149. Umapathi T, Chaudry V, Cornblath D, et al. Head drop and camptocormia. J Neurol Neurosurg Psychiatry 2002; 73: 1–7.
150. Tiple D, Fabbrini G, Colosimo C, et al. Camptocormia in Parkinson disease: an epidemiological and clinical study. J Neurol Neurosurg Psychiatry 2009; 80: 145–8.
151. Sako W, Nishio M, Maruo T, et al. Subthalamic nucleus deep brain stimulation for camptocormia associated with Parkinson's disease. Mov Disord 2009; 24: 1076–9.
152. Jankovic J. Camptocormia, head drop and other bent spine syndromes: heterogeneous etiology and pathogenesis of parkinsonian deformities. Mov Disord 2010; 25: 527–8.
153. Duvoisin RC, Marsden CD. Note on the scoliosis of parkinsonism. J Neurol Neurosurg Psychiatry 1975; 38: 787–93.
154. Grimes JD, Hassan MN, Trent G, et al. Clinical and radiographic features of scoliosis in Parkinson's disease. Adv Neurol 1987; 45: 353–5.
155. Villarejo A, Camacho A, Garcia-Ramos R, et al. Cholinergic-dopaminergic imbalance in Pisa syndrome. Clin Neuropharmacol 2003; 26: 119–21.
156. Hedrich K, Marder K, Harris J, et al. Evaluation of 50 probands with early-onset Parkinson's disease for Parkin mutations. Neurology 2002; 58: 1239–46.
157. Bozi M, Bhatia KP. Paroxysmal exercise-induced dystonia as a presenting feature of young-onset Parkinson's disease. Mov Disord 2003; 18: 1545–7.
158. Delwaide PJ, Pepin JL, Maertens de Noordhout A. Short-latency autogenic inhibition in patients with Parkinsonian rigidity. Ann Neurol 1991; 30: 83–9.
159. Mortimer JA, Webster D. Evidence for a quantitative association between EMG stretch responses and parkinsonian rigidity. Brain Res 1979; 162: 169–73.
160. Burke D. Pathophysiologic aspects of rigidity and dystonia. In: Benecke R, Conrad B, Marsden CD, eds. Motor Disturbances I. London: Academic Press, 1987: 87–100.
161. Lefaucheur JP. Motor cortex dysfunction revealed by cortical excitability studies in Parkinson's disease: influence of antiparkinsonian treatment and cortical stimulation. Clin Neurophysiol 2005; 116: 244–153.
162. Goldberg JA, Boraud T, Maraton S, et al. Enhanced synchrony among primary motor cortex neurons in the 1-methyl-4-phenyl-1,2,3,6-tetrahydropyridine primate model of Parkinson's disease. J Neurosci 2002; 22: 4639–53.
163. Delwaide PJ, Pepin JL, Maertens de Noordhout A. The audiospinal reaction in parkinsonian patients reflects functional changes in reticular nuclei. Ann Neurol 1993; 33: 63–9.
164. Berardelli A, Sabra AF, Hallett M. Physiologic mechanisms of rigidity in Parkinson's disease. J Neurol Neurosurg Psychiatry 1983; 46: 45–53.
165. Lee RG, Tatton WG. Motor responses to sudden limb displacements in primates with specific CNS lesions and in human patients with motor system disorders. Can J Neurol Sci 1975; 2: 285–93.
166. Rothwell JL, Obeso JA, Traub MM, et al. The behavior of the long-latency stretch reflex in patients with Parkinson's disease. J Neurol Neurosurg Psychiatry 1983; 76: 35–44.

167. Meyer M, Adorjani C. Quantification of the effects of muscle relaxant drugs in man by tonic stretch reflex. In: Desmedt JE, ed. Motor Control Mechanisms in Health and Disease. New York: Raven Press, 1983: 997–1012.
168. Marsden CD, Schachter M. Assessment of extrapyramidal disorders. Br J Clin Pharmacol 1981; 11: 129–151.
169. Teräväinen H, Calne DB. Quantitative assessment of parkinsonian deficits. In: Rinne UK, Klingler M, Stamm G, eds. Parkinson's Disease. Current Progress, Problems and Management. Amsterdam: Elsevier/North-Holland, 1980: 145–64.
170. Relja MA, Petravic D, Kolaj M. Quantifying rigidity with a new computerized elbow device. Clin Neuropharmacol 1996; 19: 148–56.
171. Fung VS, Burne JA, Morris JG. Objective quantification of resting and activated arkinsonian rigidity: a comparison of angular impulse and work scores. Mov Disord 2000; 15: 48–55.
172. Mak MK, Wong EC, Hui-Chan CW. Quantitative measurement of trunk rigidity in parkinsonian patients. J Neurol 2007; 254: 202–9.
173. Marusiak J, Kisiel-Sajewicz K, Jaskólska A, Jaskólski A. Higher muscle passive stiffness in Parkinson's disease patients than in controls measured by myotonometry. Arch Phys Med Rehabil 2010; 91: 800–2.
174. Endo T, Okuno R, Yokoe M, et al. A novel method for systematic analysis of rigidity in Parkinson's disease. Mov Disord 2009; 24: 2218–24.
175. Purdon-Martin J. The Basal Ganglia and Posture. Philadelphia: JB Lippincott, 1967.
176. Grimbergen YA, Langston JW, Roos RA, Bloem BR. Postural instability in Parkinson's disease: the adrenergic hypothesis and the locus coeruleus. Expert Rev Neurother 2009; 9: 279–90.
177. Gilman S, Koeppe RA, Nan B, et al. Cerebral cortical and subcortical cholinergic deficits in Parkinsonian syndromes. Neurology 2010; 74: 1416–23.
178. Thevathasan W, Aziz T. Predicting falls in Parkinson disease: a step in the right direction. Neurology 2010; 75: 107–8.
179. Traub MM, Rothwell JC, Marsden CD. Anticipatory postural reflexes in Parkinson's disease and other akinetic-rigid syndromes and in cerebellar ataxia. Brain 1980; 103: 393–412.
180. Koller WC, Glatt S, Vetere-Overfield B, Hassanein R. Falls in Parkinson's disease. Clin Neuropharmacol 1989; 12: 98–105.
181. Valkovic P, Krafczyk S, Bötzel K. Postural reactions to soleus muscle vibration in Parkinson's disease: scaling deteriorates as disease progresses. Neurosci Lett 2006; 401: 92–6.
182. Valkovic P, Krafczyk S, Saling M, et al. Postural reactions to neck vibration in Parkinson's disease. Mov Disord 2006; 21: 59–65.
183. Weiner WJ, Nora LM, Glantz RH. Elderly inpatients: postural reflex impairment. Neurology 1984; 34: 945–7.
184. Bloem BR, Grimbergen YA, van Dijk JG, Munneke M. The "posture second" strategy: a review of wrong priorities in Parkinson's disease. J Neurol Sci 2006; 248: 196–204.
185. Valkovic P, Brozová H, Bötzel K, et al. Push and Release test predicts better Parkinson fallers and nonfallers than the pull test: comparison in OFF and ON medication states. Mov Disord 2008; 1453–7.
186. Jankovic J, Nutt JG, Sudarsky L. Classification, diagnosis and etiology of gait disorders. Adv Neurol 2001; 87: 119–33.
187. Devos D, Defebvre L, Bordet R. Dopaminergic and non-dopaminergic pharmacological hypotheses for gait disorders in Parkinson's disease. Fundam Clin Pharmacol 2010; 24: 407–21.
188. Defebvre L, Kemoun G. Gait disorders in Parkinson disease. Neuroanatomic and physiologic organization of gait. Presse Med 2001; 30: 445–51.
189. Kemoun G, Defebvre L. Gait disorders in Parkinson disease. Gait freezing and falls: therapeutic management. Presse Med 2001; 30: 460–8.
190. Sarbaz Y, Gharibzadeh S, Towhidkhah F. Pathophysiology of freezing of gait and some possible treatments for it. Med Hypotheses 2012; 78: 258–61.

191. Lewis S, Barker R. A pathophysiological model of freezing of gait in Parkinson's disease. Parkinsonism Relat Disord 2009; 15: 333–8.
192. FitzGerald PM, Jankovic J. Lower body parkinsonism: evidence for vascular etiology. Mov Disord 1989; 4: 249–60.
193. Kuo SH, Kenney C, Jankovic J. Bilateral pedunculopontine nuclei stroke presenting as freezing of gait. Mov Disord 2008; 23: 616–19.
194. Jankovic J, Friedman D, Pirozzolo FJ, McCrary JA. Progressive supranuclear palsy: clinical, neurobehavioral, and neuro-ophthalmic findings. Adv Neurol 1990; 53: 293–304.
195. Winikates J, Jankovic J. Clinical correlates of vascular parkinsonism. Arch Neurol 1999; 56: 98–102.
196. Giladi N, Nieuwboer A. Understanding and treating freezing of gait in parkinsonism, proposed working definition, and setting the stage. Mov Disord 2008; 23: S423–5.
197. Morris ME, Iansek R, Galna B. Gait festination and freezing in Parkinson's disease: pathogenesis and rehabilitation. Mov Disord 2008; 23: S451–60.
198. Boghen D. Apraxia of lid opening: a review. Neurology 1997; 48: 1481–503.
199. Zarow C, Lyness SA, Mortimer JA, Chui HC. Neuronal loss is greater in the locus coeruleus than nucleus basalis and substantia nigra in Alzheimer and Parkinson diseases. Arch Neurol 2003; 60: 337–41.
200. Almeida QJ, Lebold CA. Freezing of gait in Parkinson's disease: a perceptual cause for a motor impairment? J Neurol Neurosurg Psychiatry 2010; 81: 513–18.
201. Suteerawattananon M, Morris GS, Etnyre BR, et al. Effects of visual and auditory cues on gait in individuals with Parkinson's disease. J Neurol Sci 2004; 219: 63–9.
202. Nieuwboer A. Cueing for freezing of gait in patients with Parkinson's disease: a rehabilitation perspective. Mov Disord 2008; 23: S475–81.
203. Lee MS, Kim HS, Lyoo CH. "Off" gait freezing and temporal discrimination threshold in patients with Parkinson disease. Neurology 2005; 64: 670–4.
204. Bartels AL, Balash Y, Gurevich T, et al. Relationship between freezing of gait (FOG) and other features of Parkinson's: FOG is not correlated with bradykinesia. J Clin Neurosci 2003; 10: 584–8.
205. Escola L, Michelet T, Douillard G, et al. Disruption of the proprioceptive mapping in the medial wall of parkinsonian monkeys. Ann Neurol 2002; 52: 581–7.
206. Nieuwboer A, Dom R, De Weerdt W, et al. Electromyographic profiles of gait prior to onset of freezing episodes in patients with Parkinson's disease. Brain 2004; 127: 1650–60.
207. Fahn S, Jankovic J, Hallett M. Parkinsonism: clinical features and differential diagnosis. In: Fahn S, Jankovic J, Hallett M, eds. Principles and Practice of Movement Disorders, 2nd edn. Philadelphia, PA: Elsevier, 2011: 66–93.
208. Elble RJ, Cousins R, Leffler K, Hughes L. Gait initiation by patients with lower-half parkinsonism. Brain 1996; 119: 1705–16.
209. Hunker CJ, Abbs JH, Barlow SM. The relationship between parkinsonian rigidity and hypokinesia in the orofacial system: a quantitative analysis. Neurology 1982; 32: 749–55.
210. Mehanna R, Jankovic J. Respiratory problems in neurologic movement disorders. Parkinsonism Relat Disord 2010; 16: 628–38.
211. Jankovic J. Apraxia of lid opening. Mov Disord 1995; 10: 686–7.
212. Guiloff RJ, George RJ, Marsden CD. Reversible supranuclear ophthalmoplegia associated with parkinsonism. J Neurol Neurosurg Psychiatry 1980; 43: 552–4.
213. Agostino R, Bologna M, Dinapoli L, et al. Voluntary, spontaneous, and reflex blinking in Parkinson's disease. Mov Disord 2008; 23: 669–75.
214. Brodsky H, Dat Vuong K, Thomas M, Jankovic J. Glabellar and palmomental reflexes in parkinsonian disorders. Neurology 2004; 63: 1096–8.
215. Espay AJ, Li JY, Johnston L, et al. Mirror movements in parkinsonism: evaluation of a new clinical sign. J Neurol Neurosurg Psychiatry 2005; 76: 1355–8.
216. Wu LJC, Sitburana O, Davidson A, Jankovic J. Applause sign in parkinsonian disorders and Huntington's disease. Mov Disord 2008; 23: 2307–11.
217. Wu T, Hallett M. Neural correlates of dual task performance in patients with Parkinson's disease. J Neurol Neurosurg Psychiatry 2008; 79: 760–6.

218. Zetusky WJ, Jankovic J, Pirozzolo FJ. The heterogeneity of Parkinson's disease: clinical and prognostic implications. Neurology 1985; 35: 522–6.

219. Jankovic J, Kapadia AS. Functional decline in Parkinson's disease. Arch Neurol 2001; 58: 1611–15.

220. Van Rooden SM, Heiser WJ, Kok JN, et al. The identification of Parkinson's disease subtypes using cluster analysis: a systematic review. Mov Disord 2010; 25: 969–78.

221. Marek K, Innis R, van Dyck C, et al. [123I]-CIT/SPECT imaging assessment of the rate of Parkinson's disease progression. Neurology 2001; 57: 2089–94.

222. Parkinson Study Group. Dopamine transporter brain imaging to assess the effects of pramipexole vs levodopa on Parkinson disease progression. JAMA 2002; 287: 1653–61.

223. Jankovic J. Progression of Parkinson's disease: are we making progress in charting the course? Arch Neurol 2005; 62: 351–2.

224. Lang AE. The progression of Parkinson disease: a hypothesis. Neurology 2007; 68: 948–52.

225. Maetzler W, Liepelt I, Berg D. Progression of Parkinson's disease in the clinical phase: potential markers. Lancet Neurol 2009; 8: 1158–71.

226. Brück A, Aalto S, Rauhala E, et al. A follow-up study on 6-[18F]fluoro-L-dopa uptake in early Parkinson's disease shows nonlinear progression in the putamen. Mov Disord 2009; 24: 1009–15.

227. Forsaa EB, Larsen JP, Wentzel-Larsen T, et al. Predictors and course of health-related quality of life in Parkinson's disease. Mov Disord 2008; 23: 1420–7.

228. Varrone A, Halldin C. Molecular imaging of the dopamine transporter. J Nucl Med 2010; 51: 1331–4.

229. Walker Z, Jaros E, Walker RW, et al. Dementia with Lewy bodies: a comparison of clinical diagnosis, FP-CIT single photon emission computed tomography imaging and autopsy. J Neurol Neurosurg Psychiatry 2007; 78: 1176–81.

230. O'Brien JT, McKeith IG, Walker Z, et al. DLB Study Group. Diagnostic accuracy of 123I-FP-CIT SPECT in possible dementia with Lewy bodies. Br J Psychiatry 2009; 194: 34–9.

231. Vogt T, Kramer K, Gartenschlaeger M, Schreckenberger M. Estimation of further disease progression of Parkinson's disease by dopamine transporter scan vs. clinical rating. Parkinsonism Relat Disord 2011; 17: 459–63.

232. Hubbuch M, Farmakis G, Schaefer A, et al. FP-CIT SPECT does not predict the progression of motor symptoms in Parkinson's disease. Eur Neurol 2011; 65: 187–92.

233. Booij J, Kemp P. Dopamine transporter imaging with [(123)I]FP-CIT SPECT: potential effects of drugs. Eur J Nucl Med Mol Imaging 2008; 35: 424–38.

234. Winogrodzka A, Booij J, Wolters ECh. Disease-related and drug-induced changes in dopamine transporter expression might undermine the reliability of imaging studies of disease progression in Parkinson's disease. Parkinsonism Relat Disord 2005; 11: 475–84.

235. Hoehn MM, Yahr MD. Parkinsonism: onset, progression and mortality. Neurology 1967; 17: 427–42.

236. Fahn S, Elton RL, Members of the UPDRS. Development committee: unified Parkinson's disease rating scale. In: Fahn S, Marsden CD, Calne DB, Lieberman A, eds. Recent Developments in Parkinson's Disease. Vol. II Florham Park, New Jersey: Macmillan Health Care Information, 1987: 153–63.

237. Goetz CG, Stebbins GT, Shale HM, et al. Utility of an objective dyskinesia rating scale for Parkinson's disease: inter- and intrarater reliability assessment. Mov Disord 1994; 9: 390–4.

238. Goetz CG, Stebbins GT, Chmura TA, et al. Teaching tape for the motor section of the Unified Parkinson's Disease Rating Scale. Mov Disord 1995; 10: 263–6.

239. Movement Disorder Society Task Force on Rating Scales for Parkinson's Disease. The Unified Parkinson's Disease Rating Scale (UPDRS): status and recommendations. Mov Disord 2003; 18: 738–50.

240. Goetz CG, Tilley BC, Shaftman SR, et al. Movement Disorder Society-Sponsored Revision of the Unified Parkinson's Disease Rating Scale (MDS-UPDRS): scale presentation and clinimetric testing results. Mov Disord 2008; 23: 2129–70.

241. Hagell P, Nygren C. The 39 item Parkinson's disease questionnaire (PDQ-39) revisited: implications for evidence based medicine. J Neurol Neurosurg Psychiatry 2007; 78: 1191–19.

242. Schrag A. Quality of life and depression in Parkinson's disease. J Neurol Sci 2006; 248: 151–7.
243. Luo N, Tan LC, Zhao Y, et al. Determination of the longitudinal validity and minimally important difference of the 8-item Parkinson's Disease Questionnaire (PDQ-8). Mov Disord 2009; 24: 183–7.
244. Chaudhuri KR, Martinez-Martin P, Brown RG, et al. The metric properties of a novel non-motor symptoms scale for Parkinson's disease: results from an international pilot study. Mov Disord 2007; 22: 1901–11.
245. Chaudhuri KR, Martinez-Martin P, Schapira AH, et al. International multicenter pilot study of the first comprehensive self-completed nonmotor symptoms questionnaire for Parkinson's disease: The NMSQuest study. Mov Disord 2006; 21: 916–23.
246. Wood JM, Worringham C, Kerr G, et al. Quantitative assessment of driving performance in Parkinson's disease. J Neurol Neurosurg Psychiatry 2005; 76: 176–80.
247. Thomas M, Jankovic J, Suteerawattananon M, et al. Clinical gait and balance scale (GABS): validation and utilization. J Neurol Sci 2004; 217: 89–99.
248. Hunt AL, Sethi KD. The pull test: a history. Mov Disord 2006; 21: 894–9.
249. Munhoz RP, Li JY, Kurtinecz M, et al. Evaluation of the pull test technique in assessing postural instability in Parkinson's disease. Neurology 2004; 62: 125–7.
250. Visser M, Marinus J, Bloem BR, et al. Clinical tests for the evaluation of postural instability in patients with Parkinson's disease. Arch Phys Med Rehabil 2003; 84: 1669–74.
251. Ramaker C, Marinus J, Stiggelbout AM, Van Hilten BJ. Systematic evaluation of rating scales for impairment and disability in Parkinson's disease. Mov Disord 2002; 17: 867–76.
252. Marinus J, Visser M, Stiggelbout AM, et al. A short scale for the assessment of motor impairments and disabilities in Parkinson's disease: the SPES/SCOPA. J Neurol Neurosurg Psychiatry 2004; 75: 388–95.
253. Jankovic J. Diagnosis and treatment of psychogenic parkinsonism. J Neurol Neurosurg Psychiatry 2011; 82: 1300–3.
254. Bajaj NP, Gontu V, Birchall J, et al. Accuracy of clinical diagnosis in tremulous parkinsonian patients: a blinded video study. J Neurol Neurosurg Psychiatry 2010; 81: 1223–8.
255. Schwingenschuh P, Ruge D, Edwards MJ, et al. Distinguishing SWEDDs patients with asymmetric resting tremor from Parkinson's disease: a clinical and electrophysiological study. Mov Disord 2010; 25: 560–9.
256. Wu Y, Le W, Jankovic J. Preclinical biomarkers of Parkinson disease. Arch Neurol 2011; 68: 22–30.
257. The Parkinson Progression Marker Initiative. The Parkinson Progression Marker Initiative (PPMI). Prog Neurobiol 2011; 95: 629–35.

5

Premotor symptoms

Arif Dalvi

INTRODUCTION

Parkinson's disease (PD) is clinically defined as a combination of bradykinesia with rigidity and/or tremor. These motor symptoms of PD are correlated with the deposition of Lewy bodies, the pathologic hallmark of PD, within the substantia nigra pars compacta (SNc). However, Lewy bodies are present in other regions of the brain many years, or even decades, before they are seen in the SNc (1). It stands to reason that these pathologic changes will present as symptoms depending on the structures affected. The literature documents the presence of such symptoms and postulates the presence of a premotor phase of PD. However, a consensus does not exist regarding a diagnosis of PD in this phase. Such a consensus would be invaluable should a well-defined neuroprotective therapy for PD become available. It is also of importance in understanding the genetics of PD and risk factors for the development of PD.

Changes in olfaction, constipation, sleep disorders including rapid eye movement (REM) behavior disorder (RBD), anxiety, depression, and dysautonomia can occur at any stage of PD. However, these symptoms, alone or in combination, can be markers of a developing neurodegenerative process that over time manifests as PD. These symptoms often develop in a characteristic sequence that has been correlated with pathologic staging, based on the appearance of Lewy bodies and α-synuclein deposition, called Braak staging (1). However, while this staging method provides a valid intellectual framework for understanding the progression of PD some caveats should be kept in mind. It has been noted that α-synuclein pathology may be seen in the central and autonomic system in elderly persons with no evidence of clinical neurologic disease (2). Also, a relationship between Lewy body pathology and clinical severity has not been demonstrated (3) and individuals may show late stages of α-synuclein pathology based on Braak's scheme without showing neurologic symptoms (4). Further studies combining pathologic research with imaging methods and other potential biomarkers are required to clarify our understanding of the premotor symptoms of PD.

PATHOLOGIC BASIS AND TIMELINE OF SYMPTOMS

In 1912 Friederich Lewy described the presence of eosinophilic, intracytoplasmic inclusions within substantia nigra neurons in autopsied brains of individuals affected by PD (5). These Lewy bodies have become the pathognomonic hallmark of PD, although they are not exclusive to PD and are also seen in dementia with Lewy bodies (DLB), Alzheimer's disease, and other neurodegenerative disorders such as multiple system atrophy (MSA). PD, DLB, and MSA are referred to as synucleinopathies, as the pathognomonic Lewy bodies are composed of abnormal filamentous protein inclusions with α-synuclein as their major component (6). Lewy bodies are not confined to the central nervous system (CNS) but show widespread distribution that includes autonomic nuclei, sympathetic ganglia, cardiac and pelvic plexuses, salivary glands, and skin.

Within the CNS itself, Lewy bodies are seen not only in the substantia nigra but may present in a caudal to rostral distribution as described by Braak and colleagues (1). They examined autopsy brains in three groups for Lewy bodies and related Lewy neurites. The first with a clinical diagnosis of PD ($N = 41$), the second without PD symptoms but showing Lewy bodies and neurites ($N = 69$) thus described as having incidental Lewy body disease (ILBD), and the third group with age- and gender-matched controls without any record of neurologic or psychiatric disease ($N = 58$). PD-related lesions were visualized using immunostaining for α-synuclein. Lewy pathology was observed to begin in the dorsal motor nucleus of the vagus nerve and the olfactory bulb, followed in sequence by involvement of the locus coeruleus complex and caudal raphe nuclei, the SNc, the temporal mesocortex, the prefrontal neocortex, and sensory association areas, and finally almost the entire neocortex. Each subsequent stage showed the presence of previous stages with areas affected earlier showing increasing severity of neuronal loss as later stages were reached. Motor symptoms of PD were present by history when the SNc was first affected on pathology. Based on these observations a timeline of disease progression has been suggested with symptoms such as olfactory disturbances, constipation, sleep disorders, and depression occurring in the premotor phase of the disease, the classical motor symptoms occurring when the SNc is involved, and the later stages being associated with increasing cognitive symptoms and dementia. This analysis estimates a prodromal phase of about 20 years with the clinical phase

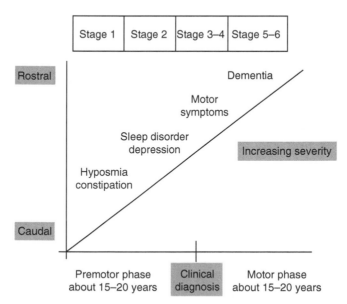

FIGURE 5.1 Timeline of symptomatic progression of Parkinson's disease. As pathologic disease spreads in a caudal to rostral direction corresponding symptoms appear. Premotor symptoms occur in Braak stages 1–2. The classical motor symptoms first appear at Braak stage 3 and progress through stage 4. Cognitive symptoms become prominent in Braak stage 5–6.

extending forward for another 20 years (7). Figure 5.1 describes the symptomatic progression of PD in the context of Braak staging.

PREMOTOR SYMPTOMS OF PARKINSON'S DISEASE

The term "premotor" in the present context relates these symptoms to established pathologic features of PD and to the later development of the classical motor symptoms of PD. Given the lack of well-defined biomarkers of PD these premotor features may be used to define the disease state very early, potentially allowing for intervention with neuroprotective strategies at a stage where they may have the most impact. Table 5.1 lists key premotor symptoms with their pathologic substrates, corresponding Braak stages, and investigational methods.

Olfactory Dysfunction

Many patients with PD will complain of hyposmia or anosmia. The pathologic correlate of this symptom is the involvement of the anterior olfactory nucleus and tract by α-synuclein aggregates seen in the earliest stages of the Braak staging scheme. Olfactory dysfunction can be readily measured clinically. Two methods are commonly used, with the first testing accuracy of odor identification called the University of Pennsylvania Smell Identification Test (UPSIT) (8) and the second testing olfactory thresholds, identification, and discrimination called the Sniffin' Sticks (9). In a multicenter study of 400 PD patients, 96.7% showed hyposmia or anosmia. However, given that olfactory dysfunction is common in the elderly population as well and in other neurodegenerative diseases, after a correction was made for age, this was reduced to 74.5% (10).

Olfactory dysfunction is insufficient as a screening tool for PD. In a study of 40 hyposmic relatives of PD patients at two years, four persons from this group were diagnosed with PD, but only one additional person received a diagnosis of PD at the five-year mark (11). Of note, all hyposmic individuals developing PD had an abnormal single photon emission computed tomography scan using a dopamine transporter ligand suggesting a combination of these tests would have a higher predictive value (11). Olfactory dysfunction is not specific for PD and may also be observed in Alzheimer's disease and the Parkinson–Dementia complex of Guam where it tends to be more severe, as well as in Huntington's disease, multi-infarct dementia, schizophrenia, and amyotrophic lateral sclerosis where it is moderate.

TABLE 5.1 Premotor Symptoms of Parkinson's Disease

Symptoms	Anatomic Correlate	Braak Staging	Diagnostic Method
Hyposmia	Olfactory bulb and anterior olfactory nucleus	1	UPSIT or Sniffin' Sticks
Constipation	Dorsal motor nucleus of vagus, myenteric plexus of intestine	1	Medical history
REM behavior disorder	Locus coeruleus and magnocellular nuclei	2	Sleep studies
Depression	Locus coeruleus and raphe nuclei	2,3	Depression scales, Transcranial sonography
Dysautonomia	Cardiac sympathetic denervation	1–3	MIBG scintigraphy, Heart rate variability

Abbreviations: MIBG, metaiodobenzylguanidine; REM, rapid eye movement; UPSIT, University of Pennsylvania Smell Identification Test.

It may also be seen following head injury and in the setting of migraine (8). Thus, while olfactory dysfunction can serve as a marker for individuals at risk for PD it is not useful in isolation for diagnosis.

Constipation

One of the earliest targets of synuclein pathology in the brain is the dorsal motor nucleus of the vagus nerve (DMNV). This nucleus provides preganglionic parasympathetic innervation to the gastrointestinal tract and thereby controls its motility. Changes in the DMNV are seen in Braak stage 1. In addition the myenteric and submucosal plexus of the intestinal tract are also affected by Lewy bodies (12). The loss of cholinergic neurons in the DMNV does not directly correlate with the presence of constipation suggesting that the involvement of the peripheral nervous system may play a more important role (13). These pathologic observations are supported by long-term studies of aging in which constipation has been shown to be a premorbid marker for PD. In the Honolulu-Asia Aging Study (HAAS) bowel habits were analyzed prospectively in 6790 elderly males none of whom had PD at enrollment but were followed for 24 years. After a mean latent period of 10 years, 96 participants were diagnosed with PD. The incidence of PD was inversely correlated with the number of bowel movements per day and was the highest in those who used laxatives frequently. The adjusted risk for PD in those with less than one bowel movement a day was 2.7-fold greater compared with those with one bowel movement per day and over fourfold greater in those with more than two bowel movements per day (14). A later work based on this dataset also revealed a similar inverse relationship between ILBD as shown on autopsy and the number of bowel movements in a day. In a case–control study of 196 PD subjects and matched controls from the Mayo Clinic the odds ratio of constipation preceding PD was 2.48 with a lag time before onset of motor symptoms of 7.9 years (15). Immunohistochemical analysis for α-synuclein of biopsy material obtained during colonoscopy may serve as a marker for PD. In a study of 29 PD patients and 10 controls, Lewy pathology was observed by immunostaining in colonic biopsies from 21 patients and in none of the controls. The extent of Lewy pathology was positively correlated with levodopa-unresponsive features and constipation (16).

Sleep Disorders

RBD is characterized by a loss of the normal atonia of REM sleep. Affected patients cry out or kick while dreaming. RBD occurs in approximately a third of patients with PD, and an additional 20% have asymptomatic loss of REM atonia (17). In contrast the incidence of RBD is not increased in essential tremor or restless legs syndrome (18).

In a prospective study one third of patients with PD met the diagnostic criteria of RBD based on polysomnography recordings. Nineteen of 33 patients with PD but only one of 16 control subjects had REM sleep without atonia. PD patients also had a lower percentage of time spent with muscle atonia during REM sleep than controls (60.1% vs. 93.2%; $P = 0.003$) (17). RBD may also predict clinical subtypes of PD and response to treatment. PD patients with coexisting RBD were less likely to be tremor predominant (14% vs. 53%; $P < 0.02$) and showed an increased frequency of falls (38% vs. 7%; $P = 0.04$). They also were less responsive to medication [Unified Parkinson's Disease Rating Scale (UPDRS) improvement 16.2% vs. 34.8%; $P = 0.049$]. Markers of overall disease severity, quantitative motor testing, and motor complications did not differ between groups (19).

Sleep disorders can appear decades before motor symptoms of PD appear (20). In a long-term study of RBD 26 of 93 patients developed a neurodegenerative disorder. The distribution of diagnoses included PD (14), Lewy body dementia (7), Alzheimer's disease (4), and MSA (1). The estimated five-year risk of neurodegenerative disease was 17.7%, the 10-year risk was 40.6%, and the 12-year risk was 52.4% (21). The pathologic basis may include a degeneration of GABAergic, glutamatergic, and cholinergic systems as a result of lesions in the laterodorsal pontine tegmentum that modulate REM sleep (pedunculopontine nucleus, lateral tegmental nucleus, locus coeruleus) and their anatomic connections. Nigrostriatal dopaminergic degeneration may play a role in the pathogenesis of RBD, but is not a sine qua non (22). The lack of correlation between RBD severity and DAT densities suggests that another pathogenic process not related to nigrostriatal dopaminergic transmission may be implicated in RBD (23). Excessive daytime somnolence (EDS) can also result from pathology in the coeruleus/subcoeruleus complex and the reticular formation, which are affected in stage 2 of Braak staging. In the HAAS study, 3000 men enrolled from 1991 to1993 and diagnosed with EDS showed a threefold increase in risk for PD 10 years later (24). This risk was not significantly reduced when adjusted for insomnia, cognitive function, depressed mood, midlife cigarette smoking, and coffee drinking.

Patients with idiopathic RBD have a risk of developing neurodegenerative disease of 19–38% at five years of follow-up and 40–65% at 10 years. About half develop PD, and half develop dementia (mostly dementia with Lewy bodies). This high risk and long latency suggest RBD as an ideal premotor marker for predicting PD (21,25). However, not every patient with PD develops RBD, and RBD appears to predict a specific clinical subtype of PD characterized by male predominance, akinetic-rigid manifestations, and a greater likelihood of dementia and autonomic symptoms.

Depression and Anxiety

Depression and anxiety occur early and often in PD. In a large registry-based study, patients with PD had a 2.4- to 3.2-fold increased risk of depression than those with osteoarthritis or diabetes (26). Depression in PD often coexists with anxiety. Two clinical subtypes have been identified in a sample of 513 patients by latent class analysis. The first is described as "anxious-depressed" and the other "depressed." However, a further large proportion of patients had relatively isolated anxiety (27).

The latency from a diagnosis of depression to a diagnosis of PD was studied in a large survey derived from the NIH-AARP Diet and Health Study. Physician-diagnosed depression and PD were stratified by the year of diagnosis in the following categories: before 1985, 1985–1994, 1995–1999, and 2000-present. Individuals with depression diagnosed after 2000 were more likely to report a concurrent diagnosis of PD than those without depression (OR = 4.7, 95% CI = 3.9, 5.7). Depression diagnosed before 2000 was also associated with higher odds of PD diagnosed after 2000 (OR = 2.0, 95% CI = 1.6, 2.4). This association was stronger for depression diagnosed in 1995–1999 (OR = 2.7, 95% CI = 2.0, 3.6), but waned with time, being lower for depression diagnosed in 1985–1994 (OR = 1.6, 95% CI = 1.1, 2.3) or before 1985 (OR = 1.7, 95% CI = 1.3, 2.3). The results confirm that depression may be a very early symptom of PD and may act as a marker 10–15 years before onset of motor symptoms (28).

In a neuropathologic study comparing depressed ($n = 11$) and nondepressed ($n = 9$) elderly PD patients a higher prevalence of pathologic features occurred in catecholamine areas of the brain in depressed PD patients. Areas affected included the locus coeruleus, dorsal vagus nerve, and the SNc. The dorsal raphe nuclei, amygdala, and cortical regions appeared to be spared (29). These areas tend to be affected first in Braak stage 2 (1).

Autonomic and Cardiac Dysfunction

Orthostatic hypotension is common in PD and is often ascribed to medication side effects. However, it may be observed independent of levodopa or dopamine agonist treatment. Multiple pathologic mechanisms have been implicated. Abnormal α-synuclein pathology in periadrenal tissues and in the adrenal gland was seen in 26.4% of elderly patients and in 11.1% of PD cases and was associated with orthostatic hypotension (30). Dysfunction of the cardiovascular autonomic system due to cardiac sympathetic denervation can occur early in PD as demonstrated by reduced tyrosine hydroxylase (TH) immunoreactivity in the cardiac nerves and myocardium. In a study of five PD patients, two ILBD cases, and seven controls a marked reduction of TH immunoreactivity was seen in four PD patients and in both individuals with ILBD. All controls showed dense TH-immunoreactivity in the cardiac nerves (31).

A novel method of assessing autonomic function is cardiac metaiodobenzyl-guanidine (MIBG) scintigraphy, which measures postganglionic sympathetic cardiac innervation. Patients with PD tend to have abnormal MIBG scintigraphy even at the earliest stages of disease (32). MIBG scintigraphy is also abnormal in Lewy Body Disease but not in Alzheimer's disease. Reduced cardiac ^{123}I-MIBG uptake is more marked in RBD than in early-stage PD. Aggregates of α-synuclein in epicardial nerve fascicles are significantly different between ILBD, PD, MSA, and controls, although degeneration of cardiac sympathetic nerves can occur in MSA. These α-synuclein aggregates are seen in the distal axons of the cardiac sympathetic nervous system before neuronal somata or neurites in the paravertebral sympathetic ganglia. This gradient of centripetal degeneration of the cardiac sympathetic nerve in PD contrasts with slight changes in MSA (33).

Patients with RBD may later develop PD. Since cardiac autonomic dysfunction is also observed in PD this could be a marker of PD. With this hypothesis in mind, heart rate variability (HRV) recorded during polysomnography evaluations was studied in patients with RBD. HRV during wakefulness was significantly decreased in patients with RBD compared with control subjects, suggesting abnormalities of both sympathetic and parasympathetic function. It was suggested that HRV measured by routine electrocardiograms could be used to screen for Lewy body disorders such as PD (34). Pupillary unrest (spontaneous change of pupil diameter in darkness) and orthostatic decreases in systolic blood pressure were greater while resting HRV was lower in PD than controls. A negative correlation between HRV and pupillary redilation velocity and a positive correlation between orthostatic change in heart rate and pupillary unrest was also noted, suggesting a simultaneous autonomic dysfunction in both pupillary and cardiac systems in PD (35).

NEUROIMAGING METHODS

Radiotracer imaging of the brain with positron emission tomography (PET) and SPECT methods has been in use for some time in the diagnosis of PD, as well as a measure of disease progression. However, a consensus has not been attained with respect to a particular methodology of evaluation (36). SPECT studies of the dopaminergic system may play a role in the premotor diagnosis of PD. These studies involve imaging of the dopamine transporter (DAT) or postsynaptic dopamine receptors. DAT SPECT in particular has been shown to be a sensitive means to detect loss of striatal DATs in early PD, and may be able to detect a dopaminergic deficit even in the premotor phase of disease (37). The loss of nigrostriatal dopaminergic cells leads to a decline of striatal DAT molecules. DAT SPECT studies in early PD patients show significant reductions in striatal DAT binding (38).

Dopaminergic PET and SPECT have a very high sensitivity and specificity for parkinsonism, but a limited ability to distinguish PD from other forms of parkinsonism. It is estimated, based on extrapolation back in time, that imaging abnormalities may first appear four to seven years before motor symptoms of PD (39,40). Asymptomatic carriers of the LRRK2 mutation showed loss of dopaminergic function on PET imaging with one case in the series progressing to clinical PD (41). Hyposmic first-degree relatives of PD patients showed dopaminergic denervation on ß-CIT SPECT imaging (42). Heterozygotes for parkin and PINK1 mutations may also show abnormalities on fluorodopa PET and raclopride binding, but it is not known if heterozygosity for these mutations is a risk factor for PD (43). The short latency of four to seven years between positive findings of PET and SPECT imaging in premotor PD and the appearance of motor symptoms limits use as a screening tool. Diagnostic accuracy in premotor stages is also not well established. SPECT imaging of DAT using [^{123}I]FP-CIT (Ioflupane I 123, DaTscan) has been recently approved by the FDA as a diagnostic tool for parkinsonism but cannot distinguish PD from atypical forms of parkinsonism (44). As this technique finds greater utilization in clinical practice, the utility of these imaging techniques in the early and premotor diagnosis of parkinsonism will be better defined.

Transcranial sonography (TCS) has been studied as a marker of depression and PD. Reduced echogenicity ("hypoechogenicity") of midbrain raphe was associated with increased risk of depression, whereas increased echogenicity ("hyperechogenicity") of the substantia nigra was felt to be a characteristic finding in PD (45). A study of normal individuals showed that those with substantia nigra hyperechogenicity also had ^{18}F-dopa uptake below normal (46) indicating a potential application in premotor diagnosis. About 40% of patients with RBD show changes on TCS. Reduced echogenicity of the midbrain raphe nuclei indicates an increased risk of depression and urinary incontinence in PD patients. This TCS finding represents degeneration of nuclei and disruption of fiber tracts of the basal limbic system in major depression and extrapyramidal disorders associated with depression (45). The simultaneous occurrence of substantia nigra hyperechogenicity and raphe hypoechogenicity in PD patients was associated with history of depression prior to onset of motor symptoms of PD. This combination in depressed subjects was associated with mild motor asymmetry suggestive of early stages of PD (47). Thus screening patients with depression and mild motor slowing with TCS may identify a subgroup at risk for PD. A limitation of TCS is the quality of temporal acoustic bone window that can limit visualization of midbrain structures in 5–10% of Caucasian subjects (47).

SCREENING FOR PD WITH PREMOTOR SYMPTOMS

Currently no therapy can slow or reverse progression of PD when diagnosed at the time of onset of motor symptoms. However, using therapies with potential neuroprotective benefit in the premotor stage could offer a way to significantly alter the natural history of PD.

The use of premotor symptoms as a screening tool to select patients for such trials must be weighed with caution. PD has a relatively low prevalence of about 100–300 per 100,000 (48). A large number of patients will need to be screened to identify subjects of interest. Screening the population at large is both expensive and has ethical perils. However, a subset of the population could be selected that has a relatively higher probability of developing PD. Thus individuals with an immediate relative with PD, especially when the affected proband has a defined genetic mutation such as the LRRK2 gene, could be selected. Individuals with environmental exposures increasing risk of PD such as exposure to pesticides or those who have a higher risk for PD based on epidemiology, such as nonsmokers could also form the basis of a selected population.

Even after combining such selection factors, the number of individuals that will need to be screened remains large and a systematic approach is necessary for a cost-effective approach to screening. Investigators in the Parkinson Associated Risk Syndrome (PARS) study have suggested such a stratified approach (49). Initial studies would evaluate premotor symptoms that can be studied by relatively inexpensive testing, such as tests for anosmia using the UPSIT. This offers a high degree of sensitivity but is nonspecific. Individuals identified by such testing can then be screened using a more expensive test offering greater specificity, such as DaTscan imaging. Others have combined olfactory testing with TCS in the Prospective validation of RIsk factors for the development of Parkinson Syndromes (PRIPS) study (50). It will be important to establish the sensitivity, specificity, and predictive value of these premotor markers to lay the basis for future clinical trials aimed at early intervention before the onset of motor symptoms of PD.

REFERENCES

1. Braak H, Del Tredici K, Rüb U, et al. Staging of brain pathology related to sporadic Parkinson's disease. Neurobiol Aging 2003; 24: 197–211.
2. Lewy FH. Paralysis agitans. I. Pathologische anatomie. In: Lewandowsky M, ed. Handbuch der Neurologie. Berlin: Springer, 1912: 920–33.
3. Jellinger KA. Formation and development of Lewy pathology: a critical update. J Neurol 2009; 256: 270–9.
4. Jellinger KA. Neuropathological spectrum of synucleinopathies. Mov Disord 2003; 18: S2–12.
5. Burke RE, Dauer WT, Vonsattel JP. A critical evaluation of the Braak staging scheme for Parkinson's disease. Ann Neurol 2008; 64: 485–91.
6. Hawkes CH, Del Tredici K, Braak H. A timeline for Parkinson's disease. Parkinsonism Relat Disord 2010; 16: 79–84.
7. Parkkinen L, Pirttilä T, Alafuzoff I. Applicability of current staging/categorization of alpha-synuclein pathology and their clinical relevance. Acta Neuropathol 2008; 115: 399–407.
8. Doty RL. The olfactory system and its disorders. Semin Neurol 2009; 29: 74–81.
9. Hummel T, Sekinger B, Wolf SR, et al. Sniffin' sticks: olfactory performance assessed by the combined testing of odor identification, odor discrimination and olfactory threshold. Chem Senses 1997; 22: 39–52.
10. Haehner A, Boesveldt S, Berendse HW, et al. Prevalence of smell loss in Parkinson's disease–a multicenter study. Parkinsonism Relat Disord 2009; 15: 490–4.
11. Ponsen MM, Stoffers D, Booij J, et al. Idiopathic hyposmia as a preclinical sign of Parkinson's disease. Ann Neurol 2004; 56: 173–81.

12. Cersosimo MG, Benarroch EE. Neural control of the gastrointestinal tract: implications for Parkinson disease. Mov Disord 2008; 23: 1065–75.
13. Benarroch EE, Schmeichel AM, Sandroni P, et al. Involvement of vagal autonomic nuclei in multiple system atrophy and Lewy body disease. Neurology 2006; 66: 378–83.
14. Abbott RD, Petrovitch H, White LR, et al. Frequency of bowel movements and the future risk of Parkinson's disease. Neurology 2001; 57: 456–62.
15. Savica R, Carlin JM, Grossardt BR, et al. Medical records documentation of constipation preceding Parkinson disease: a case-control study. Neurology 2009; 73: 1752–8.
16. Lebouvier T, Neunlist M, Bruley des Varannes S, et al. Colonic biopsies to assess the neuropathology of Parkinson's disease and its relationship with symptoms. PLoS ONE 2010; 5: e12728.
17. Gagnon JF, Bédard MA, Fantini ML, et al. REM sleep behavior disorder and REM sleep without atonia in Parkinson's disease. Neurology 2002; 59: 585–9.
18. Adler CH, Hentz JG, Shill HA, et al. Probable RBD is increased in Parkinson's disease but not in essential tremor or restless legs syndrome. Parkinsonism Relat Disord 2011; 17: 456–8.
19. Postuma RB, Gagnon JF, Vendette M, et al. REM sleep behaviour disorder in Parkinson's disease is associated with specific motor features. J Neurol Neurosurg Psychiatry 2008; 79: 1117–21.
20. Claassen DO, Josephs KA, Ahlskog JE, et al. REM sleep behavior disorder preceding other aspects of synucleinopathies by up to half a century. Neurology 2010; 75: 494–9.
21. Postuma RB, Gagnon JF, Vendette M, et al. Quantifying the risk of neurodegenerative disease in idiopathic REM sleep behavior disorder. Neurology 2009; 72: 1296–300.
22. Kim YK, Yoon IY, Kim JM, et al. The implication of nigrostriatal dopaminergic degeneration in the pathogenesis of REM sleep behavior disorder. Eur J Neurol 2010; 17: 487–92.
23. Iranzo A, Santamaria J, Tolosa E. The clinical and pathophysiological relevance of REM sleep behavior disorder in neurodegenerative diseases. Sleep Med Rev 2009; 13: 385–401.
24. Abbott RD, Ross GW, White LR, et al. Excessive daytime sleepiness and subsequent development of Parkinson disease. Neurology 2005; 65: 1442–6.
25. Iranzo A, Molinuevo JL, Santamaría J, et al. Rapid-eye-movement sleep behaviour disorder as an early marker for a neurodegenerative disorder: a descriptive study. Lancet Neurol 2006; 5: 572–7.
26. Nilsson FM, Kessing LV, Sørensen TM, et al. Major depressive disorder in Parkinson's disease: a register-based study. Acta Psychiatr Scand 2002; 106: 202–11.
27. Brown RG, Landau S, Hindle JV, et al. Depression and anxiety related subtypes in Parkinson's disease. J Neurol Neurosurg Psychiatry 2011; 82: 803–9.
28. Fang F, Xu Q, Park Y, et al. Depression and the subsequent risk of Parkinson's disease in the NIH-AARP diet and health study. Mov Disord 2010; 25: 1157–62.
29. Frisina PG, Haroutunian V, Libow LS. The neuropathological basis for depression in Parkinson's disease. Parkinsonism Relat Disord 2009; 15: 144–8.
30. Fumimura Y, Ikemura M, Saito Y, et al. Analysis of the adrenal gland is useful for evaluating pathology of the peripheral autonomic nervous system in lewy body disease. J Neuropathol Exp Neurol 2007; 66: 354–62.
31. Ghebremedhin E, Del Tredici K, Langston JW, Braak H. Diminished tyrosine hydroxylase immunoreactivity in the cardiac conduction system and myocardium in Parkinson's disease: an anatomical study. Acta Neuropathol 2009; 118: 777–84.
32. Spiegel J, Hellwig D, Farmakis G, et al. Myocardial sympathetic degeneration correlates with clinical phenotype of Parkinson's disease. Mov Disord 2007; 22: 1004–8.
33. Orimo S, Uchihara T, Nakamura A, et al. Axonal alpha-synuclein aggregates herald centripetal degeneration of cardiac sympathetic nerve in Parkinson's disease. Brain 2008; 131: 642–50.
34. Valappil RA, Black JE, Broderick MJ, et al. Exploring the electrocardiogram as a potential tool to screen for premotor Parkinson's disease. Mov Disord 2010; 25: 2296–303.
35. Jain S, Siegle GJ, Gu C, et al. Autonomic insufficiency in pupillary and cardiovascular systems in Parkinson's disease. Parkinsonism Relat Disord 2011; 17: 119–22.

36. Ravina B, Eidelberg D, Ahlskog JE, et al. The role of radiotracer imaging in Parkinson disease. Neurology 2005; 64: 208–15.
37. Booij J, Knol RJ. SPECT imaging of the dopaminergic system in (premotor) Parkinson's disease. Parkinsonism Relat Disord 2007; 13: S425–8.
38. Winogrodzka A, Bergmans P, Booij J, et al. [(123)I]beta-CIT SPECT is a useful method for monitoring dopaminergic degeneration in early stage Parkinson's disease. J Neurol Neurosurg Psychiatry 2003; 74: 294–8.
39. Vingerhoets FJ, Snow BJ, Lee CS, et al. Longitudinal fluorodopa positron emission tomographic studies of the evolution of idiopathic parkinsonism. Ann Neurol 1994; 36: 759–64.
40. Morrish PK, Rakshi JS, Bailey DL, et al. Measuring the rate of progression and estimating the preclinical period of Parkinson's disease with [18F]dopa PET. J Neurol Neurosurg Psychiatry 1998; 64: 314–19.
41. Nandhagopal R, Mak E, Schulzer M, et al. Progression of dopaminergic dysfunction in a LRRK2 kindred: a multitracer PET study. Neurology 2008; 71: 1790–5.
42. Ponsen MM, Stoffers D, Wolters ECh, et al. Olfactory testing combined with dopamine transporter imaging as a method to detect prodromal Parkinson's disease. J Neurol Neurosurg Psychiatry 2010; 81: 396–9.
43. Stoessl AJ. Positron emission tomography in premotor Parkinson's disease. Parkinsonism Relat Disord 2007; 13: S421–4.
44. Hauser RA, Grosset DG. [(123) I]FP-CIT (DaTscan) SPECT brain imaging in patients with suspected Parkinsonian syndromes. J Neuroimaging 2012; 22: 225–30.
45. Walter U, Skoloudík D, Berg D. Transcranial sonography findings related to non-motor features of Parkinson's disease. J Neurol Sci 2010; 289: 123–7.
46. Berg D, Becker G, Zeiler B, et al. Vulnerability of the nigrostriatal system as detected by transcranial ultrasound. Neurology 1999; 53: 1026–31.
47. Walter U, Hoeppner J, Prudente-Morrissey L, et al. Parkinson's disease-like midbrain sonography abnormalities are frequent in depressive disorders. Brain 2007; 130: 1799–807.
48. Baumann CR. Epidemiology, diagnosis and differential diagnosis in Parkinson's disease tremor. Parkinsonism Relat Disord 2012; 18: S90–2.
49. Stern MB, Siderowf A. Parkinson's at risk syndrome: can Parkinson's disease be predicted? Mov Disord 2010; 25: S89–93.
50. Berg D. Is pre-motor diagnosis possible? The European experience. Parkinsonism Relat Disord 2012; 18: S195–8.

6

Autonomic dysfunction and management

Richard B. Dewey Jr., Pravin Khemani,
Cherian Abraham Karunapuzha, and Shilpa Chitnis

Although Parkinson's disease (PD) is commonly regarded as a disorder of dopamine deficiency, it is actually a multisystem degenerative disorder. As nondopaminergic brain pathways are involved in the genesis of many symptoms, treatment is more extensive than merely increasing brain dopaminergic stimulation. The autonomic symptoms fall into this category, and management is often challenging. The autonomic features of PD affect cardiovascular function, gastrointestinal (GI) motility, urinary bladder function, sexual ability, and thermal regulation. A list of the common symptoms and signs of autonomic dysfunction is shown in Table 6.1. While symptoms of autonomic failure typically present later in the course of the disease, rare case reports exist of autonomic abnormalities as the presenting feature (1). This chapter will outline the common autonomic features of PD and discuss treatment approaches for each.

FREQUENCY OF AUTONOMIC DYSFUNCTION IN PD

While the focus of routine follow-up visits between PD patients and neurologists is typically on the motor symptoms of the disease, autonomic problems are frequently present, and can be identified if patients are specifically asked. In one study of 48 men with PD, 89% had at least one autonomic symptom compared with 43% of elderly control subjects (2). Autonomic symptoms seen in these men with PD included erectile dysfunction (60%), urinary urgency (46%), constipation (44%), dysphagia (23%), and orthostatism (22%), and each of these symptoms was more common in PD patients than controls. A study comparing 141 PD patients with 50 controls found that half of the PD patients felt that autonomic failure had a major impact on their daily life (3). Symptoms that were seen significantly more often in PD patients than controls included orthostatic dizziness (48% vs. 22%), bladder dysfunction (45% vs. 24%), erectile dysfunction (64% vs. 20%), and hyperhidrosis (46% vs. 22%). Fifty-six percent of the PD patients (mean Hoehn & Yahr score of 3.1) had at least two autonomic symptoms. In an effort to determine the influence of nonmotor symptoms on quality of life and to assess the detection rate of these problems during routine clinical care, 94 patients were given the Non-Motor Symptoms Questionnaire and had their clinical notes reviewed for mention of these symptoms (4). Among the most common nonmotor symptoms were autonomic problems such as nocturia, urinary urgency, hypersalivation, and constipation. Health-related quality of life in these patients correlated strongly with a scale evaluating the severity of autonomic symptoms (SCOPA-AUT). The authors found that only 44% of the nonmotor features identified by the questionnaire were documented in clinical notes, with autonomic symptoms being among the most poorly detected of all

TABLE 6.1 Autonomic Features of Parkinson's Disease

Cardiovascular
  Orthostatic hypotension
  Decreased heart rate variability
  Decreased MIBG cardiac scintigraphy
  Cardiac arrhythmias
Gastrointestinal
  Impaired swallowing
  Drooling
  Constipation
  Delayed gastric emptying
Urinary bladder
  Frequency
  Urgency
  Urge incontinence
  Nocturia
Sexual dysfunction
  Decreased desire
  Decreased arousal
Reduced attainment of orgasm
  Erectile dysfunction
  Sexual dissatisfaction
Sweating abnormalities
  Hyperhidrosis
  Anhidrosis

Abbreviation: MIBG, [123I]Metaiodobenzylguanidine.

nonmotor symptoms. Since autonomic symptoms decrease quality of life, physicians should routinely ask about these problems, so appropriate treatment can be initiated.

DIAGNOSTIC TESTING FOR AUTONOMIC DYSFUNCTION IN PD

While simple questioning can identify the presence of autonomic symptoms and lead to initiation of treatment, diagnostic testing may be helpful in confirming the presence of autonomic involvement. Certain studies can also be useful for discriminating PD from multiple system atrophy (MSA), whereas other studies are not useful in this differential diagnosis.

[123I]Metaiodobenzylguanidine Scintigraphy

[123I]Metaiodobenzylguanidine (MIBG) is a norepinephrine analog, which is transported into and stored in the terminals of sympathetic nerve endings. MIBG uptake is expressed as a ratio of single-photon emission computed tomography signal in the heart to that of the upper mediastinum. The lower the ratio, the fewer are the functioning sympathetic nerve terminals in the heart. A number of studies have looked at the sympathetic innervation of cardiac muscle in PD patients using this technique, and all have shown that MIBG uptake in myocardium is significantly less in PD than in matched controls (5). Courbon et al. compared MIBG uptake in two groups of patients with PD, those with normal autonomic function tests and those with overt dysautonomia (6). They found that patients without dysautonomia had impaired MIBG uptake, just like patients with overt autonomic symptoms. They concluded that MIBG scintigraphy is a sensitive marker of PD even in patients without autonomic symptoms. Orimo et al. used this technique to compare MIBG uptake in PD patients, normal controls, neurologic controls (essential tremor, vascular parkinsonism), and in patients with MSA (7). They found that the ratio of MIBG uptake in the heart to mediastinum was decreased in 84% of PD patients compared with normal controls. This uptake ratio was lower in more advanced compared with earlier-stage PD patients, a finding which has been replicated using fluorodopa PET scanning (8). The MIBG uptake ratio was not significantly different from controls in patients with essential tremor, vascular parkinsonism, or MSA (7). Thus, although MSA can be difficult to differentiate from PD with autonomic failure on clinical grounds, a number of studies have suggested that MIBG scintigraphy may be useful in making this distinction; PD patients have decreased uptake with MSA patients having relatively normal uptake.

In addition to being helpful at differentiating PD from mimicking conditions, autonomic involvement of the heart appears to be an early finding in PD. Spiegel et al. performed MIBG scintigraphy in 18 Hoehn & Yahr stage I, levodopa-responsive PD patients (9). They found that 13 patients (72%) had significantly reduced cardiac tracer accumulation indicating that in most PD patients, autonomic involvement of the myocardium is an early finding and might be useful in helping to differentiate PD from other conditions.

Several authors have performed pathologic studies on postmortem cardiac tissue in an effort to visualize the sympathetic denervation associated with PD. These studies have shown a near complete loss of sympathetic axons in nerve fascicles of the epicardium (10,11) with Lewy bodies being found in the cardiac plexus (12,13). In one study, five of nine patients with Lewy bodies in the sino-atrial node had atrial cardiac arrhythmias during life suggesting that the sympathetic involvement of the heart in PD might predispose to cardiac arrhythmias (13).

Autonomic Testing

An exhaustive review of the various tests of autonomic function in PD is beyond the scope of this chapter. Briefly, the tests which have been commonly employed in the study of PD autonomic failure, include heart rate variation (with deep breathing and valsalva), tilt table testing for orthostatism, sudomotor axon reflex testing, and thermoregulatory sweat testing. Abnormalities may be seen in one or more of these depending on the presenting symptoms. Several studies have suggested that as a group, autonomic failure is more severe in MSA than in PD, but these studies often use the severity of autonomic failure to help assign the diagnosis; the more severe the autonomic symptoms, the more likely the patient will be classified as having MSA. Riley and Chelimsky have noted the circular nature of this reasoning and performed a comparative study of autonomic tests in patients with PD and MSA in whom autonomic failure was not used for diagnosis (14). They found a high frequency of abnormal test results in patients with dysautonomia with both PD and MSA, and the severity of autonomic failure did not differ between the groups. They suggested that thermoregulatory sweat testing might be the most sensitive test for PD-related autonomic failure since all patients with dysautonomia with either diagnosis who received this test had abnormal results. There is some controversy on whether quantitative sudomotor axon reflex testing (QSART) is helpful for detecting sympathetic dysfunction in PD. In one study, patients with abnormal blood pressure responses to valsalva and decreased cardiac fluorodopa PET scanning (indicating sympathetic dysfunction) had normal QSART test results (15). They interpreted this finding as indicating that the sympathetic dysfunction in PD involves the loss of noradrenergic but not cholinergic function. A number of studies have confirmed that heart rate variability is decreased in patients with PD (16–19).

SYMPTOMS AND MANAGEMENT OF AUTONOMIC DYSFUNCTION IN PD
Orthostatic Hypotension

A significant drop in systolic blood pressure when moving from sitting or lying to the standing position is undoubtedly one of the most important symptoms of auto-nomic failure seen in PD. Orthostatism can be either symptomatic, in which patients complain of lightheadedness, dizziness, or actual syncope, or asymptomatic in spite of significant drops in systolic blood pressure. When symptomatic, orthostatic hypotension can lead to significant disability including wheelchair confinement.

Estimates of the frequency of orthostatic hypotension vary. A community-based study conducted in England found that 47% of a group of 89 PD patients had orthostatic hypotension as defined by a drop of 20 mmHg when standing from a supine position or to a systolic pressure of less than 90 mmHg (20). They did not find an association between PD severity and the presence of orthostatic hypotension. In a study of early untreated PD, 14% of 51 patients met similar cri-teria for orthostatic hypotension (21). The strength of this study is that all patients were followed for at least seven years, and nine of 60 patients were excluded from the analysis due to the development of other symptoms making the diagnosis of idiopathic PD insecure. Additionally, because all patients were evaluated before they began antiparkinsonian medications, the confounding effect of drugs was not a factor in this study. This is an important consideration as dopaminergic ther-apy is believed to aggravate orthostatism in patients with parkinsonism and auto-nomic failure. On the other hand, a comparative study of orthostatic blood pressure measurements in PD patients in both medication "off" and "on" states did not show a significant difference indicating that blood pressure dysregulation is due mostly to neuropathologic changes rather than to the effect of dopaminer-gic drugs (22).

The underlying mechanism of orthostatic hypotension in PD and MSA has been studied. Goldstein et al. noted that since patients with PD and orthostatic hypotension have cardiac sympathetic denervation (as shown consistently in studies of MIBG uptake) while MSA patients do not, the mechanism producing orthostatic hypotension must be different (23). They measured venous catechol-amines and metanephrines finding low levels of normetanephrine and dihydroxy-phenylglycol in patients with PD and orthostatic hypotension while in patients with MSA and orthostatic hypotension, normal levels were found. They concluded that in MSA there is dysregulation but not loss of catecholamine secreting cells in the adrenal medulla and sympathetic nervous system, while in PD there is loss of sympathetic nervous system cells with relative sparing of the adrenal medullary system.

Pathologically, studies have shown cell loss in the intermediolateral nucleus of the spinal cord in PD, with Lewy bodies being found in the hypothalamus, sym-pathetic ganglia, sacral parasympathetic nuclei, and the GI tract. This widespread distribution of cell loss in structures important for autonomic function indicates that the dysautonomia seen in PD is due to both central and peripheral autonomic nervous system involvement (24,25).

In addition to the hypotension seen in PD patients when in the upright position, the autonomic dysfunction in PD leads often to supine hypertension at night. Plaschke et al. performed 24-hour ambulatory blood pressure monitoring in PD patients with and without dysautonomia (26). They found that nocturnal mean arterial pressure was significantly higher in PD patients with dysautonomia (and in MSA patients) than in PD patients without autonomic symptoms. They suggested that supine hypertension may increase the risk of stroke in such patients.

Management of orthostatism begins with simple physical measures and progresses to drug therapy when severe. All patients with symptomatic orthostatic hypotension should be advised to raise the head off their bed by about 30 degrees. This maneuver activates the renin–angiotensin system and reduces salt excretion by the kidneys thus increasing blood pressure. Patients should also consider liberalizing dietary salt, preferably by salting their food rather than by taking salt tablets, which may pass unabsorbed through the GI tract. Rapid drinking of half a liter of water has been shown to exert an acute pressor effect in patients with orthostatism, but long-term effects of increased water drinking are not clear (27). Support hose can also be recommended, but compliance with this measure is often poor, especially in men. When orthostatic hypotension is mild, these physical measures may be sufficient. For more severe orthostatic hypotension, fludrocortisone acetate is typically recommended at a dose of 0.1–0.2 mg daily. This drug promotes salt retention by the kidney, which in turn increases plasma volume and systemic blood pressure. Patients frequently develop mild ankle edema, which is evidence that this therapy is actually working. All patients taking fludrocortisone should receive periodic testing for serum potassium, as this ion is excreted by the kidney as sodium is retained. Potassium replacement therapy should be initiated if the levels fall outside the normal range.

For those in whom physical measures and fludrocortisone are insufficient to eliminate symptomatic orthostatic hypotension, pressor agents should be considered. Examples of drugs in this class with efficacy in orthostatic hypotension include ergotamine/caffeine (28), ephedrine (29), and indomethacin (30). Midodrine hydrochloride, approved for orthostatic hypotension in 1996, has been specifically studied as a treatment for symptomatic neurogenic orthostatic hypotension in PD (31). This drug has been shown to exhibit a dose-related increase in mean systolic blood pressure with the effect peaking at one hour (32). Because of its short half-life, the drug may need to be given three times daily during the waking day at doses ranging from 2.5 to 10 mg per administration. Care should be taken not to give the drug late in the day since supine hypertension may result after the patient retires for the night. Some PD patients with milder degrees of autonomic failure may develop orthostatic hypotension only after meals, so-called postprandial hypotension. This may be related to a shunting of blood flow to the myenteric region with resulting diminished blood flow to the brain. In this case, midodrine could be administered right before a large meal to counteract this effect. Some patients find that several cups of coffee (containing caffeine) taken before or with meals may also help with postprandial orthostatic hypotension.

Pyridostigmine has been evaluated as an alternative to midodrine for supine hypertension. This agent was evaluated as a single dose of 60 mg in comparison to placebo with and without low-dose midodrine in a brief inpatient study (33). The investigation was conducted in 58 patients with neurogenic orthostatism, and while 17 had MSA, none were specifically noted to have PD with autonomic failure. They found that pyridostigmine did not cause elevation in supine systolic or diastolic pressure, it reduced the standing diastolic blood pressure fall, and it resulted in improvement in symptoms of orthostatism. In an open-label follow-up of 20 of these patients who continued pyridostigmine, five were on monotherapy, and 85% (the majority of whom were taking both pyridostigmine and midodrine) were "extremely satisfied" with their symptom control.

Droxidopa, a norepinephrine precursor not currently available in the USA, has been studied in patients with symptomatic orthostatism. In a six-week open-label study of 32 patients, most with MSA, droxidopa at a mean dose of 475 mg daily reduced the standing drop in systolic blood pressure by 17.7 mmHg and improved orthostatism in 78% of patients (34). This agent is now under clinical investigation in the USA.

Dysphagia

Swallowing difficulty is common in PD; in one small series of 13 patients, it was seen in 77% of patients (35). Potulska et al. recruited 18 PD patients for detailed swallowing studies of which 13 had symptomatic dysphagia (36). All patients, including the five who had no swallowing complaints, had prolongation of esophageal bolus transport suggesting that autonomic impairment of swallowing may occur early. Patients who complained of dysphagia had abnormalities of the oral and pharyngeal stages of swallowing. Since the oral phase of swallowing is under voluntary control, some have suggested that oral phase dysphagia is due to bradykinesia of the swallowing musculature. Evidence supporting this idea comes from a study of dyskinetic and nondyskinetic patients showing that those with dyskinesia had better swallowing efficiency, perhaps due to a more optimal dosage of levodopa (37). On the other hand, another study of 15 patients who had swallowing studies before and after a dose of levodopa showed minimal improvement following the drug, suggesting that the main problem is due to autonomic failure, not dopaminergic deficiency affecting skeletal muscle control (38).

Management of dysphagia in PD is entirely empiric. A review by the Cochrane Collaboration published in 2001 and updated in 2009 uncovered no randomized trials dealing with nonpharmacologic treatments for dysphagia in PD, and thus no recommendations for therapy could be made (39). An additional similar review of the literature shows that little progress has been made (40). Sharkawi et al. performed an uncontrolled pilot study of the Lee Silverman Voice Treatment (LSVT) for dysphagia in PD in which a modified barium swallow was done before and one month after LSVT in a group of eight patients (41). They reported that abnormalities of swallowing reduced by 51% after therapy principally by improving tongue base function during the oral and pharyngeal phases of swallowing. As this was a small uncontrolled study, further work is necessary to establish if speech therapy is helpful for dysphagia in PD. Anecdotally, it has been suggested that patients with dysphagia employ the "chin-down" posture when swallowing (42) and consider adding thickeners to liquids before drinking. Since dysphagia is a significant risk factor for aspiration pneumonia (the cause of death in many patients with advanced PD), patients should consider placement of a percutaneous gastrostomy tube when coughing during meals becomes a common occurrence.

Sialorrhea

The presence of excessive saliva in the mouth with resultant drooling is a common problem in PD with estimates of up to 77% of patients being affected (35). When severe, patients will often complain bitterly about the problem and may request drug treatment to deal with it. While the clinical impression of the physician is often that the patient has too much saliva, this turns out not to be the case. Proulx et al. studied 83 PD patients and 55 controls by collecting saliva secreted over a 5-minute period (43). They found that the PD patients secreted significantly less saliva than the normal controls, and that levodopa use was a contributor to this reduced salivary output. It has also been demonstrated that de novo patients, not yet treated with dopaminergic drugs, have decreased salivary production (44). These studies suggest that while dopaminergic drugs may exacerbate the problem, decreased salivary production may be an early sign of autonomic involvement in PD. If PD patients secrete less saliva than normal controls, why do they drool and appear to have excess saliva? The most likely explanation is that PD patients exhibit a decreased frequency of automatic swallowing, and when combined by a forward tilt of the head (common particularly in advanced PD), drooling results (43).

The treatment of drooling in PD has been attempted with anticholinergic drugs, such as benztropine, scopolamine, and glycopyrrolate; the latter having been recommended as the agent with the fewest troublesome side effects (45). A four-week, randomized crossover trial using 1 mg of glycopyrrolate three times daily showed a significant mean improvement of 0.8 points on a 9-point self-reported sialorrhea scale (46). Nine of 23 subjects with PD experienced at least a 30% improvement in drooling, which was felt to be clinically significant. The side effect more commonly seen with glycopyrrolate compared with placebo was dry mouth. Long-term studies on efficacy and tolerability of this agent for drooling in PD are not available. Several authors have reported results of botulinum toxin injections as a treatment for drooling in PD. Mancini et al. injected 450 units of botulinum toxin type-A into the parotid and submandibular glands using ultrasonographic guidance in PD and MSA patients with disabling sialorrhea (47). They reported a reduction of drooling within one week that lasted about a month and was unassociated with adverse effects such as dysphagia. Dogu et al. compared ultrasound-guided botulinum toxin type-A injections in the parotid gland with blind injections (using no guidance) and measured postinjection salivary output in the two groups (48). While subjective sialorrhea improved in both groups, the group receiving ultrasound guidance experienced a significant reduction in salivary output, whereas the blind injection group did not. The authors concluded that ultrasound guidance is necessary to ensure success with botulinum toxin injections for this purpose.

Ondo et al. evaluated the effects of botulinum toxin type-B as a treatment for sialorrhea (49). In this study, ultrasound-guided injections with 2500 units of active drug were compared with placebo injections. Efficacy was evaluated by use of a visual analog scale, questionnaires, and by salivary gland scintigraphy. The active drug group experienced significant improvement in all measures compared with the placebo group. In a more recent study of botulinum toxin type-B for sialorrhea in PD, 54 subjects were randomized to injection with placebo or 1500, 2500, or 3500 units of botulinum toxin into the submandibular and parotid glands using external anatomic landmark localization (50). They found a significant improvement in both subjective drooling scores and objectively quantified salivary flow rates in all active drug groups compared with the placebo group. The median duration of peak effect on salivary flow rate was over 100 days for active drug groups compared with 57 days for placebo. Except for dry mouth, which was more common in active drug groups, side effects were similar to placebo. Although there is considerable enthusiasm in the literature for various treatments aimed at drying up saliva, it must be kept in mind that increased salivary production is not the problem in PD, and that these patients already have reduced salivary output. Since saliva is an important component of oral health, drugs and procedures that reduce oral saliva may potentially lead to increased tooth decay (43). While this has not yet been systematically studied, caution is required in the use of these agents.

Constipation

Constipation is a very common complaint among patients with PD, and is probably multifactorial in origin. Frequency estimates vary, but in one study of 94 patients, 71% were constipated as defined by less than one bowel movement in three days (51). Although the neuropathology of PD itself is a major causative factor, these authors pointed out that in addition, PD patients have a significantly reduced water intake per day compared with controls. Further questioning of these constipated PD patients revealed that in most, decreased water drinking preceded the onset of constipation.

Braak et al. have proposed that the neuropathology of PD begins in the glossopharyngeal and vagal nerves and then spreads rostrally toward the midbrain where the substantia nigra becomes affected (52). In accordance with this finding, Singaram et al. counted neurons in the myenteric plexus of the colon and found that 9 of 11 PD patients had fewer intact dopaminergic neurons in the colon compared with controls (53). Since this is an early finding, one would expect constipation to precede the onset of motor symptoms of PD, and in fact, several careful studies have affirmed this supposition. Abbott et al. reporting on the long-term follow-up of 6790 men in the Honolulu Heart Program observed that the incidence of PD was higher in those with constipation than in those without (18.9/10,000 person-years vs. 3.8/10,000 person-years) (54,55). Patients whose constipation was resistant to treatment had the highest incidence of developing PD during the follow-up period (51.6/10,000 person-years). The main strength of this study was the elimination of recall bias through the study design, which asked patients about bowel habits an average of 12 years before they developed PD.

In addition to slowed colonic motility due to dopaminergic denervation of the GI tract, anal sphincter dysfunction has been reported in PD patients, which may contribute to constipation. Mathers et al described paradoxical anal sphincter muscle contraction during simulated defecation straining in 5 of 6 patients with PD studied with anal EMG, and they suggested, based on this finding, that functional anal outlet obstruction may contribute to constipation (56). In four of these patients, they noted improvement in the defecatory mechanism following apomorphine suggesting that this anal dyscoordination may occur on the basis of dopaminergic deficiency. Stocchi et al. confirmed the finding of impaired anal relaxation during straining in PD and added that anal sphincter EMG was normal in PD patients; by comparison sphincter EMG in MSA patients showed denervation and chronic neurogenic signs (57).

Antiparkinsonian medication has been implicated as another factor contributing to constipation in PD. The literature is conflicting on whether drugs have a significant effect on colonic motility, and perhaps the most reasonable answer is that drug therapy is not the primary cause of constipation, but in some cases, may aggravate the condition. This is probably most important for anticholinergic agents, which are known to reduce intestinal motility (58).

As the cause of constipation in PD is multifactorial, its management requires a multimodality approach. All patients should be advised to increase daily water consumption and add bulking agents to the diet such as psyllium preparations and high-fiber foods; however, rarely is this approach sufficient. Cisapride, a prokinetic agent that directly stimulates acetylcholine release in the gut, has been shown to improve constipation and shorten colonic transit time in PD (59). However, this drug was withdrawn from the market in most countries due to QT prolongation and its potential proarrhythmic effect. Mosapride citrate has a similar mechanism of action as cisapride but without known cardiac toxicity. It was studied using an open-label design in 14 patients with PD and MSA where it was well tolerated and effective in producing subjective improvement in bowel frequency and difficult defecation (60). The value of this agent in PD remains to be validated by placebo-controlled trials. Of agents that are currently available for the treatment of constipation, the osmotic laxative polyethylene glycol has been shown to be safe and effective in randomized clinical trials in non-PD populations with chronic constipation (61–63). A randomized blinded study of 14 g daily of polyethylene glycol in 57 PD patients has been reported showing that in the 47 subjects, who completed at least four weeks of treatment, both stool frequency and consistency were significantly improved compared with those in the placebo group, whereas straining at stool was unchanged (64). Side effects included nausea, diarrhea, and disagreeable taste, which led to a higher discontinuation rate in patients assigned to active drug. Lubiprostone is a new agent acting on chloride channels in the gut, which enhances fluid secretion into the intestines. Although not studied specifically in PD, it has been evaluated in a randomized, blinded study of 242 patients with chronic constipation at a dose of 24 μg twice daily compared with placebo (65). Of the 224 who underwent the four-week study, patients on active drug reported significantly improved bowel movement frequency, stool consistency, reduced straining, and reduced constipation severity. Side effects more common in the active drug group included nausea, headache, flatulence, dizziness, and abdominal pain.

For the minority of constipated PD patients in whom anal outlet obstruction is the suspected cause (presumably due to paradoxical contraction of the puborectalis muscle during straining), botulinum toxin type-A injections of 100 units into this muscle under transrectal ultrasonographic guidance have been shown to be effective in small open-label trials (66,67). In a subset of responders, patients noted recurrence of constipation after a period of four months, which responded to repeat injections with 200–300 units of botulinum toxin type-A (67). These preliminary observations need to be confirmed using randomized, controlled trials before this treatment can be recommended.

Urinary Bladder Dysfunction

The most frequent urinary complaints in PD patients are frequency, urgency, urge incontinence, and nocturia. Hobson et al. performed a community-based questionnaire survey in Wales and found that bladder problems were reported in 51% of 123 PD patients returning the survey compared with 31% of 92 controls (68). The calculated relative risk of developing bladder symptoms in PD patients compared with controls was 2.4. Lemack et al. performed a similar questionnaire-based assessment of bladder problems in PD patients, but selected early-stage patients (Hoehn & Yahr stage <2.5) to determine if bladder problems occur early in the disease (69). Men with early PD assessed using the American Urological Association Symptom Index had a mean score of 12 compared with the community sample of normal male volunteers whose mean score was 4.8. Significant differences were seen on questions for frequency, urgency, and weak urinary stream. Women completed the Urogenital Distress Inventory-6, where PD patients had a mean score of 4.8 compared with 2.1 for normal controls. There was no correlation between bladder dysfunction and any measure of motor severity of PD except for gait speed, which was significantly slower in patients with higher scores for bladder dysfunction. This observation suggests that neural pathways for gait and bladder control might be involved in parallel by the degenerative process of PD.

Urodynamic studies have been conducted in small samples of PD patients with persistent bladder complaints to elucidate the nature of the problem. Berger et al. studied 29 patients and found that detrusor hyperreflexia was present in 90%, and that incomplete sphincter relaxation during involuntary detrusor contractions as shown by EMG was present in 61% (70). Winge et al conducted detailed urodynamic studies in 32 PD patients without regard to whether they had bladder symptoms (71). Using the Danish Prostate Symptom Score (Dan-PSS), they found that 43.8% of patients met criteria for symptomatic bladder dysfunction. Irritative bladder symptoms were more commonly seen in patients with greater severity of PD as assessed by motor scoring. On urodynamic testing, bladder capacity was lower in the group with high Dan-PSS scores, and capacity increased when dopaminergic drugs were administered. Detrusor overactivity was also seen in this group, but medication administration did not impact this feature. The authors suggested that because bladder capacity improved after dopaminergic drug administration, dopamine deficiency may in part underlie the irritative bladder symptoms in PD. Whether this is due primarily to central or peripheral dopaminergic cell degeneration is unknown.

The treatment of bladder dysfunction in PD is difficult due to its often multifactorial origin. For instance, in men with irritative bladder symptoms, prostatic hypertrophy may be a contributor to outlet obstruction. For this reason, patients with symptomatic bladder dysfunction should be referred to a urologist with experience in evaluating and managing the bladder problems of PD patients. Generally, treatment will be initiated only after appropriate urodynamic testing is completed, and patients with nocturia should be advised to avoid water intake in the evening. Once a significant obstructive component has been ruled out, treatment of patients with hyperactive detrusor can begin with drugs, such as tolterodine (72), oxybutnin (73), or imipramine (74).

Other agents which have been recommended because of a presumably lower risk of CNS penetration or receptor selectivity (and thus possibly lower risk of cognitive impairment) include trospium and darifenacin (75). Sixteen PD patients with overactive bladder were followed for a year after intradetrusor injections of 500 units of botulinum toxin type-A and were evaluated using the Incontinence Quality of Life Assessment questionnaire (76). Scores on this measure improved from a mean of 32 at baseline to 11 at three months with gradual worsening to a mean score of 26 at one year. Caregiver burden improved in parallel with this subjective benefit to patients. Randomized studies of this promising modality are needed.

Sexual Dysfunction

Although PD patients rarely complain of sexual difficulties, if specifically asked, dysfunction in this area is very common. Bronner et al. performed a comprehensive assessment of sexuality in 75 patients (32 women, 43 men) with PD who did not complain of problems in this area (77). Using specific sexual function scales, they asked patients to rate their sexuality currently and retrospectively before the onset of their PD. They found that in men, 68% had erectile dysfunction, 65% were dissatisfied with their sexual life, and 40% had difficulty reaching orgasm. In women, the major problems were difficulty getting aroused (88%), difficulty reaching orgasm (75%), and decreased sexual desire (47%). Comparing scores before PD onset to the present, most patients reported a deterioration in sexual functioning with the progression of PD. Using stepwise regression, the authors found that in men associated disease, medications, and severity of PD predicted sexual dysfunction, whereas in women levodopa use appeared to decrease sexual desire. Celikel et al. evaluated sexual dysfunction in men and women and found that in men with PD, sexual function was similar to controls, whereas in women, reduced sexual drive and dissatisfaction with orgasm were problems compared with controls (78).

The underlying neuroanatomic substrate for sexual dysfunction in PD is complex and poorly understood. The central dopaminergic system is known to be important for sexual functioning, but conflicting data exist on whether dopaminergic drugs have a beneficial or harmful effect on sexual performance. Erectile dysfunction in men is probably due mainly to autonomic degeneration with the progression of PD.

Treatment of the many facets of sexual dysfunction in PD is complex, and most recommend that special attention be given to ascertaining this problem (since patients will rarely volunteer it during a routine visit) and that sexual counseling be offered to those in whom problems are identified. Erectile dysfunction in men has received specific attention in the literature, and several drugs have been tested for this problem. Sublingual apomorphine, a potent D1, D2 dopamine agonist, which is not available in the United States, has been studied and was found to be effective at improving erectile dysfunction due to several different etiologies, although it has not been specifically studied in PD patients (79). The dopamine agonist pergolide has been found to improve sexual function in PD patients, presumably also via a central dopaminergic mechanism (80).

Several studies have evaluated the effects of sildenafil in PD patients with erectile dysfunction. An open-label pilot study showed that in 10 men, sildenafil improved sexual satisfaction, erectile function, and the ability to reach orgasm (81). In a larger open-label study of 33 depressed male PD patients given a fixed dose of 50 mg of sildenafil one hour before sexual activity, 84.8% reported improved erections (82). A double-blind, placebo-controlled crossover study compared the efficacy and adverse effects of sildenafil in 12 patients with PD to 12 patients with MSA (83). Using the international index of erectile dysfunction as the primary efficacy parameter, they found that 9 of 10 PD patients completing the study had improved erectile function when assigned to active drug. There was a slight but asymptomatic decline in mean blood pressure measurements one hour after active drug ingestion in the PD patients. By contrast, although the MSA patients had improved erectile function on active drug, severe symptomatic orthostatic declines in blood pressure were seen in three patients one hour after ingestion of the active drug leading to discontinuation of recruitment of MSA patients into the study. A number of studies have evaluated the effects of sildenafil on female sexual dysfunction, but the literature is conflicting, involved various outcome measures, and often involved inappropriate statistical methods (84). There are no studies evaluating this agent in women with PD.

Sweating Dysfunction

Hyperhidrosis is a problem in some patients with PD, and when severe, this symptom can be severely disabling. Little is known about the problem due to a paucity of careful studies. A small study demonstrated that PD patients generate more sweat when exposed to heat than control patients and that excessive sweating increases with disease severity (85). Swinn et al. recruited 77 consecutive PD patients and 40 controls for a study of sweating (86). The authors designed their own questionnaire to evaluate sweating, which consisted of 41 questions. PD patients were much more likely than controls to report excess sweating, particularly episodes of whole body, drenching sweats (44% of PD patients vs. 10% of controls). Hypohidrosis was also reported, but the frequency in PD patients was not significantly different from controls. PD patients tended to experience sweating episodes when they were in the medication "off" state or "on" with dyskinesia, and 70% of patients who had dyskinesia reported excessive sweating. Sweating problems did not appear to be related to disease duration or severity. Other autonomic symptoms (urinary frequency and sialorrhea) were correlated with excess sweating. Patients who experienced drenching sweats had an impaired quality of life. In a study comparing sweat production in 16 patients with wearing off to 15 nonfluctuators, sweat production increased steadily over three hours with increasing motor scores during off states, whereas no change was seen with a similar period of observation in nonfluctuators (87).

Treatment of sweating problems in PD is difficult, and no clear guidelines or evidence-based recommendations exist. Because some episodes are associated with off periods and others with dyskinesia, efforts should be made to reduce off time as much as possible while avoiding dyskinesia by adjusting antiparkinsonian medications. While some have suggested treatment with L-dihydroxyphenylalanine or beta-blockers, no studies have been published, which evaluate these treatments in PD (88). While there is a growing literature on the treatment of focal hyperhidrosis with botulinum toxin injections (89–93), this therapy has not been studied in PD-related sweating disorders and would not be expected to be applicable to those patients with whole body drenching sweats due to the practical problem of administering the drug to the target tissue. Beyond attempted pharmacologic treatments, Swinn et al. suggest that PD patients with hyperhidrosis be counseled to avoid hot environments, overactivity, or poorly ventilated clothing (86).

SUMMARY

Autonomic symptoms are common in patients with PD, although often under-recognized. As in the case of constipation, evidence for autonomic dysfunction may precede the onset of motor features by years; however, most autonomic symptoms increase in severity with the progression of motor disability. Careful attention by treating physicians to the autonomic features of PD is necessary to recognize these problems early and begin treatment in time. As noted in a recent

American Academy of Neurology practice parameter on the treatment of nonmotor symptoms in PD, there is an urgent need for randomized controlled trials to evaluate treatments for autonomic symptoms (94).

REFERENCES

1. Kaufmann H, Nahm K, Purohit D, Wolfe D. Autonomic failure as the initial presentation of Parkinson's disease and dementia with Lewy bodies. Neurology 2004; 63: 1093–5.
2. Singer C, Weiner WJ, Sanchez-Ramos JR. Autonomic dysfunction in men with Parkinson disease. Eur Neurol 1992; 32: 134–40.
3. Magerkurth C, Schnitzer R, Braune S. Symptoms of autonomic failure in Parkinson's disease: prevalence and impact on daily life. Clin Auton Res 2005; 15: 76–82.
4. Gallagher DA, Lees AJ, Schrag A. What are the most important nonmotor symptoms in patients with Parkinson's disease and are we missing them? Mov Disord 2010; 25: 2493–500.
5. Taki J, Yoshita M, Yamada M, Tonami N. Significance of 123I-MIBG scintigraphy as a pathophysiological indicator in the assessment of Parkinson's disease and related disorders: it can be a specific marker for Lewy body disease. Ann Nucl Med 2004; 18: 453–61.
6. Courbon F, Brefel-Courbon C, Thalamas C, et al. Cardiac MIBG scintigraphy is a sensitive tool for detecting cardiac sympathetic denervation in Parkinson's disease. Mov Disord 2003; 18: 890–7.
7. Orimo S, Ozawa E, Nakade S, Sugimoto T, Mizusawa H. (123)I-metaiodobenzylguanidine myocardial scintigraphy in Parkinson's disease. J Neurol Neurosurg Psychiatry 1999; 67: 189–94.
8. Li ST, Dendi R, Holmes C, Goldstein DS. Progressive loss of cardiac sympathetic innervation in Parkinson's disease. Ann Neurol 2002; 52: 220–3.
9. Spiegel J, Mollers MO, Jost WH, et al. FP-CIT and MIBG scintigraphy in early Parkinson's disease. Mov Disord 2005; 20: 552–61.
10. Amino T, Orimo S, Itoh Y, et al. Profound cardiac sympathetic denervation occurs in Parkinson disease. Brain Pathol 2005; 15: 29–34.
11. Orimo S, Oka T, Miura H, et al. Sympathetic cardiac denervation in Parkinson's disease and pure autonomic failure but not in multiple system atrophy. J Neurol Neurosurg Psychiatry 2002; 73: 776–7.
12. Iwanaga K, Wakabayashi K, Yoshimoto M, et al. Lewy body-type degeneration in cardiac plexus in Parkinson's and incidental Lewy body diseases. Neurology 1999; 52: 1269–71.
13. Okada Y, Ito Y, Aida J, et al. Lewy bodies in the sinoatrial nodal ganglion: clinicopathological studies. Pathol Int 2004; 54: 682–7.
14. Riley DE, Chelimsky TC. Autonomic nervous system testing may not distinguish multiple system atrophy from Parkinson's disease. J Neurol Neurosurg Psychiatry 2003; 74: 56–60.
15. Sharabi Y, Li ST, Dendi R, Holmes C, Goldstein DS. Neurotransmitter specificity of sympathetic denervation in Parkinson's disease. Neurology 2003; 60: 1036–9.
16. Devos D, Kroumova M, Bordet R, et al. Heart rate variability and Parkinson's disease severity. J Neural Transm 2003; 110: 997–1011.
17. Gurevich TY, Groozman GB, Giladi N, et al. R-R interval variation in Parkinson's disease and multiple system atrophy. Acta Neurol Scand 2004; 109: 276–9.
18. Kallio M, Suominen K, Haapaniemi T, et al. Nocturnal cardiac autonomic regulation in Parkinson's disease. Clin Auton Res 2004; 14: 119–24.
19. Pursiainen V, Haapaniemi TH, Korpelainen JT, et al. Circadian heart rate variability in Parkinson's disease. J Neurol 2002; 249: 1535–40.
20. Allcock LM, Ullyart K, Kenny RA, Burn DJ. Frequency of orthostatic hypotension in a community based cohort of patients with Parkinson's disease. J Neurol Neurosurg Psychiatry 2004; 75: 1470–1.
21. Bonuccelli U, Lucetti C, Del Dotto P, et al. Orthostatic hypotension in de novo Parkinson disease. Arch Neurol 2003; 60: 1400–4.

22. Goetz CG, Lutge W, Tanner CM. Autonomic dysfunction in Parkinson's disease. Neurology 1986; 36: 73–5.

23. Goldstein DS, Holmes C, Sharabi Y, Brentzel S, Eisenhofer G. Plasma levels of catechols and metanephrines in neurogenic orthostatic hypotension. Neurology 2003; 60: 1327–32.

24. Wakabayashi K, Takahashi H. Neuropathology of autonomic nervous system in Parkinson's disease. Eur Neurol 1997; 38: 2–7.

25. Wakabayashi K, Takahashi H. The intermediolateral nucleus and Clarke's column in Parkinson's disease. Acta Neuropathol 1997; 94: 287–9.

26. Plaschke M, Trenkwalder P, Dahlheim H, Lechner C, Trenkwalder C. Twenty-four-hour blood pressure profile and blood pressure responses to head-up tilt tests in Parkinson's disease and multiple system atrophy. J Hypertens 1998; 16: 1433–41.

27. Mathias CJ, Young TM. Water drinking in the management of orthostatic intolerance due to orthostatic hypotension, vasovagal syncope and the postural tachycardia syndrome. Eur J Neurol 2004; 11: 613–19.

28. Dewey RB Jr, Rao SD, Holmburg SL, Victor RG. Ergotamine/caffeine treatment of orthostatic hypotension in parkinsonism with autonomic failure. Eur J Neurol 1998; 5: 593–9.

29. Brooks DJ, Redmond S, Mathias CJ, Bannister R, Symon L. The effect of orthostatic hypotension on cerebral blood flow and middle cerebral artery velocity in autonomic failure, with observations on the action of ephedrine. J Neurol Neurosurg Psychiatry 1989; 52: 962–6.

30. Imaizumi T, Takeshita A, Ashihara T, et al. Increase in reflex vasoconstriction with indomethacin in patients with orthostatic hypotension and central nervous system involvement. Br Heart J 1984; 52: 581–4.

31. Jankovic J, Gilden JL, Hiner BC, et al. Neurogenic orthostatic hypotension: a double-blind, placebo-controlled study with midodrine. Am J Med 1993; 95: 38–48.

32. Wright RA, Kaufmann HC, Perera R, et al. A double-blind, dose-response study of midodrine in neurogenic orthostatic hypotension. Neurology 1998; 51: 120–4.

33. Singer W, Sandroni P, Opfer-Gehrking TL, et al. Pyridostigmine treatment trial in neurogenic orthostatic hypotension. Arch Neurol 2006; 63: 513–18.

34. Mathias CJ, Senard JM, Braune S, et al. L-threo-dihydroxyphenylserine (L-threo-DOPS; droxidopa) in the management of neurogenic orthostatic hypotension: a multi-national, multi-center, dose-ranging study in multiple system atrophy and pure autonomic failure. Clin Auton Res 2001; 11: 235–42.

35. Edwards LL, Quigley EM, Harned RK, Hofman R, Pfeiffer RF. Characterization of swallowing and defecation in Parkinson's disease. Am J Gastroenterol 1994; 89: 15–25.

36. Potulska A, Friedman A, Krolicki L, Spychala A. Swallowing disorders in Parkinson's disease. Parkinsonism Relat Disord 2003; 9: 349–53.

37. Monte FS, da Silva-Junior FP, Braga-Neto P, Nobre e Souza MA, Sales de Bruin VM. Swallowing abnormalities and dyskinesia in Parkinson's disease. Mov Disord 2005; 20: 457–62.

38. Hunter PC, Crameri J, Austin S, Woodward MC, Hughes AJ. Response of parkinsonian swallowing dysfunction to dopaminergic stimulation. J Neurol Neurosurg Psychiatry 1997; 63: 579–83.

39. Deane KH, Whurr R, Clarke CE, Playford ED, Ben-Shlomo Y. Non-pharmacological therapies for dysphagia in Parkinson's disease. Cochrane Database Syst Rev 2001; CD002816.

40. Baijens LW, Speyer R. Effects of therapy for dysphagia in Parkinson's disease: systematic review. Dysphagia 2009; 24: 91–102.

41. Sharkawi AE, Ramig L, Logemann JA, et al. Swallowing and voice effects of Lee Silverman Voice Treatment (LSVT): a pilot study. J Neurol Neurosurg Psychiatry 2002; 72: 31–6.

42. Shanahan TK, Logemann JA, Rademaker AW, Pauloski BR, Kahrilas PJ. Chin-down posture effect on aspiration in dysphagic patients. Arch Phys Med Rehabil 1993; 74: 736–9.

43. Proulx M, de Courval FP, Wiseman MA, Panisset M. Salivary production in Parkinson's disease. Mov Disord 2005; 20: 204–7.

44. Bagheri H, Damase-Michel C, Lapeyre-Mestre M, et al. A study of salivary secretion in Parkinson's disease. Clin Neuropharmacol 1999; 22: 213–15.

45. Tscheng DZ. Sialorrhea: therapeutic drug options. Ann Pharmacother 2002; 36: 1785–90.

46. Arbouw ME, Movig KL, Koopmann M, et al. Glycopyrrolate for sialorrhea in Parkinson disease: a randomized, double-blind, crossover trial. Neurology 2010; 74: 1203–7.
47. Mancini F, Zangaglia R, Cristina S, et al. Double-blind, placebo-controlled study to evaluate the efficacy and safety of botulinum toxin type A in the treatment of drooling in parkinsonism. Mov Disord 2003; 18: 685–8.
48. Dogu O, Apaydin D, Sevim S, Talas DU, Aral M. Ultrasound-guided versus 'blind' intraparotid injections of botulinum toxin-A for the treatment of sialorrhoea in patients with Parkinson's disease. Clin Neurol Neurosurg 2004; 106: 93–6.
49. Ondo WG, Hunter C, Moore W. A double-blind placebo-controlled trial of botulinum toxin B for sialorrhea in Parkinson's disease. Neurology 2004; 62: 37–40.
50. Chinnapongse R, Gullo K, Nemeth P, Zhang Y, Griggs L. Safety and efficacy of botulinum toxin type B for treatment of sialorrhea in Parkinson's disease: A prospective double-blind trial. Mov Disord 2012; 27: 219–26.
51. Ueki A, Otsuka M. Life style risks of Parkinson's disease: association between decreased water intake and constipation. J Neurol 2004; 251: 18–23.
52. Braak H, Del Tredici K, Rub U, et al. Staging of brain pathology related to sporadic Parkinson's disease. Neurobiol Aging 2003; 24: 197–211.
53. Singaram C, Ashraf W, Gaumnitz EA, et al. Dopaminergic defect of enteric nervous system in Parkinson's disease patients with chronic constipation. Lancet 1995; 346: 861–4.
54. Abbott RD, Petrovitch H, White LR, et al. Frequency of bowel movements and the future risk of Parkinson's disease. Neurology 2001; 57: 456–62.
55. Abbott RD, Ross GW, White LR, et al. Environmental, life-style, and physical precursors of clinical Parkinson's disease: recent findings from the Honolulu-Asia Aging Study. J Neurol 2003; 250: 30–9.
56. Mathers SE, Kempster PA, Law PJ, et al. Anal sphincter dysfunction in Parkinson's disease. Arch Neurol 1989; 46: 1061–4.
57. Stocchi F, Badiali D, Vacca L, et al. Anorectal function in multiple system atrophy and Parkinson's disease. Mov Disord 2000; 15: 71–6.
58. Jost WH, Eckardt VF. Constipation in idiopathic Parkinson's disease. Scand J Gastroenterol 2003; 38: 681–6.
59. Jost WH, Schimrigk K. Cisapride treatment of constipation in Parkinson's disease. Mov Disord 1993; 8: 339–43.
60. Liu Z, Sakakibara R, Odaka T, et al. Mosapride citrate, a novel 5-HT4 agonist and partial 5-HT3 antagonist, ameliorates constipation in parkinsonian patients. Mov Disord 2005; 20: 680–6.
61. Cleveland MV, Flavin DP, Ruben RA, Epstein RM, Clark GE. New polyethylene glycol laxative for treatment of constipation in adults: a randomized, double-blind, placebo-controlled study. South Med J 2001; 94: 478–81.
62. Di Palma JA, Smith JR, Cleveland M. Overnight efficacy of polyethylene glycol laxative. Am J Gastroenterol 2002; 97: 1776–9.
63. DiPalma JA, DeRidder PH, Orlando RC, Kolts BE, Cleveland MB. A randomized, placebo-controlled, multicenter study of the safety and efficacy of a new polyethylene glycol laxative. Am J Gastroenterol 2000; 95: 446–50.
64. Zangaglia R, Martignoni E, Glorioso M, et al. Macrogol for the treatment of constipation in Parkinson's disease. A randomized placebo-controlled study. Mov Disord 2007; 22: 1239–44.
65. Johanson JF, Morton D, Geenen J, Ueno R. Multicenter, 4-week, double-blind, randomized, placebo-controlled trial of lubiprostone, a locally-acting type-2 chloride channel activator, in patients with chronic constipation. Am J Gastroenterol 2008; 103: 170–7.
66. Albanese A, Brisinda G, Bentivoglio AR, Maria G. Treatment of outlet obstruction constipation in Parkinson's disease with botulinum neurotoxin A. Am J Gastroenterol 2003; 98: 1439–40.
67. Cadeddu F, Bentivoglio AR, Brandara F, et al. Outlet type constipation in Parkinson's disease: results of botulinum toxin treatment. Aliment Pharmacol Ther 2005; 22: 997–1003.
68. Hobson P, Islam W, Roberts S, Adhiyman V, Meara J. The risk of bladder and autonomic dysfunction in a community cohort of Parkinson's disease patients and normal controls. Parkinsonism Relat Disord 2003; 10: 67–71.

69. Lemack GE, Dewey RB Jr, Roehrborn CG, O'Suilleabhain PE, Zimmern PE. Question-naire-based assessment of bladder dysfunction in patients with mild to moderate Parkinson's disease. Urology 2000; 56: 250–4.

70. Berger Y, Blaivas JG, DeLaRocha ER, Salinas JM. Urodynamic findings in Parkinson's disease. J Urol 1987; 138: 836–8.

71. Winge K, Werdelin LM, Nielsen KK, Stimpel H. Effects of dopaminergic treatment on bladder function in Parkinson's disease. Neurourol Urodyn 2004; 23: 689–96.

72. Serels SR, Appell RA. Tolterodine: a new antimuscarinic agent for the treatment of the overactive bladder. Expert Opin Investig Drugs 1999; 8: 1073–8.

73. Diokno AC, Appell RA, Sand PK, et al. Prospective, randomized, double-blind study of the efficacy and tolerability of the extended-release formulations of oxybutynin and tolterodine for overactive bladder: results of the OPERA trial. Mayo Clin Proc 2003; 78: 687–95.

74. Clarke B. Anticholinergic medication for the unstable bladder: prospective trials of imipramine/propantheline versus penthienate and oxybutynin versus penthienate. Int Urogynecol J Pelvic Floor Dysfunct 1996; 7: 191–5.

75. Sakakibara R, Uchiyama T, Yamanishi T, Kishi M. Genitourinary dysfunction in Parkinson's disease. Mov Disord 2010; 25: 2–12.

76. Kulaksizoglu H, Parman Y. Use of botulinum toxin-A for the treatment of overactive bladder symptoms in patients with Parkinson's disease. Parkinsonism Relat Disord 2010; 16: 531–4.

77. Bronner G, Royter V, Korczyn AD, Giladi N. Sexual dysfunction in Parkinson's disease. J Sex Marital Ther 2004; 30: 95–105.

78. Celikel E, Ozel-Kizil ET, Akbostanci MC, Cevik A. Assessment of sexual dysfunction in patients with Parkinson's disease: a case-control study. Eur J Neurol 2008; 15: 1168–72.

79. Von Keitz AT, Stroberg P, Bukofzer S, Mallard N, Hibberd M. A European multicentre study to evaluate the tolerability of apomorphine sublingual administered in a forced dose-escalation regimen in patients with erectile dysfunction. BJU Int 2002; 89: 409–15.

80. Pohanka M, Kanovsky P, Bares M, Pulkrabek J, Rektor I. Pergolide mesylate can improve sexual dysfunction in patients with Parkinson's disease: the results of an open, prospective, 6-month follow-up. Eur J Neurol 2004; 11: 483–8.

81. Zesiewicz TA, Helal M, Hauser RA. Sildenafil citrate (Viagra) for the treatment of erectile dysfunction in men with Parkinson's disease. Mov Disord 2000; 15: 305–8.

82. Raffaele R, Vecchio I, Giammusso B, et al. Efficacy and safety of fixed-dose oral sildenafil in the treatment of sexual dysfunction in depressed patients with idiopathic Parkinson's disease. Eur Urol 2002; 41: 382–6.

83. Hussain IF, Brady CM, Swinn MJ, Mathias CJ, Fowler CJ. Treatment of erectile dysfunction with sildenafil citrate (Viagra) in parkinsonism due to Parkinson's disease or multiple system atrophy with observations on orthostatic hypotension. J Neurol Neurosurg Psychiatry 2001; 71: 371–4.

84. Brown DA, Kyle JA, Ferrill MJ. Assessing the clinical efficacy of sildenafil for the treatment of female sexual dysfunction. Ann Pharmacother 2009; 43: 1275–85.

85. Turkka JT, Myllyla VV. Sweating dysfunction in Parkinson's disease. Eur Neurol 1987; 26: 1–7.

86. Swinn L, Schrag A, Viswanathan R, et al. Sweating dysfunction in Parkinson's disease. Mov Disord 2003; 18: 1459–63.

87. Pursiainen V, Haapaniemi TH, Korpelainen JT, Sotaniemi KA, Myllyla VV. Sweating in Parkinsonian patients with wearing-off. Mov Disord 2007; 22: 828–32.

88. Feddersen B, Klopstock T, Noachtar S. Hyperhidrosis in Parkinson disease. Neurology 2005; 64: 571.

89. Baumann L, Slezinger A, Halem M, et al. Pilot study of the safety and efficacy of Myobloc (botulinum toxin type B) for treatment of axillary hyperhidrosis. Int J Dermatol 2005; 44: 418–24.

90. Glaser DA. Treatment of axillary hyperhidrosis by chemodenervation of sweat glands using botulinum toxin type A. J Drugs Dermatol 2004; 3: 627–31.

91. Nelson L, Bachoo P, Holmes J. Botulinum toxin type B: a new therapy for axillary hyperhidrosis. Br J Plast Surg 2005; 58: 228–32.
92. Solish N, Benohanian A, Kowalski JW. Prospective open-label study of botulinum toxin type A in patients with axillary hyperhidrosis: effects on functional impairment and quality of life. Dermatol Surg 2005; 31: 405–13.
93. Vadoud-Seyedi J, Simonart T, Heenen M. Treatment of plantar hyperhidrosis with dermojet injections of botulinum toxin. Dermatology 2000; 201: 179.
94. Zesiewicz TA, Sullivan KL, Arnulf I, et al. Practice parameter: treatment of nonmotor symptoms of Parkinson disease: report of the Quality Standards Subcommittee of the American Academy of Neurology. Neurology 2010; 74: 924–31.

7

Sleep dysfunction

Pouya Movahed, M. Tanya Mitra, and K. Ray Chaudhuri

INTRODUCTION

The earliest description of sleep problems of Parkinson's disease (PD) dates back to the original description of PD by James Parkinson (1817) where he states, "His attendants observed, that of late the trembling would sometimes begin in his sleep, and increase until it awakened him: when he always was in a state of agitation and alarm" (1). This is probably the first description of nocturnal tremor and night-terror or confusional episodes that complicate sleep of people with PD. In spite of sleep dysfunction being a key aspect of the nonmotor symptom complex (NMS) of PD, sleep disturbances related to PD have received specific and focused diagnostic and therapeutic attention in many previous studies (2–9). The evidence base for treatment of various aspects of sleep dysfunction and its assessment by validated tools, such as the PD Sleep Scale (PDSS), have emerged in the last 10 years (10,11). Studies have also highlighted that the burden of a range of sleep dysfunction that occurs in PD is a key determinant of quality of life of patients and caregivers (12,13). Awareness has also grown that sleep problems can also affect early untreated PD and "poor nights" for people with PD may occur not only in advanced PD but also in early untreated PD or even precede the motor symptoms with a significant adverse effect on daytime functioning and functional capacity (such as driving) as well as quality of life (12–16). Certain sleep disorders may provide useful diagnostic information in differentiating between parkinsonian syndromes, such as multiple system atrophy (MSA) and progressive supranuclear palsy (PSP), and may be important prognostic indicators of neuropsychiatric disturbances and dementia, whereas others may be precipitated by the treatment of PD (17).

EPIDEMIOLOGY

Sleep dysfunction in PD is multifactorial and studies have reported that as many as 98% of patients with PD may suffer at some time from nocturnal sleep disturbances (3). The overall prevalence figures, however, are variable because of differing methodology of ascertainment and range from 25% to 98%. A community-based study reported 60% of patients with PD (144 of 239) with sleep problems, compared with 33% of healthy controls (33 of 100) with the same age and sex distribution (5), whereas Karlsen et al. (6) reported that 64% of patients with PD had a sleep disorder, compared with 33% of controls (18). The Non-Motor Symptoms Questionnaire (NMSQuest) study in 2006 observed 123 PD patients and 96 age-matched controls in an international multicenter setting. By using the validated NMSQuest it was found that symptoms such as nocturia (67%) are common in controls, whereas other sleep-related complaints, such as insomnia (41%), intense/vivid dream (31%), acting out during dreams (33%), restless legs (37%), and daytime sleepiness (28%), are more prevalent in PD. This therefore may reflect a more fundamental dysfunction of sleep-related mechanisms (Fig. 7.1). In another observational study, Hely and colleagues (2005) evaluated PD patients followed for a period of 15–18 years after being recruited to a bromocriptine versus levodopa trial (19). One third of the original cohort were evaluated and most had significant NMS, including sleep disorders, which were reported to be more troublesome and disabling for the patients than the motor symptoms or levodopa-induced dyskinesia. A multicenter study including over 1000 patients found that sleep disturbances (64%) were the second most reported symptom after psychiatric symptoms (67%) in PD patients. Interestingly, the prevalence of sleep disorders in drug-naive subjects (Hoehn and Yahr scale 1) was around 40%, which increased to approximately 82% as the condition progressed to Hoehn and Yahr scale 4–5 (20). A study by Shulman et al. reported that despite these figures, such disorders are frequently overlooked, even in specialist centers (21).

Sleep disturbances of PD may be divided into five broad categories: insomnia, parasomnias, daytime sleepiness, motor symptom-related sleep disturbances, and sleep disordered breathing (Table 7.1).

Studies of sleep architecture in PD patients show some common features such as reduced total sleep time, sleep efficiency, multiple sleep arousals, and fragmentation of sleep (8,9,22,23). A circadian variation of symptoms has been identified and as such patients can be classified into a "morning better," "morning worse," and a nonaffected group (8).

Excessive daytime somnolence (EDS) is an important aspect of sleep-related morbidity of PD and may be caused by underlying dopaminergic denervation or may be due to poor nocturnal sleep. Rapid eye movement (REM) behavior disorder (RBD), an important parasomnia is now emerging as a strong predictive nonmotor symptom of PD development (23). In the following section we review some key aspects of the pathophysiology of sleep dysfunction in PD and related sleep disorders.

PATHOPHYSIOLOGY

The pathophysiology of most sleep disturbances in PD is complex and some remain unexplained. Degeneration of central sleep regulatory neurons either directly or due to an indirect effect of dopaminergic cell loss in the brainstem and related thalamocortical pathways, is implicated (23–25). Sleep dysfunctions such as RBD

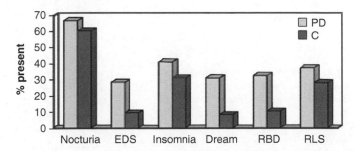

FIGURE 7.1 Sleep dysfunction in PD compared to age matched controls. NMSQuest study. *Abbreviations*: Dream, vivid dreaming; EDS, excessive daytime sleepiness; PD, Parkinson's disease; RBD, rapid eye movement behavior disorder; RLS, restless legs syndrome. *Source*: From Ref. 18.

and EDS have been suggested as possible preclinical markers of development of motor PD (26).

This clinical manifestation tends to correlate with the proposed pathologic staging of PD as proposed by Braak (27). It has been traditionally believed that the pathologic process of degeneration of dopaminergic neurons starts in the substantia nigra, while Braak proposes an alternative, as he has introduced the concept of a six-stage pathologic caudorostral process, beginning at clearly designated "induction sites" (27). In Braak stage 1 of PD, there is degeneration of the olfactory bulb and the anterior olfactory nucleus and this may clinically manifest as olfactory dysfunction. Furthermore, the intermediate reticular zone and IX/X cranial nerve nuclei are degenerated (27,28). This may not only cause sleep-related breathing problems (29) but also cause early signs of dysautonomia, which can lead to sleep dysfunction (30,31). In Braak stage 2 the pathologic process progresses rostrally to the lower brainstem and these are key areas mediating NMS, such as, sleep homeostasis and other autonomic features. The brainstem areas, particularly the raphe nucleus (serotonin), locus coeruleus (norepinephrine), and pedunculopontine nucleus (acetylcholine and glutamate) play a major role in the sleep–wake cycle and mediate the so-called flip–flop switch (Fig. 7.2) that mediates thalamocortical arousal and

TABLE 7.1   Categories of Parkinson's Disease-Related Sleep Disturbances

Insomnia
  Sleep onset
  Sleep maintenance
  Combined
Parasomnias
  REM
    REM sleep behavior disorder
    REM loss of atonia (neurophysiological)
  Non-REM
    RLS
    RLS-like syndrome
    Periodic limb movements
    Akathisia
    Confusional arousals
    Night-eating syndromes
Excessive daytime sleepiness
  Somnolence
  Sudden onset sleep
  Secondary narcolepsy without cataplexy
  Drug-induced sleep disturbance
Motor symptom-related sleep disturbances
  Nocturnal akinesia
  Tremor
  Rigor
  Early morning dystonia
Sleep disordered breathing
  Sleep apnea

Abbreviations: REM, rapid eye movement; RLS, restless leg syndrome.

sleep–wake cycle (32). The clinicopathologic correlates are becoming increasingly evident. There is strong evidence that symptoms such as olfactory dysfunction and sleep disturbances, such as RBD or excessive daytime sleepiness, may indeed precede the development of motor symptoms of PD, thus correlating with Braak stages 1 and 2 (3,28,33–35). Degeneration of the brainstem nuclei, previously mentioned, leads to dysregulation of basic REM and non-REM sleep architecture (24,25,36,37). Clinically the manifestations are insomnia, parasomnias, and EDS. The latter may be dependent on dysfunction of the flip–flop switch proposed by Saper and colleagues (Fig. 7.2) (32,38). Saper suggests that the brain can be either "off" promoting sleep by activating the ventrolateralpreoptic area (VLPO), (proposed to be a sleep-promoting centere) or "on" promoting wakefulness by activation of the tuberomamillary nucleus (TMN), which is the wake-promoting area along with locus coeruleus and the raphe nuclei (32). Regulators of the internal rhythm between the two switches are via the suprachiasmatic nucleus and also possibly mediated by, hypocretin 1 (orexin), a hypothalamic peptide (38,39). Low hypocretin-1 levels in the cerebrospinal fluid (CSF) has been shown to correlate with hypothalamic hypocretin cell loss in narcolepsy and other forms of hypersomnia (23). Hypocretin neurons project to the dopaminergic neurons in the substantia nigra, establishing a complex relationship between the systems (23). Hypocretin-1 could function as an external regulator of the flip–flop switch promoting wakefulness. Dopaminergic dysfunction caused by neuronal degeneration can destabilize this switch and its regulators, promoting rapid transitions to sleep intruding on wakefulness. Although hypocretin-1 insufficiency has not been confirmed by studies of CSF, in three patients with PD and EDS associated with dopamine agonist use, one study has reported low hypocretin-1 levels in ventricular fluid of advanced PD patients (40,41).

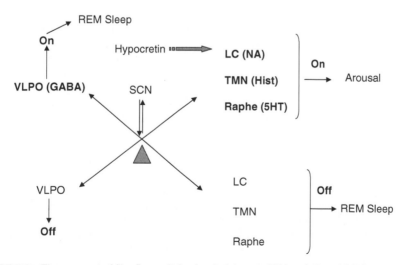

FIGURE 7.2   The concept of flip–flop switch of wakefulness. *Abbbreviations*: VLPO, ventrolateral-preoptic area; TMN, tuberomamillary nucleus; Raphe, raphe nucleus; LC, locus coeruleus; 5HT, serotonin; NA, norepinephrine; SCN, suprachiasmatic nucleus. *Source*: From Refs. 2,32.

Other nocturnal disabilities in PD arise from causes secondary to progression of disease causing "destructuring of sleep" and motor complications generated by dopaminergic treatment (42). Examples of the latter include nocturnal akinesia, early morning dystonia, and EDS. The cause of RLS in PD is unknown. Sleep disordered breathing is being increasingly recognized in PD and may reflect a combination of central and peripheral mechanisms (8,22).

SYMPTOMS
Nocturnal Akinesia
Nocturnal akinesia is perhaps the clinically most relevant symptom affecting PD patients. Nocturnal akinesia usually results from a relatively "drug free" period, as most regimes use the last dopaminergic treatment well before bedtime. Theoretically this would mean that a "wearing off" period would occur after the medication half-life expires. There is some support of this observation in the fact that some studies have reported a significant reduction in symptoms of nocturnal akinesia such as pain, spasm, and stiffness after nocturnal use of a long-acting dopamine agonist such as rotigotine, ropinirole prolonged release, or sustained infusion of apomorphine through the night (43–45). Nocturnal akinesia presents as a complex of symptoms, which range from difficulty in turning in bed to emergence of tremor (Tables 7.2 and 7.3).

Parasomnias
REM Sleep Behavior Disorder and Differential Diagnosis with Other Parasomnias
RBD was first reported by Schenck et al. in 1986 and is a parasomnia, which is typically characterized by vivid and usually frightening dreams or nightmares associated with a paradoxical simple or complex movement during REM sleep when usually muscles are atonic (17,33). RBD is thought to have a population prevalence of 0.5% and during REM sleep, patients enact their dreams, which can be vivid or unpleasant and partners report vocalizations (talking, shouting, vocal threats) and abnormal movements (arm/leg jerks, falling out of bed, violent assaults) (46–49). Typical clinical features are summarized in Table 7.4, and the criteria for diagnosis of RBD as suggested by the International Sleep Disorders Society are shown in Table 7.5 (50,51).

Although clinical history may suggest a diagnosis, in some situations, such as when there is a high risk of physical injury or loud snoring suggestive of obstructive sleep apnea is observed, confirmation of diagnosis should be obtained by a single night of polysomnography (PSG) with video telemetry. PSG would show increased electromyographic (EMG) activity during REM sleep.

Symptoms of RBD may predate the diagnosis of PD and Schenk et al. reported that in 11 of 29 men (38%) 50 years or older in whom idiopathic RBD was diagnosed, a parkinsonian disorder [i.e., MSA and dementia with Lewy bodies (DLB)] was identified after a mean interval of 3.7 ± 1.4 (SD) years following the diagnosis of RBD and 12.7 ± 7.3 years after the onset of RBD (46). There is increasing evidence that RBD tends to precede the onset of parkinsonism or dementia in patients with MSA, PD, and DLB by years or decades (47,52,53). This concept is consistent with Braak staging, which suggests that the preclinical stages 1 and 2 of PD start at the olfactory and medullary area of the brainstem, respectively (27). Although the pathologic basis of RBD is not fully understood, there is strong evidence from

TABLE 7.2 Causes of Night-Time Sleep Disruption and Daytime Sleepiness in Parkinson's Disease

Disease-related	
Insomnia	Fragmentation of sleep (sleep maintenance insomnia)
	Sleep-onset insomnia
Motor function–related	Akinesia (difficulty turning)
	Restless legs/akathisia
	Periodic limb movements of sleep
	Sensory problems (pain, paresthesia)
Urinary	Nocturia
	Nocturia with secondary postural hypotension
Neuropsychiatric/parasomnias	Depression related insomnia
	Vivid dreams and nightmares
	Nocturnal vocalizations and sleep talking
	Somnambulism
	Hallucinations
	Panic attacks
	REM behavior disorder
	Confusional awakenings
Treatment-related	
Motor	Nocturnal off-period–related tremor
	Dystonia
	Dyskinesia
	Off-period–related pain/paresthesia/muscle cramps
Urinary	Off-period–related incontinence of urine
Neuropsychiatric	Hallucinations
	Vivid dreaming
	? Off-period–related panic attacks
	? REM behavior disorder
	Akathisia
Sleep-altering medications	Alerting effect, nocturnal agitation

Abbreviations: REM, rapid eye movement; ?, possible clinical phenomenon.
Source: Adapted from Ref. 7.

TABLE 7.3 Symptoms and Signs of Nocturnal Akinesia and Night-Time Wearing Off

Difficulty in turning
Spasm/cramps in muscles
Pain
Early morning dystonia
Restless legs syndrome
Periodic limb movements
Nocturia
Tremor
Panic attacks

animal models (rat and cat) that highlight the important structures involved in the condition. Furthermore, there are a few neuroimaging and neuropathologic studies on human subjects with the condition that points toward the importance and the involvement of the same or similar structures. It has therefore been speculated that degeneration of and disturbances in brain stem nuclei, such as VLPO nucleus, LC, lateral pontine tegmentum, pedunculopontine nucleus, and sublaterodorsal (SLD) nucleus (as yet, identified in cat only), may be the key structures in the pathophysiology of RBD. These nuclei are intricately interconnected with regulatory interneurons either inhibiting or increasing the activities of one another. Projections from SLD has inhibitory effects on locomotor generators and spinal interneurons during REM sleep, thus disturbances in these nuclei may lead to lack of muscle atonia and enactment during REM sleep (53). Moreover, some valuable insights have been gained by studying different pharmacologic interventions that have been shown to be efficient in the symptomatic treatment of RBD. Clonazepam seems to be the most successful substance for the treatment of RBD symptoms (54). Melatonin also shows

TABLE 7.4 Clinical Features Characterizing REM Behavior Disorder

Predilection for male gender
Mean age of onset 50–65 yr (wide age range reported varying from 20–80 yr)
REM associated vocalizations, shouting, swearing, screaming, groaning (catathrenia)
Simple and complex motor movements:
  Muscle twitching
  Arm/leg jerking
  Kicking
  Fighting (boxing or trying to hit/strangulate partner)
  Falling out of bed
  Self and partner injury
Dreams associated with attacks by animals, humans, or insects
Behaviors are indicative of content of dreams
Occurs during the later half of sleep period (early morning)

Abbreviation: REM, rapid eye movement.
Source: Adapted from Ref. 17.

TABLE 7.5 The International Sleep Disorders Society Criteria for Diagnosis of RBD

A: The patient has a complaint of violent or injurious behavior during sleep
B: Limb or body movement is associated with dream mentation
C: At least one of the following occurs:
  1. Harmful or potentially harmful sleep behaviors
  2. Dreams appear to be acted out
  3. Sleep behaviors disrupt sleep continuity
D: Polysomnographic monitoring demonstrates at least one of the following electrophysiologic measures during rapid eye movement sleep:
  1. Excessive augmentation of chin EMG tone
  2. Excessive chin or chin or limb phasic EMG twitching, irrespective of chin EMG activity and one or more of the following:
    a. Excessive limb or body jerking
    b. Complex, vigorous, or violent behaviors
    c. Absence of epileptic activity in association with the disorder
E: The symptoms are not associated with mental disorders but may be associated with neurologic disorders
F: Other sleep disorders (e.g., sleep terrors or sleepwalking) can be present but are not the cause of the behavior

Abbreviation: EMG, electromyographic.
Source: Adapted from Refs. 50,51.

good efficacy either with or without clonazepam (55,56). The evidence for usage of other benzodiazepines is not convincing, suggesting more than a drug-class effect. Clonazepam, despite its inability to inhibit the pathologic muscle tone during REM sleep (measured by EMG) completely suppresses the symptoms of RBD (57,58). Melatonin on the other hand was able to partially restore the atonia during REM sleep in RBD patients (59). A double-blind, placebo-controlled, crossover study showed that exogenous melatonin significantly reduced REM sleep epochs without muscle atonia (60). A slow release preparation of melatonin is now available and may be an interesting candidate for future studies as conventional melatonin has a very short half-life.

A list of differential diagnoses of RBD is provided in Table 7.6. Somnambulism (sleepwalking) usually complicates early non-REM sleep and exhibits purposeful movements such as walking away from the bed, not necessarily associated with violent dreams or abrupt movements such as kicking, fighting, or jumping. Night terrors and confusional episodes occur early in sleep, unlike RBD, and may involve screaming or incoherent speech but there is no recall of the dream. Nocturnal panic attacks in PD may complicate nocturnal akinesia with dysautonomic symptoms such as palpitations, hyperhidrosis, and immediate full awareness without dream enactment. Seizure can be differentiated from RBD since it is associated with tonic–clonic posturing, tongue biting, incontinence of urine, and postictal confusion (61).

Excessive Daytime Somnolence and Sudden Onset of Sleep

EDS is a common complaint in PD patients and its prevalence has been reported to be up to 50% (62,63). Gjerstad and colleagues (2006) examined the occurrence of EDS in 232 patients of whom 138 and 89 were available for re-evaluation after four and eight years, respectively. Frequency rates of EDS increased from 5.6% in 1993 to 22.5% in 1997 and 40.8% in 2001. EDS was related to age, gender, and use of dopamine agonists. In those never having used dopamine agonists, hypersomnia was only associated with the severity of the disease according to Hoehn and Yahr staging (64). Another condition related to and co-occurring with EDS is SoS and it has been reported in up to 20% of patients (7,65–67).

EDS may manifest as patients feeling sleepy and slowly drifting off to sleep, whereas others may experience fatigue. SoS on the other hand is manifested as suddenly falling asleep without any preceding drowsiness resembling narcolepsy in some patients (23,68,69). The term sleep attacks, although discouraged, has been

TABLE 7.6 The Possible Differential Diagnosis of RBD

Parasomnias of non-REM sleep:
  Somnambulism
  Confusional arousal
  Night terrors
Nocturnal panic attacks
Nightmares
Nocturnal seizures
Severe periodic limb movements of sleep
Obstructive sleep apnea

Abbreviation: REM, rapid eye movement.

and is being used in the literature to describe the phenomenon. The causation of this sometimes disabling condition is complex and may represent a destabilization of the flip–flop switch of wakefulness due to dopaminergic denervation (32,38). In addition, the effect of poor nocturnal sleep and antiparkinsonian or other drugs may be causative (Table 7.7). As mentioned previously, the role of hypocretin/orexin neurons in the maintenance of the sleep-wake cycle and in the pathophysiology of narcolepsy has been established. However, to date, there is conflicting data describing hypocretin-1 levels in the CSF of patients with parkinsonism associated with sleep symptoms (67). Some had originally suggested the term "sleep attacks" linked to use of nonergot dopamine agonists such as pramipexole, ropinirole, and rotigotine (70). Altogether data suggest that both dopamine agonists and levodopa may increase the risk of SoS suggesting a class effect. Nevertheless, the risk seems to be significantly lower with levodopa compared with the dopamine agonists (70–73). Moreover, there seems to be some evidence of a dose-dependent relationship between EDS, SoS, and dopaminergic therapy (73). Like RBD, EDS can occur early in PD and may predate the diagnosis in some cases (34,74). However, based on a study in 15 untreated PD patients, Kaynak and colleagues (2005) reported that there is no PSG/multiple sleep latency test (MSLT) or Epworth Sleepiness Scale (ESS)-based evidence of EDS in untreated PD, but EDS occurs after treatment with dopaminergic agents (75). Although another study by Dhawan et al. suggested that EDS does occur in untreated PD (76). Arnulf and colleagues (2000) performed PSG and MSLT in PD patients with and without hallucinations (77). EDS was present in 50% of each group while sleep-onset REM periods and sleep latency below 10 minutes characteristic of narcolepsy were present mainly in the hallucinating group (77). This would suggest that a subset of PD patients may have an intrinsic susceptibility to SoS, which may be unmasked by use of some dopaminergic drugs. A study by Tan and colleagues (2002) reported that irresistible sleepiness not preceded by obvious somnolence or warning was present in 14% of a Chinese PD population compared with less than 2% in controls (78). Such subjects may, therefore, be susceptible to falling asleep while driving or operating machinery. EDS may need to be differentiated from fatigue and postprandial hypotension in PD that may unmask sleepiness and akinesia (79). Fatigue may be present in up to 43% of PD patients and is usually associated with sleepiness although tiredness is a key feature (80).

TABLE 7.7 Possible Causes of Excessive Daytime Sleepiness in Parkinson's Disease

Non–Drug Therapy-Related Reasons:
1. Advancing disease
2. Nocturnal sleep disruption
3. Parasomnias
4. Depression
Drug Therapy-Related Reasons:
1. Dopaminergic treatment in susceptible patients
2. Antihistamines
3. Hypnotics
4. Anxiolytics
5. Selective serotonin reuptake inhibitors

Source: Adapted from Ref. 7.

Driving, Excessive Daytime Sleepiness, and Sudden Onset of Sleep
The combination of motor dysfunction of PD, propensity to daytime sleepiness, and fatigue may pose a particular problem in relation to driving. A questionnaire survey of 6620 patients with 361 phone interviews by Meindorfner and colleagues (2005) suggested that 60% of this population was still driving and of those holding a driving license, 11% were implicated in the causation of at least one traffic accident in the preceding five years (66). The risk factors identified for accidents included high EDS, moderately severe motor disability of PD, and a previous history of SoS while driving. In the UK, once patients are diagnosed with PD, it is a legal requirement to inform the driving authorities.

Restless Legs Syndrome and Periodic Limb Movements
RLS and periodic limb movements (PLM) commonly occur together and can be effectively treated by dopaminergic drugs, raising speculation that there may be an underlying dopaminergic dysfunction and a link with PD. There are a few studies addressing the prevalence of RLS in PD. One observational study by Ondo et al. (2001) reported RLS to occur in PD at a rate twice the normal prevalence of RLS in the general population (68).

Other studies have suggested a prevalence rate of RLS of 21–24% in PD patients (81–83). RLS may occur across all stages of PD and even in untreated PD (84). Wetter and colleagues (2000) examined sleep and PLM patterns in drug-naive Parkinson's disease (DNPD) and MSA patients using two nights of PSG (84). They reported frequent problems with sleep disruption and increased PLM index in DNPD. These observations are in agreement with clinical findings in a study of untreated PD versus controls and advanced PD using a bedside sleep scale of PD (76). However, a confusing issue is that in some cases (more than 65% of PD patients in the study reported by Ondo et al.), RLS may emerge after the diagnosis of PD, when patients are already on dopaminergic therapy, which is thought to be first-line treatment for RLS (68). Furthermore, in PD, RLS may be confused with akathisia, which may be related to dopaminergic dyskinesia. For a formal diagnosis of PLM, overnight PSG will be useful. A syndrome mimicking RLS which may not satisfy the full clinical criteria for diagnosis of RLS, RLS-like syndrome (RLS-L) has been described from our group but needs to be confirmed in large scale observational studies.

Sleep Disordered Breathing
EDS may overlap with daytime somnolence due to sleep disordered breathing. Obstructive sleep apnea (OSA) causing sleep disordered breathing may be suggested by a history of loud crescendo snoring and irregular snoring with snorting and gasping and respiratory gaps particularly in an overweight subject. Partner corroborated history of observed apneic episodes and daytime fatigue and somnolence also suggest OSA. Formal PSG will identify sleep apnea and OSA that may occur in up to 50% of patients with PD with resultant daytime sleepiness and tiredness (22,85). Sleep apnea may co-exist with RLS, PLM, or RBD and it is important to diagnose, as treatment for RBD with clonazepam, for instance, may aggravate OSA.

Nocturia
Nocturia has been consistently shown to be one of the most common problems causing sleep disruption in PD. A survey by Stocchi et al. (2001) reported a rate of nocturia of 43% among 200 PD patients (86). An overall prevalence of 30–80% for nocturia in PD has been suggested (7,87). The validation study of the newly

developed PDSS and an independent study of the Spanish validation of the PDSS reported nocturia as the most prevalent nocturnal symptom of PD (10,88). The causation is still unclear; however, one widely accepted theory of pathogenesis suggests that the basal ganglia normally inhibits the micturition reflex via D1 receptors, and degeneration in that area results in a loss of this D1-mediated inhibition and consequently detrusor overactivity (89). Nocturia associated with nocturnal off periods may lead to incontinence of urine and bed soiling. Nocturia also appears to be a problem of advancing PD rather than early or untreated PD as indicated in a study using PDSS in untreated and advanced PD compared with controls (76).

Neuropsychiatric Comorbidites Complicating Sleep in PD

Depression is common in PD and affects sleep quality causing insomnia, usually sleep onset in type (7,8). Dementia will also lead to sleep dysfunction with evidence of RBD, insomnia, and nocturnal hallucinations. Hallucinations may complicate nocturnal sleep and some have suggested an overlap with RBD (48,77). An eight-year follow-up study of cases with RBD and PD suggested a high rate of development of visual hallucinations in those with RBD (90). Sinforiani and colleagues (2006) reported that RBD could be a risk factor for future development of hallucinations and cognitive failure based on neuropsychiatric evaluations in 110 patients (91). Additionally it has been shown that daytime sleepiness, dystonia, tremor and sleep fragmentation seem to be the important nocturnal disturbances in depressed patients with PD (92). Other neuropsychiatric disorders such as anxiety, psychotic symptoms, and dementia are prevalent and may of course have a reciprocal effect on sleep. The frequencies of these disorders have been shown to be 29% for dementia, 13% for psychotic syndromes, and 20% for anxiety. In this outpatient cohort the frequency for depression was 25% and 49% for sleep disturbances (93).

Drug Induced Sleep Disruption

Insomnia and night-time agitation may be caused by late dosing of selegiline probably as a result of its amphetamine metabolite (94). However, Lyons and colleagues (2010) were able to show that the addition of orally disintegrating selegiline with decreasing dosages of dopamine agonists substantially reduced EDS and hallucinations without compromising efficacy (95). Other drugs such as amantadine and anticholinergics may also produce an alerting effect. The post hoc subanalysis of the two studies, TEMPO and PRESTO, on the effect of rasagiline did not show any significant effects on sleep compared with placebo (96–98). Selective serotonin reuptake inhibitors (SSRIs) may need to be avoided at bedtime, as they may impair sleep onset (8). Dopamine agonists and levodopa have a variable and dose-dependent effect on sleep, either promoting or disrupting sleep. However, studies have suggested that sustained overnight dopaminergic stimulation improves sleep in PD by reducing nocturnal akinesia, RLS, and PLM (7,8).

Diagnostic Tools for Sleep Disorders in PD

Initial recognition of NMS in PD is crucial to treatment. Validated screening tools such as the NMSQuest can be used in the clinic setting to identify nonmotor symptoms a patient may not otherwise disclose. In an international, multicenter study it was found that the most frequently nondeclared nonmotor symptoms were delusions, daytime sleepiness, intense and vivid dreams, and dizziness (99).

The importance of assessment of sleep disorders in PD patients has been increasingly highlighted. In the revised version of Unified Parkinson's Disease Rating

Scale (UPDRS), an item addressing sleep disturbances has now been incorporated (100,101). In addition, various sleep scales have been reviewed by the Movement Disorder Society, to assess their suitability in PD (102). Among the existing scales only six fulfilled the criteria and were recommended for sleep disorders in PD patient populations: the Parkinson's Disease Sleep Scale (PDSS) (10), Pittsburgh Sleep Quality Index (PSQI) (103,104), the Scales for Outcomes in Parkinson's Disease (SCOPA) Sleep scale (105), the Epworth Sleepiness Scale (ESS) (106), the Inappropriate Sleep Composite Score (ISCS) (62), and the Stanford Sleepiness Scale (SSS) (107) (Table 7.8).

The PDSS (Fig. 7.3) was first validated and published in 2002 and has now been translated and used globally (10,88). The PDSS has also undergone formal linguistic validation in Italy, Spain, and Japan (88,108). It has robust test–test reliability and good discriminatory power between patients with PD and healthy controls. Patients and caregivers respond to individual questions based on their experiences in the past week, and scores for each item range from 0 (symptom severe and always experienced) to 10 (symptom free). The maximum cumulative score for the PDSS is 150 (patient is free of all symptoms). PDSS may not be suitable for screening daytime episodes of SoS, sleep apnea, RLS, or RBD. Based on this critique and the need for a treatment-measuring tool of sleep in PD, a revised version of the PDSS was created (109).

The current revised version (PDSS-2) (Fig. 7.4) is extended so that it encompasses several previously unmet needs in evaluating certain sleep disturbances in PD, such as those caused by nocturnal RLS, akinesia, pain, and sleep apnea. Daytime sleepiness and so-called sleep attacks were considered daytime problems with complex regulation in PD patients (110) and were completely removed from the

TABLE 7.8 The Items Listed in the SCOPA Sleep Scale

Night-time Sleep:
  Difficulty falling asleep
  Being awake too often
  Lying awake too long
  Waking too early
  Having too little sleep
Overall sleep quality (0–6)
Daytime sleepiness:
  Falling asleep unexpectedly
  Falling asleep while sitting
  Falling asleep watching TV
  Falling asleep while talking
  Difficulty staying awake
  Sleepiness problematic
Other Sleep Parameters:
  Using sleep medications, no. (%)
  Sleep initiation time, min
  Time awake per night, h
  Actual sleep per night, h
  Sleep in daytime, min
  Planned naps, no. (%)
  Unplanned naps, no. (%)
  Unexpected sleep, no. (%)

Source: Adapted from Ref. 105.

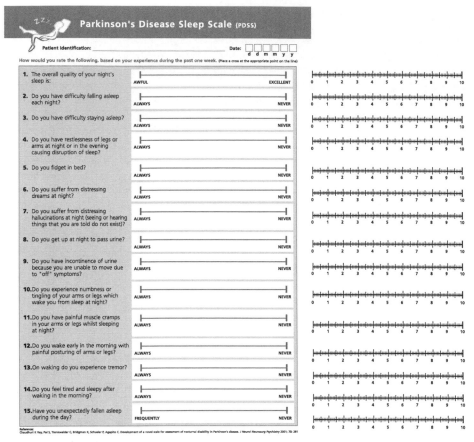

FIGURE 7.3 The Parkinson's Disease Sleep Scale. The scale on the right is on a transparency and needs to be applied on the printed scale after the scale has been scored by placing a cross mark on each 10 cm-line by patient/partner.

questionnaire. Nevertheless, a combination of subitems correlated well with EDS measured by the ESS (111).

In clinical practice, PDSS-1 would be useful for screening as well as epidemiologic studies while PDSS-2 is more suited to studies addressing treatment. Additionally sleep architecture studied by using PSG and MSLT provide measures of alertness. These studies are not routinely required for assessment of sleep in PD. However, in cases where OSA or severe PLM is suspected, PSG is essential. In cases of severe RBD or other parasomnias, PSG is useful for confirmation of diagnosis. A pathologic MSLT result (sleep latency < 10 min) in a PD patient may also suggest a propensity to SoS. However, SoS can occur despite normal alertness measured by MSLT (112).

Recently a single question item (RBD1Q) has been validated (sensitivity 93.8%, specificity 87.2%) for diagnosis of RBD (133).

Treatment

There is a poor evidence base for treatment of sleep problems in PD and the issue is complicated by the fact that treatment of sleep problems in PD needs to take into

Parkinson's Disease Sleep Scale (PDSS)

Please rate the severity of the following based on your experiences during the past week (7 days). Please make a cross in the answer box

	Very often (This means 6 to 7 days a week)	Often (This means 4 to 5 days a week)	Sometimes (This means 2 to 3 days a week)	Occasionally (This means 1 day a week)	Never
1) Overall, did you sleep well during the last week?	☐ 4	☐ 3	☐ 2	☐ 1	☐ 0
2) Did you have difficulty falling asleep each night?	☐ 4	☐ 3	☐ 2	☐ 1	☐ 0
3) Did you have difficulty staying asleep?	☐ 4	☐ 3	☐ 2	☐ 1	☐ 0
4) Did you have restlessness of legs or arms at nights causing disruption of sleep?	☐ 4	☐ 3	☐ 2	☐ 1	☐ 0
5) Was your sleep disturbed due to an urge to move your legs or arms?	☐ 4	☐ 3	☐ 2	☐ 1	☐ 0
6) Did you suffer from distressing dreams at night?	☐ 4	☐ 3	☐ 2	☐ 1	☐ 0
7) Did you suffer from distressing hallucinations at night (seeing or hearing things that you are told do not exist)?	☐ 4	☐ 3	☐ 2	☐ 1	☐ 0
8) Did you get up at night to pass urine?	☐ 4	☐ 3	☐ 2	☐ 1	☐ 0
9) Did you feel uncomfortable at night because you were unable to turn around in bed or move due to immobility?	☐ 4	☐ 3	☐ 2	☐ 1	☐ 0
10) Did you feel pain in your arms or legs which woke you up from sleep at night?	☐ 4	☐ 3	☐ 2	☐ 1	☐ 0
11) Did you have muscle cramps in your arms or legs which woke you up whilst sleeping at night?	☐ 4	☐ 3	☐ 2	☐ 1	☐ 0
12) Did you wake early in the morning with painful posturing of arms and legs?	☐ 4	☐ 3	☐ 2	☐ 1	☐ 0
13) On waking, did you experience tremor?	☐ 4	☐ 3	☐ 2	☐ 1	☐ 0
14) Did you feel tired and sleepy after waking in the morning?	☐ 4	☐ 3	☐ 2	☐ 1	☐ 0
15) Did you wake up at night due to snoring or difficulties with breathing?	☐ 4	☐ 3	☐ 2	☐ 1	☐ 0

FIGURE 7.4 PDSS-2: self-rating questionnaire. *Abbreviation*: PDSS, Parkinson's Disease Sleep Scale. (PDSS-2 is protected by international copyright, with all rights reserved to Claudia Trenkwalder and Ray Chaudhuri. Do not use without permission. For information on, or permission to use PDSS-2, please contact: contact@mapi-trust.org.)

account the multifactorial nature of sleep disturbance in PD. A review by the Movement Disorders Society reported that there were no robust trials of dopaminergic agents for treatment of nonmotor symptoms in PD, including sleep (113). Although sparse, there are some trials that have addressed different aspects of sleep disturbances in PD. These will be dealt within each section below and a summary of management strategies for sleep disturbances related to PD is outlined in Table 7.9.

The use of the PDSS (1 or 2) enables the clinician to adopt a systematic and pragmatic approach to treatment of night-time symptoms. An example would be that patients with low scores for questions 10–13 (<6) in the PDSS-1, indicating nocturnal motor disabilities due to wearing off, might benefit from extending the action of levodopa by combining levodopa with entacapone, or using a long-acting dopamine agonist. Low scores in response to questions 6 and 7, indicating hallucinations, might warrant withdrawal of night-time dopamine agonists or treatment with clonazepam if RBD is suspected.

TABLE 7.9 Management Strategies for Symptoms Contributing to Nocturnal Disturbance in Parkinson's Disease

---

Insomnia-related symptoms
  Fragmented sleep with difficulty in sleep onset and sleep maintenance
    Nonpharmacologic measures
      Avoidance of night-time alcohol, caffeine, tobacco
      Increase in daytime physical activity and ensuring exposure to daylight
      Psychologic therapies: relaxation training, cognitive therapies, biofeedback training
    Pharmacologic strategies
      Short-acting benzodiazepines
      Nonbenzodiazepine hypnotics: zopiclone
      Tricyclic antidepressants: amitriptyline (may help nocturia but may aggravate RLS and tremor) (May interact with MAO inhibitors)

Motor symptoms
  Fidgeting, painful cramps, and posturing, tremor, akinesia, RLS-type symptoms
    Nonpharmacologic measures
      Use of satin bed sheets and bed straps to help moving in bed
      Bed rails
    Pharmacologic strategies (based on case series and open-label trials)
      Sustained dopaminergic stimulation (night-time dosing of):
        CR levodopa ± COMT inhibitor, carbidopa/levodopa/entacapone
        Long-acting dopamine agonists, e.g., transdermal rotigotine and ropinirole prolonged release (44)
        Nocturnal apomorphine infusion (severe RLS/PLM/dystonia/cramps)
      Practical measures to aid bioavailability of dopaminergic medications
        Avoidance of high-protein meals at night
        Domperidone if delayed gastric emptying

REM behavior disorder:
  Clonazepam (usually first choice)
  Melatonin (alone or in combination with clonazepam)
  Other options (weak evidence): pramipexole, carbamazepine, donepezil, levodopa
  Circadin (Long acting version of melatonin)

Urinary symptoms
  Nocturia (Incontinence of urine because of inability to move during "off" phase)
    Non-pharmacologic measures
      Reduction of evening fluid intake
      Emptying bladder before bed
      Use of condom catheters/bedside commode
      If associated with postural hypotension, head-up tilt of bed
    Pharmacologic strategies
      Low-dose amitriptyline
      Possible role for transdermal rotigotine patch (2)
      If associated with detrusor instability: oxybutinin, tolterodine (Beware of anticholinergic side effect)
      If associated with morning hypotension: desmopressin nasal spray; avoidance of evening diuretics, antihypertensives, vasodilators

---

Abbreviations: CR, controlled-release; COMT, catechol O-methyl-transferase; MSA, multiple system atrophy; LBD, Lewy body dementia; PSP, progressive supranuclear gaze palsy; RLS, restless legs syndrome; PLM, Periodic Limb Movement. *Source*: Adapted from Refs. 7,8.

Sleep Hygiene
Sleep benefit is a common phenomenon of variable duration ranging from 30 minutes to 3 hours seen in PD and implies improvement in mobility and motor state the morning after drug intake at night (8). The mechanism of sleep benefit is unknown and possible causes may include (*i*) recovery of dopaminergic function and storage during sleep, (*ii*) a circadian rhythm–related phenomenon, or (*iii*) a pharmacologic hypothesis that may involve drug-induced motor-fluctuations and/or mechanisms relating to the variability of the transport of levodopa through the blood–brain barrier (8,40). Good sleep hygiene is useful as well. Activities such as a hot bath about 2 hours before bedtime, maximizing daytime activity, ensuring bright light exposure, having a hot sweet drink or a light snack at bedtime, use of handrails in bed and/or stain sheets to enable easier turning in bed, flexible bed times, and reclining armchair for some, and avoiding stimulants such as tea or coffee at bedtime are part of good sleep hygiene (114).

Nocturia
Nocturia remains one of the most common causes of sleep disruption in PD and needs to be tackled by avoiding diuretics or tea/coffee at bedtime and use of nasal spray of desmopressin in some patients (87). Some have suggested the use of combined D2/D1 receptor dopamine agonists such as pergolide, but this has not been established in clinical trials (115). In cases with risk of urinary incontinence, condom catheters or a bedside urinal is essential to ensure a good quality sleep with minimal interruption.

Nocturnal Akinesia
Nocturnal akinesia is usually caused by night-time wearing off and strategies promoting overnight dopaminergic stimulation may be helpful. Sustained-release levodopa/benserazide significantly ($P < 0.016$) improved night-time akinesia (ability to turn in bed) and total time awake (significantly decreased from 2.13 to 0.67 hours, $P = 0.046$) in a 12-month open-label, noncomparative trial, including 15 patients with PD and distressing nocturnal symptoms (116). In a recently published study on ropinirole prolonged release given once-daily, the PDSS ≤ 100 subgroup (i.e., troublesome nocturnal symptoms) demonstrated treatment benefits for PDSS groupings of motor symptoms on waking and global quality of sleep (44). Furthermore, another study using PDSS-2 showed beneficial effects for patients with early-morning motor dysfunction and better control of both motor function and nocturnal sleep disturbances with 24-hour transdermal delivery of rotigotine sustained at 12 months open label follow up (RECOVER study) (45). Overnight apomorphine infusion also has been reported to be beneficial for nocturnal motor and nonmotor symptoms of advanced PD patients (43).

Excessive Daytime Sleepiness
In PD, severe EDS needs treatment and firstly concurrent medications that may be sedating should be eliminated or reduced (Table 7.7). Modafinil (100–400 mg/day), a nonaddictive sleep–wake cycle activator is nonstimulating and the only drug that has shown efficacy in improving EDS in double-blind, placebo-controlled trials (117,118). A seven-week double-blind, placebo crossover study of 200 mg of modafinil followed by a four-week open-label extension (200 and 400 mg) study by Adler et al. (2003) showed significant improvement in EDS with modafinil and improvement in clinical global impression scores for wakefulness in the open-label

arm (118). Those with high ESS scores and a history of SoS should be advised not to drive alone or for long distances. Dopamine agonists when started should be titrated up slowly, especially in older patients. There is some evidence that an inverse histamine H_3 agonist, sodium oxybate, adenosine A2A receptor antagonists, and caffeine may contribute to the treatment of EDS (119–121). Caffeine in doses of 100–200 mg BID is being particularly investigated.

Neuropsychiatric Problems
Depression affects approximately 40% of patients with PD and may contribute to sleep disturbances necessitating active treatment with sedating antidepressants (e.g., trazodone or low-dose mirtazapine) or SSRIs. Panic attacks can occur in both "on" and "off" periods, and "off" related panic can be overcome by sustained dopaminergic stimulation. Successful treatment of the depression often leads to improvement of sleep quality in PD. However, there is lack of evidence for the most commonly used group of agents, that is, the SSRIs mainly due to flaws in study design (122). Nevertheless, there is sparse evidence for the use of tricyclic agents, such as desipramine (123) and nortriptyline (124). In 2010, Barone and colleagues conducted a placebo-controlled, randomized trial. They used the dopamine agonist pramipexole and reported small but significant improvements that could not be fully explained by associated improvement in motor symptoms (125).

The management of other neuropsychiatric problems such as anxiety and psychotic syndromes should predominantly be based on the severity of the problem and the effect on the patient and/or the caregiver. For instance, not all perceptual disorders need pharmacologic intervention. However, some nonpharmacologic and pharmacologic treatment strategies are outlined in Table 7.9. Furthermore, it is of great importance that the effect of the intervention is regularly evaluated in order to achieve the delicate balance of effect versus side effects.

REM Behavior Disorder
The effectiveness of clonazepam and melatonin has already been mentioned. Even though clonazepam remains the most efficient drug for RBD, there is still no controlled trial confirming its effect (17) and it should be used with caution in patients with dementia, gait disorders, or concomitant OSA. Its use should be monitored carefully over time as RBD appears to be a precursor to neurodegenerative disorders with dementia in some patients (54). Other suggested therapies include other benzodiazepines (temazepam and alprazolam) and benzodiazepine-like drugs, such as zopiclone, even though the evidence base is rather poor (54,126).

Although polypharmacy is generally discouraged, some patients could benefit from the combination of melatonin or zopiclone with a "lower" dose of clonazepam. For further reading on other drugs in the therapeutic arsenal, see Ref. 54. Night-time dosing with drugs such as selegiline may aggravate RBD (127). Others have reported a paradoxic worsening of RBD during deep brain stimulation (DBS) of the subthalamic nucleus (STN) (128).

The dopamine agonists have shown good efficacy in the treatment of RLS in several studies (129). A study with the transdermal rotigotine patch given to PD patients showed significant improvement in PDSS-2 items addressing RLS (45), whereas surprisingly, ropinirole prolonged release given to patients with advanced PD did not significantly improve RLS (44). In severe cases, hospital admission with overnight apomorphine infusion may be required (43).

Deep Brain Stimulation
DBS has been used for treatment of medication-resistant motor complications for over 20 years. Data from these interventions, through mainly case series and reports have given us the opportunity for better understanding the effect of neuromodulation upon sleep disturbances in PD patients (130). Arnulf et al. (2000) monitored the effects of bilateral DBS in 10 PD patients with sleep problems. They found that stimulation decreased nocturnal and early morning dystonia and increased sleep efficiency. However, there was no effect on PLM or RBD. The positive findings have been reproduced in several other studies, showing improvement in not only the motor signs of PD but also in sleep architecture (128,131,132). In addition, there are some reports that have detected improvement in sleep architecture and daytime sleepiness with DBS in the pedunculopontine nucleus. The value of stimulation of this nucleus for sleep disturbances needs to be further investigated (132).

The Future
The natural history and much of the pathophysiology of sleep disorders of PD remain unknown and treatment of several aspects of sleep disorders in PD lacks a robust evidence base. These areas will need investigation and research in the future. Another key area of interest is likely to focus on unraveling the role of hypocretin in the causation of sleep–wake cycle-related dysfunctions in PD. Pathophysiologic and observational studies will also help devise better treatment strategies for nocturnal parasomnias, such as RBD, RLS, and sleep disordered breathing.

CONCLUSION
Sleep disorders in patients with PD are common, are a key component of the non-motor symptom complex of PD, and remain underdiagnosed and undertreated. Sleep problems may arise from uncontrolled motor symptoms, degeneration of the neuroanatomic substrates responsible for the sleep–wake cycle, or unwanted medication side effects. Routine assessment of patients with PD should include inquiry regarding the quality of sleep and sleep-related symptoms. Use of validated clinical tools, such as the PDSS, SCOPA-sleep, and ESS, offers a robust way to assess the presence or absence of sleep disruption and also to guide treatment. Uncontrolled nocturnal motor symptoms may be ameliorated by long-acting dopaminergic agents, while other sleep disruptions, such as hallucinations or RBD, require a different approach. In resistant cases patients may need to undergo polysomnography and/or multiple sleep latency tests. Targeted night-time treatment should result in improved sleep for patients with PD.

REFERENCES
1. Parkinson J. An essay on the shaking palsy 1817. J Neuropsychiatry Clin Neurosci 2002; 14: 223–36; discussion 222.
2. Chaudhuri KR, Schapira AH. Non-motor symptoms of Parkinson's disease: dopaminergic pathophysiology and treatment. Lancet Neurol 2009; 8: 464–74.
3. Chaudhuri KR, Healy DG, Schapira AH. Non-motor symptoms of Parkinson's disease: diagnosis and management. Lancet Neurol 2006; 5: 235–45.
4. Lees AJ, Blackburn NA, Campbell VL. The nighttime problems of Parkinson's disease. Clin Neuropharmacol 1988; 11: 512–19.
5. Tandberg E, Larsen JP, Karlsen K. Excessive daytime sleepiness and sleep benefit in Parkinson's disease: a community-based study. Mov Disord 1999; 14: 922–7.

6. Karlsen K, Larsen JP, Tandberg E, et al. Fatigue in patients with Parkinson's disease. Mov Disord 1999; 14: 237–41.
7. Chaudhuri KR. Nocturnal symptom complex in PD and its management. Neurology 2003; 61:S17–23.
8. Garcia-Borreguero D, Larrosa O, Bravo M. Parkinson's disease and sleep. Sleep Med Rev 2003; 7: 115–29.
9. Adler CH, Thorpy MJ. Sleep issues in Parkinson's disease. Neurology 2005; 64: S12–20.
10. Chaudhuri KR, Pal S, DiMarco A, et al. The Parkinson's disease sleep scale: a new instrument for assessing sleep and nocturnal disability in Parkinson's disease. J Neurol Neurosurg Psychiatry 2002; 73: 629–35.
11. Zesiewicz TA, Sullivan KL, Arnulf I, et al. Practice parameter: treatment of nonmotor symptoms of Parkinson disease: report of the Quality Standards Subcommittee of the American Academy of Neurology. Neurology 2010; 74: 924–31.
12. Karlsen KH, Larsen JP, Tandberg E, et al. Influence of clinical and demographic variables on quality of life in patients with Parkinson's disease. J Neurol Neurosurg Psychiatry 1999; 66: 431–5.
13. Aarsland D, Larsen JP, Tandberg E, et al. Predictors of nursing home placement in Parkinson's disease: a population-based, prospective study. J Am Geriatr Soc 2000; 48: 938–42.
14. Findley L, Aujla M, Bain PG, et al. Direct economic impact of Parkinson's disease: a research survey in the United Kingdom. Mov Disord 2003; 18: 1139–45.
15. Bosanquet N, May J, Johnson N. Alzheimer's disease in the United Kingdom. Burden of disease and future care. Health Policy Review Paper. London: Health Policy Unit, Imperial College School of Medicine, 1998.
16. Hilker R, Razai N, Ghaemi M, et al. [18F]fluorodopa uptake in the upper brainstem measured with positron emission tomography correlates with decreased REM sleep duration in early Parkinson's disease. Clin Neurol Neurosurg 2003; 105: 262–9.
17. Boeve BF, Silber MH, Ferman TJ, et al. Association of REM sleep behavior disorder and neurodegenerative disease may reflect an underlying synucleinopathy. Mov Disord 2001; 16: 622–30.
18. Chaudhuri KR, Martinez-Martin P, Schapira AH, et al. International multicenter pilot study of the first comprehensive self-completed nonmotor symptoms questionnaire for Parkinson's disease: the NMSQuest study. Mov Disord 2006; 21: 916–23.
19. Hely MA, Morris JG, Reid WG, et al. Sydney Multicenter Study of Parkinson's disease: non-L-dopa-responsive problems dominate at 15 years. Mov Disord 2005; 20: 190–9.
20. Barone P, Antonini A, Colosimo C, et al. The PRIAMO study: A multicenter assessment of nonmotor symptoms and their impact on quality of life in Parkinson's disease. Mov Disord 2009; 24: 1641–9.
21. Shulman LM, Taback RL, Rabinstein AA, et al. Non-recognition of depression and other non-motor symptoms in Parkinson's disease. Parkinsonism Relat Disord 2002; 8: 193–7.
22. Arnulf I, Konofal E, Merino-Andreu M, et al. Parkinson's disease and sleepiness: an integral part of PD. Neurology 2002; 58: 1019–24.
23. Rye DB, Jankovic J. Emerging views of dopamine in modulating sleep/wake state from an unlikely source: PD. Neurology 2002; 58: 341–6.
24. Shouse MN, Siegel JM. Pontine regulation of REM sleep components in cats: integrity of the pedunculopontine tegmentum (PPT) is important for phasic events but unnecessary for atonia during REM sleep. Brain Res 1992; 571: 50–63.
25. Lai YY, Siegel JM. Physiological and anatomical link between Parkinson-like disease and REM sleep behavior disorder. Mol Neurobiol 2003; 27: 137–52.
26. Lang AE. A critical appraisal of the premotor symptoms of Parkinson's disease: potential usefulness in early diagnosis and design of neuroprotective trials. Mov Disord 26: 775–83.
27. Braak H, Del Tredici K, Rub U, et al. Staging of brain pathology related to sporadic Parkinson's disease. Neurobiol Aging 2003; 24: 197–211.
28. Kingsbury AE, Bandopadhyay R, Silveira-Moriyama L, et al. Brain stem pathology in Parkinson's disease: an evaluation of the Braak staging model. Mov Disord 2010; 25: 2508–15.

29. Celle S, Peyron R, Faillenot I, et al. Undiagnosed sleep-related breathing disorders are associated with focal brainstem atrophy in the elderly. Hum Brain Mapp 2009; 30: 2090–7.
30. Braak H, Braak E. Pathoanatomy of Parkinson's disease. J Neurol 2000; 247: II3–10.
31. Zaccai J, Brayne C, McKeith I, et al. Patterns and stages of alpha-synucleinopathy: relevance in a population-based cohort. Neurology 2008; 70: 1042–8.
32. Saper CB, Chou TC, Scammell TE. The sleep switch: hypothalamic control of sleep and wakefulness. Trends Neurosci 2001; 24: 726–31.
33. Schenck CH, Mahowald MW. REM sleep behavior disorder: clinical, developmental, and neuroscience perspectives 16 years after its formal identification in SLEEP. Sleep 2002; 25: 120–38.
34. Abbott RD, Ross GW, White LR, et al. Excessive daytime sleepiness and subsequent development of Parkinson disease. Neurology 2005; 65: 1442–6.
35. Ross GW, Petrovitch H, Abbott RD, et al. Association of olfactory dysfunction with risk for future Parkinson's disease. Ann Neurol 2008; 63: 167–73.
36. Parent A, Hazrati LN. Functional anatomy of the basal ganglia. I. The cortico-basal ganglia-thalamo-cortical loop. Brain Res Brain Res Rev 1995; 20: 91–127.
37. Karachi C, Yelnik J, Tande D, et al. The pallidosubthalamic projection: an anatomical substrate for nonmotor functions of the subthalamic nucleus in primates. Mov Disord 2005; 20: 172–80.
38. MacMahon D. Why excessive daytime sleepiness is an important issue in Parkinson's disease. Adv Clin Neurol Rehabil 2005; 5: 46–9.
39. Nishino S, Ripley B, Overeem S, et al. Hypocretin (orexin) deficiency in human narcolepsy. Lancet 2000; 355: 39–40.
40. Ripley B, Overeem S, Fujiki N, et al. CSF hypocretin/orexin levels in narcolepsy and other neurological conditions. Neurology 2001; 57: 2253–8.
41. Drouot X, Moutereau S, Nguyen JP, et al. Low levels of ventricular CSF orexin/hypocretin in advanced PD. Neurology 2003; 61: 540–3.
42. Diederich NJ, Vaillant M, Mancuso G, et al. Progressive sleep 'destructuring' in Parkinson's disease. A polysomnographic study in 46 patients. Sleep Med 2005; 6: 313–18.
43. Reuter I, Ellis CM, Ray Chaudhuri K. Nocturnal subcutaneous apomorphine infusion in Parkinson's disease and restless legs syndrome. Acta Neurol Scand 1999; 100: 163–7.
44. Chaudhuri K, Martinez-Martin P, Rolfe KA, et al. Improvements in nocturnal symptoms with ropinirole prolonged release in patients with advanced Parkinson's disease. Eur J Neurol 2012; 19: 105–13.
45. Trenkwalder C, Kies B, Rudzinska M, et al. Rotigotine effects on early morning motor function and sleep in Parkinson's disease: a double-blind, randomized, placebo-controlled study (RECOVER). Mov Disord 2011; 26: 90–9.
46. Schenck CH, Bundlie SR, Mahowald MW. Delayed emergence of a parkinsonian disorder in 38% of 29 older men initially diagnosed with idiopathic rapid eye movement sleep behaviour disorder. Neurology 1996; 46: 388–93.
47. Olson EJ, Boeve BF, Silber MH. Rapid eye movement sleep behaviour disorder: demographic, clinical and laboratory findings in 93 cases. Brain 2000; 123: 331–9.
48. Fantini ML, Ferini-Strambi L, Montplaisir J. Idiopathic REM sleep behavior disorder: toward a better nosologic definition. Neurology 2005; 64: 780–6.
49. Comella CL, Nardine TM, Diederich NJ, et al. Sleep-related violence, injury, and REM sleep behavior disorder in Parkinson's disease. Neurology 1998; 51: 526–9.
50. International Classification of Sleep Disorders, revised. Diagnostic and coding manual. Rochester, Minnesota: American Sleep Disorders Association, 1997: 177–80.
51. Mahowald MW, Schenck CH. REM sleep behaviour disorder. In: Kryger M, Dement W, eds. Principles and Practice of Sleep Medicine, R.T. Philadelphia: W B Saunders, 2000: 724–41.
52. Stiasny-Kolster K, Doerr Y, Möller JC, et al. Combination of 'idiopathic' REM sleep behaviour disorder and olfactory dysfunction as possible indicator for alpha-synucleinopathy demonstrated by dopamine transporter FP-CIT-SPECT. Brain 2005; 128: 126–37.
53. Boeve BF, Silber MH, Saper CB, et al. Pathophysiology of REM sleep behaviour disorder and relevance to neurodegenerative disease. Brain 2007; 130: 2770–88.

54. Aurora RN, Zak RS, Maganti RK, et al. Best practice guide for the treatment of REM sleep behavior disorder (RBD). J Clin Sleep Med 2010; 6: 85–95.
55. Boeve BF, Silber MH, Ferman TJ. Melatonin for treatment of REM sleep behavior disorder in neurologic disorders: results in 14 patients. Sleep Med 2003; 4: 281–4.
56. Kunz D, Bes F. Melatonin as a therapy in REM sleep behavior disorder patients: an open-labeled pilot study on the possible influence of melatonin on REM-sleep regulation. Mov Disord 1999; 14: 507–11.
57. Lapierre O, Montplaisir J. Polysomnographic features of REM sleep behavior disorder: development of a scoring method. Neurology 1992; 42: 1371–4.
58. Schenck CMM. Polysomnographic, neurologic, psychiatric, and clinical utcome report on 70 consecutive cases with REM sleep behavior disorder (RBD): Sustained clonazepam efficacy in 89.5% of 57 treated patients. Cleveland Clin J Med 1990; 57: S9–S23.
59. Takeuchi N, Uchimura N, Hashizume Y, et al. Melatonin therapy for REM sleep behavior disorder. Psychiatry Clin Neurosci 2001; 55: 267–9.
60. Kunz D, Mahlberg R. A two-part, double-blind, placebo-controlled trial of exogenous melatonin in REM sleep behaviour disorder. J Sleep Res 2010; 19: 591–6.
61. Mahowald MW, Schenck CH. Insights from studying human sleep disorders. Nature 2005; 437: 1279–85.
62. Hobson DE, Lang AE, Martin WR, et al. Excessive daytime sleepiness and sudden-onset sleep in Parkinson disease: a survey by the Canadian Movement Disorders Group. JAMA 2002; 287: 455–63.
63. Factor SA, McAlarney T, Sanchez-Ramos JR, et al. Sleep disorders and sleep effect in Parkinson's disease. Mov Disord 1990; 5: 280–5.
64. Gjerstad MD, Alves G, Wentzel-Larsen T, et al. Excessive daytime sleepiness in Parkinson disease: is it the drugs or the disease? Neurology 2006; 67: 853–8.
65. Korner Y, Meindorfner C, Moller JC, et al. Predictors of sudden onset of sleep in Parkinson's disease. Mov Disord 2004; 19: 1298–305.
66. Meindorfner C, Korner Y, Moller JC, et al. Driving in Parkinson's disease: mobility, accidents, and sudden onset of sleep at the wheel. Mov Disord 2005; 20: 832–42.
67. Haq IZ, Naidu Y, Reddy P, et al. Narcolepsy in Parkinson's disease. Expert Rev Neurother 2010; 10: 879–84.
68. Ondo WG, Dat Vuong K, Khan H, et al. Daytime sleepiness and other sleep disorders in Parkinson's disease. Neurology 2001; 57: 1392–6.
69. Olanow CW, Schapira AH, Roth T. Waking up to sleep episodes in Parkinson's disease. Mov Disord 2000; 15: 212–15.
70. Frucht S, Rogers JD, Greene PE, et al. Falling asleep at the wheel: motor vehicle mishaps in persons taking pramipexole and ropinirole. Neurology 1999; 52: 1908–10.
71. Andreu N, Chale JJ, Senard JM, et al. L-Dopa-induced sedation: a double-blind cross-over controlled study versus triazolam and placebo in healthy volunteers. Clin Neuropharmacol 1999; 22: 15–23.
72. Ferreira JJ, Galitzky M, Montastruc JL, et al. Sleep attacks and Parkinson's disease treatment. Lancet 2000; 355: 1333–4.
73. Paus S, Brecht HM, Koster J, et al. Sleep attacks, daytime sleepiness, and dopamine agonists in Parkinson's disease. Mov Disord 2003; 18: 659–67.
74. Fabbrini G, Barbanti P, Aurilia C, et al. Excessive daytime sleepiness in de novo and treated Parkinson's disease. Mov Disord 2002; 17: 1026–30.
75. Kaynak D, Kiziltan G, Kaynak H, et al. Sleep and sleepiness in patients with Parkinson's disease before and after dopaminergic treatment. Eur J Neurol 2005; 12: 199–207.
76. Dhawan V, Dhoat S, Williams AJ, et al. The range and nature of sleep dysfunction in untreated Parkinson's disease (PD). A comparative controlled clinical study using the Parkinson's disease sleep scale and selective polysomnography. J Neurol Sci 2006; 248: 158–62.
77. Arnulf I, Bonnet AM, Damier P, et al. Hallucinations, REM sleep, and Parkinson's disease: a medical hypothesis. Neurology 2000; 55: 281–8.
78. Tan EK, Lum SY, Fook-Chong SM, et al. Evaluation of somnolence in Parkinson's disease: comparison with age- and sex-matched controls. Neurology 2002; 58: 465–8.

79. Chaudhuri KR, Ellis C, Love-Jones S, et al. Postprandial hypotension and parkinsonian state in Parkinson's disease. Mov Disord 1997; 12: 877–84.
80. van Hilten JJ, Weggeman M, van der Velde EA, et al. Sleep, excessive daytime sleepiness and fatigue in Parkinson's disease. J Neural Transm Park Dis Dement Sect 1993; 5: 235–44.
81. Peralta CM, Frauscher B, Seppi K, et al. Restless legs syndrome in Parkinson's disease. Mov Disord 2009; 24: 2076–80.
82. Ondo WG, Vuong KD, Jankovic J. Exploring the relationship between Parkinson disease and restless legs syndrome. Arch Neurol 2002; 59: 421–4.
83. Gomez-Esteban JC, Zarranz JJ, Tijero B, et al. Restless legs syndrome in Parkinson's disease. Mov Disord 2007; 22: 1912–16.
84. Wetter TC, Collado-Seidel V, Pollmacher T, et al. Sleep and periodic leg movement patterns in drug-free patients with Parkinson's disease and multiple system atrophy. Sleep 2000; 23: 361–7.
85. Diederich NJ, Vaillant M, Leischen M, et al. Sleep apnea syndrome in Parkinson's disease. A case-control study in 49 patients. Mov Disord 2005; 20: 1413–18.
86. Stocchi F, Vacca L, Valente M, et al. Sleep disorders in Parkinson's disease. Adv Neurol 2001; 86: 289–93.
87. Grandas F, Iranzo A. Nocturnal problems occurring in Parkinson's disease. Neurology 2004; 63: S8–11.
88. Martinez-Martin P, Salvador C, Menendez-Guisasola L, et al. Parkinson's Disease Sleep Scale: validation study of a Spanish version. Mov Disord 2004; 19: 1226–32.
89. Blackett H, Walker R, Wood B. Urinary dysfunction in Parkinson's disease: a review. Parkinsonism Relat Disord 2009; 15: 81–7.
90. Onofrj M, Thomas A, D'Andreamatteo G, et al. Incidence of RBD and hallucination in patients affected by Parkinson's disease: 8-year follow-up. Neurol Sci 2002; 23: S91–4.
91. Sinforiani E, Zangaglia R, Manni R, et al. REM sleep behavior disorder, hallucinations, and cognitive impairment in Parkinson's disease. Mov Disord 2006; 21: 462–6.
92. Suzuki K, Miyamoto M, Miyamoto T, et al. Correlation between depressive symptoms and nocturnal disturbances in Japanese patients with Parkinson's disease. Parkinsonism Relat Disord 2009; 15: 15–19.
93. Riedel O, Klotsche J, Spottke A, et al. Frequency of dementia, depression, and other neuropsychiatric symptoms in 1,449 outpatients with Parkinson's disease. J Neurol 257: 1073–82.
94. Heinonen EH, Myllyla V. Safety of selegiline (deprenyl) in the treatment of Parkinson's disease. Drug Saf 1998; 19: 11–22.
95. Lyons KE, Friedman JH, Hermanowicz N, et al. Orally disintegrating selegiline in Parkinson patients with dopamine agonist-related adverse effects. Clin Neuropharmacol 2010; 33: 5–10.
96. Elmer L, Schwid S, Eberly S, et al. Rasagiline-associated motor improvement in PD occurs without worsening of cognitive and behavioral symptoms. J Neurol Sci 2006; 248: 78–83.
97. Parkinson Study Group. A controlled trial of rasagiline in early Parkinson disease: the TEMPO Study. Arch Neurol 2002; 59: 1937–43.
98. Chen JJ, Swope DM, Dashtipour K. Comprehensive review of rasagiline, a second-generation monoamine oxidase inhibitor, for the treatment of Parkinson's disease. Clin Ther 2007; 29: 1825–49.
99. Chaudhuri KR, Prieto-Jurcynska C, Naidu Y. The nondeclaration of nonmotor symptoms of Parkinson's disease to health care professionals: an international study using the nonmotor symptoms questionnaire. Mov Disord 2010; 25: 704–9.
100. Goetz CG, Tilley BC, Shaftman SR, et al. Movement Disorder Society-sponsored revision of the Unified Parkinson's Disease Rating Scale (MDS-UPDRS): scale presentation and clinimetric testing results. Mov Disord 2008; 23: 2129–70.
101. Goetz CG, Fahn S, Martinez-Martin P, et al. Movement Disorder Society-sponsored revision of the Unified Parkinson's Disease Rating Scale (MDS-UPDRS): process, format, and clinimetric testing plan. Mov Disord 2007; 22: 41–7.

102. Hogl B, Arnulf I, Comella C, et al. Scales to assess sleep impairment in Parkinson's disease: critique and recommendations. Mov Disord 2010; 25: 2704–16.
103. Buysse DJ, Reynolds CF, Monk TH, et al. The Pittsburgh Sleep Quality Index: a new instrument for psychiatric practice and research. Psychiatry Res 1989; 28: 193–213.
104. Uemura Y, Nomura T, Inoue Y, et al. Validation of the Parkinson's disease sleep scale in Japanese patients: a comparison study using the Pittsburgh sleep quality index, the epworth sleepiness scale and Polysomnography. J Neurol Sci 2009; 287: 36–40.
105. Martinez-Martin P, Visser M, Rodriguez-Blazquez C, et al. SCOPA-sleep and PDSS: two scales for assessment of sleep disorder in Parkinson's disease. Mov Disord 2008; 23: 1681–8.
106. Johns MW. A new method for measuring daytime sleepiness: the Epworth sleepiness scale. Sleep 1991; 14: 540–5.
107. Hoddes E, Zarcone V, Smythe H, et al. Quantification of sleepiness: a new approach. Psychophysiology 1973; 10: 431–6.
108. Abe K, Hikita T, Sakoda S. Sleep disturbances in Japanese patients with Parkinson's disease--comparing with patients in the UK. J Neurol Sci 2005; 234: 73–8.
109. Trenkwalder C, Kohnen R, Hogl B, et al. Parkinson's disease sleep scale--validation of the revised version PDSS-2. Mov Disord 2011; 26: 644–52.
110. Arnulf I, Leu S, Oudiette D. Abnormal sleep and sleepiness in Parkinson's disease. Curr Opin Neurol 2008; 21: 472–7.
111. Chaudhuri KR, Pal S, Bridgman K, et al. Achieving 24-hour control of Parkinson's disease symptoms: use of objective measures to improve nocturnal disability. Eur Neurol 2001; 46: 3–10.
112. Moller JC, Rethfeldt M, Korner Y, et al. Daytime sleep latency in medication-matched Parkinsonian patients with and without sudden onset of sleep. Mov Disord 2005; 20: 1620–2.
113. Goetz CG, Poewe W, Rascol O, et al. Evidence-based medical review update: pharmacological and surgical treatments of Parkinson's disease: 2001 to 2004. Mov Disord 2005; 20: 523–39.
114. Schapira AH. Present and future drug treatment for Parkinson's disease. J Neurol Neurosurg Psychiatry 2005; 76: 1472–8.
115. Yoshimura N, Mizuta E, Kuno S, et al. The dopamine D1 receptor agonist SKF 38393 suppresses detrusor hyperreflexia in the monkey with parkinsonism induced by 1-methyl-4-phenyl-1,2,3,6-tetrahydropyridine (MPTP). Neuropharmacology 1993; 32: 315–21.
116. Van den Kerchove M, Jacquy J, Gonce M, De Deyn PP. Sustained-release levodopa in parkinsonian patients with nocturnal disabilities. Acta Neurol Belg 1993; 93: 32–9.
117. Hogl B, Saletu M, Brandauer E, et al. Modafinil for the treatment of daytime sleepiness in Parkinson's disease: a double-blind, randomized, crossover, placebo-controlled polygraphic trial. Sleep 2002; 25: 905–9.
118. Adler CH, Caviness JN, Hentz JG, et al. Randomized trial of modafinil for treating subjective daytime sleepiness in patients with Parkinson's disease. Mov Disord 2003; 18: 287–93.
119. Lin JS, Dauvilliers Y, Arnulf I, et al. An inverse agonist of the histamine H(3) receptor improves wakefulness in narcolepsy: studies in orexin-/- mice and patients. Neurobiol Dis 2008; 30: 74–83.
120. Schwartz JC. The histamine H3 receptor: from discovery to clinical trials with pitolisant. Br J Pharmacol 2011; 163: 713–21.
121. Knie B, Mitra MT, Logishetty K, et al. Excessive daytime sleepiness in patients with Parkinson's disease. CNS Drugs 2011; 25: 203–12.
122. Shabnam GN, Th C, Kho D, et al. Therapies for depression in Parkinson's disease. Cochrane Database Syst Rev 2003: CD003465.
123. Devos D, Dujardin K, Poirot I, et al. Comparison of desipramine and citalopram treatments for depression in Parkinson's disease: a double-blind, randomized, placebo-controlled study. Mov Disord 2008; 23: 850–7.

124. Menza M, Dobkin RD, Marin H, et al. A controlled trial of antidepressants in patients with Parkinson disease and depression. Neurology 2009; 72: 886–92.
125. Barone P, Poewe W, Albrecht S, et al. Pramipexole for the treatment of depressive symptoms in patients with Parkinson's disease: a randomised, double-blind, placebo-controlled trial. Lancet Neurol 2010; 9: 573–80.
126. Anderson KN, Shneerson JM. Drug treatment of REM sleep behavior disorder: the use of drug therapies other than clonazepam. J Clin Sleep Med 2009; 5: 235–9.
127. Louden MB, Morehead MA, Schmidt HS Activation by selegiline (Eldepryle) of REM sleep behavior disorder in parkinsonism. W V Med J 1995; 91: 101.
128. Krack P, Batir A, Van Blercom N, et al. Five-year follow-up of bilateral stimulation of the subthalamic nucleus in advanced Parkinson's disease. N Engl J Med 2003; 349: 1925–34.
129. Oertel W, Trenkwalder C, Benes H, et al. Long-term safety and efficacy of rotigotine transdermal patch for moderate-to-severe idiopathic restless legs syndrome: a 5-year open-label extension study. Lancet Neurol 2011; 10: 710–20.
130. Arnulf I, Bejjani BP, Garma L, et al. Improvement of sleep architecture in PD with sub-thalamic nucleus stimulation. Neurology 2000; 55: 1732–4.
131. Hjort N, Ostergaard K, Dupont E. Improvement of sleep quality in patients with advanced Parkinson's disease treated with deep brain stimulation of the subthalamic nucleus. Mov Disord 2004; 19: 196–9.
132. Amara AW, Watts RL, Walker HC. The effects of deep brain stimulation on sleep in Parkinson's disease. Ther Adv Neurol Disord 2011; 4: 15–24.
133. Postuma RB, Arnulf I, Hogl B, et al. A single-question screen for rapid eye movement sleep behavior disorder: a multicenter validation study. Mov Disord 2012; 27: 913–6.

8 Neuropsychological aspects

Julie A. Fields and Alexander I. Tröster

INTRODUCTION

This chapter provides the reader with a basic understanding of the role of neuropsychology in the evaluation of cognition and behavior in Parkinson's disease (PD), with an emphasis on patterns of neurobehavioral functioning, measures used to assess these functions, and evidence-based research supporting potential underlying mechanisms. In this context, current findings regarding the emerging and controversial concept of "mild cognitive impairment" in PD are presented. Challenges and limitations encountered in test administration and interpretation of results are also enumerated. The pathophysiology of PD is described briefly in order to provide a framework for understanding the hypothesized neurobehavioral processes and heterogeneity in cognitive profiles. Treatment options and associated side effects relevant to neuropsychological and psychiatric status are discussed. Finally, similarities and differences in Parkinson-plus syndromes and the utility of neuropsychological assessment in differential diagnoses are presented.

ROLE OF NEUROPSYCHOLOGY IN PARKINSON'S DISEASE

Neuropsychology is the study of brain–behavior relationships, serving an important role in clinical practice as well as research. Neuropsychological assessment provides patients, families, caregivers, and healthcare professionals with helpful information regarding an individual's cognitive and emotional status that is used to:

- determine the presence and pattern of deficits in order to help identify, confirm, or clarify the diagnosis of neurologic disorders;
- assess the risk of developing a neurodegenerative disease;
- delineate strengths and weaknesses to help guide the patient and family in making appropriate accommodations to work, home, and social environment;
- establish a baseline prior to intervention that allows the critical evaluation of candidacy for a particular treatment and subsequent measurement of treatment outcomes;
- provide insight into the patient's capacity for important decision-making and consent to treatment; and
- predict and monitor cognitive trajectory.

PD is the second most common neurodegenerative disease after Alzheimer's disease (AD) (1), afflicting more than 4 million people worldwide over the age of 50 years (2). Motor disability in PD is often compounded by cognitive and behavioral changes, impacting not only patients but also their caregivers. In fact, these changes have been associated with reduced life expectancy in PD (3). Neuropsychology thus can make an important contribution to the management of PD patients. Additionally, since there is considerable heterogeneity in the cognitive phenotypes of PD, neuro-psychological assessment can help differentiate PD from diseases that share patho-logic features, such as AD, Lewy body disease (LBD), and other Parkinson-plus syndromes (4), which becomes particularly salient for treatment planning and pre-dicting prognosis.

Evaluating patients with PD can be challenging. Motor difficulties (e.g., tremor, rigidity, bradykinesia, on–off fluctuations) as well as nonmotor symptoms (e.g., depression, anxiety, apathy, fatigue, medication side-effects) can interfere with testing, and type and length of test batteries must be planned accordingly. Since so many aspects of life are affected by PD, a comprehensive battery is desirable. How-ever, this may not always be feasible, and one must often weigh answering the referral question and obtaining enough data to make practical recommendations against minimizing the patient's discomfort (and possibly suboptimal performance) and financial burden. A detailed interview with both the patient and an informant is imperative, especially in cases where only minimal testing can realistically be performed. Neurobehavioral assessment should take place as soon as symptoms occur or when concern is raised so that treatment recommendations and accommo-dations can be made early enough to effectively impact quality of life.

If only a brief assessment is undertaken, a global measure of cognitive func-tioning should be administered. This allows one to measure overall level of cogni-tive impairment, which can be used to estimate functional disability (5). In addition, brief self-report measures of depression, anxiety, apathy, sleep, and quality of life will be beneficial in making appropriate recommendations for treatment and psy-chosocial accommodations.

Notwithstanding the challenges noted above, a more comprehensive assess-ment battery is preferable, and should not be compromised in certain situations. For example, surgical treatment of PD is not without cognitive and psychiatric mor-bidity. Screening measures designed to detect cognitive decline in AD are com-monly used but are typically poorly sensitive to mild subcortical dementias, such as in PD (6). Alternatively, thorough baseline testing can delineate existing difficulties, such as predementia syndromes or prominent psychiatric or behavioral phenom-ena that are harbingers of further decline and poor neurobehavioral outcomes post-surgically. In cases of significant preexisting impairment, surgical decision-making can become an ethical dilemma. Quite often, patients are so distressed by their debilitating motor dysfunction that they are willing to consent to treatment without fully understanding how nonmotor symptoms can negatively impact their lives and the lives of their caregivers. In some circumstances, they do not have the mental capacity to understand the consequences. Screening instruments are generally insufficient to assess the executive functioning deficits that some studies show are associated with decision-making capacity (7) and should be avoided.

Comprehensive assessments are also recommended when it becomes appar-ent that a patient's cognitive difficulties are interfering with his/her ability to carry out fundamental and/or instrumental activities of daily living. This is especially important when consideration is being given to restricting an individual's daily activities and independence, such as with driving, or when determining the level of care a patient may need. Finally, more detailed testing is necessary for tracking cog-nitive change over time, especially when there is concern for an evolving dementia. See Table 8.1 for commonly used neuropsychological tests in PD. A comprehensive battery should measure a variety of abilities in each cognitive domain.

TABLE 8.1 Commonly Used Neuropsychological Tests by Cognitive Domain Assessed

Premorbid estimates	Barona Demographic Equations; North American Adult Reading Test (NAART); Wechsler Test of Adult Reading (WTAR); Wide Range Achievement Test (WRAT)
Neuropsychological screening	Mattis Dementia Rating Scale (DRS); Mini-Mental State Examination (MMSE); Repeatable Battery for the Assessment of Neuropsychological Status (RBANS)
Intelligence	Kaufman Brief Intelligence Test (KBIT); Raven's Progressive Matrices; Wechsler Abbreviated Scale of Intelligence (WASI); Wechsler Adult Intelligence Scale (WAIS)
Attention and working memory	Auditory Consonant Trigrams (ACT); Brief Test of Attention (BTA); Continuous Performance Tests (CPT); Digit and Visual Span subtests (Wechsler Memory Scale); Paced Auditory Serial Addition Test (PSAT); Stroop test[a]
Executive function	Cognitive Estimation Test (CET); Delis–Kaplan Executive Function Scale (DKEFS); Halstead Category Test; Trail Making Test (TMT)[a]; Wisconsin Card Sorting Test (WCST); Tower of Toronto; Tower of London; DKEFS Tower Test[a]
Memory	Benton Visual Retention Test (BVRT-R); California Verbal Learning Test (CVLT); Rey Auditory Verbal Learning Test (RAVLT); Selective Reminding Test; Rey Complex Figure Test (RCFT)[a]; Wechsler Memory Scale (WMS)[a]; Hopkins Verbal Learning Test (HVLT)
Language	Boston Naming Test (BNT); Controlled Oral Word Association Test (COWAT); Sentence Repetition; Token Test; Complex Ideational Material
Visuoperception	Benton Facial Recognition Test; Benton Judgment of Line Orientation (JLO); Hooper Visual Organization Test (HVOT)
Motor and sensory perception	Finger Tapping[a]; Grooved Pegboard[a]; Hand Dynamometer[a]; Sensory-Perceptual Examination (SPE)
Mood state and personality	Beck Anxiety Inventory (BAI); State-Trait Anxiety Inventory (STAI); Hospital Anxiety and Depression Scale (HDAS); Beck Depression Inventory (BDI); Hamilton Depression Rating Scale (HDRS); Patient Health Questionnaire (PDQ-9); Mood Disorder Questionnaire (MDQ); Montgomery–Asberg Depression Rating Scale; Profile of Mood States (POMS); Starkstein Apathy Scale; Maudsley Obsessional-Compulsive Inventory; Yale–Brown Obsessive Compulsive Scale; Neuropsychiatric Inventory (NPI); Minnesota Multiphasic Personality Inventory (MMPI); Personality Assessment Inventory (PAI)
Quality of life, coping and stressors	Parkinson's Disease Questionnaire (PDQ); Medical Outcomes Study 26-item short form (SF-36); Sickness Impact Profile (SIP); Linear Analog Self Assessment (LASA); Coping Responses Inventory (CRI); Ways of Coping Questionnaire; Life Stressors and Social Resources Inventory (LISRES)

[a]*Note*: Test may not be appropriate for patients with marked speech and/or motor impairment.
Source: Adapted from Ref. 12.

TESTING CONSIDERATIONS

Several methodologic issues pertinent to interpretation of neuropsychological test results and research findings warrant brief mention. The first is that the use of demographically adjusted norms (e.g., age, education, and ethnicity) can enhance positive predictive value (8), that is, the probability that diminished test scores truly reflect that an individual is or will become diseased, and lower the probability of misdiagnosis. Misdiagnosis can also result when an individual's premorbid level of functioning is not taken into consideration. IQ has been shown to predict neuropsychological test performance, especially among those with average IQ or less (9). This means that patients with "normally" low premorbid intellectual functioning who achieve low scores on objective testing may be incorrectly classified as impaired if baseline IQ is not taken into account, and similarly, those who are functioning at a high level premorbidly may actually be showing decline when scores "fall" into the average range and can be misclassified as normal.

What constitutes meaningful cognitive change must also be considered. In order to monitor cognitive and disease trajectory or to evaluate change posttreatment, one must undergo serial assessment(s). Multiple assessments can produce practice effects that may falsely suggest improvement or mask decline. In addition, disease progression or fluctuations, measurement error, and regression to the mean can also cloud interpretation. One can gain reasonable confidence that an observed change is real and significant by applying methods, such as a Reliable Change Index, based on the expected course of PD and modified for practice effects (10).

PATHOPHYSIOLOGY OF NEUROBEHAVIORAL DYSFUNCTION IN PARKINSON'S DISEASE

PD is a hypokinetic movement disorder associated primarily with dysfunction of the basal ganglia and frontostriatal circuits. The dorsolateral, orbitofrontal, and cingulate circuits are particularly important in the regulation of cognition, affect, and motivation, respectively (11), and the complex interactions of these frontostriatal circuits are probably responsible for the neurobehavioral changes in PD (12,13). Specifically, neurobehavioral changes have been linked to the nigrostriatal depletion of dopamine in mesocortical and mesolimbic pathways (14,15), as well as cell loss in nondopaminergic neurotransmitter systems in other brain regions (16,17), including the locus coeruleus, dorsal raphe nuclei, nucleus basalis of Meynert, and dorsal vagal nucleus, the substrates of noradrenergic, serotonergic, and cholinergic systems. Additionally, there is evidence that nigral, brainstem, limbic, and neocortical Lewy bodies contribute to the cognitive deficits observed in PD (18). In the later stages of PD, the amygdala, hippocampi, and frontal and temporoparietal association cortices are involved (19). Thus, dementia in PD (PDD) probably evolves from the progressive involvement of neurochemical and structural changes.

Naturally, given what is understood about the pathophysiology of PD, research on cognition has traditionally centered on frontostriatal dysfunction. Cognitive impairment in PD presents in what is commonly described as a "subcortical" pattern of deficits (20), that is, reduced attention, executive functioning, processing speed, and visuospatial abilities, although the distinction between cortical and subcortical functioning remains controversial. However, there is considerable heterogeneity in cognitive profiles in PD, and other aspects of cognition are frequently affected as well. The reason for this heterogeneity is unclear, but is likely multifactorial. For instance, in addition to cognitive changes that occur as a function of aging and disease progression, uneven dopamine loss across basal ganglia circuitry (21), changes in dopamine receptor sensitivity and concentrations (22), and/or the emergence of cortical Lewy bodies and other non-PD pathologies (23) may interact to produce diverse profiles. There has been some suggestion that there may be different subtypes of cognitive profiles in PD, one with mainly frontal-executive deficits and one with mainly temporal-amnestic deficits (24,25), and structural imaging studies have consistently shown parietotemporal lobe and prefrontal cortex atrophy in PDD (26–28).

NEUROBEHAVIORAL PROFILE OF PARKINSON'S DISEASE

Studies in community-based cohorts show that between 17% and 30% of PD patients without dementia have cognitive impairment (1), which may already be present at the time of diagnosis (29,30). Estimates vary due to methodologic differences, but Aarsland et al. (31) pooled data from eight cohorts using similar definitions and impairment criteria and found that roughly 26% of patients with PD were classified as having mild cognitive impairment. These investigators also found a twofold risk of mild cognitive impairment in untreated PD patients as compared with healthy elderly controls (29). Early changes in PD include bradyphrenia, deficiencies in working memory, executive functioning, language, visuospatial skills, learning and recall, and mood disturbance (20,32–34). Psychosis is rare in untreated PD (35), but hallucinations may occur in as many as 40% of treated patients (36).

Estimates of PDD also vary widely due to ascertainment methods and diagnostic criteria. A systematic review found that the point prevalence of PDD is more than 30% (37), whereas longitudinal estimates of cumulative prevalence within the PD population range from 75% to 90% (38,39). Although 80% or more of patients with PD may ultimately develop dementia (38,39), it appears that the time course from the onset of cognitive symptoms to dementia may be prolonged as much as 20 years (39,40). PDD shares characteristics with the "subcortical" changes in early PD, yet whether it is just a more severe form of cognitive change with disease progression or whether it follows a different pathway is unclear. Longitudinal studies indicate a course of decline in most cognitive domains, with more rapid decline in attention and psychomotor speed, but also significant declines in memory, executive functioning, and visuospatial abilities (41). See Table 8.2 for risk factors for dementia in PD. Interestingly, Janvin et al. (42) applied Petersen and colleagues' (43) diagnostic criteria for mild cognitive impairment (MCI) to a PD sample and found that single- and multiple-domain nonmemory subtypes were associated with the later development of dementia, whereas the amnestic MCI subtype was not. From a practical standpoint, the value of predicting prognosis when there is no disease-altering treatment lies in symptom management (e.g., whether to undergo brain surgery) and planning for future needs (e.g., independent vs. assisted living). In fact, PDD predicts nursing home placement (44) and has been associated with mortality (3).

Attention/Working Memory

Simple attentional skills (i.e., digit span) are relatively preserved in nondemented PD (45,46). However, impairments become more evident as task complexity increases (31) and more demands are placed on working memory (i.e., the ability to attend to, hold, and manipulate information in formulating responses) (47), such as when mentally sequencing and repeating a string of numbers presented in random order (48), or when divided or selective attention is required (49–51). Poor performance on visual search and cancellation tasks requiring selective attention and vigilance has also been reported, even after accounting for motor impairment (52).

TABLE 8.2 Risk Factors Associated with Dementia in Parkinson's Disease

Demographic Variables
  Older age
  Later age of PD onset
Disease Variables
  Severity of motor symptoms
  Longer duration of PD symptoms
  Akinetic-dominant type
  Axial impairment
  Presence of ApoE2 and ApoE4 alleles
Neurobehavioral Variables
  Presence of hallucinations or psychosis
  Depression
  Lower MMSE at baseline
  Declines in cognitive test performance:
    Executive/attention
    Verbal fluency
    Visuoperceptual
    List learning

Abbreviation: PD, Parkinson's disease.

In fact, visual attention deficits, particularly important for visual search and object recognition, have been identified as predictors of poor driving performance and safety errors (53). Taylor et al. (54) calculated a "power of attention" score using mean choice reaction time, simple reaction time, and digit vigilance reaction time scores and demonstrated that poor baseline attentional function, when present, is associated with more rapid cognitive decline.

Attention is impaired in PDD, not only on complex attentional tasks that require the self-allocation of attentional resources, divided attention, and selective attention (55,56), but in the later stages on less-demanding tasks in which external cues are provided (57). Attention also appears to fluctuate in PDD, although to a lesser extent than observed in LBD (58). Studies examining attentional processes in PDD have found that vigilance and focused attention are important determinants of ADL functions (59).

Executive Functioning

Executive functioning deficits, for example, higher-order processes involving cognitive flexibility, planning, working memory, and learning, are evident early in the course of PD and are similar to those observed in patients with frontal lobe lesions (17). Findings such as this have led to the concept of frontostriatal dysexecutive syndrome in PD, which is supported by reports that these functions can improve with dopamine-enhancing medications that restore dopamine concentrations to dorsal frontal regions (60,61). Functional neuroimaging data bolster these findings. Positron emission tomography studies have shown reduced blood flow in the globus pallidus (62) as well as the caudate and dorsolateral frontal cortex of PD patients during an executive functioning task as compared with controls, with normalization in dorsolateral frontal cortex and performance after levodopa administration (63).

It is postulated that executive dysfunction underlies other cognitive changes in PD (13,20), but it is unlikely that executive deficits alone explain the range of cognitive changes observed in PD (64,65). A recent meta-analysis (66) of executive functioning studies in early-stage, nondemented PD patients revealed cognitive difficulties in five areas examined, that is, cognitive flexibility (verbal fluency), set switching (Trails B and Wisconsin Card Sorting Test), inhibition (Stroop), selective attention/working memory (digit span backward), and concept formation (Wisconsin Card Sorting Test). However, owing to the fact that one neuropsychological test rarely, if ever, measures one single construct, comparison among studies is challenging. That is, the same tests may be described as measuring different functions in different studies, for example, verbal fluency may be classified as an executive function in some studies but as a measure of language in others. Slowness in problem solving (67) and diminished planning accuracy (68) have been observed on tower tests. Deficits have also been observed on gambling tasks that evaluate decision making, judgment, and impulsivity (69), but this may be related to dopaminergic therapy (70).

Evidence suggests that executive functioning impairments are impaired in patients with PDD and have been shown to predict incipient dementia in PD (71–73). Woods and Tröster (73) generated receiver–operating characteristic curves and predictive values for list learning, recognition discriminability, perseverative errors, and working memory in initially nondemented patients who met diagnostic criteria for dementia one year later and found that impairment on two or more of these measures provided high sensitivity and positive predictive value (89% and 85%, respectively) in discriminating between demented and nondemented PD groups.

Performance on measures of executive functioning has important implications to daily life, such as consenting for medical treatment (7) and engaging in instrumental daily activities (74), such as shopping, taking medications, and driving. Neuropsychologists are frequently asked to make recommendations about a patient's driving capacity based on cognitive testing, and performance on tests of attention and executive functioning may provide insight. For example, Trails B, a measure of divided attention and mental flexibility, is associated with increased risk of reduced driving abilities (53).

Language

Verbal fluency and visual confrontation naming are typically preserved early in the course of PD (12,75). Frank aphasias are rare (76), although comprehension of complex syntax may be reduced (77). Language impairments in PD are not a universal finding, but deficits in semantic fluency (29,32), verb (action) naming fluency (78,79), phonemic fluency (53,80), and alternating fluency (81) have been demonstrated. One hypothesis for verbal fluency deficits, when they are observed, is that they are secondary to executive dysfunction (80), since generation of words from designated categories or beginning with certain letters requires efficient organization of verbal material, self-monitoring of responses previously given, effortful self-initiation, and inhibition of responses based on specified rules (82). Successful verbal fluency performance relies on efficient clustering and switching strategies, that is, grouping responses within a dimension and switching efficiently to another dimension as appropriate, such as naming zoo animals until the category is exhausted and then switching to farm animals. Clustering appears to be relatively preserved in PD and PDD, but switching impairments have been observed in PDD (83). A meta-analysis conducted by Henry et al. (82) found that semantic fluency deficits are more commonly reported than phonemic fluency deficits, and an alternative hypothesis could be that semantic memory deficits result from temporal lobe dysfunction rather than frontal lobe dysfunction. In a 20-year Sydney Multicenter Study, significant declines in lexical and semantic fluency emerged in patients with late-onset PD (i.e., dementia appeared 10 or more years after PD diagnosis) at the 20-year point that were not present at baseline and were only modestly present at 10-year follow-up (40). Confrontation naming deficits, when they do occur, tend to present later in the disease course when cognitive impairment or PDD is more pronounced (84).

Impaired semantic fluency has been identified as a significant predictor of PDD, without an association for phonemic fluency or other frontally based tasks (85). These authors hypothesized that the dementing process (and subsequent decline in semantic fluency) in PD is related to tau, whereas frontal-executive dysfunction evolves independently and is more related to dopaminergic processes, with better prognosis. In contrast, findings from earlier studies show an association between phonemic fluency and incident dementia (71,72,86). This discrepancy again alludes to the possibility of different underlying mechanisms for cognitive phenotypes in PD and PDD.

Visuospatial Functioning

Visuoperceptual impairments are one of the earliest and most observable cognitive deficits in PD (87), including difficulties in judging line orientations (42,50,53), facial recognition (88), form discrimination (88), picture completion (72), block construction (53), figure copy (53), spatial reasoning (50), and memory for spatial location (89). Although motor dysfunction undoubtedly contributes to impaired performance on tasks with high motor demands, the observation that deficits are present even on tasks free of or with minimal motor demands argues against this being the sole explanation (90). Furthermore, there is neuroanatomic evidence over and above basal ganglia dysfunction to support neurobehavioral findings. Neuroimaging suggests that visuoperceptual and visuospatial deficits in PD may arise from gray matter changes in temporoparietal cortical regions, specifically, fusiform, parahippocampal, and middle occipital regions (88) as well as functional changes in occipital and posterior parietal regions (91).

Substantial visuoperceptual deficits are observed in PDD. Visual discrimination, space-motion, and object-form perception, have been noted to a greater degree in PDD compared with PD or AD, and resemble those of LBD (92). Furthermore, evidence suggests that visuospatial impairments are precursors of PDD. For example, poor performance on a picture completion test that involves inhibiting irrelevant stimuli predicted dementia in one study (72). Visuoperceptual tasks involving construction/drawing abilities tend to show marked impairment in PDD, especially with more severe dementia (56), but it is unclear how much of this is due to motor and/or executive demands. Additionally, the presence of visual hallucinations in conjunction with visuoperceptual deficits may increase the risk of progression to PDD and may follow a more rapid course. Ramirez-Ruiz et al. (93) reported that nearly half of their nondemented hallucinating PD patients developed dementia during a one-year period between baseline and follow-up evaluations. Although almost 70% showed impairments in multiple cognitive domains, mainly visual memory for faces and visuoperceptive–visuospatial functions were affected.

From a practical standpoint, measurement of visuospatial abilities can help determine whether an individual can navigate the environment or safely operate a vehicle, and this may be relevant even before dementia emerges. Uc et al. (53) found that nondemented drivers with PD identified fewer landmarks and traffic signs and committed more at-fault safety errors than neurologically normal controls, and the most important predictors were performance on a test of visual attention and a complex figure-copy test.

Learning and Memory
Deficits in memory are a less frequent finding in PD, although data from a multicenter pooled analysis of studies in mild cognitive impairment from eight cohorts of well-defined PD patients indicated that memory was more commonly affected than executive/attention or visuospatial domains (31). Other studies have also reported deficits in verbal memory, including impairments in immediate and delayed story recall (50) as well as immediate and delayed word-list learning (29,50). Memory dysfunction in PD typically involves a slowness to learn new information (94), resulting in difficulty retrieving newly learned information from memory stores as indicated by mild impairments in free recall but relatively intact recognition (55,95,96) (the "retrieval deficit hypothesis"). However, this concept has been challenged by others who have demonstrated impaired recognition in PD (97). One explanation for this discrepancy among studies is that retrieval deficits may be observed more frequently in PD when there is a frontal-executive phenotype, but when the temporal-amnestic phenotype predominates, recognition and recall are both impaired. It has been proposed that memory deficits observed in PD may be, at least in part, secondary to frontal/executive dysfunction (13,90,98). However, even when executive dysfunction is controlled for, there is some evidence that memory deficits are still present (31,98). This would be consistent with hypotheses of distinct cognitive phenotypes (24,25), and provide some explanation for the cognitive heterogeneity in PD. In particular, it has been shown that there may be different memory subtypes—one with an impaired retrieval profile with disruption of dorsolateral prefrontal activity and one with an encoding deficit profile with disruption in anterior hippocampal activity (99,100).

Visuospatial memory impairments have also been observed (101) and may be differentially affected by disease severity. Remote memory is generally preserved in early PD (102), although may decline as the disease progresses (103). Few studies have examined prospective memory in PD, but there is some evidence of impairment (104). This involves remembering to complete a planned task at some time point in the future, and is likely associated with planning and executive working memory (104), functions thought to be subserved by the frontal lobe (105). Finally, procedural memory, or the "how-to" memory programs that one performs automatically without conscious thought, appears to be task dependent and may or may not be impaired (106,107).

Levy et al. (71) found that impaired immediate and delayed recall scores on the Selective Reminding Test at baseline in a nondemented PD sample were associated with incident dementia. Evidence indicates that memory deficits in PD are less severe and are distinguishable from those observed in AD, but as PDD progresses, broader memory deficits, including deficient encoding and consolidation, become apparent and the memory profiles of AD and PDD converge (108).

PARKINSON'S DISEASE VERSUS LEWY BODY DEMENTIA
LBD is the second most common form of dementia (after AD) in individuals over the age of 75 years and is associated with increased functional impairment and a

higher risk of mortality as compared with AD (109). LBD and PDD share many clinical and pathologic features, and according to the most current criteria, the differentiation between them is based on a temporal association between PD motor symptoms and dementia onset. A diagnosis of PDD requires the presence of parkinsonism at least one year prior to onset of dementia, whereas if dementia precedes parkinsonism by at least one year a diagnosis of LBD is made (110). However, examination of the cardinal features of LBD suggests that cognitive changes may not be the earliest markers of LBD (4,111). LBD is often accompanied by visual hallucinations, cognitive fluctuations, and rapid eye movement (REM) sleep behavior (17,109). Hallucinations have been associated with visuoperceptual impairment and are a core feature of LBD (112). Approximately 75% of LBD patients experience hallucinations and 50% experience delusions (113).

Neuropsychological studies have not been able to distinguish between PDD and LBD (12,25), and in conjunction with pathophysiologic similarities, it is possible that PDD and LBD may fall on a continuum rather than represent distinct entities. Similar to PDD, LBD generally follows a subcortical pattern and is typically associated with deficits in attention, frontal-executive functioning, letter fluency, and visuospatial and constructional abilities (20,114,115), which can be differentiated from the cortical pattern of AD by showing significantly better naming and memory performance (115). Noe et al. (56) compared patients with AD, PDD, and LBD matched for severity of dementia and found that PDD and LBD patients performed significantly worse on measures of attention but better on tests of memory than AD patients. LBD patients also performed worse on tests of visual memory, visuoperceptive, and visuoconstructional tasks than AD patients, but there were no differences between PD and LBD groups on any cognitive measure. It has been noted, however, that a subgroup of patients with LBD may have cortical and hippocampal changes that present with a more cortical profile rather than predominantly frontosubcortical changes (25).

EFFECTS OF EMOTIONAL FUNCTIONING ON COGNITION IN PARKINSON'S DISEASE

Neurobehavioral manifestations are observed in a large proportion of patients with PD, often predating motor symptoms, and may be precursors for the disease itself and further decline in mood and cognition. The mechanisms are not completely understood, but neuroimaging, neuropathologic, neuropsychologic, and behavioral evidence suggests a complex interaction of biologic, psychological, and environmental factors underlying the evolution and presentation of symptoms. Emotional dysfunction deserves attention because there is mounting evidence that nonmotor symptoms contribute to poor health status in PD, and in fact one study examining nonmotor factors in 462 patients found that depression had more than twice the impact on health status in PD than motor symptoms and that anxiety was also a significant determinant (116).

Depression and Apathy

Behavioral disturbances are quite common in PD and PDD and can negatively impact cognitive functioning as well as quality of life. Depression and apathy are among the most common behavioral disturbances observed and often coexist. However, there is a subset of patients who experience one without the other, indicating that they are distinct entities. Prevalence rates of depression in PD vary widely, partially due to differences in assessment settings as well as overlap in symptoms on diagnostic instruments, but 30–40% is commonly reported (117). Depression may predate PD by several years (118), and in fact is a risk factor for PD and PDD (119). Depression significantly affects cognition and hastens cognitive decline in PD (120), likely due in large part to the common frontal subcortical pathways and biologic correlates they share (121). Effects of depression on cognition include impairments in executive functions and memory (122,123), especially in the later stages of PD.

Apathy has been defined as "diminished motivation not attributable to decreased level of consciousness, cognitive impairment, or emotional distress" (124). Perhaps for this reason, the reported prevalence rates of apathy in PD range widely from 17% to 70%, influenced by the assessment tool being used, the rater, and the extent of coexisting depression and/or cognitive decline (117). Recently, Ziropadja et al. (125) found in a series of 360 patients at various disease stages that apathy coexisted with depression in 36.9% of PD patients, compared with depression without apathy in 4.4%, apathy without depression in 23%, and neither apathy nor depression in 35.2%. Measurement of cognitive decline attributable to apathy is confounded by its frequent coexistence with depression, but it appears that nondepressed PD patients with apathy exhibit decreased working memory, poor planning and abstract reasoning, and recall as compared with patients without apathy regardless of whether or not they have depression (126), possibly reflecting frontostriatal dysfunction causing inefficient cognitive strategies that disrupt recall. Similarly, in other studies apathy in PD has been associated with bradyphrenia, global cognitive impairment, executive dysfunction, and memory impairment (127–130). Like depression, apathy appears to be predictive of dementia in PD (131) and leads to increased functional decline and debility (127).

Anxiety

Anxiety affects up to 40% of patients with PD (117), and similar to depression and apathy, may present before motor symptoms are evident (118). Anxiety also coexists with depression, and as many as 75% of patients with PD and depression also have an anxiety disorder (132). This includes episodic (e.g., panic attacks, often associated with off-periods), generalized anxiety syndromes, and phobias (133,134). Despite a high prevalence of anxiety in PD, few studies have systematically examined the relationship between anxiety and cognitive functioning in PD, and this may be due to measurement difficulty given its comorbidity with depression as well as overlap with motor symptoms (135). Ryder et al. (136) found that self-reported symptoms of trait anxiety were negatively related to performance on a neuropsychological screening battery in male PD patients. Bogdanova et al. (137) recently examined apathy and anxiety in relation to laterality of PD symptoms in a nondemented sample and found a dissociation between these two emotional states and cognitive domains. Specifically, in patients with left-sided PD symptoms, apathy was associated with performance on nonverbally mediated executive function and visuospatial tasks (consistent with right hemisphere dysfunction), whereas in patients with right-sided PD symptoms (left hemisphere dysfunction), anxiety was significantly correlated with performance on verbally mediated tasks.

EFFECTS OF PHARMACOLOGIC AND SURGICAL TREATMENT ON COGNITION AND BEHAVIOR IN PARKINSON'S DISEASE

Pharmacologic Treatments

Pharmacotherapy provides relief for the debilitating motor symptoms of PD via a variety of mechanisms directed toward correcting the dopamine depletion that is characteristic of the disease. While many medications have proven efficacy in improving both motor and nonmotor symptoms of PD, the same medications may paradoxically also have deleterious effects (Table 8.3). One hypothesis for ensuing neurobehavioral impairments may be that the brain regions with less dopamine depletion initially (138), such as the caudate nucleus and the ventral striatum, particularly the nucleus accumbens and associated frontostriatal loops with the orbitofrontal cortex, may be subject to dopamine overdose (61,139). A review by Kehagia et al. (17) enumerates amelioration of deficits on tasks of planning, switching between well-learned tasks, digit span, response inhibition, and working memory, whereas deterioration was noted in concurrent learning, probabilistic reversal learning, weather prediction classification, gambling and decision making, and responding with distraction after dopamine replacement. An increase in visual hallucinations was also noted.

Findings concerning the impact of *levodopa* on cognitive functioning are inconsistent, with some studies showing improvements, some decrements, and others an absence of significant change. There has been some suggestion that the effects may depend on task demands and striatal dopamine levels (140). One of the most frequent behavioral findings with dopamine replacement, especially *dopamine agonists*, is the development of impulse control disorders, such as pathologic gambling, compulsive spending, and hypersexuality (Table 8.3). There is some evidence to suggest that male sex, young age at onset, novelty-seeking behavior, high impulsivity, and a family or personal history of addictive behavior are associated with the neurobehavioral side effects of dopamine agonists (141,142). Dopamine agonists may afford some benefit for depressive symptoms, but have limited or negative effects on cognition. Some improvements in cognitive skills have been demonstrated with *catechol-O-methyl-transferase inhibitors*. Findings are again mixed with regard to *monoamine oxidase-B inhibitors*, some studies showing improvement in aspects of cognition and others no effect. *Glutamate-blocking agents* may improve cognition, but may put patients at risk for psychotic symptoms.

Anticholinergics lead to motor improvement in PD; however, these improvements are accompanied by impairments in memory, executive functioning, and global cognitive abilities. Confusional states have also been induced by anticholinergics. Treatment of nonmotor symptoms of PD include the class of *cholinesterase inhibitors*, initially avoided due to concern of worsening of motor symptoms (143), now being used more frequently with the recognition of beneficial effects not only on cognition, but on psychiatric symptoms in both PDD and LBD.

Neurosurgical Interventions

Neurosurgical interventions for the treatment of the debilitating motor symptoms of PD are sought when pharmacotherapy is no longer effective at controlling motor complications. Postsurgical neurobehavioral changes are difficult to measure and compare across studies due to methodologic differences, but it is now recognized that although these surgical procedures are generally deemed "relatively safe," they are in many cases not without cognitive and psychiatric morbidity. It is therefore

TABLE 8.3 Neurobehavioral Effects of Medications Used to Treat Motor Symptoms of Parkinson's Disease

Drug Category	Generic Name	Trade Name	Neurobehavioral Effects	
			Positive	Negative
Dopamine replacement	carbidopa/ levodopa	Sinemet Atamet Lodosyn Larodopa Parcopa Stalevo (+ COMT)	Transient improvements in learning and memory, visuoperception, and executive functions; improvements in planning accuracy, visuospatial working memory, prospective memory, and verbal fluency; poorer working memory and aspects of executive functioning *after* levodopa *withdrawal*	Hallucinations, delusions, confusion, depression, anxiety, agitation, nightmares; hedonistic homeostatic dysregulation syndrome; depression and psychosis with Stalevo
Dopamine agonists	pramipexole ropinirole bromocriptine pergolide rotigotine apomorphine	Mirapex Requip Parlodel Permax Neupro (patch) Apokyn (injection)	Some improvement in depressive symptoms with pramipexole, ropinirole, and pergolide	Deficits in verbal fluency, executive function, and verbal short-term memory with pramipexole; minimal effect on cognition with bromocriptine and pergolide; development of impulse control disorders, including increased impulsivity, compulsive gambling, increased sexual behaviors; hallucinations, delusions, depression, and confusion with apomorphine
Catechol O-methyltransferase (COMT) Inhibitors	entacapone tolcapone	Comtan Tasmar	Improvement in attention, memory, and constructional skills	Hallucinations

Monoamine Oxidase-B (MAO-B) Inhibitors	selegiline rasagiline	Eldepryl Deprenyl Carbex Zelapar Azilect	Improvements in global cognitive functioning, P300 latencies, and memory or no change	Depression and hallucinations
Glutamate (NMDA) Blocking Drugs	amantadine memantine	Symmetrel Namenda Akatinol	Improvement in global cognition and rate of mental decline, speed of attention, verbal fluency and a frontal assessment battery; decrease in disinhibition, irritability, anxiety, and hallucinations	Hallucinations and confusion in advanced disease
Anticholinergics	benztropine trihexyphenidyl	Cogentin Artane		Memory impairment and executive dysfunction; confusion; sedation and delirium
Cholinesterase Inhibitors	rivastigmine donepezil galantamine	Exelon Aricept Razadyne	Improvement in attention, verbal fluency, and global cognitive functioning; reduction in sleep disturbance, anxiety, and hallucinations	

important to carefully evaluate surgical candidates' preoperative cognitive and psychiatric status to assess risk for unfavorable surgical outcomes, for example, as a result of preexisting dementia, depression, or impulse control disorders. Postoperative assessment is also important in order to optimize motor benefit with stimulation and/or medication adjustments without unduly compromising neurobehavioral functioning and quality of life as well as to address psychiatric and functional complications that may arise.

Ablation

Surgical lesioning techniques include thalamotomy, subthalamotomy, and pallidotomy, targeting the ventral-intermediate nucleus of the thalamus (VIM), the subthalamic nucleus (STN), and the globus pallidus internus (GPi), respectively. Ablative surgeries, given the irreversibility of neurologic deficits should they occur, have been largely supplanted by deep brain stimulation (DBS). However, ablative therapy is still considered an effective alternative for a select group of patients (144), such as those with a history of infection related to previous DBS implantation, those with limited access to centers specializing in DBS surgery, and those not willing or able to have implantable hardware requiring long-term follow-up for programming and maintenance.

Modern thalamotomy is associated with less cognitive morbidity than observed in earlier studies, which commonly found impairments in language and memory (145). Subthalamotomy appears to be safe from a cognitive standpoint (146,147) and may even be associated with improvements on measures of initiation/perseveration, attention, executive functioning, and semantic fluency (148). Investigations following unilateral pallidotomy have yielded inconsistent findings, with many studies showing no significant change (149,150), whereas others show transient (151) or persistent changes (152,153). Bilateral pallidotomy has been associated with a higher incidence of cognitive morbidity compared with unilateral surgery, although findings are again inconsistent and based on small sample sizes or mixed procedures.

Deep Brain Stimulation

DBS is the most frequently implemented surgical technique for PD because it brings with it (i) the potential for reversibility should surgical procedures fail to provide adequate benefit, (ii), the ability to optimize benefit with the adjustment of stimulation parameters, and (iii) in many cases a reduction in medication. It has also been associated with diminished cognitive morbidity compared with ablative procedures. In general, DBS is considered "relatively safe," yet is often accompanied by neurobehavioral sequelae (154).

Few studies have examined cognitive changes following VIM DBS for PD, but thalamic stimulation does not appear to be associated with changes in overall cognitive functioning (155,156) or the verbal fluency and memory changes that are sometimes observed after thalamotomy, and in fact, improvements on tasks of problem solving, verbal fluency, naming, and delayed recall have been observed up to 12 months postoperatively (156,157). When verbal fluency declines are observed, they are more likely to occur after left-sided VIM DBS (158).

Pallidal stimulation is associated with relatively little risk of cognitive decline overall, regardless of whether stimulation is unilateral or bilateral. Many studies have found no significant change in cognitive functioning (159–161), and changes observed in visuoconstructional ability and/or semantic verbal fluency in other studies (162,163) were rarely of clinical significance. Another study, however, comparing staged bilateral GPi or STN DBS did find declines in verbal fluency and working memory regardless of surgical site (164). Since it appears to carry less risk of cognitive and behavioral decline than STN, some researchers have proposed that bilateral GPi DBS is a safe and effective treatment for PD patients for whom STN DBS is contraindicated, such as those with preexisting cognitive impairment or psychiatric disturbance (165), but this requires further investigation.

The effect of STN stimulation on cognitive and behavioral functioning is debated, with some studies showing no significant cognitive morbidity (166,167). On the other hand, Parsons et al. (168) conducted a meta-analysis of 28 studies and found small but significant declines in executive function, verbal learning and memory, and verbal fluency. Declines in both phonemic and semantic fluency are the most frequently reported sequelae after STN DBS. Controlled studies have reported greater declines in verbal fluency, color naming, selective attention, verbal memory, and response inhibition (169–172) compared with nonsurgical PD controls. Similarly, a multicenter randomized controlled trial of 121 patients undergoing bilateral STN or GPi DBS versus 134 patients receiving best medical therapy found that DBS patients declined on measures of working memory, processing speed, phonemic fluency, and visual delayed recall, whereas the best medical therapy group showed slight improvements on these measures (173).

Perhaps of equal or greater concern is the frequency with which increased psychiatric and mood disturbances are observed after STN DBS, including depression (174), apathy (175), suicide (176,177), and impulse control disorders (178). These findings underscore the importance of carefully selecting patients for surgery as well as monitoring cognitive and psychiatric changes postsurgery (179).

Transplantation
There are few studies examining neurobehavioral outcomes following fetal mesencephalic transplant, and those studies that have reported outcomes differed in technical procedures, target regions, and included small numbers of patients. Although most individuals have not shown significant cognitive changes after surgery (180), some cognitive decline may occur in patients with preoperative deficits (181).

NEUROPSYCHOLOGICAL ASPECTS OF PARKINSON-PLUS SYNDROMES
Neuropsychological assessment complements neurologic examination and diagnostic tests in the differential diagnosis of diseases that share similar underlying or mixed pathologies but have different phenotypic presentations, for example, progressive supranuclear palsy (PSP), multiple system atrophy (MSA), and corticobasal degeneration (CBD). A summary of key neurobehavioral features is presented in Table 8.4.

Progressive Supranuclear Palsy
The prevalence rates of dementia in PSP are difficult to estimate because frequently studies do not report cognitive functioning since cognitive impairment is considered a supportive feature (NINDS-SPSP) in the diagnosis of PSP rather than a primary diagnostic criterion (182). The current estimates range from 10% to 52%

TABLE 8.4 Comparison of Neurobehavioral Features of Parkinson's Disease with Dementia and Parkinson-Plus Syndromes

Neurobehavioural Features	PDD	LBD	CBD	PSP	MSA
Attention	-	--	-	-	--
Executive (e.g., problem-solving, conceptualization, planning, flexibility)	--	--	-	--	0/-
Language					
Letter fluency	--	--	-	-/--	-
Category fluency	--	--	-	-	-
Visual confrontation naming	0/-	-/--	0/-	0	0
Memory					
Recall of new information	--	-/--	0/-	0/-	0/-
Recall of remote information	-	?	?	0	0
Recognition	0/-	-	0	0	0
Visuoperceptual/visuoconstruction	-	--	-	-	-
Fluctuating cognition	0/-	--	0	0	0
Praxis	0/-	0/-	--	0/-	0
Alien-hand syndrome	0	0	-/--	0	0
Depression	--	--	-	0/-	0/-
Apathy	-	-	-	--	--

Abbreviations: 0, impairment absent; -, mild-to-moderate impairment; --, moderate to severe impairment; ?, questionable; PDD, Parkinson's disease with dementia; LBD, Lewy body dementia; CBD, corticobasal degeneration; PSP, progressive supranuclear palsy; MSA, multiple system atrophy.

(183,184). Estimates using diagnostic criteria requiring cognitive impairment may be as high as 71% (185). There may be subtypes of cognitive impairment in PSP, but the typical pattern follows that of "subcortical dementia," with early and prominent executive dysfunction and profound slowed information processing speed (186,187). As compared to patients with PD, cognitive slowing and executive dysfunction in PSP emerges earlier in the disease course, is more severe, and progresses more rapidly (188,189). Verbal fluency, especially phonemic, is greatly reduced (190,191) in PSP and may be sensitive to the differentiation of PD, PSP, and MSA (191), although Brown et al. (182) found that when matched for overall level of cognitive functioning, verbal fluency did not distinguish between PSP and MSA. Memory complaints are mild, consisting of impaired free recall and accelerated rates of forgetting but preserved recognition memory (192,193). The early presence of cognitive impairment distinguishes PSP from MSA (194).

Multiple System Atrophy

MSA is a sporadic, progressive neurodegenerative syndrome that encompasses three conditions, including olivopontocerebellar atrophy (OPCA), striatonigral degeneration (SND), and Shy–Drager syndrome (SDS). Hallmark features include dysautonomia, parkinsonism, cerebellar ataxia, and pyramidal signs (195), with two clinically predominant motor presentations (196). The parkinsonian presentation (MSA-P) corresponds most closely to SND and the cerebellar presentation (MSA-C) to OPCA (12). Cognitive deficits are generally subtle or late appearing in MSA, and in fact, significant cognitive decline is an exclusionary feature according to current MSA diagnostic criteria (196). However, approximately 10% of patients with parkinsonism have MSA (197), and dementia has been reported in 14–16% of MSA cases (184,198). Cognitive symptoms in MSA are qualitatively similar to PD and PSP, but less severe than those observed in PSP (182), although verbal fluency (often subsumed under the rubric of executive functioning) has been found to be more impaired in MSA compared with age- and disease severity–matched PD patients (189,199). MSA-P impairments include verbal fluency, visual search and attention, executive functions, and verbal memory (199,200), whereas MSA-C may involve mild deficits in verbal fluency and verbal memory (201). Patients with MSA-P may have more severe and widespread cognitive dysfunction than patients with MSA-C (202), although dementia may be more prevalent in familial than sporadic OPCA (203).

Corticobasal Degeneration

The prevalence and incidence of CBD are unknown, probably owing to poor diagnostic accuracy related to its clinical and pathologic overlap with PSP and frontotemporal dementia. CBD is characterized by progressive asymmetric rigidity and apraxia (typically ideomotor, that is, inability to use, name, or mimic tool use) (193,204), often accompanied by myoclonus, cortical sensory loss, alien limb behavior (i.e., cortical dysfunction) as well as bradykinesia, dystonia, and tremor (i.e., subcortical basal ganglia dysfunction) (205,206). It is now recognized that cognitive impairment is part of that constellation of symptoms and may even precede motor symptoms (207,208). Progressive aphasia, most frequently the nonfluent type (206), may be a presenting feature of CBD and may help distinguish it from PSP, MSA, and PD. One of the most consistent findings in CBD is impairment on tests of frontal lobe functioning and verbal fluency (193,209–212). Other impairments commonly observed in CBD include visuospatial skills (212,213), constructional apraxia (211), handwriting (214), spelling (212), and acalculia (209,211,214). Results on tests of naming are variable. Several studies have shown preserved naming (212), whereas others have found impairments (209). When naming impairments are found, significant benefit from cuing suggests a retrieval rather than a semantic memory deficit (209). Findings with regard to episodic memory are also inconsistent, with some studies showing relatively preserved performance (208) and others finding impairments (193). Episodic memory impairments are associated with encoding and retrieval deficits believed to arise from deficient frontally mediated strategic processes, differing qualitatively from AD.

REFERENCES

1. Aarsland D, Bronnick K, Fladby T. Mild cognitive impairment in Parkinson's disease. Curr Neurol Neurosci Rep 2011; 11: 371–8.
2. Dorsey ER, Constantinescu R, Thompson JP, et al. Projected number of people with Parkinson disease in the most populous nations, 2005 through 2030. Neurology 2007; 68: 384–6.
3. Levy G, Tang MX, Louis ED, et al. The association of incident dementia with mortality in PD. Neurology 2002; 59: 1708–13.
4. Fields JA, Ferman TJ, Boeve BF, et al. Neuropsychological assessment of patients with dementing illness. Nat Rev Neurol 2011; 7: 677–87.
5. Fields JA, Machulda M, Aakre J, et al. Utility of the DRS for predicting problems in day-to-day functioning. Clin Neuropsychol 2010; 24: 1167–80.
6. McKeith IG. Spectrum of Parkinson's disease, Parkinson's dementia, and Lewy body dementia. Neurol Clin 2000; 18: 865–902.

7. Dymek MP, Atchison P, Harrell L, et al. Competency to consent to medical treatment in cognitively impaired patients with Parkinson's disease. Neurology 2001; 56: 17–24.

8. Smith GE, Ivnik RJ. Normative neuropsychology. In: Petersen R, ed. Mild Cognitive Impairment. New York: Oxford University Press, 2003: 63–88.

9. Diaz-Asper CM, Schretlen DJ, Pearlson GD. How well does IQ predict neuropsychological test performance in normal adults? J Int Neuropsychol Soc 2004; 10: 82–90.

10. Tröster AI, Woods SP, Morgan EE. Assessing cognitive change in Parkinson's disease: development of practice effect-corrected reliable change indices. Arch Clin Neuropsychol 2007; 22: 711–18.

11. Middleton FA, Strick PL. Basal ganglia output and cognition: evidence from anatomical, behavioral, and clinical studies. Brain Cogn 2000; 42: 183–200.

12. Tröster AI, Fields JA. Parkinson's disease, progressive supranuclear palsy, corticobasal degeneration and related disorders of the frontostriatal system. In: Morgan JE, Ricker JH, eds. Textbook of Clinical Neuropsychology. New York: Psychology Press, 2008: 536–77.

13. Zgaljardic DJ, Borod JC, Foldi NS, et al. A review of the cognitive and behavioral sequelae of Parkinson's disease: relationship to frontostriatal circuitry. Cogn Behav Neurol 2003; 16: 193–210.

14. Blonder LX, Slevin JT. Emotional dysfunction in Parkinson's disease. Behav Neurol 2011; 24: 201–17.

15. Mattay VS, Tessitore A, Callicott JH, et al. Dopaminergic modulation of cortical function in patients with Parkinson's disease. Ann Neurol 2002; 51: 156–64.

16. Dubois B, Pilon B, Lhermitte F, et al. Cholinergic deficiency and frontal dysfunction in Parkinson's disease. Ann Neurol 1990; 28: 117–21.

17. Kehagia AA, Barker RA, Robbins TW. Neuropsychological and clinical heterogeneity of cognitive impairment and dementia in patients with Parkinson's disease. Lancet Neurol 2010; 9: 1200–13.

18. Kaufer DL, Tröster AI. Neuropsychology of dementia with Lewy bodies. In: Miller BL, Goldenberg G, eds. Handbook of Clinical Neurology: Neuropsychology and Behavior, Part I, 3rd edn. Amsterdam: Elsevier, 2008.

19. Braak H, Del Tredici K, Rub U, et al. Staging of brain pathology related to sporadic Parkinson's disease. Neurobiol Aging 2003; 24: 197–211.

20. Dubois B, Pillon B. Cognitive deficits in Parkinson's disease. J Neurol 1997; 244: 2–8.

21. Lewis SJ, Barker RA. Understanding the dopaminergic deficits in Parkinson's disease: insights into disease heterogeneity. J Clin Neurosci 2009; 16: 620–5.

22. Goldman-Rakic PS, Muly EC 3rd, Williams GV. D(1) receptors in prefrontal cells and circuits. Brain Res Brain Res Rev 2000; 31: 295–301.

23. Kempster PA, O'Sullivan SS, Holton JL, et al. Relationships between age and late progression of Parkinson's disease: a clinico-pathological study. Brain 2010; 133: 1755–62.

24. Aarsland D, Kurz MW. The epidemiology of dementia associated with Parkinson's disease. Brain Pathol 2010; 20: 633–9.

25. Janvin CC, Larsen JP, Salmon DP, et al. Cognitive profiles of individual patients with Parkinson's disease and dementia: comparison with dementia with lewy bodies and Alzheimer's disease. Mov Disord 2006; 21: 337–42.

26. Jokinen P, Bruck A, Aalto S, et al. Impaired cognitive performance in Parkinson's disease is related to caudate dopaminergic hypofunction and hippocampal atrophy. Parkinsonism Relat Disord 2009; 15: 88–93.

27. Kenny ER, Burton EJ, O'Brien JT. A volumetric magnetic resonance imaging study of entorhinal cortex volume in dementia with lewy bodies. A comparison with Alzheimer's disease and Parkinson's disease with and without dementia. Dement Geriatr Cogn Disord 2008; 26: 218–25.

28. Lyoo CH, Ryu YH, Lee MS. Topographical distribution of cerebral cortical thinning in patients with mild Parkinson's disease without dementia. Mov Disord 2010; 25: 496–9.

29. Aarsland D, Bronnick K, Larsen JP, et al. Cognitive impairment in incident, untreated Parkinson disease: the Norwegian ParkWest study. Neurology 2009; 72: 1121–6.

30. Foltynie T, Brayne CE, Robbins TW, et al. The cognitive ability of an incident cohort of Parkinson's patients in the UK. The CamPaIGN study. Brain 2004; 127: 550–60.

31. Aarsland D, Bronnick K, Williams-Gray C, et al. Mild cognitive impairment in Parkinson disease: a multicenter pooled analysis. Neurology 2010; 75: 1062–9.
32. Benito-Leon J, Louis ED, Posada IJ, et al. Population-based case-control study of cognitive function in early Parkinson's disease (NEDICES). J Neurol Sci 2011; 310: 176–82.
33. Bondi MW, Tröster AI. Neurobehavioral consequences of basal ganglia dysfunction. In: Nussbaum PD, ed. Handbook of Neuropsychology and Aging. New York: Plenum, 1997: 216–45.
34. Pillon B, Boller F, Levy R, et al. Cognitive deficits and dementia in Parkinson's disease. In: Boller F, Cappa SF, eds. Handbook of Neuropsychology. Amsterdam: Elsevier, 2001: 311–71.
35. Cummings JL. Neuropsychiatric complications of drug treatment in Parkinson's disease. In: Huber S, Cummings JL, eds. Parkinson's Disease: Neurobehavioral Aspects. New York: Oxford University Press, 1992: 313–27.
36. Fenelon G, Mahieux F, Huon R, et al. Hallucinations in Parkinson's disease: prevalence, phenomenology and risk factors. Brain 2000; 123: 733–45.
37. Aarsland D, Zaccai J, Brayne C. A systematic review of prevalence studies of dementia in Parkinson's disease. Mov Disord 2005; 20: 1255–63.
38. Buter TC, van den Hout A, Matthews FE, et al. Dementia and survival in Parkinson disease: a 12-year population study. Neurology 2008; 70: 1017–22.
39. Hely MA, Reid WG, Adena MA, et al. The Sydney multicenter study of Parkinson's disease: the inevitability of dementia at 20 years. Mov Disord 2008; 23: 837–44.
40. Reid WG, Hely MA, Morris JG, et al. Dementia in Parkinson's disease: a 20-year neuropsychological study (Sydney Multicentre Study). J Neurol Neurosurg Psychiatry 2011; 82: 1033–7.
41. Muslimovic D, Post B, Speelman JD, et al. Cognitive decline in Parkinson's disease: a prospective longitudinal study. J Int Neuropsychol Soc 2009; 15: 426–37.
42. Janvin CC, Larsen JP, Aarsland D, et al. Subtypes of mild cognitive impairment in Parkinson's disease: progression to dementia. Mov Disord 2006; 21: 1343–9.
43. Petersen RC, Doody R, Kurz A, et al. Current concepts in mild cognitive impairment. Arch Neurol 2001; 58: 1985–92.
44. Aarsland D, Larsen JP, Tandberg E, et al. Predictors of nursing home placement in Parkinson's disease: a population-based, prospective study. J Am Geriatr Soc 2000; 48: 938–42.
45. Bublak P, Muller U, Gron G, et al. Manipulation of working memory information is impaired in Parkinson's disease and related to working memory capacity. Neuropsychology 2002; 16: 577–90.
46. Green J, McDonald WM, Vitek JL, et al. Neuropsychological and psychiatric sequelae of pallidotomy for PD: clinical trial findings. Neurology 2002; 58: 858–65.
47. Cooper JA, Sagar HJ, Jordan N, et al. Cognitive impairment in early, untreated Parkinson's disease and its relationship to motor disability. Brain 1991; 114: 2095–122.
48. Stebbins GT, Gabrieli JD, Masciari F, et al. Delayed recognition memory in Parkinson's disease: a role for working memory? Neuropsychologia 1999; 37: 503–10.
49. Lee SS, Wild K, Hollnagel C, et al. Selective visual attention in patients with frontal lobe lesions or Parkinson's disease. Neuropsychologia 1999; 37: 595–604.
50. Muslimovic D, Post B, Speelman JD, et al. Motor procedural learning in Parkinson disease. Brain 2007; 130: 2887–97.
51. Uc EY, Rizzo M, Anderson SW, et al. Visual dysfunction in Parkinson's disease without dementia. Neurology 2005; 65: 1907–13.
52. Filoteo JV, Williams BJ, Rilling LM, et al. Performance of Parkinson's disease patients on the visual search and attention test: impairment in single-feature but not dual-feature visual search. Arch Clin Neuropsychol 1997; 12: 621–34.
53. Uc EY, Rizzo M, Anderson SW, et al. Impaired visual search in drivers with Parkinson's disease. Ann Neurol 2006; 60: 407–13.
54. Taylor JP, Rowan EN, Lett D, et al. Poor attentional function predicts cognitive decline in patients with non-demented Parkinson's disease independent of motor phenotype. J Neurol Neurosurg Psychiatry 2008; 79: 1318–23.

55. Brown RG, Marsden CD. Internal versus external cues and the control of attention in Parkinson's disease. Brain 1988; 111: 323–45.
56. Noe E, Marder K, Bell KL, et al. Comparison of dementia with Lewy bodies to Alzheimer's disease and Parkinson's disease with dementia. Mov Disord 2004; 19: 60–7.
57. Yamada T, Izyuuinn M, Schulzer M, et al. Covert orienting attention in Parkinson's disease. J Neurol Neurosurg Psychiatry 1990; 53: 593–6.
58. Ballard CG, Aarsland D, McKeith I, et al. Fluctuations in attention: PD dementia vs DLB with parkinsonism. Neurology 2002; 59: 1714–20.
59. Bronnick K, Ehrt U, Emre M, et al. Attentional deficits affect activities of daily living in dementia-associated with Parkinson's disease. J Neurol Neurosurg Psychiatry 2006; 77: 1136–42.
60. Cooper JA, Sagar HJ, Doherty SM, et al. Different effects of dopaminergic and anticholinergic therapies on cognitive and motor function in Parkinson's disease. A follow-up study of untreated patients. Brain 1992; 115: 1701–25.
61. Gotham AM, Brown RG, Marsden CD. 'Frontal' cognitive function in patients with Parkinson's disease 'on' and 'off' levodopa. Brain 1988; 111: 299–21.
62. Owen AM, Doyon J, Dagher A, et al. Abnormal basal ganglia outflow in Parkinson's disease identified with PET. Implications for higher cortical functions. Brain 1998; 121: 949–65.
63. Cools R, Stefanova E, Barker RA, et al. Dopaminergic modulation of high-level cognition in Parkinson's disease: the role of the prefrontal cortex revealed by PET. Brain 2002; 125: 584–94.
64. Stefanova ED, Kostic VS, Ziropadja LJ, et al. Declarative memory in early Parkinson's disease: serial position learning effects. J Clin Exp Neuropsychol 2001; 23: 581–91.
65. Tröster AI, Fields JA. Frontal cognitive function and memory in Parkinson's disease: toward a distinction between prospective and declarative memory impairments? Behav Neurol 1995; 8: 59–74.
66. Kudlicka A, Clare L, Hindle JV. Executive functions in Parkinson's disease: Systematic review and meta-analysis. Mov Disord 2011; 26: 2305–15.
67. Morris RG, Downes JJ, Sahakian BJ, et al. Planning and spatial working memory in Parkinson's disease. J Neurol Neurosurg Psychiatry 1988; 51: 757–66.
68. Owen AM, Sahakian BJ, Hodges JR, et al. Dopamine-dependent fronto-striatal planning deficits in early Parkinson's disease. Neuropsychology 1995; 9: 126–40.
69. Bechara A, Damasio AR, Damasio H, et al. Insensitivity to future consequences following damage to human prefrontal cortex. Cognition 1994; 50: 7–15.
70. Cools R, Barker RA, Sahakian BJ, et al. L-Dopa medication remediates cognitive inflexibility, but increases impulsivity in patients with Parkinson's disease. Neuropsychologia 2003; 41: 1431–41.
71. Levy G, Jacobs DM, Tang MX, et al. Memory and executive function impairment predict dementia in Parkinson's disease. Mov Disord 2002; 17: 1221–6.
72. Mahieux F, Fenelon G, Flahault A, et al. Neuropsychological prediction of dementia in Parkinson's disease. J Neurol Neurosurg Psychiatry 1998; 64: 178–83.
73. Woods SP, Tröster AI. Prodromal frontal/executive dysfunction predicts incident dementia in Parkinson's disease. J Int Neuropsychol Soc 2003; 9: 17–24.
74. Cahn-Weiner DA, Farias ST, Julian L, et al. Cognitive and neuroimaging predictors of instrumental activities of daily living. J Int Neuropsychol Soc 2007; 13: 747–57.
75. Gunzler SA, Schoenberg MR, Riley DE, et al. Parkinson's disease and other movement disorders. In: Schoenberg MR, Scott JG, eds. The Little Black Boof of Neuropsychology: A Syndrome-Based Approach. New York: Springer, 2011: 567–646.
76. Levin BE, Katzen HL. Early cognitive changes and nondementing behavioral abnormalities in Parkinson's disease. Adv Neurol 2005; 96: 84–94.
77. Skeel RL, Crosson B, Nadeau SE, et al. Basal ganglia dysfunction, working memory, and sentence comprehension in patients with Parkinson's disease. Neuropsychologia 2001; 39: 962–71.
78. Piatt AL, Fields JA, Paolo AM, et al. Lexical, semantic, and action verbal fluency in Parkinson's disease with and without dementia. J Clin Exp Neuropsychol 1999; 21: 435–43.

79. McDowd J, Hoffman L, Rozek E, et al. Understanding verbal fluency in healthy aging, Alzheimer's disease, and Parkinson's disease. Neuropsychology 2011; 25: 210–25.
80. Flowers KA, Robertson C, Sheridan MR. Some characteristics of word fluency in Parkinson's disease. J Neurolinguistics 1995; 9: 33–46.
81. Zec RF, Landreth ES, Fritz S, et al. A comparison of phonemic, semantic, and alternating word fluency in Parkinson's disease. Arch Clin Neuropsychol 1999; 14: 255–64.
82. Henry JD, Crawford JR. Verbal fluency deficits in Parkinson's disease: a meta-analysis. J Int Neuropsychol Soc 2004; 10: 608–22.
83. Tröster AI, Fields JA, Testa JA, et al. Cortical and subcortical influences on clustering and switching in the performance of verbal fluency tasks. Neuropsychologia 1998; 36: 295–304.
84. Frank EM, McDade HL, Scott WK. Naming in dementia secondary to Parkinson's, Huntington's, and Alzheimer's diseases. J Commun Disord 1996; 29: 183–97.
85. Williams-Gray CH, Evans JR, Goris A, et al. The distinct cognitive syndromes of Parkinson's disease: 5 year follow-up of the CamPaIGN cohort. Brain 2009; 132: 2958–69.
86. Jacobs DM, Marder K, Cote LJ, et al. Neuropsychological characteristics of preclinical dementia in Parkinson's disease. Neurology 1995; 45: 1691–6.
87. Passafiume D, Boller F, Keefe MC. Neuropsychological impairment in patients with Parkinson's disease. In: Grant I, Adams KM, eds. Neuropsychological Assessment of Neuropsychiatric Disorders. New York: Oxford University Press, 1986: 374–83.
88. Pereira JB, Junque C, Marti MJ, et al. Neuroanatomical substrate of visuospatial and visuoperceptual impairment in Parkinson's disease. Mov Disord 2009; 24: 1193–9.
89. Pillon B, Ertle S, Deweer B, et al. Memory for spatial location is affected in Parkinson's disease. Neuropsychologia 1996; 34: 77–85.
90. Tröster AI. Neuropsychological characteristics of dementia with Lewy bodies and Parkinson's disease with dementia: differentiation, early detection, and implications for "mild cognitive impairment" and biomarkers. Neuropsychol Rev 2008; 18: 103–19.
91. Abe Y, Kachi T, Kato T, et al. Occipital hypoperfusion in Parkinson's disease without dementia: correlation to impaired cortical visual processing. J Neurol Neurosurg Psychiatry 2003; 74: 419–22.
92. Mosimann UP, Mather G, Wesnes KA, et al. Visual perception in Parkinson disease dementia and dementia with Lewy bodies. Neurology 2004; 63: 2091–6.
93. Ramirez-Ruiz B, Junque C, Marti MJ, et al. Cognitive changes in Parkinson's disease patients with visual hallucinations. Dement Geriatr Cogn Disord 2007; 23: 281–8.
94. Faglioni P, Saetti MC, Botti C. Verbal learning strategies in Parkinson's disease. Neuropsychology 2000; 14: 456–70.
95. Raskin SA, Borod JC, Tweedy J. Neuropsychological aspects of Parkinson's disease. Neuropsychol Rev 1990; 1: 185–221.
96. Taylor AE, Saint-Cyr JA, Lang AE. Frontal lobe dysfunction in Parkinson's disease. The cortical focus of neostriatal outflow. Brain 1986; 109: 845–83.
97. Higginson CI, Wheelock VL, Carroll KE, et al. Recognition memory in Parkinson's disease with and without dementia: evidence inconsistent with the retrieval deficit hypothesis. J Clin Exp Neuropsychol 2005; 27: 516–28.
98. Bronnick K, Alves G, Aarsland D, et al. Verbal memory in drug-naive, newly diagnosed Parkinson's disease. The retrieval deficit hypothesis revisited. Neuropsychology 2011; 25: 114–24.
99. Saykin AJ, Johnson SC, Flashman LA, et al. Functional differentiation of medial temporal and frontal regions involved in processing novel and familiar words: an fMRI study. Brain 1999; 122: 1963–71.
100. Weintraub D, Moberg PJ, Culbertson WC, et al. Evidence for impaired encoding and retrieval memory profiles in Parkinson disease. Cogn Behav Neurol 2004; 17: 195–200.
101. Owen AM, Beksinska M, James M, et al. Visuospatial memory deficits at different stages of Parkinson's disease. Neuropsychologia 1993; 31: 627–44.
102. Leplow B, Dierks C, Herrmann P, et al. Remote memory in Parkinson's disease and senile dementia. Neuropsychologia 1997; 35: 547–57.
103. Freedman M, Rivoira P, Butters N, et al. Retrograde amnesia in Parkinson's disease. Can J Neurol Sci 1984; 11: 297–301.

104. Katai S, Maruyama T, Hashimoto T, et al. Event based and time based prospective memory in Parkinson's disease. J Neurol Neurosurg Psychiatry 2003; 74: 704–9.
105. Bondi MW, Kaszniak AW, Bayles KA, et al. Contributions of frontal system dysfunction to memory and perceptual abilities in Parkinson's disease. Neuropsychology 1993; 7: 89–102.
106. Ferraro FR, Balota DA, Connor LT. Implicit memory and the formation of new associations in nondemented Parkinson's disease individuals and individuals with senile dementia of the Alzheimer type: a serial reaction time (SRT) investigation. Brain Cogn 1993; 21: 163–80.
107. Kuzis G, Sabe L, Tiberti C, et al. Explicit and implicit learning in patients with Alzheimer disease and Parkinson disease with dementia. Neuropsychiatry Neuropsychol Behav Neurol 1999; 12: 265–9.
108. Stern Y, Marder K, Tang MX, et al. Antecedent clinical features associated with dementia in Parkinson's disease. Neurology 1993; 43: 1690–2.
109. Racine CA. Dementia with Lewy bodies. In: Miller BL, Boeve BF, eds. The Behavioral Neurology of Dementia. New York: Cambridge University Press, 2009: 7–26.
110. Emre M, Aarsland D, Brown R, et al. Clinical diagnostic criteria for dementia associated with Parkinson's disease. Mov Disord 2007; 22: 1689–707; quiz 837.
111. Smith GE, Boeve B, Pankratz S, et al. Time course of diagnostic features of Lewy body disease. Neurology 2009; 72: A246.
112. McKeith IG, Dickson DW, Lowe J, et al. Diagnosis and management of dementia with Lewy bodies: third report of the DLB Consortium. Neurology 2005; 65: 1863–72.
113. Aarsland D, Ballard C, Larsen JP, et al. A comparative study of psychiatric symptoms in dementia with Lewy bodies and Parkinson's disease with and without dementia. Int J Geriatr Psychiatry 2001; 16: 528–36.
114. Collerton D, Burn D, McKeith I, et al. Systematic review and meta-analysis show that dementia with Lewy bodies is a visual-perceptual and attentional-executive dementia. Dement Geriatr Cogn Disord 2003; 16: 229–37.
115. Ferman TJ, Boeve BF, Smith GE, et al. Dementia with Lewy bodies may present as dementia and REM sleep behavior disorder without parkinsonism or hallucinations. J Int Neuropsychol Soc 2002; 8: 907–14.
116. Hinnell C, Hurt CS, Landau S, et al. Nonmotor versus motor symptoms: How much do they matter to health status in Parkinson's disease? Mov Disord 2012; 27.
117. Aarsland D, Marsh L, Schrag A. Neuropsychiatric symptoms in Parkinson's disease. Mov Disord 2009; 24: 2175–86.
118. Ishihara L, Brayne C. A systematic review of depression and mental illness preceding Parkinson's disease. Acta Neurol Scand 2006; 113: 211–20.
119. Hubble JP, Cao T, Hassanein RE, et al. Risk factors for Parkinson's disease. Neurology 1993; 43: 1693–7.
120. Sano M, Stern Y, Williams J, et al. Coexisting dementia and depression in Parkinson's disease. Arch Neurol 1989; 46: 1284–6.
121. Fields JA, Norman S, Straits-Tröster KA, et al. The impact of depression on memory in neurodegenerative disease. In: Tröster AI, ed. Memory in Neurodegenerative Disease: Biological, Cognitive, and Clinical Perspectives. Cambridge: Cambridge University Press, 1998: 314–37.
122. Kuzis G, Sabe L, Tiberti C, et al. Cognitive functions in major depression and Parkinson disease. Arch Neurol 1997; 54: 982–6.
123. Norman S, Tröster AI, Fields JA, et al. Effects of depression and Parkinson's disease on cognitive functioning. J Neuropsychiatry Clin Neurosci 2002; 14: 31–6.
124. Marin RS. Differential diagnosis and classification of apathy. Am J Psychiatry 1990; 147: 22–30.
125. Ziropadja L, Stefanova E, Petrovic M, et al. Apathy and depression in Parkinson's disease: the Belgrade PD study report. Parkinsonism Relat Disord 2012; 18: 339–42.
126. Varanese S, Perfetti B, Ghilardi MF, et al. Apathy, but not depression, reflects inefficient cognitive strategies in Parkinson's disease. PLoS One 2011; 6: e17846.
127. Aarsland D, Larsen JP, Lim NG, et al. Range of neuropsychiatric disturbances in patients with Parkinson's disease. J Neurol Neurosurg Psychiatry 1999; 67: 492–6.

128. Dujardin K, Sockeel P, Devos D, et al. Characteristics of apathy in Parkinson's disease. Mov Disord 2007; 22: 778–84.
129. Pluck GC, Brown RG. Apathy in Parkinson's disease. J Neurol Neurosurg Psychiatry 2002; 73: 636–42.
130. Starkstein SE, Mayberg HS, Preziosi TJ, et al. Reliability, validity, and clinical correlates of apathy in Parkinson's disease. J Neuropsychiatry Clin Neurosci 1992 Spring; 4: 134–9.
131. Dujardin K, Sockeel P, Delliaux M, et al. Apathy may herald cognitive decline and dementia in Parkinson's disease. Mov Disord 2009; 24: 2391–7.
132. Schiffer RB, Kurlan R, Rubin A, et al. Evidence for atypical depression in Parkinson's disease. Am J Psychiatry 1988; 145: 1020–2.
133. Mondolo F, Jahanshahi M, Grana A, et al. Evaluation of anxiety in Parkinson's disease with some commonly used rating scales. Neurol Sci 2007; 28: 270–5.
134. Walsh K, Bennett G. Parkinson's disease and anxiety. Postgrad Med J 2001; 77: 89–93.
135. Higginson CI, Fields JA, Koller WC, et al. Questionnaire assessment potentially overestimates anxiety in Parkinson's disease. J Clin Psychol Med Settings 2001; 8: 95–9.
136. Ryder KA, Gontkovsky ST, McSwan KL, et al. Cognitive function in Parkinson's disease: association with anxiety but not depression. Aging Neuropsychol Cogn 2002; 9: 77–84.
137. Bogdanova Y, Cronin-Golomb A. Neurocognitive correlates of apathy and anxiety in Parkinson's disease. Parkinsons Dis 2012; 2012: 793076.
138. Kish SJ, Shannak K, Hornykiewicz O. Uneven pattern of dopamine loss in the striatum of patients with idiopathic Parkinson's disease. Pathophysiologic and clinical implications. N Engl J Med 1988; 318: 876–80.
139. Swainson R, Rogers RD, Sahakian BJ, et al. Probabilistic learning and reversal deficits in patients with Parkinson's disease or frontal or temporal lobe lesions: possible adverse effects of dopaminergic medication. Neuropsychologia 2000; 38: 596–612.
140. Cools R. Dopaminergic modulation of cognitive function-implications for L-DOPA treatment in Parkinson's disease. Neurosci Biobehav Rev 2006; 30: 1–23.
141. Antonini A, Cilia R. Behavioural adverse effects of dopaminergic treatments in Parkinson's disease: incidence, neurobiological basis, management and prevention. Drug Saf 2009; 32: 475–88.
142. Voon V, Thomsen T, Miyasaki JM, et al. Factors associated with dopaminergic drug-related pathological gambling in Parkinson disease. Arch Neurol 2007; 64: 212–16.
143. Richard IH, Justus AW, Greig NH, et al. Worsening of motor function and mood in a patient with Parkinson's disease after pharmacologic challenge with oral rivastigmine. Clin Neuropharmacol 2002; 25: 296–9.
144. Bronstein JM, Tagliati M, Alterman RL, et al. Deep brain stimulation for Parkinson disease: an expert consensus and review of key issues. Arch Neurol 2011; 68: 165.
145. Tröster AI, Fields JA. The role of neuropsychological evaluation in the neurosurgical treatment of movement disorders. In: Tarsy D, Vitek JL, Lozano AM, eds. Surgical Treatment of Parkinson's Disease and Other Movement Disorders. Totowa, NJ: Humana Press, 2003: 213–40.
146. Alvarez L, Macias R, Pavon N, et al. Therapeutic efficacy of unilateral subthalamotomy in Parkinson's disease: results in 89 patients followed for up to 36 months. J Neurol Neurosurg Psychiatry 2009; 80: 979–85.
147. Bickel S, Alvarez L, Macias R, et al. Cognitive and neuropsychiatric effects of subthalamotomy for Parkinson's disease. Parkinsonism Relat Disord 2010; 16: 535–9.
148. Alvarez L, Macias R, Lopez G, et al. Bilateral subthalamotomy in Parkinson's disease: initial and long-term response. Brain 2005; 128: 570–83.
149. Gironell A, Kulisevsky J, Rami L, et al. Effects of pallidotomy and bilateral subthalamic stimulation on cognitive function in Parkinson disease. A controlled comparative study. J Neurol 2003; 250: 917–23.
150. Smeding HM, Esselink RA, Schmand B, et al. Unilateral pallidotomy versus bilateral subthalamic nucleus stimulation in PD--a comparison of neuropsychological effects. J Neurol 2005; 252: 176–82.
151. Alegret M, Valldeoriola F, Tolosa E, et al. Cognitive effects of unilateral posteroventral pallidotomy: a 4-year follow-up study. Mov Disord 2003; 18: 323–8.

152. Hariz MI, Bergenheim AT. A 10-year follow-up review of patients who underwent Leksell's posteroventral pallidotomy for Parkinson disease. J Neurosurg 2001; 94: 552–8.
153. Strutt AM, Lai EC, Jankovic J, et al. Five-year follow-up of unilateral posteroventral pallidotomy in Parkinson's disease. Surg Neurol 2009; 71: 551–8.
154. Voon V, Kubu C, Krack P, et al. Deep brain stimulation: neuropsychological and neuropsychiatric issues. Mov Disord 2006; S305–27.
155. Hugdahl K, Wester K. Neurocognitive correlates of stereotactic thalamotomy and thalamic stimulation in Parkinsonian patients. Brain Cogn 2000; 42: 231–52.
156. Tröster AI, Fields JA, Wilkinson SB, et al. Neuropsychological functioning before and after unilateral thalamic stimulating electrode implantation in Parkinson's disease. Neurosurgical Focus 1997; 2: 1–6.
157. Woods SP, Fields JA, Lyons KE, et al. Neuropsychological and quality of life changes following unilateral thalamic deep brain stimulation in Parkinson's disease: a one-year follow-up. Acta Neurochir (Wien) 2001; 143: 1273–7; discussion 8.
158. Schuurman PR, Bruins J, Merkus MP, et al. A comparison of neuropsychological effects of thalamotomy and thalamic stimulation. Neurology 2002; 59: 1232–9.
159. Fields JA, Tröster AI, Wilkinson SB, et al. Cognitive outcome following staged bilateral pallidal stimulation for the treatment of Parkinson's disease. Clin Neurol Neurosurg 1999; 101: 182–8.
160. Ghika J, Villemure JG, Fankhauser H, et al. Efficiency and safety of bilateral contemporaneous pallidal stimulation (deep brain stimulation) in levodopa-responsive patients with Parkinson's disease with severe motor fluctuations: a 2-year follow-up review. J Neurosurg 1998; 89: 713–18.
161. Trepanier LL, Kumar R, Lozano AM, et al. Neuropsychological outcome of GPi pallidotomy and GPi or STN deep brain stimulation in Parkinson's disease. Brain Cogn 2000; 42: 324–47.
162. Tröster AI, Fields JA, Wilkinson SB, et al. Unilateral pallidal stimulation for Parkinson's disease: neurobehavioral functioning before and 3 months after electrode implantation. Neurology 1997; 49: 1078–83.
163. Volkmann J. Deep brain stimulation for the treatment of Parkinson's disease. J Clin Neurophysiol 2004; 21: 6–17.
164. Rothlind JC, Cockshott RW, Starr PA, et al. Neuropsychological performance following staged bilateral pallidal or subthalamic nucleus deep brain stimulation for Parkinson's disease. J Int Neuropsychol Soc 2007; 13: 68–79.
165. Rouaud T, Dondaine T, Drapier S, et al. Pallidal stimulation in advanced Parkinson's patients with contraindications for subthalamic stimulation. Mov Disord 2010; 25: 1839–46.
166. Fraraccio M, Ptito A, Sadikot A, et al. Absence of cognitive deficits following deep brain stimulation of the subthalamic nucleus for the treatment of Parkinson's disease. Arch Clin Neuropsychol 2008; 23: 399–408.
167. Heo JH, Lee KM, Paek SH, et al. The effects of bilateral subthalamic nucleus deep brain stimulation (STN DBS) on cognition in Parkinson disease. J Neurol Sci 2008; 273: 19–24.
168. Parsons TD, Rogers SA, Braaten AJ, et al. Cognitive sequelae of subthalamic nucleus deep brain stimulation in Parkinson's disease: a meta-analysis. Lancet Neurol 2006; 5: 578–88.
169. Mikos A, Zahodne L, Okun MS, et al. Cognitive declines after unilateral deep brain stimulation surgery in Parkinson's disease: a controlled study using Reliable Change, part II. Clin Neuropsychol 2010; 24: 235–45.
170. Witt K, Daniels C, Reiff J, et al. Neuropsychological and psychiatric changes after deep brain stimulation for Parkinson's disease: a randomised, multicentre study. Lancet Neurol 2008; 7: 605–14.
171. York MK, Dulay M, Macias A, et al. Cognitive declines following bilateral subthalamic nucleus deep brain stimulation for the treatment of Parkinson's disease. J Neurol Neurosurg Psychiatry 2008; 79: 789–95.
172. Zahodne LB, Okun MS, Foote KD, et al. Cognitive declines one year after unilateral deep brain stimulation surgery in Parkinson's disease: a controlled study using reliable change. Clin Neuropsychol 2009; 23: 385–405.

173. Weaver FM, Follett K, Stern M, et al. Bilateral deep brain stimulation vs best medical therapy for patients with advanced Parkinson disease: a randomized controlled trial. JAMA 2009; 301: 63–73.
174. Tan SK, Hartung H, Sharp T, et al. Serotonin-dependent depression in Parkinson's disease: a role for the subthalamic nucleus? Neuropharmacology 2011; 61: 387–99.
175. Funkiewiez A, Ardouin C, Caputo E, et al. Long term effects of bilateral subthalamic nucleus stimulation on cognitive function, mood, and behaviour in Parkinson's disease. J Neurol Neurosurg Psychiatry 2004; 75: 834–9.
176. Burkhard PR, Vingerhoets FJ, Berney A, et al. Suicide after successful deep brain stimulation for movement disorders. Neurology 2004; 63: 2170–2.
177. Voon V, Krack P, Lang AE, et al. A multicentre study on suicide outcomes following subthalamic stimulation for Parkinson's disease. Brain 2008; 131: 2720–8.
178. Broen M, Duits A, Visser-Vandewalle V, et al. Impulse control and related disorders in Parkinson's disease patients treated with bilateral subthalamic nucleus stimulation: a review. Parkinsonism Relat Disord 2011; 17: 413–17.
179. Lang AE, Houeto JL, Krack P, et al. Deep brain stimulation: preoperative issues. Mov Disord 2006; 21: S171–96.
180. Trott CT, Fahn S, Greene P, et al. Cognition following bilateral implants of embryonic dopamine neurons in PD: a double blind study. Neurology 2003; 60: 1938–43.
181. Thompson LL, Cullum CM, O'Neill S, et al. Effects of fetal cell transplantation on cognitive and psychological functioning in Parkinson's disease. Arch Clin Neuropsychol 1997; 12: 416.
182. Brown RG, Lacomblez L, Landwehrmeyer BG, et al. Cognitive impairment in patients with multiple system atrophy and progressive supranuclear palsy. Brain 2010; 133: 2382–93.
183. Josephs KA, Dickson DW. Diagnostic accuracy of progressive supranuclear palsy in the society for progressive supranuclear palsy brain bank. Mov Disord 2003; 18: 1018–26.
184. O'Sullivan SS, Massey LA, Williams DR, et al. Clinical outcomes of progressive supranuclear palsy and multiple system atrophy. Brain 2008; 131: 1362–72.
185. Pillon B, Dubois B, Ploska A, et al. Severity and specificity of cognitive impairment in Alzheimer's, Huntington's, and Parkinson's diseases and progressive supranuclear palsy. Neurology 1991; 41: 634–43.
186. McMonagle P, Kertesz A. Cognition in corticobasal degeneration and progressive supranuclear palsy. In: Miller BL, Boeve BF, eds. The Behavioral Neurology of Dementia. New York: Cambridge University Press, 2009: 288–301.
187. Millar D, Griffiths P, Zermansky AJ, et al. Characterizing behavioral and cognitive dysexecutive changes in progressive supranuclear palsy. Mov Disord 2006; 21: 199–207.
188. Dubois B, Pillon B, Legault F, et al. Slowing of cognitive processing in progressive supranuclear palsy. A comparison with Parkinson's disease. Arch Neurol 1988; 45: 1194–9.
189. Soliveri P, Monza D, Paridi D, et al. Neuropsychological follow up in patients with Parkinson's disease, striatonigral degeneration-type multisystem atrophy, and progressive supranuclear palsy. J Neurol Neurosurg Psychiatry 2000; 69: 313–18.
190. Bak TH, Crawford LM, Hearn VC, et al. Subcortical dementia revisited: similarities and differences in cognitive function between progressive supranuclear palsy (PSP), corticobasal degeneration (CBD) and multiple system atrophy (MSA). Neurocase 2005; 11: 268–73.
191. Lange KW, Tucha O, Alders GL, et al. Differentiation of parkinsonian syndromes according to differences in executive functions. J Neural Transm 2003; 110: 983–95.
192. Grafman J, Litvan I, Stark M. Neuropsychological features of progressive supranuclear palsy. Brain Cogn 1995; 28: 311–20.
193. Pillon B, Blin J, Vidailhet M, et al. The neuropsychological pattern of corticobasal degeneration: comparison with progressive supranuclear palsy and Alzheimer's disease. Neurology 1995; 45: 1477–83.
194. Testa D, Monza D, Ferrarini M, et al. Comparison of natural histories of progressive supranuclear palsy and multiple system atrophy. Neurol Sci 2001; 22: 247–51.

195. Bhidayasiri R, Ling H. Multiple system atrophy. Neurologist 2008; 14: 224–37.
196. Gilman S, Wenning GK, Low PA, et al. Second consensus statement on the diagnosis of multiple system atrophy. Neurology 2008; 71: 670–6.
197. Vanacore N. Epidemiological evidence on multiple system atrophy. J Neural Transm 2005; 112: 1605–12.
198. Wenning GK, Ben-Shlomo Y, Hughes A, et al. What clinical features are most useful to distinguish definite multiple system atrophy from Parkinson's disease? J Neurol Neurosurg Psychiatry 2000; 68: 434–40.
199. Dujardin K, Defebvre L, Krystkowiak P, et al. Executive function differences in multiple system atrophy and Parkinson's disease. Parkinsonism Relat Disord 2003; 9: 205–11.
200. Monza D, Soliveri P, Radice D, et al. Cognitive dysfunction and impaired organization of complex motility in degenerative parkinsonian syndromes. Arch Neurol 1998; 55: 372–8.
201. Burk K, Daum I, Rub U. Cognitive function in multiple system atrophy of the cerebellar type. Mov Disord 2006; 21: 772–6.
202. Kawai Y, Suenaga M, Takeda A, et al. Cognitive impairments in multiple system atrophy: MSA-C vs MSA-P. Neurology 2008; 70: 1390–6.
203. Berciano J. Olivopontocerebellar atrophy. A review of 117 cases. J Neurol Sci 1982; 53: 253–72.
204. Pharr V, Uttl B, Stark M, et al. Comparison of apraxia in corticobasal degeneration and progressive supranuclear palsy. Neurology 2001; 56: 957–63.
205. Boeve BF. Early clinical features of the parkinsonian-related dementias. In: Miller BL, Boeve BF, eds. The Behavioral Neurology of Dementia. New York: Cambridge University Press, 2009: 197–212.
206. Graham NL, Bak TH, Hodges JR. Corticobasal degeneration as a cognitive disorder. Mov Disord 2003; 18: 1224–32.
207. Grimes DA, Lang AE, Bergeron CB. Dementia as the most common presentation of cortical-basal ganglionic degeneration. Neurology 1999; 53: 1969–74.
208. Murray R, Neumann M, Forman MS, et al. Cognitive and motor assessment in autopsy-proven corticobasal degeneration. Neurology 2007; 68: 1274–83.
209. Beatty WW, Scott JG, Wilson DA, et al. Memory deficits in a demented patient with probable corticobasal degeneration. J Geriatr Psychiatry Neurol 1995; 8: 132–6.
210. Dubois B, Slachevsky A, Litvan I, et al. The FAB: a Frontal Assessment Battery at bedside. Neurology 2000; 55: 1621–6.
211. Frisoni GB, Pizzolato G, Zanetti O, et al. Corticobasal degeneration: neuropsychological assessment and dopamine D2 receptor SPECT analysis. Eur Neurol 1995; 35: 50–4.
212. Graham NL, Bak T, Patterson K, et al. Language function and dysfunction in corticobasal degeneration. Neurology 2003; 61: 493–9.
213. Bak TH, Caine D, Hearn VC, et al. Visuospatial functions in atypical parkinsonian syndromes. J Neurol Neurosurg Psychiatry 2006; 77: 454–6.
214. Arvanitakis Z, Graff-Radford N. Focal degenerative dementia syndromes. Clin Geriatr Med 2001; 17: 303–18.

9 Management of anxiety and depression

Jack J. Chen

INTRODUCTION

Anxiety and depressive disturbances have become recognized as common nonmotor, psychiatric comorbidities in idiopathic Parkinson's disease (PD), which contribute to additional disability, such as significant impairments of cognitive, functional, motor, and social performance. This leads to reductions in quality of life, high levels of care dependency, and increased caregiver distress (1–8). Preliminary data suggest that depression may be an independent predictor of mortality in patients with PD (9). However, these affective disturbances are under-recognized and under-treated in patients with PD due to diagnostic imprecision, symptom overlap with motor and cognitive features of PD, complexity of diagnosis, health care access and resources, and under-reporting of symptoms by patients and caregivers (10–12).

In the presence of other comorbid psychiatric conditions, depressive symptoms, quality of life, and functional domains are further worsened. In PD, anxiety and depressive symptoms can occur as isolated disorders or can coexist (i.e., anxious-depressed phenotype) (13). The presence of anxiety with depression has been found to increase the severity of depressive symptoms and to delay the response to psychotropic treatment. Therefore, effective detection and treatment of anxiety and depression are important aspects of PD management. This chapter discusses the epidemiology, possible mechanisms, recognition, and management of these affective disorders in idiopathic PD.

ANXIETY
Epidemiology

In James Parkinson's original monograph, *An Essay on the Shaking Palsy*, only a brief mention was made of the nonmotor symptoms of anxiety and depression (14). However, it is now known that clinically significant anxiety symptoms occur in 20% to greater than 50% of PD patients, a frequency greater than that found in community dwelling age-matched controls (3,8,15,16). Notably, anxiety and depressive syndromes are frequently comorbid findings. Menza et al. (17) reported a depressive disorder in 92% of PD patients diagnosed with an anxiety disorder, and an anxiety disorder was present in 67% of depressed PD patients. This is consistent with results by Starkstein et al. (18), reporting depression in 76% of patients with PD and anxiety.

In addition to generalized anxiety disorder (GAD), patients with PD regardless of gender also experience panic disorders and social phobias with a prevalence of approximately 30%. (19–21). Some persons with PD may perceive themselves as "disfigured" and may experience significant distress in social interaction and develop social anxiety secondary to PD (22). The presence of anxiety not only contributes to mental and somatic discomfort, but may also contribute to existing motor symptoms or fluctuations. For example, patients will report that episodic states of anxiety will aggravate pre-existing tremor or dyskinesia, and fear of falling has been associated with impaired postural stability. Additionally, an "internal tremor" is frequently associated with anxiety. Consequently, in patients with high levels of anxiety or significant episodic anxiety, the initiation of appropriate anxiolytic therapy may improve motor symptoms as well as mental and psychosocial functioning.

Mechanisms

Several theories have been proposed to explain the occurrence of anxiety in PD, but overall, little is known. Anxiety in PD is attributed to a combination of medical, neurochemical, and psychosocial phenomena. In a subset of patients, anxiety disorders are a "reactive" response secondary to the diagnosis of PD. However, when compared with non-PD patients with chronic illnesses and similar disability, patients with PD have significantly more severe anxiety (23). Epidemiologic observations indicate that patients with PD are at greater risk of developing anxiety disorders before the diagnosis of PD (24,25). These findings suggest that anxiety may be an early nonmotor phenotype of PD and that disability, although it may contribute to anxiety, is not the sole etiologic determinant.

Anxiety has been associated with motor fluctuations (26–28). During medication "off " phases, patients may experience feelings of despair, hopelessness, and panic that dissipate during the "on" phases (21). Frequency of freezing is also highly correlated with the presence of panic disorders and secondary panic attacks (29). However, emotional fluctuations do not always correlate temporally with motor state (30,31). In a study of 87 patients with PD, 29% had fluctuations in anxiety, 24% in motor, and 21% in mood (30). Of the patients with motor fluctuations, 75% had mood and/or anxiety fluctuations that did not necessarily correlate with motor state. Although the pattern of anxiety or mood fluctuations can be heterogeneous, adjustment of antiparkinson medications to minimize the motor fluctuations can be beneficial.

Neurochemically, degeneration of subcortical nuclei and ascending dopamine, norepinephrine, and serotonin (5-HT) pathways within the basal ganglia–frontal circuits may be responsible for symptoms of anxiety (32–35). Remy et al. (35) utilized [^{11}C]RTI-32 positron emission tomography (PET), an in vivo marker of both dopamine and norepinephrine transporter binding, to localize differences between eight depressed and 12 nondepressed patients with PD matched for age, disease duration, and antiparkinsonian medication. Exploratory analyses revealed that the severity of anxiety in the PD patients was inversely correlated with binding of [^{11}C]RTI-32 in the amygdala, locus coeruleus, and thalamus. These results suggest that anxiety in PD might be associated with a specific loss of dopaminergic and noradrenergic innervation in the locus coeruleus and the limbic system.

Detection and Recognition

An attentive and careful history is vital for recognition of anxiety disturbances in PD. Specific inquiry about symptoms should occur, especially when the history provided by the patient or family suggests that anxiety phenomena are prominent in the context of day-to-day function or in relationship to medication effects, as with "on-off" non-motor fluctuations. While the fundamental feature of an anxiety disorder is unwarranted apprehension or anxiety, establishing the diagnosis of an anxiety disorder can be challenging in patients with PD. Diagnostic imprecision may occur because several symptoms of anxiety overlap with mental and somatic symptoms commonly associated with PD and many patients have clinically significant anxiety that does not correspond directly to the *Diagnostic and Statistical Manual of Mental Disorders-Fourth Edition (DSM-IV)* criteria (36). For example, generalized anxiety disorder in the general population includes a period of at least six months with prominent tension, worry, and feelings of apprehension about everyday events and problems, along with the presence of at least three of six other symptoms, including sleep disturbance, difficulty concentrating, muscle tension, and three others. Panic attacks require unprovoked episodes of severe apprehension accompanied by at least four of 22 various autonomic, psychic, and somatic symptoms (36). However, since several of the accompanying symptoms, such as tremor, concentration difficulties, dizziness, muscle aches, and numbness or tingling, are also commonly attributed to PD, they may not be recognized as components of an anxiety disorder.

Given that anxiety appears to be common over the course of PD, periodic assessment would significantly enhance detection. In a clinic-based study, Shulman et al. (16) reported that recognition of anxiety more than doubled (from 19% to 39%) when patients were screened with the Beck Anxiety Inventory (BAI). The BAI, the Hamilton Anxiety Rating Scale and Hospital Anxiety and Depression Scale-anxiety subscale (HADS-A) have demonstrated variable clinimetric performance in the PD population (37–43). Because anxiety and depressive symptoms are frequently comorbid in PD, a finding of anxiety should also prompt a screening for depression.

Treatment
Agents that possess anxiolytic properties include benzodiazepines, buspirone, mirtazapine, nefazodone, selective serotonin reuptake inhibitors (SSRIs), trazodone, tricyclic antidepressants (TCAs), and venlafaxine. Although several agents, including bromazepam, buspirone, citalopram, paroxetine, and sertraline, have been specifically evaluated for the treatment of anxiety in PD (44–48), overall there is relatively limited evidence available on pharmacotherapy. Nonpharmacologic therapies, including cognitive and behavioral therapies (with or without pharmacotherapy) may be particularly effective and warrant additional investigation.

Benzodiazepines
Although benzodiazepines are commonly used in the management of anxiety, only one randomized controlled trial addressed this in the PD population (44). Bromazepam, a long-acting benzodiazepine, was reported to improve psychic and somatic (i.e., tremor) symptoms of anxiety. Anecdotally, other benzodiazepines have also been noted to be effective. Clonazepam was reported to be effective in a patient with anxiety and panic attacks that were refractory to alprazolam, lorazepam, and numerous antidepressants (49). Although benzodiazepines may be effective, long-term use, especially in the elderly or frail patient, may be associated with unfavorable effects on alertness, cognition, and gait, and an increased risk of falls (50). Therefore, benzodiazepines should be used judiciously with careful evaluation of potential risks and benefits.

Selective Serotonin Reuptake Inhibitors
Results from uncontrolled studies suggest that SSRIs are effective for anxiety in PD (46–48). In an open-label study ($n = 10$), Menza et al. (46) reported that citalopram

(mean dose 19 mg/day) improved anxiety in depressed PD patients. In a study of 30 patients, paroxetine (20 mg twice daily) reduced psychic and somatic anxiety symptoms, as well as depressive symptoms after six weeks (47). Sertraline was also found to have anxiolytic effects in PD patients (48). Although these data are derived from uncontrolled studies, many specialists prefer to use SSRIs for managing anxiety and depression in PD (51).

The SSRIs are relatively well tolerated, although acute, treatment-emergent side effects, such as agitation, diarrhea/loose stools, insomnia, nausea, and sedation, may occur. Occasionally, SSRIs may worsen tremor, and chronic use is associated with an increased risk of developing endocrinologic and metabolic adverse effects, such as hyponatremia, sexual dysfunction, and weight gain (Table 9.1) (52). Reversible SSRI-induced worsening of parkinsonism has also been reported but is uncommon (53–55). For patients on a concomitant monoamine oxidase-B (MAO-B) inhibitor (e.g., rasagiline, selegiline) for PD and SSRIs, there is a theoretic concern for occurrence of 5-HT syndrome. In one survey-based study, the frequency of 5-HT syndrome in patients on concomitant selegiline was 0.24%, with 0.04% of patients experiencing serious symptoms (56). In a review of several studies that assessed the combination of rasagiline with antidepressant therapy in PD, the combination was well tolerated and no 5-HT syndrome was detected (57). Abrupt discontinuation of SSRIs after extended treatment may precipitate a withdrawal or discontinuation

TABLE 9.1   Comparison of Selected Antidepressant Side Effects

	Sedation	Antimuscarinic	Hypotension	Weight Gain	Sexual Dysfunction
TCAs					
Amitriptyline	+++	+++	++	+++	+
Doxepin	++	+++	++	++	+
Imipramine	++	++	+++	++	+
Desipramine	+	+	+	+	0
Nortriptyline	+	+	+	+	0
SSRIs					
Citalopram	+	+	0	+	++
Escitalopram	+	+	0	+	++
Fluoxetine	0	0	0	+	+++
Fluvoxamine	0	0	0	++	++
Paroxetine	+	+	0	++	+++
Sertraline	0	0	0	+	+++
Other					
Bupropion	0	+	0	0	0
Desvenlafaxine	+	+	0	+	+
Duloxetine	+	++	0	0	++
Mirtazapine	++[a]	+	++	+++[a]	++
Nefazodone	++	0	++	0	+
Venlafaxine	+	+	0	+	+++

[a]At low doses.
Abbreviations: +, minor; ++, moderate; +++, major; 0, nonsignificant; SSRIs, selective serotonin reuptake inhibitors; TCAs, tricyclic antidepressants.
Source: From Ref. 52.

syndrome, characterized by somatic and psychological symptoms that resemble anxiety (58). Therefore, if discontinuation is required, a gradual tapering of the dosage is recommended, particularly with short half-life agents, such as paroxetine.

Miscellaneous Agents

Buspirone, an anxiolytic with partial 5-HT agonism and low sedative potential, has not been evaluated in a controlled manner for the management of anxiety in PD. However, in a 12-week randomized, controlled study ($n = 16$) evaluating the effect of buspirone on PD motor symptoms, moderate doses (10–40 mg/day) of buspirone were associated with a modest beneficial effect on anxiety (45). Higher daily doses (i.e., 100 mg) of buspirone significantly enhanced anxiety and worsened parkinsonism. In a three-week randomized, controlled study ($n = 10$) evaluating the effect of low-dose buspirone on levodopa-induced dyskinesia, no significant effect on anxiety was noted (59). However, since the therapeutic onset of buspirone requires up to six weeks, the short duration of this study may not have been sufficient to detect any significant anxiolytic effect.

DEPRESSION
Epidemiology

Depressive symptomatology may occur at any stage of PD and is a major factor related to poor quality of life for both patients and caregivers, with caregiver distress highly correlated with the patient's severity of depression (6,10,60,61). Depressive symptoms and disorders are common in PD. In a community-based study, the prevalence of depressive symptomatology in PD patients was six times that of healthy age- and gender-matched controls (62). In a registry-based study of 211,245 patients, Nilsson et al. (63) compared the incidence of depression in PD patients ($n = 11,698$) with non-PD patients with diabetes ($n = 91,318$) and non-PD patients with osteoarthritis ($n = 10,822$) who were matched for degree of disability. An increased probability of developing a depressive episode was found for patients with PD when compared with the diabetes and osteoarthritis groups. Nilsson et al. (64) also showed that patients with an affective disorder (depression or mania) had an increased risk of being diagnosed with PD (odds ratio 2.2) when compared with patients having osteoarthritis or diabetes.

In an analysis of 10 studies that used DSM-III criteria to define depression, an aggregate prevalence of 42% was reported for depressive disorders in PD (65). The prevalence rates of dysthymia, minor depression, and major depression in PD patients were 22.5%, 36.6%, and 24.8%, respectively. Studies using DSM-IV criteria and a structured clinical interview reported similar results, with the prevalence of major depression ranging from 20% to 25% in PD (12,66–68). Additionally, depression or depressive symptoms appear to occur more frequently in the presence of advanced disease, anxiety, cognitive impairment, and psychosis (15,62,69,70).

In an international survey of over 1000 PD patients, more than 50% of patients displayed clinically significant depressive symptomatology (6). In a clinic-based study of over 350 patients with PD, clinically significant depressive symptomatology was present in 57% of patients, with 40.2% considered mildly to moderately depressed and 16.7% classified as moderately to severely depressed (69).

Patients with PD may also suffer from depressive symptoms that do not meet criteria for major depression, minor depression, or dysthymic disorder, but nonetheless seem to have clinical relevance. Subsyndromal depression is defined as the presence of two or more depressive symptoms at subthreshold levels (i.e., short duration or not present most of the day or nearly every day) (71). Patients with depressive symptoms only during medication "off " states may be classified as having subsyndromal depression. With the inclusion of clinically important subsyndromal depressive disorders, the prevalence of clinically significant depressive symptomatology is present in greater than 40% of patients with PD (6,12,16,62,69).

Mechanisms

The underlying mechanism for depression in PD remains poorly understood, but the phenotypic expression of depressive disorders has been attributed to a combination of medical, neurochemical, and psychosocial phenomena. Depression may be a "reactive" response or demoralization phenomenon associated with the diagnosis of PD and its relative disability. However, when compared with patients with other chronic disabling conditions matched for functional disability, patients with PD exhibit greater depressive symptomatology (72). Additionally, in patients with PD, depression often precedes the onset of motor symptoms (26,73,74), and the natural history of depression in PD does not parallel the progression of physical symptoms, suggesting that it is an independent process (75,76). In comparison with control subjects, patients with PD are approximately twice as likely to experience a mood disorder (anxiety, depression, nervousness, overstrain) in the 10 years preceding onset of motor symptoms (73). These findings suggest that, in a subset of patients, depression may be an early nonmotor phenotype of PD and that disability, although it may contribute to depressive symptoms in PD, is not the sole etiologic determinant (77). As with anxiety, mood fluctuations are sometimes associated with medication "on" and "off " states. Levodopa-induced elevations in plasma homocysteine levels in patients with PD were associated with greater depressive symptomatology, as well as impaired performance on a battery of cognitive tests (78). The association between elevated homocysteine levels and psychiatric symptomatology requires further investigation.

Affective and behavioral changes (e.g., aggression, depression, mania) have also been reported as complications of deep brain stimulation (DBS), especially subthalamic nucleus (STN) DBS (79–82). In contrast, depression or worsening depression is infrequent after thalamic and pallidal DBS. Although the STN itself is unlikely to directly influence the serotonergic midbrain system (e.g., dorsal raphe nucleus), STN stimulation may result in serotonin inhibition via interconnecting pathways and regions (e.g., substantia nigra pars reticulata, medial prefrontal cortex, ventral pallidum) (83). Mood disturbances induced by STN DBS could be the result of stimulation spreading to adjacent nonmotor circuits, aberrant electrode placement, or activation of inappropriate contacts, resulting in stimulation of adjacent cells or fiber tracts. In some cases, alteration of the contact selection reverses the depression (84,85) Additionally, anxiety or depressive symptoms may be due to exacerbation or unmasking of previously existing disorders (86). It is also possible that depressive or anxiety symptoms may be a reactive response if the procedure was less successful than anticipated and, in some cases, depressive symptoms may be part of a "dopaminergic withdrawal syndrome" that occurs secondary to postprocedure dose-reduction of dopamimetic agents.

Pathologic degeneration of mesolimbic dopamine, norepinephrine, and 5-HT pathways in conjunction with degeneration of orbital–frontal circuits and subcortical structures, such as the locus coeruleus, dorsal raphe nuclei, and ventral tegmental area, are postulated to be associated with the expression of depressive symptoms (35,87–92). Morphologic and functional neuroimaging studies demonstrate that in PD, depression is correlated with reduced activity in depression-related neural networks, including prefrontal lobes (e.g., inferior and medial), thalamus, anterior and posterior cingulate (91). An in vivo single photon emission computed tomography study with [^{123}I] β-carboxymethoxy-iodophenyl tropane (β-CIT) demonstrated that in patients with PD, disruption of the brainstem raphe 5-HT system is highly correlated with mood and mentation (92). Overall, the studies on the functional anatomy of depression in PD demonstrate that deficits in serotoninergic and noradrenergic innervations to cortical and subcortical components are involved.

Detection and Assessment

Recognition of depressive disturbances in PD requires awareness and specific inquiry about symptoms, especially when the history provided by the patient or family is suggestive that depressive phenomena are prominent in the context of day-to-day function. The recognition of depressive symptoms in PD and diagnostic issues remain an active area of refinement in PD research (11). In a clinic-based study, nearly two-thirds of patients with clinically significant depressive symptomatology were not receiving antidepressant therapy (12). Older individuals often under-report depressive symptoms and are likely to focus on somatic or vegetative complaints (e.g., fatigue or loss of energy, reduced sexual desire or functioning, pain, sleep changes, or appetite changes), which are the prominent features of mood disorders as well as PD (93). Patients may simply attribute any mood symptoms to their PD, even when their PD has been relatively stable and the mood changes are relatively acute. In one study, over half the patients who had clinically significant depressive symptoms did not consider themselves depressed (12).

The assessment and recognition of depression has been ranked highly as an indicator for improving care of PD patients (94). All PD patients should be screened periodically to detect clinically significant depressive symptomatology. However, follow-up and availability of mental health services must be available. In a clinic-based study, the detection of depressive symptomatology in patients with PD more than doubled (21–44%) when patients were screened using the Beck Depression Inventory (BDI) (16). If self-reported disability is out of proportion to findings on the neurologic examination, depression should be suspected. Caregivers or family members are often valuable sources of information about the patient's psychological well-being, especially when self-report may be unreliable.

The DSM-IV diagnostic criteria for major depression includes the persistent presence of five of the following nine symptoms: anhedonia, depressed mood, diminished ability to think or concentrate, fatigue or loss of energy, feelings of worthlessness or inappropriate guilt, insomnia or hypersomnia, psychomotor agitation or retardation, recurrent thoughts of death, and significant weight gain or loss (36). Although the core features of a depressive syndrome (i.e., anhedonia, diminished interest level, sadness) are requisite features for diagnosing DSM-IV depression, the assessment of depression in patients with PD is not always straightforward and uncertainties remain (11). Both anhedonia and decreased interest along with several of the additional depressive symptoms overlap with features of PD. This is highlighted by a study demonstrating that anergy, early morning awakening, and psychomotor retardation are common and similarly frequent in both depressed and nondepressed patients with PD (95). Despite overlap of symptomatology, the core affective features of depression (i.e., anhedonia, diminished interest level, sadness) should be present (96).

Clinician-completed symptom rating scales can be used as a screening tool to provide a measure of symptom severity or response to treatment. Examples include the Hamilton Depression Rating Scale (HAMD) and the Montgomery–Asberg Depression Rating Scale that have been validated for use in the PD population (68,97–99).

Despite the issue of overlapping somatic complaints of depression from underlying medical illnesses or consequence of aging, key psychological symptoms of depression, such as anhedonia, sad mood, decreased interest in normally pleasurable activities or social avoidance, remain helpful for screening and assessment. The United States Preventive Services Task Force (USPST) has recommended screening for depression in all adults, regardless of medical comorbidities (100). For routine clinical purposes, the USPST recommends asking the patient two questions: "Over the past two weeks, have you felt down or hopeless?" and "Over the past two weeks, have you felt little interest in doing things?" A "yes" to either question is a positive screen and warrants additional investigation. If depression screening is implemented, there should be access to mental health support.

If there is adequate follow-up assessment and treatment of patients, self-report instruments may be an effective means of screening for depressive symptomatology in patients with PD. Several standardized, self-report instruments that are easily and rapidly administered in the outpatient setting are available and can be scored by physicians or allied health professionals. Examples include the BDI, Geriatric Depression Scale (GDS), HADS, Zung Self-Rating Scale, and the Center for Epidemiologic Studies Depression Scale (42,101–104). Although the 21-item BDI contains several somatic items, it has been determined to be a valid and internally consistent instrument for screening depression in the PD population if the cutoff score is modified (105–107). Instruments that are free of somatic items include the 30-item GDS (GDS-30) (103), the 15-item GDS (GDS-15) (108), and the seven -item depression component of the HADS (42), all of which have been found to be clinimetrically suitable for use in the PD population (43,109–113). A 12-item shortform BDI, which excludes somatic items, has also been used to assess depression in PD (114).

A physical examination and laboratory screening (e.g., complete blood count, liver function, serum testosterone level, serum vitamin B12, thyroid function) should be performed to exclude potential systemic causes of depressive symptomatology. Testosterone deficiency is also associated with depressive symptomatology (e.g., anhedonia, fatigue, and sexual dysfunction) and, likewise, symptoms of hypothyroidism (e.g., anxiety, difficulty with concentration, dysphoria, fatigue, irritability, and motor retardation) resemble depressive symptomatology. It is also important to ensure that patients are on optimal doses of antiparkinson drugs to minimize motor fluctuations that may contribute to mood fluctuations.

Treatment

Depression in PD patients often persists or worsens longitudinally, and untreated minor depression commonly progresses to major depression. Therefore, even mild depressive disturbances should be considered clinically significant and should warrant monitoring if not definitive treatment. The efficacy and safety of various antidepressants in the management of depression in patients with PD has been addressed in numerous uncontrolled (46,55,115–132) and controlled studies (133–149). A review and meta-analysis of 10 studies, demonstrated uncertainty and a lack of strong randomized evidence supporting the clinical benefit of SSRIs or TCAs for depression in PD (150). However, despite limited randomized evidence to support the efficacy of antidepressants in PD depression, the SSRIs are generally well tolerated and a trial of these agents is warranted. An evidence-based review by the Movement Disorder Society concluded that the secondary amine TCAs (i.e., desipramine, nortriptyline) are likely efficacious and possibly useful but side effects are common (151).

Pharmacologic Treatment
Selective Serotonin Reuptake Inhibitors
The SSRIs are the most commonly prescribed antidepressants in patients with PD (152). This is presumably due to better tolerability over other antidepressants. The SSRIs inhibit the synaptosomal reuptake of 5-HT and are generally preferred over the TCAs because of better overall tolerability (Table 9.1). For the management of depression in patients with PD, all currently available SSRIs have been studied; albeit the numbers of patients in most trials have been relatively small. Results from uncontrolled retrospective and prospective studies suggest that citalopram (46,55,119–121), escitalopram (122), fluoxetine (55,123), fluvoxamine (55), paroxetine (47,124–126), and sertraline (55,127–129) are effective for the treatment of depression in PD, with the majority of studies investigating citalopram or sertraline. In a prospective, open-label study ($n = 62$) examining the efficacy of four SSRIs (citalopram, fluoxetine, fluvoxamine, and sertraline) for the treatment of PD depression, all agents were similarly effective (55). Taken together, the data from uncontrolled studies in depressed PD patients suggest that the efficacy of SSRIs may be a class effect.

As with the uncontrolled studies, a variety of SSRIs have been evaluated in a controlled manner for depression in PD (133–144). However, results are mixed. In a randomized, placebo-controlled trial (n = 52), sponsored by the National Institutes of Health, paroxetine (controlled-release) failed to demonstrate superiority over placebo (141). However, in the same study, nortriptyline demonstrated an antidepressant effect. Other studies have also reported no significant difference between SSRIs and placebo (136,138). However, in other controlled studies, both SSRIs and TCAs have demonstrated an antidepressant effect with comparable effect size (133,139,140) and several studies comparing one SSRI to another have reported similar magnitude of clinical antidepressant effect (135,138,142,143). Thus, based solely on the available scientific evidence, the efficacy of SSRIs for the management of depression in PD appears favorable yet remains unclear. Furthermore, many PD patients remain depressed despite long-term treatment with an SSRI (12). This may be related to use of an inadequate antidepressant dosage, limited efficacy, or poor adherence to medication.

Tricyclic Antidepressants
The TCAs inhibit synaptosomal reuptake of dopamine, norepinephrine and, to a lesser extent, 5-HT. The TCAs also possess antimuscarinic and antihistaminic properties. Amitriptyline (133,137,139), desipramine (140,145), imipramine (146), and nortriptyline (141,147) have all demonstrated antidepressive effects in randomized, controlled trials involving parkinsonian patients. In a randomized, double-blinded,

placebo-controlled trial (n = 48), desipramine and citalopram both improved depressive symptoms compared with placebo (140). However, side effects were more common in the desipramine group. In another randomized, double-blinded, placebo-controlled trial (n = 52), sponsored by the National Institutes of Health, nortriptyline demonstrated an antidepressant effect over placebo (141). In the same study, paroxetine failed to demonstrate superiority over placebo. In two studies conducted in the prelevodopa era, desipramine and imipramine improved parkinsonian motor symptoms, as well as symptoms of anxiety and depression (145,146). Uncontrolled studies have reported favorably on the efficacy of imipramine in treating PD depression (131,132). There are no published data on doxepin for the management of depression in PD.

The tertiary amine TCAs (e.g., amitriptyline and imipramine) are associated with clinically significant central and peripheral side effects (e.g., antimuscarinic effects, confusion, hallucinations, hypotension, sedation, sexual dysfunction, and weight gain) that are often undesirable and/or intolerable for patients (Table 9.1), especially the elderly. However, in a subset of patients, such as those with overactive bladder or drooling, the antimuscarinic activity of TCAs may be of added benefit. In nondemented patients, sedating TCAs (e.g., amitriptyline) may be helpful for insomnia. The secondary amine TCAs (e.g., desipramine and nortriptyline) are associated with a milder degree of side effects and are preferable if potent antimuscarinic effects are not desired. Lastly, the TCAs rarely have been associated with treatment-emergent extrapyramidal symptoms (153,154).

Miscellaneous Agents

In addition to SSRIs and TCAs, several other antidepressants are available, including bupropion, desvenlafaxine, duloxetine, milnacipran, mirtazapine, moclobemide, nefazodone, reboxetine, selegiline, trazodone, and venlafaxine. Of these other antidepressants, only mirtazapine, moclobemide, and nefazodone have been evaluated in a controlled manner for the management of depression in PD (135,148,149). In terms of natural products, high-dose S-adenosyl-methionine was found to be effective for PD depression in a 10-week, open-label, pilot study involving 13 patients (155).

Bupropion, a dopamine reuptake inhibitor, may be effective in PD depression (118). Common side effects include agitation, constipation, dry mouth, excessive sweating, tremor, and weight loss. Uncommon side effects include psychosis and seizures at high dosages.

Mirtazapine is a dual-action antidepressant that augments noradrenergic and serotonergic transmission via antagonism of central α_2-autoreceptors. The drug also has antihistaminic properties. In a randomized, double-blind, placebo-controlled study involving 20 depressed PD patients, mirtazapine 30 mg/day in combination with brief psychotherapy was superior to placebo in reducing depression (148). Common side effects include constipation, dry mouth, orthostasis, sedation, and weight gain. The incidence of sedation was inversely correlated with dosage. Additionally, uncontrolled data suggest that mirtazapine attenuates parkinsonian tremor and levodopa-induced dyskinesia (156,157). Uncommon side effects include agranulocytosis, hypercholesterolemia, hepatic impairment, hallucinations/psychosis, and rapid eye movement sleep behavior disorder.

Moclobemide (not available in the United States) is a reversible inhibitor of monoamine oxidase type A (MAO-A), and selegiline is an irreversible, selective inhibitor of monoamine oxidase type B (MAO-B). Inhibition of brain MAO-A activity increases norepinephrine and serotonin concentrations. One small controlled trial (n = 10) compared moclobemide to moclobemide plus selegiline in PD patients with major depression and found a greater benefit with combination of moclobemide–selegiline treatment (149). To date, no published data are available on the efficacy and safety of transdermal selegiline for the treatment of depression in patients with PD.

Nefazodone and trazodone possess antidepressive and anxiolytic properties. Both agents antagonize 5-HT receptors and modestly inhibit the reuptake of norepinephrine and 5-HT. In a controlled comparative study (n = 16), nefazodone and fluoxetine were similarly effective at improving depression, with nefazodone also producing a notable improvement in motor symptoms (135). However, the use of nefazodone may be limited by reports of hepatoxicity and significant hepatic CYP450 3A4-mediated drug–drug interactions. Trazodone has not been studied in PD depression; however, low-dose trazodone is commonly used as a sedative/hypnotic. Of note, a metabolite of trazodone, m-chlorophenylpiperazine, is anxiogenic and a subset of patients may experience irritability and enhanced anxiety, especially if trazodone is used in the presence of a potent CYP450 2D6 isoenzyme inhibitor (e.g., fluoxetine and paroxetine) (158). Common side effects of both nefazodone and trazodone include dizziness, orthostatic hypotension, and sedation.

Desvenlafaxine, duloxetine, milnacipran, and venlafaxine are dual-action antidepressants that selectively inhibit norepinephrine and 5-HT reuptake. Atomoxetine and reboxetine are selective norepinephrine reuptake inhibitors. To date, there are no published reports on the use of desvenlafaxine or duloxetine for managing depression in PD. In a randomized, placebo-controlled study, atomoxetine did not demonstrate efficacy for depression in PD (159). Preliminary reports on milnacipran and reboxetine (not available in the United States) suggest that these antidepressants may be effective in PD patients (115–117). Open-label and controlled data demonstrate that venlafaxine is well tolerated and improves depressive symptoms in patients with PD (128,142). In a larger randomized, double-blinded, placebo-controlled study ($N = 115$), venlafaxine extended-release was found to be as effective as paroxetine for improving depression in PD (142). At low doses, the pharmacologic activity of venlafaxine resembles that of an SSRI and, therefore, an anxiolytic effect can also be expected. At higher doses, norepinephrine reuptake activity becomes more pronounced and an activating effect can be expected. Venlafaxine-induced hypertension has also been observed at higher dosages; therefore, blood pressure should be monitored periodically.

Dopamine Agonists

Pramipexole and ropinirole have been reported to have antidepressant properties in patients with PD (160–165). In a large, randomized, double-blinded, placebo-controlled trial (n = 323), pramipexole was found to improve depressive symptoms independent of changes in motor function (163). In an eight-month, prospective, randomized study ($n = 41$) comparing the antidepressant effects of pramipexole and pergolide, as an add-on to levodopa in depressed patients with PD, a significant improvement in depressive symptoms was only observed in the pramipexole-treated patients (161). In a prospective, observational study of 657 pramipexole-treated patients with PD, the frequency of anhedonia and depression was significantly reduced during treatment with pramipexole (162). In a relatively small study, adjunctive ropinirole improved both anxiety and depressive symptoms in PD patients with motor fluctuations (164). The preliminary evidence suggesting beneficial antidepressive effects of dopamine agonists in PD is interesting, however, there is currently insufficient evidence to recommend dopamine agonists as treatment of depressive symptoms in patients with PD.

Assessment of Efficacy

Overall, based on reported clinical experience and the available scientific data, SSRIs and TCAs (in particular the secondary amines) may be considered possibly useful for the treatment of depression in PD, and the agent that provides the best overall clinical benefit-to-risk profile should be selected. Amoxapine and lithium should be avoided, given the propensity of these agents to worsen motor symptoms and the availability of safer agents (166,167). Additionally, the nonselective MAO inhibitors (e.g., isocarboxazid, phenelzine, and tranylcypromine) should be avoided in levodopa-treated patients due to the risk of hypertensive crisis. Several antidepressants, such as bupropion, fluoxetine, fluvoxamine, nefazodone, and paroxetine, are potent in vivo inhibitors of various cytochrome P450 (CYP450) drug-metabolizing isoenzymes and may increase the risk for adverse drug interactions.

Before initiating therapy, it is important to insure that adequate follow-up and mental health services are available. For the antidepressant-treated patient who fails therapy at maximal, tolerated doses, the antidepressant should be discontinued and replaced by another from a different pharmacologic class. For example, if a patient fails to respond to an SSRI, a switch to a dual action antidepressant (e.g., venlafaxine) could be made. When anxiety is present with depression, there may initially be a slowed response to antidepressant therapy. Since depression is a potentially recurrent disorder, once depressive symptoms have improved or recovery has been achieved, it is recommended that maintaining treatment at the effective dose should continue for at least six months to reduce the risk for relapse. Persisting symptoms of concurrent anxiety have been found to increase the risk for relapse of depression. Treatment discontinuation should occur with a slow tapering of medication. Patients coming off medications need to be seen more often to monitor for treatment response or symptom relapse.

Nonpharmacologic Treatment

Cognitive behavior therapy (CBT) is based on the construct that depressed people hold distorted cognitions. The aim of CBT is to provide a structured approach to help people to identify maladaptive thoughts contributing to emotional discomfort and to replace them with more enabling alternatives. Preliminary evidence suggests that CBT improves depressive symptoms in patients with PD (168–171). In a randomized, controlled study of 80 patients with PD and depression, in-person CBT was found to be a viable approach (170). A study using telephone-based CBT demonstrated results comparable to those of in-person CBT treatment studies (171).

In cases of severe pharmacologically refractory major depression, serial electroconvulsive therapy (ECT) may be effective for improving depressive symptoms and may also provide transient improvement in motor symptoms (172,173). However, common adverse effects of ECT include delirium and cognitive impairment, and its long-term utility is limited. Preliminary data suggest that repetitive transcranial magnetic stimulation (rTMS), a less invasive physical intervention than ECT, may improve depressive symptoms as well as cognitive and motor symptoms in PD patients (147,174–176). The role of rTMS in management of depression in PD warrants further evaluation.

Lastly, application of a structured, supervised physical therapy program improves depressive symptomatology in patients with PD (177,178).

CONCLUSION

Anxiety and depression are prevalent nonmotor features in patients with PD. These affective disorders contribute to the accelerated disability and functional morbidity in patients with PD, and are correlated with poor quality of life and increased caregiver distress. Various instruments may be utilized to facilitate screening, diagnosis, and assessment of anxiety and depression. However, despite attempts to improve the sensitivity and specificity of these instruments for use in the PD population, uncertainties remain. The best approach may be to remain vigilant, to have a low threshold for intervention, and to utilize an individualized approach. Before initiating therapy, adequate follow-up and mental health services should be available. The scientific data on the efficacy of nonpharmacologic and pharmacologic treatments for the treatment of anxiety and depression in the PD population are relatively sparse with the majority of studies characterized by relatively small sample size. Despite the lack of strong evidence demonstrating the efficacy of antidepressants in PD patients, the available data suggest that the SSRIs and secondary amine TCAs may possibly be efficacious for the PD population and that the SSRIs are better tolerated. Clinicians should rely on empiric assessments of known risks and putative benefits to guide treatment decisions. Additionally, a targeted and individualized multimodal approach utilizing psychotherapeutic interventions along with pharmacologic therapies should be considered.

REFERENCES

1. Hanna KK, Cronin-Golomb A. Impact of anxiety on quality of life in Parkinson's disease. Parkinsons Dis 2012; 2012: 640707.
2. Riedel O, Dodel R, Deuschl G, et al. Depression and care-dependency in Parkinson's disease: Results from a nationwide study of 1449 outpatients. Parkinsonism Relat Disord 2012; 18: 598–601.
3. Pontone GM, Williams JR, Anderson KE, et al. Anxiety and self-perceived health status in Parkinson's disease. Parkinsonism Relat Disord 2011; 17: 249–54.
4. Weintraub D, Moberg PJ, Duda JE, et al. Effect of psychiatric and other nonmotor symptoms on disability in Parkinson's disease. J Am Geriatr Soc 2004; 52: 784–8.
5. Mathias JL. Neurobehavioral functioning of persons with Parkinson's disease. Appl Neuropsychol 2003; 10: 57–68.
6. Global Parkinson's Disease Survey (GPDS) Steering Committee. Factors impacting on quality of life in Parkinson's disease: results from an international survey. Mov Disord 2002; 17: 60–7.
7. Cubo E, Bernard B, Leurgans S, et al. Cognitive and motor function in patients with Parkinson's disease with and without depression. Clin Neuropharmacol 2000; 23: 331–4.
8. Richard IH, Schiffer RB, Kurlan R. Anxiety and Parkinson's disease. J Neuropsychiatry Clin Neurosci 1996; 8: 383–92.
9. Hughes TA, Ross HF, Mindham RHS, et al. Mortality in Parkinson's disease and its association with dementia and depression. Acta Neurol Scand 2004; 110: 118–23.
10. Gallagher DA, Lees AJ, Schrag A. What are the most important nonmotor symptoms in patients with Parkinson's disease and are we missing them? Mov Disord 2010; 25: 2493–500.

11. Marsh L, McDonald WM, Cummings J, et al. Provisional diagnostic criteria for depression in Parkinson's disease: Report of an NINDS/NIMH Work Group. Mov Disord 2006; 21: 148–58.
12. Weintraub D, Moberg PJ, Duda JE, et al. Recognition and treatment of depression in Parkinson's disease. J Geriatr Psychiatry Neurol 2003; 16: 178–83.
13. Brown RG, Landau S, Hindle JV, et al. PROMS-PD Study Group. Depression and anxiety related subtypes in Parkinson's disease. J Neurol Neurosurg Psychiatry 2011; 82: 803–9.
14. Ostheimer AJ. An essay on the shaking palsy, by James Parkinson, MD, Member of the Royal College of Surgeons. Arch Neurol Psychiatry 1922; 7: 681–710.
15. Dissanayaka NN, Sellbach A, Matheson S, et al. Anxiety disorders in Parkinson's disease: prevalence and risk factors. Mov Disord 2010; 25: 838–45.
16. Shulman LM, Taback RL, Rabinstein AA, et al. Non-recognition of depression and other non-motor symptoms in Parkinson's disease. Parkinsonism Relat Disord 2002; 8: 193–7.
17. Menza MA, Robertson-Hoffman DE, Bonapace AS. Parkinson's disease and anxiety: comorbidity with depression. Biol Psychiatry 1993; 34: 465–70.
18. Starkstein SE, Robinson RG, Leiguardia R, et al. Anxiety and depression in Parkinson's disease. Behav Neurol 1993; 6: 151–4.
19. Stein MB, Heuser IJ, Juncos JL, et al. Anxiety disorders in patients with Parkinson's disease. Am J Psychiatry 1990; 147: 217–20.
20. Nuti A, Ceravolo R, Piccinni A, et al. Psychiatric comorbidity in a population of Parkinson's disease patients. Eur J Neurol 2004; 11: 315–20.
21. Vazquez A, Jimenez-Jimenez FJ, Garcia-Ruiz P, Garcia-Urra D. "Panic attacks" in Parkinson's disease: a long-term complication of levodopa therapy. Acta Neurol Scand 1993; 87: 14–18.
22. Bolluk B, Ozel-Kizil ET, Akbostanci MC, Atbasoglu EC. Social anxiety in patients with Parkinson's disease. J Neuropsychiatry Clin Neurosci 2010; 22: 390–4.
23. Schiffer RB, Kurlan R, Rubin A, et al. Evidence for atypical depression in Parkinson's disease. Am J Psychiatry 1988; 145: 1020–2.
24. Weisskopf MG, Chen H, Schwarzschild MA, et al. Prospective study of phobic anxiety and risk of Parkinson's disease. Mov Disord 2003; 18: 646–51.
25. Shiba M, Bower JH, Maraganore DM, et al. Anxiety disorders and depressive disorders preceding Parkinson's disease: a case-control study. Mov Disord 2000; 15: 669–77.
26. Racette BA, Hartlein JM, Hershey T, et al. Clinical features and comorbidity of mood fluctuations in Parkinson's disease. J Neuropsychiatry Clin Neurosci 2002; 14: 438–42.
27. Witjas T, Kaphan E, Azulay JP, et al. Nonmotor fluctuations in Parkinson's disease: frequent and disabling. Neurology 2002; 59: 408–13.
28. Friedenberg DL, Cummings JL. Parkinson's disease, depression, and the on-off phenomenon. Psychosomatics 1989; 30: 94–9.
29. Lauterbach EC, Freeman A, Vogel RL. Correlates of generalized anxiety and panic attacks in dystonia and Parkinson disease. Cogn Behav Neurol 2003; 16: 225–33.
30. Richard IH, Frank S, McDermott MP, et al. The ups and downs of Parkinson disease: a prospective study of mood and anxiety fluctuations. Cogn Behav Neurol 2004; 17: 201–7.
31. Nissenbaum H, Quinn NP, Brown RG, et al. Mood swings associated with the "on-off" phenomenon in Parkinson's disease. Psychol Med 1987; 17: 899–904.
32. Prediger RD, Matheus FC, Schwarzbold ML, et al. Anxiety in Parkinson's disease: a critical review of experimental and clinical studies. Neuropharmacology 2012; 62: 115–24.
33. Kano O, Ikeda K, Cridebring D, et al. Neurobiology of depression and anxiety in Parkinson's disease. Parkinsons Dis 2011; 2011: 143547.
34. Kerenyi LK, Ricaurte GA, Schretlen DJ, et al. Positron emission tomography of striatal serotonin transporters in Parkinson's disease. Arch Neurol 2003; 60: 1223–9.
35. Remy P, Doder M, Lees A, et al. Depression in Parkinson's disease: loss of dopamine and noradrenaline innervation in the limbic system. Brain 2005; 128: 1314–22.

36. American Psychiatric Association Diagnostic and Statistical Manual of Mental Disorders DSM-IV-TR, 4th edn. Text Revised. Washington, DC: American Psychiatric Association Press, 2000.
37. Leentjens AF, Dujardin K, Marsh L, et al. Anxiety rating scales in Parkinson's disease: a validation study of the Hamilton anxiety rating scale, the Beck anxiety inventory, and the hospital anxiety and depression scale. Mov Disord 2011; 26: 407–15.
38. Rodriguez-Blazquez C, Frades-Payo B, Forjaz MJ, de Pedro-Cuesta J, Martinez-Martin P. Longitudinal Parkinson's disease Patient Study Group. Psychometric attributes of the hospital anxiety and depression scale in Parkinson's disease. Mov Disord 2009; 24: 519–25.
39. Forjaz MJ, Rodriguez-Blázquez C, Martinez-Martin P; Longitudinal Parkinson's disease Patient Study Group. Rasch analysis of the hospital anxiety and depression scale in Parkinson's disease. Mov Disord 2009; 24: 526–32.
40. Mondolo F, Jahanshahi M, Granà A, et al. Evaluation of anxiety in Parkinson's disease with some commonly used rating scales. Neurol Sci 2007; 28: 270–5.
41. Beck AT, Epstein N, Brown G, et al. An inventory for measuring clinical anxiety: psychometric properties. J Consult Clin Psychol 1988; 56: 893–7.
42. Zigmond AS, Snaith RP. The hospital anxiety and depression scale. Acta Psychiatr Scand 1983; 67: 361–70.
43. Marinus J, Leentjens AF, Visser M, et al. Evaluation of the hospital anxiety and depression scale in patients with Parkinson's disease. Clin Neuropharmacol 2002; 25: 318–24.
44. Casacchia M, Zamponi A, Squitieri G, et al. Treatment of anxiety in Parkinson's disease with bromazepam [in Italian]. Riv Neurol 1975; 45: 326–38.
45. Ludwig CL, Weinberger DR, Bruno G, et al. Buspirone, Parkinson's disease, and the locus ceruleus. Clin Neuropharmacol 1986; 9: 373–8.
46. Menza M, Marin H, Kaufman K, et al. Citalopram treatment of depression in Parkinson's disease: the impact on anxiety, disability, and cognition. J Neuropsychiatry Clin Neurosci 2004; 16: 315–19.
47. Tarczy MI, Szombathelyi E. Depression in Parkinson's disease with special regard to anxiety: experiences with paroxetine treatment [abstr]. Mov Disord 1998; 13: 275.
48. Shulman LM, Singer C, Liefert R, Mellman T, Weiner WJ. Therapeutic effects of sertraline in patients with Parkinson's disease [abstr]. Mov Disord 1996; 11: 12.
49. Chuang C, Fahn S. Dramatic benefit with clonazepam treatment of intractable anxiety and panic attacks in Parkinson's disease [abstr]. Mov Disord 2001; 16: S35.
50. Cumming RG, Le Couteur DG. Benzodiazepines and risk of hip fractures in older people: a review of the evidence. CNS Drugs 2003; 17: 825–37.
51. Richard IH, Kurlan R. A survey of antidepressant drug use in Parkinson's disease. Neurology 1997; 49: 1168–70.
52. Anon Drug Facts and Comparisons. St. Louis: Facts and Comparisons, 2011.
53. Gony M, Lapeyre-Mestre M, Montastruc JL. Risk of serious extrapyramidal symptoms in patients with Parkinson's disease receiving antidepressant drugs: a pharmacoepidemiologic study comparing serotonin reuptake inhibitors and other antidepressant drugs. Clin Neuropharmacol 2003; 26: 142–5.
54. van de Vijver DA, Roos RA, Jansen PA, et al. Start of a selective serotonin reuptake inhibitor (SSRI) and increase of antiparkinsonian drug treatment in patients on levodopa. Br J Clin Pharmacol 2002; 54: 168–70.
55. Dell'Agnello G, Ceravolo R, Nuti A, et al. SSRIs do not worsen Parkinson's disease: evidence from an open-label, prospective study. Clin Neuropharmacol 2001; 24: 221–7.
56. Richard IH, Kurlan R, Tanner C, et al. Serotonin syndrome and the combined use of deprenyl and an antidepressant in Parkinson's disease. Neurology 1997; 48: 1070–7.
57. Chen JJ. Pharmacologic safety concerns in Parkinson's disease: facts and insights. Int J Neurosci 2011; 121: 45–52.
58. Black K, Shea C, Dursun S, et al. Selective serotonin reuptake inhibitor discontinuation syndrome: proposed diagnostic criteria. J Psychiatry Neurosci 2000; 25: 255–61.
59. Bonifati V, Fabrizio E, Cipriani R, et al. Buspirone in levodopa-induced dyskinesias. Clin Neuropharmacol 1994; 17: 73–82.

60. Slawek J, Derejko M, Lass P. Factors affecting the quality of life of patients with idiopathic Parkinson's disease-a cross-sectional study in an outpatient clinic attendees. Parkinsonism Relat Disord 2005; 11: 465–8.

61. Miller E, Berrios GE, Politynska BE. Caring for someone with Parkinson's disease: factors that contribute to distress. Int J Geriatr Psychiatry 1996; 11: 263–8.

62. Tandberg E, Larsen JP, Aarsland D, et al. The occurrence of depression in Parkinson's disease: a community based study. Arch Neurol 1996; 53: 175–9.

63. Nilsson FM, Kessing LV, Sorensen TM, et al. Major depressive disorder in Parkinson's disease: a register-based study. Acta Psychiatr Scand 2002; 106: 202–11.

64. Nilsson FM, Kessing LV, Bolwig TG. Increased risk of developing Parkinson's disease for patients with major affective disorder: a register study. Acta Psychiatr Scand 2001; 104: 380–6.

65. Slaughter JR, Slaughter KA, Nichols D, et al. Prevalence, clinical manifestations, etiology, and treatment of depression in Parkinson's disease. J Neuropsychiatry Clin Neurosci 2001; 13: 187–96.

66. Leentjens AF, Marinus J, Van Hilten JJ, et al. The contribution of somatic symptoms to the diagnosis of depressive disorder in Parkinson's disease: a discriminant analytic approach. J Neuropsychiatry Clin Neurosci 2003; 15: 74–7.

67. Naarding P, Leentjens AF, van Kooten F, et al. Disease-specific properties of the Hamilton Rating Scale for depression in patients with stroke, Alzheimer's dementia, and Parkinson's disease. J Neuropsychiatry Clin Neurosci 2002; 14: 329–34.

68. Leentjens AF, Verhey FR, Lousberg R, et al. The validity of the Hamilton and Montgomery-Asberg Depression Rating Scales as screening and diagnostic tools for depression in Parkinson's disease. Int J Geriatr Psychiatry 2000; 15: 644–9.

69. Rojo A, Aguilar M, Garolera MT, et al. Depression in Parkinson's disease: clinical correlates and outcome. Parkinsonism Relat Disord 2003; 10: 23–8.

70. Gotham AM, Brown RG, Marsden CD. Depression in Parkinson's disease: a quantitative and qualitative analysis. J Neurol Neurosurg Psychiatry 1986; 49: 381–9.

71. Judd MM, Rapaport M, Paulus MB. Subsyndromal symptomatic depression: a new mood disorder? J Clin Psychiatry 1994; 55(Suppl): 18–28.

72. Ehmann TS, Beninger RJ, Gawel MJ, et al. Depressive symptoms in Parkinson's disease: a comparison with disabled control subjects. J Geriatr Psychiatry Neurol 1990; 3: 3–9.

73. Brown R, Jahanshahi M. Depression in Parkinson's disease: a psychosocial viewpoint. Adv Neurol 1995; 65: 61–84.

74. Huber SJ, Freidenberg DL, Paulson GW, et al. The pattern of depressive symptoms varies with progression of Parkinson's disease. J Neurol Neurosurg Psychiatry 1990; 53: 275–8.

75. Gonera EG, van't Hof M, Berger HJ, et al. Symptoms and duration of the prodromal phase in Parkinson's disease. Mov Disord 1997; 12: 871–6.

76. Leentjens AF, Van den Akker M, Metsemakers JF, et al. Higher incidence of depression preceding the onset of Parkinson's disease: a register study. Mov Disord 2003; 18: 414–18.

77. Jacob EL, Gatto NM, Thompson A, et al. Occurrence of depression and anxiety prior to Parkinson's disease. Parkinsonism Relat Disord 2010; 16: 576–81.

78. O'Suilleabhain PE, Sung V, Hernandez C, et al. Elevated plasma homocysteine level in patients with Parkinson disease: motor, affective, and cognitive associations. Arch Neurol 2004; 61: 865–8.

79. Bronstein JM, Tagliati M, Alterman RL, et al. Deep brain stimulation for Parkinson disease: an expert consensus and review of key issues. Arch Neurol 2011; 68: 165–71.

80. Okun MS, Wu SS, Foote KD, et al. Do stable patients with a premorbid depression history have a worse outcome after deep brain stimulation for Parkinson's disease? Neurosurgery 2011; 69: 357–260.

81. Thobois S, Ardouin C, Lhommée E, et al. Non-motor dopamine withdrawal syndrome after surgery for Parkinson's disease: predictors and underlying mesolimbic denervation. Brain 2010; 133: 1111–27.

82. Follett KA, Weaver FM, Stern M, et al. CSP 468 Study Group. Pallidal versus subthalamic deep-brain stimulation for Parkinson's disease. N Engl J Med 2010; 362: 2077–91.

83. Tan SK, Hartung H, Sharp T, Temel Y. Serotonin-dependent depression in Parkinson's disease: a role for the subthalmic nucleus? Neuropharmacology 2011; 61: 387–99.

84. Okun MS, Green J, Saben R, et al. Mood changes with deep brain stimulation of STN and GPi: results of a pilot study. J Neurol Neurosurg Psychiatry 2003; 74: 1584–6.

85. Doshi PK, Chhaya N, Bhatt MH. Depression leading to attempted suicide after bilateral subthalamic nucleus stimulation for Parkinson's disease. Mov Disord 2002; 17: 1084–5.

86. Houeto JL, Mesnage V, Mallet L, et al. Behavioural disorders, Parkinson's disease and subthalamic stimulation. J Neurol Neurosurg Psychiatry 2002; 72: 701–7.

87. Ballanger B, Klinger H, Eche J, et al. Role of serotonergic 1A receptor dysfunction in depression associated with Parkinson's disease. Mov Disord 2012; 27: 84–9.

88. Kostić VS, Filippi M. Neuroanatomical correlates of depression and apathy in Parkinson's disease: magnetic resonance imaging studies. J Neurol Sci 2011; 310: 61–3.

89. Kostić VS, Agosta F, Petrović I, et al. Regional patterns of brain tissue loss associated with depression in Parkinson's disease. Neurology 2010; 75: 857–63.

90. Politis M, Wu K, Loane C, et al. Depressive symptoms in PD correlate with higher 5-HT binding in raphe and limbic structures. Neurology 2010; 75: 1920–7.

91. Benoit M, Robert PH. Imaging correlates of apathy and depression in Parkinson's disease. J Neurol Sci 2011; 310: 58–60.

92. Murai T, Muller U, Werheid K, et al. In vivo evidence for differential association of striatal dopamine and midbrain serotonin systems with neuropsychiatric symptoms in Parkinson's disease. J Neuropsychiatry Clin Neurosci 2001; 13: 222–8.

93. Gallo JJ, Rabins PV. Depression without sadness: alternative presentations of depression in late life. Am Fam Physician 1999; 60: 820–6.

94. Cheng EM, Siderowf A, Swarztrauber K, et al. Development of quality of care indicators for Parkinson's disease. Mov Disord 2004; 19: 136–50.

95. Starkstein SE, Preziosi TJ, Forrester AW, et al. Specificity of affective and autonomic symptoms of depression in Parkinson's disease. J Neurol Neurosurg Psychiatry 1990; 53: 869–73.

96. Starkstein S, Dragovic M, Jorge R, et al. Diagnostic criteria for depression in Parkinson's disease: a study of symptom patterns using latent class analysis. Mov Disord 2011; 26: 2239–45.

97. Reijnders JS, Lousberg R, Leentjens AF. Assessment of depression in Parkinson's disease: the contribution of somatic symptoms to the clinimetric performance of the Hamilton and Montgomery-Asberg rating scales. J Psychosom Res 2010; 68: 561–5.

98. Williams J. A structured interview guide for the Hamilton Depression Rating Scale. Arch Gen Psychiatry 1988; 45: 742–7.

99. Montgomery SA, Asberg M. A new depression scale, designed to be sensitive to change. Br J Psychiatry 1979; 134: 382–9.

100. Pignone MP, Gaynes BN, Rushton JL, et al. Screening for depression in adults: a summary of the evidence for the U.S. Preventive Services Task Force. Ann Intern Med 2002; 136: 765–76.

101. Beck A, Steer R, Brown G. Manual for the Beck Depression Inventory, 2nd edn. San Antonio: The Psychological Corporation, 1996.

102. Radloff L. The CES-D scale: a self-report depression scale for research in the general population. Appl Psychol Meas 1977; 1: 385–401.

103. Yesavage JA. Geriatric depression scale. Psychopharmacol Bull 1988; 24: 709–10.

104. Zung W. A self-rating depression scale. Arch Gen Psychiatry 1965; 12: 63–70.

105. Visser M, Leentjens AF, Marinus J, et al. Reliability and validity of the Beck depression inventory in patients with Parkinson's disease. Mov Disord 2006; 21: 668–72.

106. Leentjens AF, Verhey FR, Luijckx GJ, et al. The validity of the Beck Depression Inventory as a screening and diagnostic instrument for depression in patients with Parkinson's disease. Mov Disord 2000; 15: 1221–4.

107. Levin BE, Llabre MM, Weiner WJ. Parkinson's disease and depression: psychometric properties of the Beck Depression Inventory. J Neurol Neurosurg Psychiatry 1988; 51: 1401–4.

108. Sheikh JI, Yesavage JA. Geriatric Depression Scale (GDS): recent evidence and development of a shorter version. In: Brink TL, ed. Clinical Gerontology: a Guide to Assessment and Intervention. New York: Haworth Press, 1986.
109. Weintraub D, Oehlberg KA, Katz IR, et al. Test characteristics of the 15-item geriatric depression scale and hamilton depression rating scale in Parkinson disease. Am J Geriatr Psychiatry 2006; 14: 169–75.
110. Ertan FS, Ertan T, Kiziltan G, et al. Reliability and validity of the Geriatric Depression Scale in depression in Parkinson's disease. J Neurol Neurosurg Psychiatry 2005; 76: 1445–7.
111. Thompson AW, Liu H, Hays RD, et al. Diagnostic accuracy and agreement across three depression assessment measures for Parkinson's disease. Parkinsonism Relat Disord 2011; 17: 40–5.
112. Mondolo F, Jahanshahi M, Granà A, et al. The validity of the hospital anxiety and depression scale and the geriatric depression scale in Parkinson's disease. Behav Neurol 2006; 17: 109–15.
113. Rodriguez-Blazquez C, Frades-Payo B, Forjaz MJ, et al. Longitudinal Parkinson's disease Patient Study Group. Psychometric attributes of the hospital anxiety and depression scale in Parkinson's disease. Mov Disord 2009; 24: 519–25.
114. Scheinthal SM, Steer RA, Giffin L, et al. Evaluating geriatric medical outpatients with the Beck Depression Inventory-Fast screen for medical patients. Aging Ment Health 2001; 5: 143–8.
115. Pintor L, Bailles E, Valldeoriola F, et al. Response to 4-month treatment with reboxetine in Parkinson's disease patients with a major depressive episode. Gen Hosp Psychiatry 2006; 28: 59–64.
116. Lemke MR. Effect of reboxetine on depression in Parkinson's disease patients. J Clin Psychiatry 2002; 63: 300–4.
117. Takahashi H, Kamata M, Yoshida K, et al. Remarkable effect of milnacipran, a serotoninnoradrenalin reuptake inhibitor (SNRI), on depressive symptoms in patients with Parkinson's disease who have insufficient response to selective serotonin reuptake inhibitors (SSRIs): two case reports. Prog Neuropsychopharmacol Biol Psychiatry 2005; 29: 351–3.
118. Leentjens AF, Verhey FR, Vreeling FW. Successful treatment of depression in a Parkinson disease patient with bupropion [in Dutch]. Ned Tijdschr Geneeskd 2000; 144: 2157–9.
119. Rampello L, Chiechio S, Raffaele R, et al. The SSRI, citalopram, improves bradykinesia in patients with Parkinson's disease treated with L-dopa. Clin Neuropharmacol 2002; 25: 21–4.
120. Aarsland D, Larsen JP, Lim NG, et al. 2-Adrenoreceptor antagonism and serotonin reup-take inhibiton in patients with Parkinson's disease and depression. Nord J Psychiatry 2000; 54: 411–15.
121. Rihmer Z, Satori M, Pestality P. Selegiline-citalopram combination in patients with Parkinson's disease and major depression. Int J Psychiatry Clin Pract 2000; 4: 123–5.
122. Weintraub D, Taraborelli D, Duda JE, et al. Escitalopram for the treatment of major depression in Parkinson's disease: impact on depression, cognition, and motor function. Mov Disord 2004; 19: S188.
123. Montastruc JL, Fabre N, Blin O, et al. Does fluoxetine aggravate Parkinson's disease? A pilot prospective study. Mov Disord 1995; 10: 355–7.
124. Ceravolo R, Nuti A, Piccinni A, et al. Paroxetine in Parkinson's disease: effects on motor and depressive symptoms. Neurology 2000; 55: 1216–18.
125. Tesei S, Antoini A, Canesi M, et al. Tolerability of paroxetine in Parkinson's disease: a prospective study. Mov Disord 2000; 15: 986–9.
126. Wittgens W, Donath O, Trenckmann U. Treatment of depressive syndromes in Parkinson's disease (P.D.) with paroxetine [abstr]. Mov Disord 1997; 12: 128.
127. Bayulkem K, Torun F. Effectiveness of sertraline in treatment of depression with Parkinson's disease [abstr]. Mov Disord 2002; 17: S74.
128. Bayulkem K, Torun F. Therapeutic efficiency of venlafaxine in depressive patients with Parkinson's disease [abstr]. Mov Disord 2002; 7: S75.

129. Hauser RA, Zesiewicz TA. Sertraline for the treatment of depression in Parkinson's disease. Mov Disord 1997; 12: 756–9.
130. Meara RJ, Bhowmick BK, Hobson JP. An open uncontrolled study of the use of sertraline in the treatment of depression in Parkinson's disease. J Serotonin Res 1996; 4: 243–9.
131. Mandell AJ, Markham C, Fowler W. Parkinson's syndrome, depression and imipramine: a preliminary report. Calif Med 1961; 95: 12–14.
132. Strauss H. Office treatment of depressive states with a new drug (imipramine). N Y State J Med 1959; 59: 2906–10.
133. Antonini A, Zecchinelli A, Tesei S, et al. A randomized single-blind study of sertraline vs. amitriptyline for the treatment of depression in patients with Parkinson's disease. Mov Disord 2004; 19: S263.
134. Fregni F, Santos CM, Myczkowski ML, et al. Repetitive transcranial magnetic stimulation is as effective as fluoxetine in the treatment of depression in patients with Parkinson's disease. J Neurol Neurosurg Psychiatry 2004; 75: 1171–4.
135. Avila A, Cardona X, Martin-Baranera M, et al. Does nefazodone improve both depression and Parkinson disease?: a pilot randomized trial. J Clin Psychopharmacol 2003; 23: 509–13.
136. Leentjens AF, Vreeling FW, Luijckx GJ, et al. SSRIs in the treatment of depression in Parkinson's disease. Int J Geriatr Psychiatry 2003; 18: 552–4.
137. Serrano-Duenas M. A comparison between low doses of amitriptyline and low doses of fluoxetin used in the control of depression in patients suffering from Parkinson's disease [in Spanish]. Rev Neurol 2002; 35: 1010–14.
138. Wermuth L, Sorensen PS, Timm B, et al. Depression in idiopathic Parkinson's disease treated with citalopram:a placebo-controlled trial. Nordic J Psychiatry 1998; 52: 163–9.
139. Rabey JM, Orlov E, Korczyn AD. Comparison of fluvoxamine versus amitriptyline for treatment of depression in Parkinson's disease [abstr]. Neurology 1996; 46: A374.
140. Devos D, Dujardin K, Poirot I, et al. Comparison of desipramine and citalopram treatments for depression in Parkinson's disease: a double-blind, randomized, placebo-controlled study. Mov Disord 2008; 23: 850–7.
141. Menza M, Dobkin RD, Marin H, et al. A controlled trial of antidepressants in patients with Parkinson disease and depression. Neurology 2009; 72: 886–92.
142. Richard IH. A multicenter randomized, double-blind, placebo-controlled trial of paroxetine and venlafaxine extended release for depression in Parkinson's disease [abstract P19.8]. Presented at the 2nd World Parkinson Congress, 2010.
143. Marino S, Sessa E, Di Lorenzo G, et al. Sertraline in the treatment of depressive disorders in patients with Parkinson's disease. Neurol Sci 2008; 29: 391–5.
144. Barone P, Scarzella L, Marconi R, et al. Depression/Parkinson Italian Study Group. Pramipexole versus sertraline in the treatment of depression in Parkinson's disease: a national multicenter parallel-group randomized study. J Neurol 2006; 253: 601–7.
145. Laitinen L. Desipramine in treatment of Parkinson's disease. Acta Neurol Scand 1969; 45: 109–13.
146. Strang RR. Imipramine in treatment of Parkinson's disease: a double-blind placebo study. BMJ 1965; 2: 33–4.
147. Andersen J, Aabro E, Gulmann N, et al. Antidepressive treatment in Parkinson's disease:a controlled trial of the effect of nortriptyline in patients with Parkinson's disease treated with L-dopa. Acta Neurol Scand 1980; 62: 210–19.
148. Weiser R, Hernandez-Rojas J, Flores J, et al. Efficacy, tolerability and safety of mirtazapine in the treatment of major depressive disorder due to Parkinson's disease. Mov Disord 2004; 19: S205.
149. Steur EN, Ballering LA. Moclobemide and selegiline in the treatment of depression in Parkinson's disease. J Neurol Neurosurg Psychiatry 1997; 63: 547.
150. Skapinakis P, Bakola E, Salanti G, et al. Efficacy and acceptability of selective serotonin reuptake inhibitors for the treatment of depression in Parkinson's disease: a systematic review and meta-analysis of randomized controlled trials. BMC Neurol 2010; 10: 49.
151. Seppi K, Weintraub D, Coelho M, et al. The Movement Disorder Society Evidence-Based Medicine Review Update: Treatments for the non-motor symptoms of Parkinson's disease. Mov Disord 2011; 26: S42–80.

152. Chen P, Kales HC, Weintraub D, et al. Antidepressant treatment of veterans with Parkinson's disease and depression: analysis of a national sample. J Geriatr Psychiatry Neurol 2007; 20: 161–5.
153. Gill HS, DeVane CL, Risch SC. Extrapyramidal symptoms associated with cyclic antidepressant treatment: a review of the literature and consolidating hypothesis. J Clin Psychopharmacol 1997; 17: 377–89.
154. Vandel P, Bonin B, Leveque E, et al. Tricyclic antidepressant-induced extrapyramidal side effects. Eur Neuropsychopharmacol 1997; 7: 207–12.
155. Di Rocco A, Rogers JD, Brown R, et al. S-Adenosyl-methionine improves depression in patients with Parkinson's disease in an open-label clinical trial. Mov Disord 2000; 15: 1225–9.
156. Gordon PH, Pullman SL, Louis ED, et al. Mirtazapine in parkinsonian tremor. Parkinsonism Relat Disord 2002; 9: 125–6.
157. Meco G, Fabrizio E, Di Rezze S, et al. Mirtazapine in L-dopa-induced dyskinesias. Clin Neuropharmacol 2003; 26: 179–81.
158. Bagdy G, Graf M, Anheuer ZE, et al. Anxiety-like effects induced by acute fluoxetine, sertraline or m-CPP treatment are reversed by pretreatment with the 5-HT2C receptor antagonist SB-242084 but not the 5-HT1A receptor antagonist WAY-100635. Int J Neuropsychopharmacol 2001; 4: 399–408.
159. Weintraub D, Mavandadi S, Mamikonyan E, et al. Atomoxetine for depression and other neuropsychiatric symptoms in Parkinson disease. Neurology 2010; 75: 448–55.
160. Reichmann H, Brecht MH, Koster J, et al. Pramipexole in routine clinical practice: a prospective observational trial in Parkinson's disease. CNS Drugs 2003; 17: 965–73.
161. Rektorova I, Rektor I, Bares M, et al. Pramipexole and pergolide in the treatment of depression in Parkinson's disease: a national multicentre prospective randomized study. Eur J Neurol 2003; 10: 399–406.
162. Lemke MR, Brecht HM, Koester J, et al. Anhedonia, depression, and motor functioning in Parkinson's disease during treatment with pramipexole. J Neuropsychiatry Clin Neurosci 2005; 17: 214–20.
163. Barone P, Poewe W, Albrecht S, et al. Pramipexole for the treatment of depressive symptoms in patients with Parkinson's disease: a randomised, double-blind, placebo-controlled trial. Lancet Neurol 2010; 9: 573–80.
164. Rektorova I, Balaz M, Svatova J, et al. Effects of ropinirole on nonmotor symptoms of Parkinson's disease: a prospective multicenter study. Clin Neuropharmacol 2008; 31: 261–6.
165. Leentjens AF. The role of dopamine agonists in the treatment of depression in patients with Parkinson's disease: a systematic review. Drugs 2011; 71: 273–86.
166. Sa DS, Kapur S, Lang AE. Amoxapine shows an antipsychotic effect but worsens motor function in patients with Parkinson's disease and psychosis. Clin Neuropharmacol 2001; 24: 242–3.
167. Coffey CE, Ross DR, Massey EW, et al. Dyskinesias associated with lithium therapy in parkinsonism. Clin Neuropharmacol 1984; 7: 223–9.
168. Cole K, Vaughan F. Brief cognitive behavioural therapy for depression associated with Parkinson's disease. A single case series. Behav Cogn Psychother 2005; 33: 89–102.
169. Dreisig H, Beckmann JM, Wermuth L, et al. Psychological effects of structure cognitive psychotherapy in young patients with Parkinson disease: a pilot study. Nordic J Psychiatry 1999; 53: 217–21.
170. Dobkin RD, Menza M, Allen LA, et al. Cognitive-behavioral therapy for depression in Parkinson's disease: a randomized, controlled trial. Am J Psychiatry 2011; 168: 1066–74.
171. Dobkin RD, Menza M, Allen LA, et al. Telephone-based cognitive-behavioral therapy for depression in Parkinson disease. J Geriatr Psychiatry Neurol 2011; 24: 206–14.
172. Moellentine C, Rummans T, Ahlskog JE, et al. Effectiveness of ECT in patients with parkinsonism. J Neuropsychiatry Clin Neurosci 1998; 10: 187–93.
173. Popeo D, Kellner CH. ECT for Parkinson's disease. Med Hypotheses 2009; 73: 468–9.
174. Boggio PS, Fregni F, Bermpohl F, et al. Effect of repetitive TMS and fluoxetine on cognitive function inpatients with Parkinson's disease and concurrent depression. Mov Disord 2005; 20: 1178–84.

175. Dragasevic N, Potrebic A, Damjanovic A, et al. Therapeutic efficacy of bilateral prefrontal slow repetitive transcranial magnetic stimulation in depressed patients with Parkinson's disease: an open study. Mov Disord 2002; 17: 528–32.
176. Pal E, Nagy F, Aschermann Z, Balazs E, Kovacs N. The impact of left prefrontal repetitive transcranial magnetic stimulation on depression in Parkinson's disease: a randomized, double-blind, placebo-controlled study. Mov Disord 2010; 25: 2311–17.
177. Pellecchia MT, Grasso A, Biancardi LG, et al. Physical therapy in Parkinson's disease: an open long-term rehabilitation trial. J Neurol 2004; 251: 595–8.
178. Dereli EE, Yaliman A. Comparison of the effects of a physiotherapist-supervised exercise programme and a self-supervised exercise programme on quality of life in patients with Parkinson's disease. Clin Rehabil 2010; 24: 352–62.

Management of psychosis and dementia

Thien Thien Lim, Kelvin L. Chou, and Hubert H. Fernandez

INTRODUCTION

James Parkinson in his original observations on Parkinson's disease (PD) commented mainly on tremor and gait abnormality (1); however, it has become increasingly evident that PD patients can have cognitive and behavioral changes, and that these changes, most notably psychosis and dementia, can affect motor function. Furthermore, pharmacotherapy of psychosis and dementia can limit optimal treatment of the motor symptoms through dopamine antagonism and can even contribute to cognitive and behavioral dysfunction in PD. This makes it complicated to differentiate which features are medication side effects and which are intrinsic to PD.

It is essential to identify both psychosis and dementia in PD. Those with concomitant dementia are more prone to the development of dopamine-induced confusion, agitation, and psychosis, limiting treatment of the motor symptoms. Psychosis in PD is a risk factor for nursing home placement (2,3) and is associated with a higher mortality rate (4,5). Moreover, psychosis is the single greatest stress for caregivers. Dementia in PD also contributes to caregiver stress (6) and leads to a more rapid motor and functional decline (7,8), early institutionalization (2,9), and increased mortality (10–12). As the manifestations of psychosis and dementia are potentially treatable, recognition and treatment may enable the PD patient to live at home for a longer period and decrease caregiver stress.

PSYCHOSIS

Psychosis is a disorder characterized by hallucinations, delusions, or disorganized thinking (13), and is estimated to occur in 20–40% of PD patients (14,15). The most common manifestations of psychosis in PD are visual hallucinations (14,16–18). Although visual hallucinations are a common feature of patients with dementia with Lewy bodies (DLB), and may occasionally occur in demented PD patients who are not taking medications, the vast majority of PD patients who develop psychotic symptoms do so on antiparkinsonian therapy, and may return to their nonpsychotic baseline if the PD medications are discontinued (19–21). All antiparkinsonian drugs, not just dopaminergic agents, have been demonstrated to cause psychosis (22–25). Visual hallucinations in PD may occur at any time, and may be vivid and realistic, or out of focus. Patients may experience "presence" hallucinations (the sensation that someone or something is in the room) or "passage" hallucinations (brief visions seen in the peripheral field of vision) (14). Auditory hallucinations are the second most common, with tactile and olfactory hallucinations occurring less commonly (18). Nonvisual hallucinations mainly occur in people who already suffer from visual ones (14,18,26,27).

Delusions, or beliefs that do not have a foundation in reality, occur less frequently in PD. The phenomenology of delusions in PD overlaps with those seen in other dementias (28) and usually carries a paranoid theme. However, most types of delusions occur with relatively equal frequency (18). Thought broadcasting, ideas of reference, loosened associations, and "negative" symptoms are generally uncommon in PD.

There is no gold standard rating scale for the severity of psychosis in PD. Many different scales have been used to assess psychosis in PD studies, including the Neuropsychiatric Inventory (NPI) (29), Brief Psychiatric Rating Scale (BPRS) (30), Behave-AD (31), Positive and Negative Symptom Scale (PANSS) (32), Scale for the Assessment of Positive Symptoms (33), Clinical Global Impression Scale (CGIS) (34), and the Parkinson Psychosis Rating Scale (PPRS) (35). Many of these scales were developed for use in Alzheimer's disease (AD) or schizophrenia. As psychosis in PD manifests generally as "positive" symptoms such as hallucinations and delusions (18), and "negative" symptoms, such as conceptual disorganization are not present, scales such as the BPRS and the PANSS assess many nonrelevant items. Only one scale, the PPRS, has been validated in the PD population. However, some items on the PPRS, such as sexual preoccupation, may not be that prominent in PD psychosis. There is only one item each on hallucinations, delusions, and illusions, which may not fully explore and track the phenomenology of PD psychosis. It has also not been tested in a longitudinal fashion, and its ability to track changes due to treatment has not been studied. A Movement Disorder Society Task Force on Rating Scales in Psychosis for PD evaluated the existing scales and felt that none were ideal in clinical practice, although some could be useful in clinical trials or PD psychosis research (36). The majority of the respondents felt that an ideal scale would take less than 10 minutes to administer, have a reliable caregiver/observer that contributed to the history/information obtained, would capture illusions and sense of presence hallucinations, would be able to differentiate drug-induced psychosis from delirium, could be administered by a nonphysician and reflected the severity of psychosis over the last 7–14 days. This task force felt that a scale to adequately assess psychosis in PD was warranted.

Pathophysiology of Psychosis and Risk Factors
The pathophysiology of psychosis in PD is poorly understood, but dopaminergic and serotonergic mechanisms have been proposed. One theory is that chronic excessive stimulation of dopamine receptors, particularly in the mesolimbic/mesocortical pathways, causes hypersensitization, resulting in psychosis when patients are treated with dopaminergic agents (37). However, exogenous dopamine supplementation by itself is not the only factor in the development of psychosis since all PD medications (anticholinergics, dopaminergics, and amantadine) can induce hallucinations despite their different mechanisms of action (25), and PD psychosis was described prior to the use of levodopa (38). Serotonin has been implicated because the atypical antipsychotic drugs are purported to work through their high affinity for 5-HT2 compared with D2 receptors. However, PD patients with psychosis have decreased serotonin content in the brainstem at autopsy (39). Potential explanations for this finding include postsynaptic serotonergic hypersensitivity as a result of decreased central serotonin activity (40) and/or increases in serotonin activity from levodopa administration (41).

The precise anatomic substrate of hallucinations and psychosis is unknown, but may be due in part to visual dysfunction. PD patients who hallucinate perform slightly worse on visual acuity testing (mean visual acuity 20/45) than nonhallucinators (20/33) (17) and have greater impairment in color vision and contrast sensitivity (42). Furthermore, visual evoked potentials are abnormal in PD patients with visual hallucinations (43). Other structures in the brain may also be involved. One reported patient experienced formed visual hallucinations after bilateral subthalamic nucleus (STN) deep brain stimulation (DBS) surgery only when the stimulators were turned on (44), leading the authors to hypothesize that this resulted from stimulation of limbic fibers near the STN. Finally, a functional magnetic resonance imaging study demonstrated greater activation in the frontal lobe in PD patients with chronic visual hallucinations compared with nonhallucinators (45). The exact contribution of these neurotransmitters and structures to the genesis of psychosis is unclear.

The presence of dementia, advancing age, impaired vision, depression, sleep disorders, and longer disease duration have all been associated with the development of drug-induced psychosis (15,46–49). Although psychosis has been reported to occur with all of the antiparkinsonian medications (22–25), the dopamine agonists are more likely to cause psychosis than levodopa (50,51). The duration or dose of antiparkinsonian drug therapy, however, has not been found to be associated with an increased risk for psychosis (46,52,53).

There have been no genetic correlates of psychotic symptoms and PD. A study by Factor et al. showed that there was no association between psychotic symptoms and polymorphisms in the apoprotein, alpha-synuclein or microtuble-associated protein tau genes (54). However, the same study found an association between freezing of gait (but not tremor or postural instability) and psychotic symptoms leading the authors to conclude that patients with freezing of gait need to be monitored closely for psychotic symptoms.

General Treatment of Psychosis

The management of the psychotic PD patient begins by searching for correctable causes, including infection, metabolic derangements, social stress, and drug toxicity. Infections may not always cause fevers in the geriatric population, so a search for urinary tract infections or pneumonias is warranted. Some PD patients who did not manifest psychotic symptoms at home may decompensate upon moving into the hospital environment. In many of these cases, moving the patient into a secure familiar environment or treating the underlying medical illness may ameliorate psychotic symptoms (19). Finally, medications with central nervous system (CNS) effects may cause or exacerbate psychosis in PD and are often overlooked. These medications include pain or sleeping medications, such as narcotics, anxiolytics, hypnotics, and antidepressants.

If psychotic symptoms persist despite identification and correction of the above factors, antiparkinsonian medications are slowly reduced and if possible discontinued. Antiparkinsonian drugs should be reduced and discontinued in the following order: anticholinergic agents, amantadine, MAO-B inhibitors, dopamine agonists, catechol-O-methyltransferase inhibitors and, finally, levodopa (55). If psychosis improves, the patient is then maintained on the lowest possible dose of antiparkinsonian medications. If psychosis persists, and further reductions in antiparkinsonian medications cause intolerable motor function, the use of an atypical antipsychotic agent is warranted.

Specific Treatments for Psychosis
Atypical Antipsychotics
Atypical antipsychotics are typically used to treat psychosis in PD. Table 10.1 provides a summary of atypical antipsychotic studies in PD. The United States Food and Drug Administration (FDA) has required all atypical antipsychotic manufacturers to have a boxed warning on their product labels, saying that atypical antipsychotics, when used in elderly patients with dementia, were associated with a higher risk of mortality (56). However, since the deaths were primarily due to cardiovascular or infectious causes, it is unclear how the atypical antipsychotics cause increased mortality. Since psychosis can be difficult to treat in PD, it is likely that these agents will continue to be utilized until a direct cause and effect relationship is uncovered.

Clozapine
Clozapine was the first atypical antipsychotic approved by the FDA, and is the only atypical antipsychotic that has been demonstrated to have better efficacy than typical neuroleptics (77). Double-blind placebo-controlled and open-label studies with clozapine have shown that the drug effectively treats psychosis in PD without worsening motor function (55,58,59). The first double-blind, placebo-controlled trial of clozapine in PD resulted in the only negative study (57). It was a small study of six patients at a single site. Three patients completed the study and three had worsened parkinsonism. However, the authors titrated clozapine using a schizophrenia titration schedule and went as high as 250 mg/day. This resulted in subjects complaining of severe sedation, which may have partly manifested as worsened parkinsonism. We now know that doses as small as 6.25 mg daily can result in improvement of psychosis in PD patients.

Two randomized, double-blind, placebo-controlled trials of low-dose clozapine have been published (58,78). One trial was conducted in the United States and one in France. In the U.S. trial, clozapine, at a mean dose of 25 mg/day, resulted in a significant benefit on four measures of psychosis. Motor function did not decline, and tremor improved significantly. Only one subject suffered a decline in white blood cell (WBC) count requiring termination, which was reversed within one week after stopping clozapine. The most commonly used dose was 6.25 mg/day. The French study reported similar results, with patients taking a mean dose of 35 mg/day.

In terms of long-term efficacy and safety, a retrospective analysis of 39 parkinsonian patients on a mean dose of 47 mg/day of clozapine for 60 months showed that 85% had continued response to the medication, whereas 13% had complete resolution of psychosis (79). A second study reported a five-year follow-up of 32 patients with PD and psychosis, 14 of whom had dementia (80). Nineteen of these patients were still taking clozapine at a mean dose of 20 mg/day. Nine subjects had stopped clozapine because of improvement in their psychosis, but three patients discontinued the drug due to somnolence.

Unfortunately, with clozapine, there is concern about agranulocytosis. Therefore, weekly WBC monitoring for six months, biweekly monitoring for the next six months, and monthly monitoring thereafter is mandated. This complication is not dose related, so monitoring must be performed in all patients on clozapine. Although agranulocytosis had been thought to occur in 1–1.5% of patients, the actual incidence of agranulocytosis was only 0.38% in an analysis of over 99,000 U.S. patients with schizophrenia (81). Sedation, orthostatic hypotension, and sialorrhea

TABLE 10.1 Double-Blind and Selected Open-Label Reports of Atypical Antipsychotics in Parkinson's Disease

Agent	Design	Number of Patients	Dosage (mg/day)	Number with Improved Psychosis	Number with Worsened PD
Clozapine					
Wolters et al. (57)	Double-Blind	6	75–250	3	3
Parkinson Study Group (58)	Double-Blind	60	24.7	Improved mean BPRS	0
Pollak et al. (59)	Double-blind with open-label follow up	60	36	Improved mean CGIS, positive subscore of PANSS	0
Risperidone					
Meco et al. (60)	Open-label	6	0.67	6	0
Ford et al. (61)	Open-label	6	1.5	6	6
Rich et al. (62)	Open-label	6	0.5–4	4	5
Workman et al. (63)	Open-label	9	1.9	9	0
Meco et al. (64)	Open-label	10	0.73	9	3
Leopold (65)	Open-label	39	1.1	33	6
Mohr et al. (66)	Open-label	17	1.1	16	1
Ellis et al. (67)	Double blind	5	1.2	Improved mean BPRS	Worsening on UPDRS motor subscale, but no significant difference with clozapine group
Olanzapine					
U.S. Olanzapine trial (68)	Double-blind	41	4.2	Improved total BPRS, NPI, and CGIS psychosis scores	Worsening of total and motor UPDRS scores
European Olanzapine trial (68)	Double-blind	49	4.1	Improved total BPRS, NPI, and CGIS Psychosis Scores	Worsening of total and motor UPDRS scores
Ondo et al. (69)	Double-blind	16	4.6	No significant improvement overall	Worsened UPDRS motor scores

Quetiapine

Study	Design				
Fernandez et al. (70)	Double-blind	16	58.3	Improved on hallucination subscale of BPRS ($P = 0.02$) and on CGIS	3
Ondo et al. (71)	Double-blind	21	75–200	No significant improvement in BPRS scores	No significant worsening of UPDRS scores
Rabey et al. (72)	Double-blind	30	119.2	No difference compared to placebo	No difference compared to placebo
Reddy et al. (73)	Retrospective	43	54	32	5
Fernandez et al. (74)	Retrospective	103	60.8	84	13

Aripiprazole

Fernandez et al. (75)	Open-label	8	12.8	4	3
Friedman et al. (76)	Open-label	14	1–5	6	5

Abbreviations: BPRS, Brief Psychosis Rating Scale; CGIS, Clinical Global Impression of Severity; NPI, Neuropsychiatric Inventory; PANSS, Positive and Negative Syndrome Scale; PD, Parkinson's disease; UPDRS, Unified Parkinson's Disease Rating Scale.

are other common side effects of clozapine (59), but anticholinergic side effects have not been a major problem in PD (58). The use of atypical antipsychotics has been associated with a "metabolic syndrome" (insulin resistance, weight gain, dyslipidemia, and abnormal glucose metabolism) in schizophrenic patients (82). This has not been shown to occur in PD patients. The prevalence of diabetes in 44 parkinsonian subjects was similar to that of an age-matched group in the general population (79). This may be because subjects in this study were on a smaller dose of clozapine (50.6 mg/day) when compared with doses used in schizophrenic patients (300–900 mg/day). In summary, low-dose clozapine is safe and effective for psychosis in PD patients. However, due to stringent monitoring, the search for a more practical and "low-maintenance" treatment for psychosis in PD remains an important goal.

Thomas and Friedman published a retrospective chart review of patients treated with clozapine (83). Clozapine was indicated for psychosis in 39 patients, for tremor in 19 and for both tremor and psychosis in an additional six patients. Fifty (82%) of 61 patients reported an improvement or resolution of their symptoms with clozapine treatment. Thirty patients reported improvement in psychotic symptoms, 15 reported improvement in tremor and five reported improvement in both psychosis and tremor. Thirty-six patients (59%) reported adverse effects, including sedation, weakness, and worsening of motor symptoms, hallucinations, weight gain, increased blood glucose level, constipation, confusion or behavioral disturbance, drooling, and myoclonus. Two patients developed a drop in WBC count below 3.5 mm^3 × 10^9/L, of which one was transient and the other patient's blood count recovered to normal after discontinuing the medication. None had started on new diabetes medications or cholesterol-lowering agents while on clozapine. None of the patients reported a cardiac event while on clozapine. Although 11 patients died while on clozapine, none were thought to be related to clozapine use.

Risperidone

Risperidone is chemically distinct from clozapine and was found to behave more like "typical" neuroleptics, with a dose-dependent incidence of extrapyramidal side effects (84,85). In PD, all but one report of risperidone were open-label (Table 10.1).

Although risperidone was effective for psychosis in general, some reports describe the complete absence of motor side effects (60,63,86), whereas others report severe motor worsening in each patient who took the drug (61,87). The few studies that reported no worsening of parkinsonism followed small numbers of patients for a short period of time. Five open-label studies of risperidone reported 78 PD patients on doses ranging from 0.5 to 4.0 mg/day, with 21 having worsening of motor features (61,62,64–66), although in the largest open-label study (39 patients), five of the six patients that worsened were thought to have DLB, rather than PD (65).

In the only double-blind study of risperidone (67), the efficacy and safety of risperidone and clozapine were compared. Ten subjects with PD psychosis were enrolled. The mean motor Unified Parkinson's Disease Rating Scale (UPDRS) score worsened in the risperidone group and improved in the clozapine group, although this difference did not reach statistical significance. On the contrary, risperidone improved psychosis, whereas clozapine did not.

It is unclear why the results of risperidone studies in PD are so mixed; maybe multiple factors are responsible. Most of the studies were open-label and differ in terms of speed of medication titration and duration of the observations. However, given the results in the PD population thus far, it is unlikely that a double-blind placebo-controlled trial will be performed, and many movement disorder specialists are reluctant to place patients on this agent.

Olanzapine

Olanzapine has a chemical structure similar to clozapine. It offered more promise than risperidone, because it induced catalepsy at higher doses than would be used in humans (88) and did not cause significant prolactin secretion, a feature seen with risperidone (89). The first open-label study of olanzapine in PD showed that it was effective for drug-induced psychosis in 15 nondemented patients, at a mean dose of 6.5 mg/day, without worsening motor function (90). However, all subsequent open-label studies of olanzapine in PD showed that approximately 40% of subjects had motor decline (91). Four double-blind trials of olanzapine have been published, three of which were placebo-controlled and one which compared olanzapine with clozapine (68,69,92). The clozapine trial was prematurely stopped because six of seven olanzapine-treated subjects had significant motor decline (92). All three of the placebo-controlled trials reported that olanzapine had no effect on psychosis in PD and exacerbated parkinsonism (68,69). In addition, sedation and weight gain were common undesirable side effects. An evidence-based review of the treatment of psychosis in PD concluded that "there is insufficient evidence to demonstrate efficacy of olanzapine" and "olanzapine carries an unacceptable risk of motor deterioration" at low doses (93).

Quetiapine

Of all the atypical antipsychotics, quetiapine has the closest structural resemblance to clozapine. It has a strong affinity for the serotonin 5-HT2 receptor and moderate affinity for the dopamine D2 receptor (94). It also has low affinity for the muscarinic receptor, and thus anticholinergic effects are not seen. Agranulocytosis has not been reported with quetiapine.

There have been multiple open-label studies of quetiapine for drug-induced psychosis in PD—the two largest reports have been retrospective analyses. Reddy et al. (73) found that 35 of 43 PD patients treated with quetiapine had improved psychosis. Five patients (13%), all of whom were demented, experienced mild worsening of motor symptoms but not significant enough to discontinue treatment. Fernandez et al. (74) reported 106 parkinsonian patients treated with quetiapine. Seventy-eight out of 106 (74%) remained on quetiapine for a mean duration of 15 months at an average dose of 60 mg/day. Eighty-seven (82%) patients had partial or complete resolution of their psychosis, whereas 19 (18%) patients had no improvement. Motor decline was noted in 34 (32%) patients, but rarely warranted quetiapine discontinuation. Demented subjects had a 12-fold increased risk of nonresponse.

Patients experiencing visual hallucinations tend to have lower sleep efficiency and reduced total REM sleep time and percentage compared with those without visual hallucinations (95). A double-blind, placebo-controlled study of 16 patients by Fernandez et al. (70) showed that quetiapine improves visual hallucinations in PD, but not through normalization of sleep architecture. Patients randomized to quetiapine improved in the CGIS ($P = 0.03$) and the hallucination item of the BPRS compared with placebo. However, the change in the total BPRS was not significant between the two arms ($P = 0.78$). The UPDRS scores improved slightly in the quetiapine arm but did not reach statistical significance. Although the length of REM stage increased in the treatment arm and decreased in the placebo arm, it was not statistically significant ($P = 0.19$). The study is limited by the small sample size and high drop out rate (four in the quetiapine group and one in the placebo arm).

A double-blind, randomized, comparison trial of 40 PD patients placed on either quetiapine or clozapine found that both medications improved psychosis (96). There was no difference between the two groups in any parameters, either behaviorally or motorically, and the investigators concluded that both medications were equally efficacious. However, in two double-blind, placebo-controlled trials, quetiapine was not found to be efficacious for PD psychosis (71,72). In one trial (71), 31 subjects with PD psychosis were randomized in a 2:1 double-blind fashion to quetiapine or placebo. The final dose of quetiapine ranged from 75 to 200 mg/day, but the trial may not have been adequately powered to detect an effect. The second double-blind, placebo-controlled trial randomized 30 patients to quetiapine (mean dose 119 mg/day) and 28 patients to placebo (72). Fifteen patients in the quetiapine group discontinued the medication, 10 of them because of lack of efficacy. The authors postulated that the large dropout rate might have influenced their results. The results of these two trials are surprising, given that the available open-label studies of over 400 patients suggest that quetiapine appears to be well tolerated and effective. Future double-blind studies with larger numbers of subjects are needed.

Atypical antipsychotics have been associated with reports of new-onset diabetes mellitus. A retrospective study done by Fernandez et al. (97) showed a prevalence of 22.6% (12/53) of new-onset diabetes mellitus, slightly higher than the reported age-matched general population (17.3%) (98). The authors commented that they did not consider the body weight and fasting blood glucose prior to the study, which could have influenced the results.

Ziprasidone

Ziprasidone has a much higher affinity for serotonin 5-HT2 than dopamine D2 receptors and other atypical agents (99). Ziprasidone prolongs the QT interval, which has limited its use. However, there have been no cases of ziprasidone causing torsades de pointes (100). There have been only two case series reported on ziprasidone in PD. The first was a small open-label, 12-week trial in 12 PD patients (mean age 72.1 years) with psychosis (101). Mean doses of ziprasidone were 24 mg at one month and 32 mg at 12 weeks, with an improvement in psychosis of 58% after one month and 72% at 12 weeks. Although two patients had a slight worsening of motor symptoms, the UPDRS motor scores did not significantly worsen over the course of the trial. Two patients had to withdraw from the study, one because of sedation and the other due to gait deterioration. The second open-label report investigated an intramuscular preparation of ziprasidone for the emergency treatment of psychosis in PD (102). Five patients were given gluteal intramuscular injections of either 10 or 20 mg of ziprasidone. The mean BPRS score before injection was 72 and improved to 48 two hours after injection. During the 24 hours following the injections, there was no worsening of parkinsonian symptoms. On the basis of these studies, it appears that ziprasidone may be helpful for psychotic symptoms in PD without worsening parkinsonism. Furthermore, it is available in an intramuscular preparation, which can be useful, especially in delusional patients who refuse to take oral medications. However, on the basis of a review of the available data on ziprasidone in schizophrenia, it was concluded that its extrapyramidal symptom profile is "the same as olanzapine but not quite as good as quetiapine or clozapine" in one review (103), whereas in another review, ziprasidone was reported to produce "slightly more extrapyramidal side effects than olanzapine" (104).

Aripiprazole

Aripiprazole differs from the other agents in that it is a partial agonist at the D2 and 5HT1 receptors and an antagonist at the 5HT2a receptors. Aripiprazole also has a high 5HT/D2 affinity ratio, which theoretically makes it less likely to cause extrapyramidal symptoms. The data on aripiprazole in PD are scarce. An initial open-label study showed that aripiprazole improved psychosis completely in two out of eight subjects with PD, whereas the other six subjects discontinued the medication: two due to lack of efficacy, two due to motor worsening, one due to lack of motor improvement, and one due to intolerable restlessness and confusion (75). Another study of 14 PD subjects with drug-induced psychosis showed that aripiprazole (dose range 1–5 mg/day) improved psychosis in six patients, worsened psychosis in four, and caused no significant change in four (76). Eight subjects in this study withdrew: three because of worsened parkinsonism, two because of increased psychosis, two due to both worsened parkinsonism and psychosis, and one because of lack of efficacy. Although these studies were open-label and preliminary, they suggest that aripiprazole has a variable effect on psychotic symptoms, causes a high dropout rate due to adverse effects, and therefore should be used with caution in the PD population.

Odansetron

Odansetron is a selective 5HT-3 receptor antagonist. Although odansetron was ineffective for psychosis in schizophrenic patients (105), there have been reports of its success in the PD population. Zoldan et al. (106,107) reported two open-label trials with improvement of psychosis in a total of 40 PD patients. One patient had headache and seven had constipation. These positive findings have not been reproduced by others (108).

Cholinesterase Inhibitors

In multiple AD trials, cholinesterase inhibitors had mild-to-moderate benefits in both cognition and psychosis (109,110). Cholinesterase inhibitors are also effective for psychosis in DLB patients and are a potential alternative to the atypical antipsychotics for PD psychosis. An early open-label study with tacrine showed that five of seven demented PD patients had complete resolution of psychotic symptoms (111); however, the use of this drug has been limited because of hepatic toxicity.

Fabbrini et al. (112) administered donepezil (5 mg qhs) to eight nondemented PD patients with visual hallucinations, with or without delusions. At the end of two months, subjects had decreased PPRS scores with hallucinations and paranoid ideation, being the most responsive. However, two patients experienced clinically significant motor decline. Another small open-label study enrolled six patients with PD, dementia, and psychotic symptoms and treated them with 10 mg/day of donepezil (113). Five patients showed moderate-to-significant improvement in psychosis and one showed minimal improvement. None had worsening of motor symptoms. Finally, Kurita et al. (114) reported three PD patients who had improvement of visual hallucinations with 5 mg/day of donepezil without worsening of motor function, but one patient had treatment emergent delusions that resolved, after donepezil was discontinued. Only one placebo-controlled trial of donepezil has been reported for PD psychosis (115). This was a randomized, crossover trial in 22 subjects with PD and dementia. There was no difference in BPRS scores between patients on donepezil and patients on placebo; however, the trial excluded patients with severe psychosis.

Rivastigmine can also improve hallucinations in PD patients (116,117). In a 24-week, double-blind, placebo-controlled, randomized trial of 541 PD patients with dementia (118), patients on rivastigmine showed a mean improvement of 2.0 on the NPI, from a baseline mean score of 12.7.

There is one open-label study of galantamine on psychosis in PD (119). Seven of the nine patients with hallucinations improved, three of whom had complete amelioration of psychosis. However, three patients experienced increased tremor.

Pimavanserin (ACP-103)

Pimavanserin is an inverse agonist on the $5-HT_{2A}$ with 10 times selectivity over $5-HT_{2C}$ and no significant affinity or activity at $5-HT_{2B}$ and dopamine receptors (120). Through the selective serotonin activity, pimavanserin is expected to improve psychosis and possibly sleep in PD patients without deleterious effects on motor function. In September 2009, the first Phase III Parkinson's Disease Psychosis (PDP) trial (-012 Study) (121) was announced. The study did not meet its primary end-point of antipsychotic efficacy, although it showed that the 40 mg pimavanserin arm consistently demonstrated signals of efficacy across a number of measures. The study met the secondary endpoint of motoric tolerability and was safe, having similar frequency of adverse events to placebo. A double-blind, randomized, multi-center, 28-day study on the tolerability and efficacy of pimavanserin showed that pimavanserin-treated patients showed significantly greater improvement in some but not all measures of psychosis, including Scale for Assessment of Positive Symptoms (SAPS) global measures of hallucinations and delusions, persecutory delusions, and the UPDRS measure of delusions and hallucinations at a dose which did not impair motor function, or cause sedation or hypotension (122).

Patterns, Trends, and Recommendations in Antipsychotic Prescribing for Parkinson's Disease Psychosis

A study by Weintraub et al. (123) examined the frequency and characteristics, including changes over time, of antipsychotic use in a large cohort of patients with PD. Data were derived from national Department of Veterans Affairs (VA) databases for patients seen in fiscal years 2002 and 2008. There were about 60,000 patients in the VA system with the diagnosis of PD. Patients with the diagnosis of secondary parkinsonism and DLB were excluded. A total of 9504 patients were included, 2597 with PD and psychosis and 6907 with dementia and psychosis without PD. In 2008, 50% of patients with PD and psychosis were prescribed an antipsychotic. Quetiapine was most commonly prescribed (33% of all patients or 65.9% of treated patients), followed by risperidone (8.6% or 17.3%), aripiprazole (6.0% or 12.1%) and olanzapine (5.7% or 11.5%). Clozapine (0.9% or 1.8%) was rarely prescribed. Overall antipsychotic use was greater with PD and psychosis with dementia than in patients with dementia and psychosis without PD ($P < 0.001$). As compared to 2002, the re-evaluation in 2008 revealed: (*i*) persistence in risperidone and olanzapine use in both groups despite the warnings and guidelines set forth by the American Academy of Neurology (AAN) and Movement Disorder Society; (*ii*) the frequent use of aripiprazole, despite some reports of worsening of motor function; and (*iii*) the very infrequent use of clozapine, the gold-standard treatment for PD psychosis. The predictors of antipsychotic use in patients with PD includes younger age ($P < 0.001$) and absence of dementia ($P < 0.001$).

The AAN guideline (124) has recommended clozapine (Level B) and quetiapine (Level C) for patients with PD and psychosis with the recommendation of monitoring of absolute neutrophil count in patients on clozapine. Olanzapine should not be routinely considered based on the guideline.

Electroconvulsive Therapy

Electroconvulsive therapy (ECT) is an effective treatment for primary psychiatric disorders, especially treatment-resistant depression. Experience with ECT for PD psychosis, however, is limited to case studies. ECT has been demonstrated to be beneficial in PD patients with psychosis (125–127), and can transiently improve parkinsonian motor symptoms, but may require a period of hospitalization and result in significant confusion. ECT should only be considered when patients are resistant to pharmacologic therapies.

Long-Term Outcome of Treatment for Psychosis

Goetz and Stebbins (5) described 11 PD patients in a nursing home with hallucinations, all of whom were never discharged from the nursing home and died within two years. In an open-label extension of the U.S. double-blind clozapine trial, only 25% of subjects who were followed up till the end of the study died over a 26-month observational period. Forty-two percent were in nursing homes, 68% were demented, and 69% were still psychotic (4). A separate study of 39 parkinsonian patients, treated with clozapine for psychosis, found that only 15% had died over a span of five years and 33% had been admitted to nursing homes (128).

There are very few studies looking at whether or not patients can be weaned off their antipsychotic medications. Fernandez et al. (129) tried to wean off clozapine or quetiapine in psychiatrically stable PD patients with a history of drug-induced psychosis. Unfortunately, the study had to be aborted after enrolling only six patients, who had all been on their antipsychotics for an average of 20 months. Five experienced worsened psychosis, and three of these patients had a more severe psychosis than at baseline, suggesting the possibility of a "rebound psychosis." In contrast, a five-year follow-up of 32 PD patients with psychosis on clozapine found that nine were able to discontinue the clozapine without recurrence of psychosis (80). More research in this area is needed, but a six-year longitudinal study of PD patients with hallucinations found that hallucinators at baseline continued to have hallucinations at the end of study observation (16). Therefore, once patients start antipsychotic medications, it is likely that they will require treatment indefinitely.

DEMENTIA

A substantial number of patients with PD will develop dementia. There were no formal criteria for the diagnosis of PD dementia until the Movement Disorder Society Task Force published their proposed clinical diagnostic criteria (Table 10.2) (130). They defined two categories: probable and possible PD dementia. In order to have probable PD dementia, patients must have the presence of two core features: a diagnosis of PD per the Queen Square Brain Bank criteria (131,132) plus a

TABLE 10.2 Criteria for The Diagnosis of Probable and Possible PD Dementia

Probable PD Dementia
A. Core features: Both must be present
B. Associated clinical features:
  • Typical profile of cognitive deficits, including impairment in at least two of the four core cognitive domains (impaired attention which may fluctuate, impaired executive functions, impairment in visuospatial functions, and impaired free recall memory which usually improves with cueing)
  • The presence of at least one behavioral symptom (apathy, depressed or anxious mood, hallucinations, delusions, excessive daytime sleepiness) supports the diagnosis of probable PD dementia, lack of behavioral symptoms, however, does not exclude the diagnosis
C. None of the group III features present
D. None of the group IV features present

Possible PD Dementia
A. Core features: Both must be present
B. Associated clinical features:
  • Atypical profile of cognitive impairment in one or more domains, such as prominent or receptive-type (fluent) aphasia, or pure storage-failure type amnesia (memory does not improve with cueing or in recognition tasks) with preserved attention
  • Behavioral symptoms may or may not be present
OR
C. One or more of the group III features present
D. None of the group IV features present

Abbreviation: PD, Parkinson's disease.
Source: Adapted from Ref. 134.

dementia syndrome, characterized by slow onset and decline in cognition in at least one cognitive domain, interfering with daily life and representing a decline from a premorbid level. The following associated features also must be present: documented impairment in at least two of four core cognitive domains (attention, executive function, memory, visuospatial) and behavioral features (apathy, hallucinations, delusions, excessive daytime sleepiness) (Table 10.3) (130). Finally, there cannot be any confounding factors, such as the presence of vascular disease that could contribute to cognitive impairment, or other disorders, such as delirium, that could explain the cognitive impairment. For possible PD dementia, the two core features must be present and there can be no other disorders responsible for the cognitive impairment, but the associated features criteria do not have to be met. The Movement Disorder Society Task Force also recommended two levels of tests to implement these definitions. Level I (Table 10.4) is a practical set that can be used by any clinician without expertise in neuropsychological methods. Level II (Table 10.5) employs a more detailed method for greater descriptive documentation suitable for research purposes (133).

Complicating the picture of dementia in PD is the clinical entity of DLB, a dementing illness characterized by parkinsonism, visual hallucinations, and fluctuating cognition (136). There are multiple clinical (parkinsonism, visual hallucinations, attention deficits, executive dysfunction) and pathologic similarities (Lewy bodies in the limbic and neocortex) between the two disorders, leading to the hypothesis that the two conditions could be considered as opposite ends of the spectrum of one illness (137,138). From a neuropsychological view, PD dementia and DLB are more readily distinguished from AD than each other, although there

TABLE 10.3   Features of Dementia Associated with Parkinson's Disease

I. Core features

1. Diagnosis of Parkinson's disease according to Queen Square Brain Bank criteria
2. A dementia syndrome with insidious onset and slow progression, developing within the context of established Parkinson's disease and diagnosed by history, clinical, and mental examination, defined as:
   - Impairment in more than one cognitive domain
   - Representing a decline from premorbid level
   - Deficits severe enough to impair daily life (social, occupational, or personal care), independent of the impairment ascribable to motor or autonomic symptoms

II. Associated clinical features

1. Cognitive features:
   - Attention: Impaired. Impairment in spontaneous and focused attention, poor performance in attentional tasks; performance may fluctuate during the day and from day to day
   - Executive functions: Impaired. Impairment in tasks requiring initiation, planning, concept formation, rule finding, set shifting or set maintenance; impaired mental speed (bradyphrenia)
   - Visuospatial functions: Impaired. Impairment in tasks requiring visual-spatial orientation, perception, or construction
   - Memory: Impaired. Impairment in free recall of recent events or in tasks requiring learning new material, memory usually improves with cueing, recognition is usually better than free recall
   - Language: Core functions largely preserved. Word finding difficulties and impaired comprehension of complex sentences may be present
2. Behavioral features:
   - Apathy: decreased spontaneity; loss of motivation, interest, and effortful behavior
   - Changes in personality and mood including depressive features and anxiety
   - Hallucinations: mostly visual, usually complex, formed visions of people, animals or objects
   - Delusions: usually paranoid, such as infidelity, or phantom boarder (unwelcome guests living in the home) delusions
   - Excessive daytime sleepiness

III. Features which do not exclude PD dementia, but make the diagnosis uncertain

   - Co-existence of any other abnormality which may by itself cause cognitive impairment, but judged not to be the cause of dementia, e.g. presence of relevant vascular disease in imaging
   - Time interval between the development of motor and cognitive symptoms not known

IV. Features suggesting other conditions or diseases as cause of mental impairment, which, when present make it impossible to reliably diagnose PD dementia

Cognitive and behavioral symptoms appearing solely in the context of other conditions such as:
   - Acute confusion due to
     a. Systemic diseases or abnormalities
     b. Drug intoxication
   - Major depression according to DSM-IV
   - Features compatible with "Probable Vascular dementia" criteria according to NINDS-AIREN (dementia in the context of cerebrovascular disease as indicated by focal signs in neurologic exam such as hemiparesis, sensory deficits, and evidence of relevant cerebrovascular disease by brain imaging AND a relationship between the two as indicated by the presence of one or more of the following: onset of dementia within three months after a recognized stroke, abrupt deterioration in cognitive functions, and fluctuating, stepwise progression of cognitive deficits)

Abbreviations: DSM-IV, Diagnostic and Statistical Manual of Mental Disorders, 4th edition; NINDS-AIREN, National Institute of Neurological Disorders and Stroke and Association Internationale pour la Recherché et l'Enseignement en Neurosciences; PD, Parkinson's disease.
Source: Adapted from Ref. 134.

TABLE 10.4   Algorithm for Diagnosing PD Dementia at Level I

---

1. A diagnosis of PD based on the Queen's Square Brain Bank criteria for PD
2. PD developed prior to the onset of dementia
3. MMSE below 26
4. Cognitive deficits severe enough to impact daily living (Caregiver interviews or Pill Questionnaire)
5. Impairment in at least two of the following tests:
   a. Months reversed or Seven backwards
   b. Lexical fluency or Clock drawing
   c. MMSE pentagons
   d. Three-Word recall
The presence of one of the following behavioral symptoms: apathy or depressed mood or delusion or excessive daytime sleepiness may support the diagnosis of probably PD dementia.
The presence of major depression or delirium or any other abnormality may by itself cause significant cognitive impairment makes the diagnosis uncertain.

Abbreviations: MMSE, Mini-Mental State Examination; PD, Parkinson's disease.
Source: Adapted from Ref. 135.

may be more severe impairment on tasks involving attention, working memory, and verbal fluency in DLB than in PD dementia (139).

Clinical criteria for distinguishing DLB from PD dementia have also been published (130,137). Patients whose disease begins with cognitive impairment are diagnosed with DLB, whereas patients who first develop parkinsonism and meet the criteria for a diagnosis of idiopathic PD are diagnosed with PD dementia when dementia occurs (140). This definition of PD dementia is consistent temporally with the Movement Disorder Society Task Force definition mentioned earlier (130). However, long-term studies with neuropathologic follow-up will be essential in determining whether this clinical distinction correlates with the underlying pathologic substrate.

Incidence, Prevalence, and Risk Factors

Estimates of incidence and prevalence of dementia in PD vary widely because of different definitions, methods of ascertainment, and study designs. The prevalence rates of dementia in hospital or clinic-based cohort studies range from 11% to 22% (141–143), whereas population-based estimates are somewhat higher, ranging from 18% to 44% (9,144–147), perhaps reflecting referral bias. A systematic review of the literature estimated that the prevalence of dementia in PD ranges from 25% to 31% (148). This review also found that dementia in PD accounted for 3–4% of the total dementia population.

Incidence rates for PD dementia range from 4% to 11% per year, with a relative risk for the development of dementia in PD of 2–6 (12,147,149–151). Age and severity of extrapyramidal symptoms were associated with an overall risk of developing dementia. One study demonstrated that age and severity of disease by themselves were not associated with a greater risk of dementia, but the combination of these two features resulted in an almost 10-fold greater risk (152), suggesting a combined effect. Later age of onset of PD, longer duration of PD symptoms, the presence of hallucinations, depressive symptoms, and a family history of dementia have also been reported to be risk factors for dementia in PD, although less consistently.

Some common risk factors for the development of AD, including head injury, hypertension, and diabetes mellitus, are not predictors for the development of

TABLE 10.5 Summary of Tests at Level II Testing for PD Dementia

Global Efficiency Executive Functions	Mattis DRS
Working memory	Digit span
	Spatial span (CANTAB)
	Digit ordering test
Conceptualization	Similarities (WAIS-III)
	Wisconsin CST
Set activation	Verbal fluency (C, F, L)
Set shifting	TMT
Set maintenance	Stroop test
	Odd man out test
Behavioral control	Prehension behavior
Memory	
	RAVLT
	Free and cued recall test
Instrumental functions	
Language	
Visuo-constructive	Boston naming test
Visuo-spatial	Copy of the clock
	Benton line orientation test
	Cube analysis (VOSP)
Visuo-perceptive	Benton face recognition test
	Fragmented letters (VOSP)
Neuropsychiatric functions	
Apathy	Apathy scale
Depression	MADRS
	Hamilton
	Beck depression inventory
	GDS-15
Visual hallucination	PPQ6
Psychosis	NPI

Abbreviations: CST, Card Sorting Test; DRS, Dementia Rating Scale; MADRS, Montgomery–Asberg Depression Rating Scales; NPI, The Neuropsychiatric Inventory; PPQ, Parkinson Psychosis Questionnaire; PD, Parkinson's disease; RAVLT, Rey Auditory Verbal Learning Test; TMT, Trail Making Test; VOSP, Visual Object and Space Perception Battery; WAIS, Wechsler Adult Intelligence Scale.

dementia in PD (153). However, smoking might protect against cognitive decline and dementia in PD (154,155), although there is a study which did not show an association (156). In addition, amantadine (an NMDA antagonist) use may delay the onset of dementia in PD patients and reduce the severity of dementia (157).

The epsilon 4 isoform of the apolipoprotein E gene (APO-E4) and butyrylcho-linesterase-K (BuChE-K) alleles have been associated with an increased risk for AD. APO-E4 has also been shown to correlate with an increased risk of dementia in PD (12,158,159). Some PD dementia patients may also carry both the APO-E4 allele and the BuChE-K alelle, which appears to result in more rapid cognitive deterioration (160,161). The epsilon 2 allele (APO-E2) has also been reported to be associated with the development of dementia in PD patients (12,158), although the effect of all these genotypes on PD dementia remains controversial. In patients with mild PD without dementia, there seems to be a role for catecholaminergic metabolism and its modulation by the COMT Val158Met polymorphism in executive function (162–164). COMT genotype might affect performance on tasks sensitive to fronto-striatal dysfunction, such as the Tower of London test, reflecting cortical dopamine modulation. However, the COMT genotype does not seem to be a risk factor for dementia (165). Dementia has been reported in genetic forms of PD and glucocerebrosidase mutations implicated in Lewy body formation may also increase the risk of PD dementia (166,167). The risk of developing dementia in the early stage of the disease is higher among carriers of mutations in the alpha-synuclein gene (168,169).

Clinical Features and Progression of PD Dementia

In many PD patients, mild cognitive impairment (MCI) is present, even at the time of diagnosis (170,171). Executive function deficits are usually the earliest cognitive signs in PD, although the visuospatial and memory domains may also be affected (28,172,173). The concept of PD-MCI is an evolving one, and there are no universally accepted criteria for PD-MCI. There are reported criteria for MCI in general, requiring subjective cognitive complaints, along with objective evidence of cognitive impairment without functional impairment (174). However, this definition is not specific to PD. Identifying subjective cognitive impairment in PD patients without dementia has been difficult, and many studies looking at MCI may not include this feature as part of their MCI definition. Nevertheless, some studies have indicated that the presence of MCI confers an increased risk of developing dementia in PD (175,176).

PD patients with dementia have difficulties in the domains of executive function, memory, attention, and visuospatial function. Unlike AD, language deficits are uncommon in PD dementia. In the domain of executive dysfunction, verbal fluency problems are common (177). Although memory complaints are common, the memory deficits in PD are considered to be problems with retrieval, rather than encoding, as seen in AD. Thus recognition memory recall is less affected than free recall in PD dementia (130). Fluctuating attention is a common feature of DLB, but is also present in PD dementia patients, who perform more poorly on tests of attention compared with AD patients (178).

The rate of cognitive decline in PD can be variable depending on the population subset. A community-based study estimated that the mean overall annual rate of cognitive decline in PD patients was one point on the Mini-Mental State Examination (MMSE) (179). However, patients with PD and dementia declined faster, at a rate of 2.3 points, whereas PD patients who did not develop dementia progressed at the same rate as age-matched controls. The mean duration of PD before dementia develops is approximately 10 years, although this varies widely between individuals (144,149). In the Sydney Multicenter Study (180), after 20 years follow-up of newly diagnosed PD patients, 25 of 30 (83%) surviving patients were demented, leading the authors to suggest that the development of dementia in PD was inevitable.

Pathophysiology of PD Dementia
Pathology and Imaging

There is controversy regarding which features are the primary contributors to dementia in PD. PD is characterized by cell loss in the substantia nigra pars compacta (SNc), resulting in loss of dopaminergic input into the striatum. Several pathologic and functional imaging studies have shown that in PD, there is greater depletion in the lateral compartment of the SNc, which projects to the putamen, than in the medial compartment, which projects to the caudate (181–183). Cognitive impairment is associated with loss of dopaminergic projections to the caudate (184). This functional division of the striatum is, perhaps, the main reason for the predominance of motor, over cognitive symptoms in PD and is likely why dopaminergic agents do not markedly improve cognition in PD (185).

A relationship between cholinergic deficiency and dementia in PD has also been reported (186). Striking cell loss is seen in the nucleus basalis of Meynert, which provides projections to the amygdala and neocortex (186,187). Additionally, choline acetyltransferase activity has consistently been reported to be decreased to approximately 40–60% of control values in frontal, temporal, and hippocampal cortex (188–190), and correlates with cognitive impairment. Loss of neurons in the locus ceruleus and corresponding noradrenergic deficiency may also be associated with cognitive impairment in PD, but this has not been consistently shown (191,192).

Studies of brain metabolism have shown hypoperfusion in the occipital, temporo-parietal, and prefrontal cortex in patients with DLB and PD dementia. Normal controls and patients with PD without dementia in general do not show significant changes (193).

Multiple autopsy series have shown that the presence of AD pathology correlates with dementia in PD (194,195). However, because some demented PD patients can have minimal numbers of plaques and neurofibrillary tangles, the assertion that AD pathology is responsible for PD dementia remains controversial (131,196,197). Positron emission tomography (PET) studies using [11C]PIB, a marker of brain amyloid deposition, have found that amyloid load is significantly raised in over 80% of DLB subjects but only 15% in the PD dementia subjects (150).

Much of the literature has focused on the presence of Lewy bodies in the cortex and limbic system, and their association with cognitive impairment. Hurtig et al. (196), in a clinicopathologic study of 22 demented and 20 nondemented PD patients, discovered that cortical Lewy bodies were highly sensitive (91%) and specific (90%) neuropathologic markers of dementia in PD. In contrast, the presence of AD pathology (senile plaques and neurofibrillary tangles) was only 64% sensitive and between 70% and 75% specific for dementia. In another study, Apaydin et al. (198) looked at the brains of 13 PD patients with dementia compared with nine PD patients without dementia. The authors found that 12 of the 13 demented PD patients had a 10-fold increase in Lewy body counts compared with the nondemented group. In seven of these patients, Lewy bodies were primarily present in the limbic areas, whereas in the other five, the Lewy bodies were widespread.

Biomarkers
Because of the large amount of clinical overlap between PD dementia and DLB, and pathologic overlap between these two Lewy body disorders and AD pathology, groups have looked at whether cerebrospinal fluid (CSF) biomarkers could help distinguish between these disorders. Parnetti et al. (199) showed that CSF levels of Aβ42 and total tau differ between DLB and PD dementia patients. CSF Aβ42 (a marker inversely related to senile plaque density), was remarkably low in DLB compared with PD dementia. In addition, CSF total tau (a marker of axonal damage), was higher in DLB as compared with PD dementia. Levels of CSF p-tau (a CSF biomarker of neurofibrillary tangles and elevated in AD) did not significantly differ between DLB and PD dementia. These CSF biomarkers may have the potential to aid in differentiating these different disorders, but unfortunately reports have been inconsistent in the literature. For example, CSF total tau levels have not been

reported to be increased in all studies of DLB (200), and was reported to be increased in PD dementia in one study (201).

General Treatment of Dementia

Similar to the guidelines governing the general treatment of psychosis, any sudden change in cognition or behavior is most likely due to a medical cause. Therefore, infections, metabolic and endocrine derangements, and hypoperfusion states should be considered and treated if present. A switch to an unfamiliar environment may also precipitate an acute deterioration in cognitive status, and can be helped to a small degree with reassurance and frequent orientation. Substance abuse, including reliance on over-the-counter preparations containing antihistamines, is another factor that may be commonly overlooked. A review of the medication list is necessary and medications with CNS effects (sedatives, narcotics, antidepressants, anxiolytics, and antihistamines) should be discontinued, or used sparingly. The clinician should also be aware that other commonly prescribed medications, including antiemetics, antispasmodics for the bladder, H_2 receptor antagonists, antiarrhythmic agents, antihypertensive agents, and nonsteroidal anti-inflammatory agents, may also cause cognitive impairment.

Treatment for Dementia
Cholinesterase Inhibitors

Four cholinesterase inhibitors have been approved by the FDA for the treatment of AD: tacrine (1993), donepezil (1995), rivastigmine (2000), and galantamine (2001), but only rivastigmine has been approved for PD dementia (2006). They are all postulated to help correct the cholinergic deficit seen in PD dementia by increasing the amount of acetylcholine (ACh) available for binding to cholinergic receptors in the synaptic cleft. For all the cholinesterase inhibitors, the most common side effects are gastrointestinal distress (nausea, diarrhea, vomiting), fatigue, insomnia, and muscle cramps (202). Rivastigmine tends to also be associated with weight loss and dizziness.

Although all these medications inhibit the action of acetylcholinesterase (AChE), there are subtle differences between these agents, especially with regard to butyrylcholinesterase (BuChE) inhibition and effect on the nicotinic receptors (Table 10.6). BuChE also breaks down ACh in the synaptic cleft, so inhibition of both BuChE and AChE may theoretically have greater clinical effect in dementia than inhibition of AChE alone. Both tacrine and rivastigmine inhibit BuChE. Cholinergic nicotinic receptor binding is reduced in PD and directly parallels the degree of dementia (203). Galantamine is also an allosteric modulator of presynaptic nicotinic cholinergic receptors. Therefore, by potentiating cholinergic nicotinic transmission, galantamine may be more suited for patients with PD dementia. However, despite these differences between the cholinesterase inhibitors, there have been no comparison trials to suggest that one is superior over another for PD dementia.

Hutchinson and Fazzini (111) reported an open-label trial of tacrine in seven patients with PD dementia. All patients had improvement in hallucinations: five with complete resolution and two with partial improvement. They also had a 7.1-point improvement in mean MMSE scores and an improvement in motor scores. These results suggested that cholinesterase inhibitors could improve neuropsychiatric features in PD without motor deterioration. However,

TABLE 10.6 Properties of the Cholinesterase Inhibitors

Property	Tacrine	Donepezil	Rivastigmine	Galantamine
Chemical class	Acridine	Piperidine	Carbamate	Phenanthrene alkaloid
Cholinesterase selectivity	AChE and BuChE	AChE	AChE and BuChE	AChE
Nicotinic ACh receptor action	Modulator	–	–	Allosteric modulation
Type of cholinesterase inhibition	Noncompetitive reversible	Noncompetitive reversible	Noncompetitive reversible; most potent	Competitive reversible; least potent
Dose range (mg)	5–160	2.5–10	1.5–12	4–32
Dosing frequency	qid	qd	bid	Bid or qd with sustained release preparation

Abbreviations: ACh, acetylcholine; AChE, acetylcholinesterase; BuChE, butyrylcholinesterase.

in other studies, tacrine was associated with fulminant hepatotoxicity, which has limited its use.

The accumulation of evidence that cholinesterase inhibitors were effective for the cognitive and behavioral sequelae of DLB without significant motor side effects rejuvenated interest in these compounds for treating dementia in PD (204–208). Subsequently, multiple open-label reports in PD dementia emerged and are summarized in Table 10.7 (111,113,114,116,117,119,209–211). Unfortunately, variability in the trial designs, inclusion criteria, and assessment measures make it difficult to compare studies. Overall, however, it appears that the cholinesterase inhibitors result in mild improvements in cognition without change in parkinsonian features. The few studies that reported motor deterioration noticed an effect mainly on tremor.

In a randomized, double-blind, placebo-controlled trial (212), 14 individuals with PD and cognitive impairment received either donepezil (5 or 10 mg/day) or placebo in a cross-over design of two sequential periods lasting 10 weeks each. Patients had a history of cognitive decline at least one year after the onset of parkinsonism (3.0 ± 2.6 years) to decrease the likelihood of enrolling patients with DLB. The entire cohort had a mean age of 71 years, average duration of PD 10.8 years, and a mean levodopa dose of 485 mg/day. Patients had to have a MMSE score between 16 and 26. In addition, all patients had to have a decline in memory and at least one other category of cognitive function. After 10 weeks of treatment, donepezil improved the MMSE score by 2.1 points, but the placebo group did not improve (0.3). Furthermore, the clinician's interview-based impression of change (CIBIC) was greater for the donepezil group when compared with placebo. Motor function did not worsen during donepezil treatment, and no carry-over effect was noted.

There have been two other double-blind, placebo-controlled trials of donepezil in PD patients. Leroi et al. (213) randomized 16 patients to donepezil (2.5–10 mg/day) or placebo. Patients had to meet Diagnostic and Statistical Manual of Mental

TABLE 10.7 Summary of Open-label Studies of Cholinesterase Inhibitors for Dementia in Parkinson's Disease

Study	Drug	N	Age	Length PD	Cognitive Outcome	Motor Response
Hutchinson and Fazzini (111)	Tacrine	7	74	8	Improved MMSE, VH reduced	UPDRS markedly improved
Werber and Rabey (211)	Tacrine/ Donepezil	7/4	75	10	ADAS-cog improved, MMSE nonsignificant improvement	SPES unchanged overall but 5 patients had motor improvement
Bergman and Lerner (113)	Donepezil	6	69	5	Improvement on SAPS (5/6)	SAS unchanged
Kurita et al. (114)	Donepezil	3	70	12	MMSE improved in 1 patient 16 to 21	Unchanged in 2 patients, tremor worsened in 1
Minett et al. (210)	Donepezil	11 (PDD) 8 (DLB)	ND	ND	Improved MMSE in both groups, no significant change in NPI	No change in mean UPDRS motor scores, 7 patients reported tremor
Reading et al. (117)	Rivastigmine	12	71	12	Improved NPI and MMSE	UPDRS unchanged
Bullock and Cameron (116)	Rivastigmine	5	75	ND	Cognition improved in 2 and stabilized in 2. 1 patient did not have dementia	Not formally tested. 2 patients worsened, 1 improved slightly
Giladi et al. (209)	Rivastigmine	28	75	7	Improved ADAS-cog scores, but not MMSE	UPDRS mildly improved
Aarsland et al. (119)	Galantamine	16	76	13	Global cognitive improvement in 8 patients, worse in 4	6 Patients improved, 4 had no change, 3 had worsened tremor

Abbreviations: ADAS-cog, Alzheimer's Disease Assessment Scale-cognitive subscale; DLB, dementia with Lewy bodies; MMSE, Mini-Mental State Examination; ND, not described; PDD, Parkinson's disease with dementia; SAPS, Scale for the Assessment of Positive Symptoms; SAS, Simpson–Angus Scale; UPDRS, Unified Parkinson's Disease Rating Scale; SPES, Short Parkinson Evaluation Scale.

Disorders, 4th edition (DSM-IV) criteria for either dementia or cognitive impairment secondary to PD. Seven patients were placed on donepezil therapy for a mean duration of 15.2 weeks. There was no difference between the two groups at the final visit in terms of MMSE or DRS scores, but the donepezil group had a 60% improvement in the DRS memory subscore, compared with a 12.5% improvement in the placebo arm. Four of the donepezil-treated patients withdrew from the study, one from worsening parkinsonism. However, there were no significant group differences in the UPDRS scores from baseline to the final visit. The second trial used a crossover design in 22 PD subjects with dementia (115). Patients had to have an MMSE score between 17 and 26, and meet DSM-IV criteria for dementia in order to be included in the study. Each treatment period was 10 weeks with a six-week washout between the two periods. Patients on donepezil had a nonsignificant improvement in their ADAS-cog scores (primary outcome measure), but had a two-point improvement on their MMSE score and on overall clinical impression. The FDA has approved a high dose of donepezil (23 mg) for the treatment of moderate-to-severe AD, but this dose has not been studied in PD dementia patients.

There are no placebo-controlled trials reported for galantamine at this time. However, a large double-blind, placebo-controlled trial of rivastigmine for dementia in PD has been reported (118). This study enrolled 541 patients with mild-to-moderate dementia and PD, and randomized them to rivastigmine (mean dose 8.6 mg/d) or placebo for 24 weeks. About 410 subjects completed the study with dropouts primarily due to nausea, vomiting, and tremor. There was a significant improvement in the primary outcome measures for the rivastigmine group: ADAS-cog score at 24 weeks (2.1 ± 8.2) and the overall clinical impression. Secondary efficacy variables, Alzheimer's Disease Cooperative Study–Activities of Daily Living Scale, NPI-10, MMSE, verbal fluency, Cognitive Drug Research Computerized Assessment System power of attention tests, and the Clock-Drawing test also improved in the rivastigmine group. In a 24-week open extension of this trial (214), patients on rivastigmine in the original trial maintained their improvement at week 48 of treatment, whereas patients who were previously taking placebo and placed on rivastigmine (mean 7.7 mg/day) experienced a 2.8 point improvement in ADAS-cog scores at the end of 24 weeks.

In summary, there are emerging data that cholinesterase inhibitors produce a mild-to-moderate benefit on cognition in PD dementia. Although direct comparison between the different drugs is difficult, rivastigmine is the only approved medication for PD dementia. Other possible approaches to improving cholinergic function in the brain, such as dietary supplementation with cholinergic precursors (lecithin) and administration of cholinergic receptor agonists (bethanechol, milameline, tasaclidine), have not been found to be useful in AD and are unlikely to be tried in patients with PD dementia.

NMDA Antagonists

Memantine, an N-methyl-D-aspartate antagonist, has been approved for AD but not for PD dementia. There have been two randomized, double-blind placebo-controlled trials for memantine in patients with PD dementia reported. Aarsland et al. (215) performed a parallel-group, 24-week, randomized, controlled study of memantine (20 mg per day) versus placebo in patients with PD dementia or DLB. Seventy two patients with PD dementia or DLB were randomly assigned to memantine (34) or placebo (38) and 56 (78%) completed the study. The withdrawals were similar in both groups owing to adverse events. At 24 weeks, the memantine group had better CGIS compared with placebo. The subgroup analysis showed no difference in the mean Clinical Global Impression of Change, Last Observation Carried Forward method (CGIC LOCF) in patients with DLB (mean difference −0.1, −1.1 to 1.3) but a more pronounced global response in patients with PD dementia (mean difference 1.4, 0.6 to 2.2).

Another randomized, double-blind, placebo-controlled trial of memantine in PD dementia/DLB was reported by Emre et al. (216). This study enrolled 199 subjects. Thirty-four subjects with DLB and 62 with PD dementia were given memantine, and 41 with DLB and 58 with PD dementia were given placebo. There were 159 (80%) patients that completed the study with 80 in the memantine group and 79 in the placebo group. In the PD dementia group, the Alzheimer's Disease Cooperative Study-Clinical Global Impression of Change (ADCS-CGIC) score and NPI scores were not significantly different between the memantine and placebo groups at week 24 or at any time point. The study showed that there was improvement in the ADCS-CGIC and NPI scores in the DLB group who received memantine when compared with placebo. Thus, it remains unclear if memantine is beneficial in patients with PD dementia.

Other Pharmacologic Agents

Few other pharmacologic strategies for specifically treating dementia in PD have been reported. Because noradrenergic depletion could contribute to executive dysfunction in PD, Bedard et al. (217) conducted a trial of naphtoxazine (SDZ-NVI-085), a selective noradrenergic alpha 1 agonist, versus placebo in nondemented patients with PD. The results of the study demonstrated improved performance on tasks of set-shifting and cognitive flexibility, such as the Stroop and Odd-Man-Out tests. Furthermore, specific evoked potentials (Nd1 and Nd2 curves), thought to reflect attentional processes and known to be affected in PD, were improved with naphtoxazine.

The effect of estrogen replacement therapy (ERT) on the risk of development of dementia was investigated in 87 women with PD without dementia, 80 women with PD with dementia, and 989 nondemented healthy women. ERT did not affect the risk of PD, but appeared to be protective for the development of dementia, arising within the setting of PD [odds ratio 0.22, 95% confidence interval (95% CI) 0.05–1.0] (218). Furthermore, a survey of PD patients residing in nursing homes in five U.S. states demonstrated that female residents on ERT were less cognitively impaired than patients not taking ERT (219).

Simvastatin, a 3-hydroxy-3-methylglutaryl-coenzyme (HMG coA) reductase inhibitor, was shown to reduce the incidence of dementia and PD in subjects 65 years and older (220). Data from the decision support system of the U.S. Veterans Affairs database were analyzed for 4.5 million subjects. The hazard ratio for incidence of dementia for simvastatin and atorvastatin were 0.46 (CI 0.44–0.48, $P < 0.0001$) and 0.91 (CI 0.80–1.02, $P = 0.11$), respectively. Lovastatin was not associated with reduction in the incidence of dementia. Simvastatin also exhibited a reduced hazard ratio (HR) for newly acquired PD (HR 0.51, CI 0.4–0.55, $P < 0.0001$). The authors concluded that the effect of simvastatin, as compared with lovastatin and atorvastatin could be partly due to the strong efficacy with intermediate permeability to the blood–brain barrier. Further studies are required to determine if these findings are due to a biologic action of simvastatin or a statistical effect.

REFERENCES

1. Parkinson J. An Essay on the Shaking Palsy. London: Sherwood, Neely, & Jones, 1817.
2. Aarsland D, Larsen JP, Tandberg E, et al. Predictors of nursing home placement in Parkinson's disease: a population-based, prospective study. J Am Geriatr Soc 2000; 48: 938–42.
3. Goetz CG, Stebbins GT. Risk factors for nursing home placement in advanced Parkinson's disease. Neurology 1993; 43: 2227–9.
4. Factor SA, Feustel PJ, Friedman JH, et al. Longitudinal outcome of Parkinson's disease patients with psychosis. Neurology 2003; 60: 1756–61.
5. Goetz CG, Stebbins GT. Mortality and hallucinations in nursing home patients with advanced Parkinson's disease. Neurology 1995; 45: 669–71.
6. Aarsland D, Larsen JP, Karlsen K, et al. Mental symptoms in Parkinson's disease are important contributors to caregiver distress. Int J Geriatr Psychiatry 1999; 14: 866–74.
7. Louis ED, Tang MX, Cote L, et al. Progression of parkinsonian signs in Parkinson disease. Arch Neurol 1999; 56: 334–7.
8. Marras C, Rochon P, Lang AE. Predicting motor decline and disability in Parkinson disease: a systematic review. Arch Neurol 2002; 59: 1724–8.
9. Aarsland D, Tandberg E, Larsen JP, et al. Frequency of dementia in Parkinson disease. Arch Neurol 1996; 53: 538–42.
10. Fernandez HH, Lapane KL. Predictors of mortality among nursing home residents with a diagnosis of Parkinson's disease. Med Sci Monit 2002; 8: CR241–6.
11. Hughes TA, Ross HF, Mindham RH, et al. Mortality in Parkinson's disease and its association with dementia and depression. Acta Neurol Scand 2004; 110: 118–23.
12. de Lau LM, Schipper CM, Hofman A, et al. Prognosis of Parkinson disease: risk of dementia and mortality: the Rotterdam Study. Arch Neurol 2005; 62: 1265–9.
13. American Psychiatric Association. Diagnostic and Statistical Manual of Mental Disorders, 4th edn. (DSM-IV), 4th edn. Washington, DC: American Psychiatric Association, 1994.
14. Fenelon G, Mahieux F, Huon R, et al. Hallucinations in Parkinson's disease: prevalence, phenomenology and risk factors. Brain 2000; 123: 733–45.
15. Sanchez-Ramos JR, Ortoll R, Paulson GW. Visual hallucinations associated with Parkinson disease. Arch Neurol 1996; 53: 1265–8.
16. Goetz CG, Wuu J, Curgian LM, et al. Hallucinations and sleep disorders in PD: six-year prospective longitudinal study. Neurology 2005; 64: 81–6.
17. Holroyd S, Currie L, Wooten GF. Prospective study of hallucinations and delusions in Parkinson's disease. J Neurol Neurosurg Psychiatry 2001; 70: 734–8.
18. Chou KL, Messing S, Oakes D, et al. Drug-induced psychosis in Parkinson disease: phenomenology and correlations among psychosis rating instruments. Clin Neuropharmacol 2005; 28: 215–19.
19. Factor SA, Molho ES, Podskalny GD, et al. Parkinson's disease: drug-induced psychiatric states. Adv Neurol 1995; 65: 115–38.
20. Greene P, Cote L, Fahn S. Treatment of drug-induced psychosis in Parkinson's disease with clozapine. Adv Neurol 1993; 60: 703–6.
21. Marsh L, Williams JR, Rocco M, et al. Psychiatric comorbidities in patients with Parkinson disease and psychosis. Neurology 2004; 63: 293–300.
22. Cummings JL. Behavioral complications of drug treatment of Parkinson's disease. J Am Geriatr Soc 1991; 39: 708–16.
23. Fernandez HH, Friedman JH. The role of atypical antipsychotics in the treatment of movement disorders. CNS Drugs 1999; 11: 467–83.
24. Fischer P, Danielczyk W, Simanyi M, et al. Dopaminergic psychosis in advanced Parkinson's disease. Adv Neurol 1990; 53: 391–7.
25. Goetz CG, Tanner CM, Klawans HL. Pharmacology of hallucinations induced by long-term drug therapy. Am J Psychiatry 1982; 139: 494–7.
26. Inzelberg R, Kipervasser S, Korczyn AD. Auditory hallucinations in Parkinson's disease. J Neurol Neurosurg Psychiatry 1998; 64: 533–5.
27. Tousi B, Frankel M. Olfactory and visual hallucinations in Parkinson's disease. Parkinsonism Relat Disord 2004; 10: 253–4.

28. Cahn-Weiner DA, Grace J, Ott BR, et al. Cognitive and behavioral features discriminate between Alzheimer's and Parkinson's disease. Neuropsychiatry Neuropsychol Behav Neurol 2002; 15: 79–87.
29. Cummings JL. The Neuropsychiatric inventory: assessing psychopathology in dementia patients. Neurology 1997; 48: S10–16.
30. Overall JE, Gorham DR. The brief psychiatric rating scale. Psychol Rep 1962; 10: 799–812.
31. Reisberg B, Borenstein J, Salob SP, et al. Behavioral symptoms in Alzheimer's disease: phenomenology and treatment. J Clin Psychiatry 1987; 48(Suppl): 9–15.
32. Kay SR, Opler LA, Lindenmayer JP. The Positive and Negative Syndrome Scale (PANSS): rationale and standardisation. Br J Psychiatry 1989; 155: 59–67.
33. Andreasen NC. Scale for the Assessment of Positive Symptoms (SAPS). Iowa City: University of Iowa, 1984.
34. Guy W. ECDEU Assessment Manual for Psychopharmacology. Revised. Rockville, Md: Alcohol, Drug Abuse and Mental Health Administration, 1976.
35. Friedberg G, Zoldan J, Weizman A, et al. Parkinson psychosis rating scale: a practical instrument for grading psychosis in Parkinson's disease. Clin Neuropharmacol 1998; 21: 280–4.
36. Fernandez HH, Aarsland D, Fénelon G, et al. Scales to assess psychosis in Parkinson's disease: critique and recommendations. Mov Disord 2008; 23: 484–500.
37. Klawans HL, Goetz C, Nausieda PA, et al. Levodopa-induced dopamine receptor hyper-sensitivity. Trans Am Neurol Assoc 1977; 102: 80–3.
38. Rondot P, de Recondo J, Coignet A, et al. Mental disorders in Parkinson's disease after treatment with L-DOPA. Adv Neurol 1984; 40: 259–69.
39. Birkmayer W, Riederer P. Responsibility of extrastriatal areas for the appearance of psychotic symptoms (clinical and biochemical human post-mortem findings). J Neural Transm 1975; 37: 175–82.
40. Nausieda PA, Tanner CM, Klawans HL. Serotonergically active agents in levodopa-induced psychiatric toxicity reactions. Adv Neurol 1983; 37: 23–32.
41. Melamed E, Zoldan J, Friedberg G, et al. Involvement of serotonin in clinical features of Parkinson's disease and complications of L-DOPA therapy. Adv Neurol 1996; 69: 545–50.
42. Diederich NJ, Goetz CG, Raman R, et al. Poor visual discrimination and visual hallucinations in Parkinson's disease. Clin Neuropharmacol 1998; 21: 289–95.
43. Matsui H, Udaka F, Tamura A, et al. The relation between visual hallucinations and visual evoked potential in Parkinson disease. Clin Neuropharmacol 2005; 28: 79–82.
44. Diederich NJ, Alesch F, Goetz CG. Visual hallucinations induced by deep brain stimulation in Parkinson's disease. Clin Neuropharmacol 2000; 23: 287–9.
45. Stebbins GT, Goetz CG, Carrillo MC, et al. Altered cortical visual processing in PD with hallucinations: an fMRI study. Neurology 2004; 63: 1409–16.
46. Aarsland D, Larsen JP, Cummins JL, et al. Prevalence and clinical correlates of psychotic symptoms in Parkinson disease: a community-based study. Arch Neurol 1999; 56: 595–601.
47. Arnulf I, Bonnet AM, Damier P, et al. Hallucinations, REM sleep, and Parkinson's disease: a medical hypothesis. Neurology 2000; 55: 281–8.
48. Barnes J, David AS. Visual hallucinations in Parkinson's disease: a review and phenomenological survey. J Neurol Neurosurg Psychiatry 2001; 70: 727–33.
49. Comella CL, Tanner CM, Ristanovic RK. Polysomnographic sleep measures in Parkinson's disease patients with treatment-induced hallucinations. Ann Neurol 1993; 34: 710–14.
50. Parkinson Study Group. Pramipexole vs levodopa as initial treatment for Parkinson disease: A randomized controlled trial. JAMA 2000; 284: 1931–8.
51. Rascol O, Brooks DJ, Korczyn AD, et al. 056 Study Group. A five-year study of the incidence of dyskinesia in patients with early Parkinson's disease who were treated with ropinirole or levodopa. N Engl J Med 2000; 342: 1484–91.
52. Klein C, Kompf D, Pulkowski U, et al. A study of visual hallucinations in patients with Parkinson's disease. J Neurol 1997; 244: 371–7.

53. Merims D, Shabtai H, Korczyn AD, et al. Antiparkinsonian medication is not a risk factor for the development of hallucinations in Parkinson's disease. J Neural Transm 2004; 111: 1447–53.
54. Factor SA, Steenland NK, Higgins DS, et al. Disease-related and correlates of psychotic symptoms in Parkinson's disease. Mov Disord 2011; 26: 2190–5.
55. Friedman JH, Factor SA. Atypical antipsychotics in the treatment of drug-induced psychosis in Parkinson's disease. Mov Disord 2000; 15: 201–11.
56. Schneider LS, Dagerman KS, Insel P. Risk of death with atypical antipsychotic drug treatment for dementia: meta-analysis of randomized placebo-controlled trials. JAMA 2005; 294: 1934–43.
57. Wolters EC, Hurwitz TA, Mak E, et al. Clozapine in the treatment of parkinsonian patients with dopaminomimetic psychosis. Neurology 1990; 40: 832–4.
58. Parkinson Study Group. Low-dose clozapine for the treatment of drug-induced psychosis in Parkinson's disease. N Engl J Med 1999; 340: 757–63.
59. Pollak P, Tison F, Rascol O, et al. Clozapine in drug induced psychosis in Parkinson's disease: a randomised, placebo controlled study with open follow up. J Neurol Neurosurg Psychiatry 2004; 75: 689–95.
60. Meco G, Alessandria A, Bonifati V, et al. Risperidone for hallucinations in levodopa-treated Parkinson's disease patients. Lancet 1994; 343: 1370–1.
61. Ford B, Lynch T, Greene P. Risperidone in Parkinson's disease. Lancet 1994; 344: 681.
62. Rich SS, Friedman JH, Ott BR. Risperidone versus clozapine in the treatment of psychosis in six patients with Parkinson's disease and other akinetic-rigid syndromes. J Clin Psychiatry 1995; 56: 556–9.
63. Workman RH Jr, Orengo CA, Bakey AA, et al. The use of risperidone for psychosis and agitation in demented patients with Parkinson's disease. J Neuropsychiatry Clin Neurosci 1997; 9: 594–7.
64. Meco G, Alessandri A, Giustini P, et al. Risperidone in levodopa-induced psychosis in advanced Parkinson's disease: an open-label, long-term study. Mov Disord 1997; 12: 610–12.
65. Leopold NA. Risperidone treatment of drug-related psychosis in patients with parkinsonism. Mov Disord 2000; 15: 301–4.
66. Mohr E, Mendis T, Hildebrand K, et al. Risperidone in the treatment of dopamine-induced psychosis in Parkinson's disease: an open pilot trial. Mov Disord 2000; 15: 1230–7.
67. Ellis T, Cudkowicz ME, Sexton PM, et al. Clozapine and risperidone treatment of psychosis in Parkinson's disease. J Neuropsychiatry Clin Neurosci 2000; 12: 364–9.
68. Breier A, Sutton VK, Feldman PD, et al. Olanzapine in the treatment of dopamimetic-induced psychosis in patients with Parkinson's disease. Biol Psychiatry 2002; 52: 438–45.
69. Ondo WG, Levy JK, Vuong KD, et al. Olanzapine treatment for dopaminergic-induced hallucinations. Mov Disord 2002; 17: 1031–5.
70. Fernandez HH, Okun MS, Rodriguez RL, et al. Quetiapine improves visual hallucinations in Parkinson's disease but not through normalization of sleep architecture: results from a double-blind clinical-polysomnography study. Int J Neurosci 2009; 119: 2196–205.
71. Ondo WG, Tintner R, Voung KD, et al. Double-blind, placebo-controlled, unforced titration parallel trial of quetiapine for dopaminergic-induced hallucinations in Parkinson's disease. Mov Disord 2005; 20: 958–63.
72. Rabey JM, Prokhorov T, Miniovich A, et al. The effect of quetiapine in Parkinson's disease (PD) psychotic patients: A double-blind labeled study of three months duration. Mov Disord 2005; 20: S46.
73. Reddy S, Factor SA, Molho ES, et al. The effect of quetiapine on psychosis and motor function in parkinsonian patients with and without dementia. Mov Disord 2002; 17: 676–81.
74. Fernandez HH, Trieschmann ME, Burke MA, et al. Long-term outcome of quetiapine use for psychosis among Parkinsonian patients. Mov Disord 2003; 18: 510–14.

75. Fernandez HH, Trieschmann ME, Friedman JH. Aripiprazole for drug-induced psychosis in Parkinson disease: preliminary experience. Clin Neuropharmacol 2004; 27: 4–5.
76. Friedman JH, Berman RM, Carson W, et al. Low dose aripiprazole for the treatment of drug induced psychosis in Parkinson's disease patients. Mov Disord 2005; 20: S92.
77. Baldessarini RJ, Frankenburg FR; Clozapine. A novel antipsychotic agent. N Engl J Med 1991; 324: 746–54.
78. French Clozapine Parkinson Study Group. Clozapine in drug-induced psychosis in Parkinson's disease. Lancet 1999; 353: 2041–2.
79. Fernandez HH, Friedman JH, Lansang MC, et al. Diabetes mellitus among parkinsonian patients treated chronically with clozapine. Parkinsonism Relat Disord 2004; 10: 439–41.
80. Klein C, Gordon J, Pollak L, et al. Clozapine in Parkinson's disease psychosis: 5-year follow-up review. Clin Neuropharmacol 2003; 26: 8–11.
81. Honigfeld G, Arellano F, Sethi J, et al. Reducing clozapine-related morbidity and mortality: 5 years of experience with the Clozaril National Registry. J Clin Psychiatry 1998; 59: 3–7.
82. Holt RI, Peveler RC, Byrne CD. Schizophrenia, the metabolic syndrome and diabetes. Diabet Med 2004; 21: 515–23.
83. Thomas AA, Friedman JH. Current use of Clozapine in Parkinson's disease and related disorders. Clin Neuropharmacol 2010; 33: 14–16.
84. Katz IR, Jeste DV, Mintzer JE, et al. Risperidone Study Group. Comparison of risperidone and placebo for psychosis and behavioral disturbances associated with dementia: a randomized, double-blind trial. J Clin Psychiatry 1999; 60: 107–15.
85. Rosebush PI, Mazurek MF. Neurologic side effects in neuroleptic-naive patients treated with haloperidol or risperidone. Neurology 1999; 52: 782–5.
86. Allen RL, Walker Z, D'Ath PJ, et al. Risperidone for psychotic and behavioural symptoms in Lewy body dementia. Lancet 1995; 346: 185.
87. McKeith IG, Ballard CG, Harrison RW. Neuroleptic sensitivity to risperidone in Lewy body dementia. Lancet 1995; 346: 699.
88. Moore NA, Tye NC, Axton MS, et al. The behavioral pharmacology of olanzapine, a novel "atypical" antipsychotic agent. J Pharmacol Exp Ther 1992; 262: 545–51.
89. Beasley CM Jr, Tollefson GD, Tran PV. Efficacy of olanzapine: an overview of pivotal clinical trials. J Clin Psychiatry 1997; 58: 7–12.
90. Wolters EC, Jansen EN, Tuynman-Qua HG, et al. Olanzapine in the treatment of dopaminomimetic psychosis in patients with Parkinson's disease. Neurology 1996; 47: 1085–7.
91. Fernandez HH, Trieschmann ME, Friedman JH. Treatment of psychosis in Parkinson's disease: safety considerations. Drug Saf 2003; 26: 643–59.
92. Goetz CG, Blasucci LM, Leurgans S, et al. Olanzapine and clozapine: comparative effects on motor function in hallucinating PD patients. Neurology 2000; 55: 789–94.
93. Goetz CG, Koller WC, Poewe W, et al. Management of Parkinson's disease. Mov Disord 2002; 17: S120–7.
94. Saller CF, Salama AI. Seroquel: biochemical profile of a potential atypical antipsychotic. Psychopharmacology (Berl) 1993; 112: 285–92.
95. Comella CL, Tanner CM, Ristanovic RK. Polysomnographic sleep measures in Parkinson's disease patients with treatment-induced hallucinations. Ann Neurol 1993; 34: 710–14.
96. Morgante L, Epifanio A, Spina E, et al. Quetiapine and clozapine in parkinsonian patients with dopaminergic psychosis. Clin Neuropharmacol 2004; 27: 153–6.
97. Fernandez HH, McCown KM, Romrell J, et al. New-onset diabetes mellitus among Parkinsonian patients treated with long term quetiapine. Drug Target Insights 2008; 3: 27–9.
98. CDC. National Health and Nutrition Examination Survey 1999-2000 data files. [Available from: http://www.cdc.gov/nchs/data/hhis/earlyrelease/2004]
99. Stahl SM, Shayegan DK. The psychopharmacology of ziprasidone: receptor-binding properties and real-world psychiatric practice. J Clin Psychiatry 2003; 64: 6–12.

100. Glassman AH. Schizophrenia, antipsychotic drugs, and cardiovascular disease. J Clin Psychiatry 2005; 66: 5–10.
101. Gomez-Esteban JC, Zarranz JJ, Velasco F, et al. Use of ziprasidone in parkinsonian patients with psychosis. Clin Neuropharmacol 2005; 28: 111–14.
102. Oechsner M, Korchounov A. Parenteral ziprasidone: a new atypical neuroleptic for emergency treatment of psychosis in Parkinson's disease? Hum Psychopharmacol 2005; 20: 203–5.
103. Weiden PJ, Iqbal N, Mendelowitz AJ, et al. Best clinical practice with ziprasidone: update after one year of experience. J Psychiatr Pract 2002; 8: 81–97.
104. Komossa K, Rummel-Kluge C, Hunger H, et al. Cochrane Schizophrenia Group. Ziprasidone versus other atypical antipsychotics for schizophrenia. Cochrane Database Syst Rev 2009; 4: CD006627.
105. White A, Corn TH, Feetham C, et al. Ondansetron in treatment of schizophrenia. Lancet 1991; 337: 1173.
106. Zoldan J, Friedberg G, Goldberg-Stern H, et al. Ondansetron for hallucinosis in advanced Parkinson's disease. Lancet 1993; 341: 562–3.
107. Zoldan J, Friedberg G, Livneh M, et al. Psychosis in advanced Parkinson's disease: treatment with ondansetron, a 5-HT3 receptor antagonist. Neurology 1995; 45: 1305–8.
108. Eichhorn TE, Brunt E, Oertel WH. Ondansetron treatment of L-dopa-induced psychosis. Neurology 1996; 47: 1608–9.
109. Rogers SL, Farlow MR, Doody RS, et al. A 24-week, double-blind, placebo-controlled trial of donepezil in patients with Alzheimer's disease. Donepezil Study Group. Neurology 1998; 50: 136–45.
110. Tariot PN, Solomon PR, Morris JC, et al. The Galantamine USA-10 Study Group. A 5-month, randomized, placebo-controlled trial of galantamine in AD. Neurology 2000; 54: 2269–76.
111. Hutchinson M, Fazzini E. Cholinesterase inhibition in Parkinson's disease. J Neurol Neurosurg Psychiatry 1996; 61: 324–5.
112. Fabbrini G, Barbanti P, Aurilia C, et al. Donepezil in the treatment of hallucinations and delusions in Parkinson's disease. Neurol Sci 2002; 23: 41–3.
113. Bergman J, Lerner V. Successful use of donepezil for the treatment of psychotic symptoms in patients with Parkinson's disease. Clin Neuropharmacol 2002; 25: 107–10.
114. Kurita A, Ochiai Y, Kono Y, et al. The beneficial effect of donepezil on visual hallucinations in three patients with Parkinson's disease. J Geriatr Psychiatry Neurol 2003; 16: 184–8.
115. Ravina B, Putt M, Siderowf A, et al. Donepezil for dementia in Parkinson's disease: a randomised, double blind, placebo controlled, crossover study. J Neurol Neurosurg Psychiatry 2005; 76: 934–9.
116. Bullock R, Cameron A. Rivastigmine for the treatment of dementia and visual hallucinations associated with Parkinson's disease: a case series. Curr Med Res Opin 2002; 18: 258–64.
117. Reading PJ, Luce AK, McKeith IG. Rivastigmine in the treatment of parkinsonian psychosis and cognitive impairment: preliminary findings from an open trial. Mov Disord 2001; 16: 1171–4.
118. Emre M, Aarsland D, Albanese A, et al. Rivastigmine for dementia associated with Parkinson's disease. N Engl J Med 2004; 351: 2509–18.
119. Aarsland D, Hutchinson M, Larsen JP. Cognitive, psychiatric and motor response to galantamine in Parkinson's disease with dementia. Int J Geriatr Psychiatry 2003; 18: 937–41.
120. Vanover KE, Weiner DM, Makhay M, et al. Pharmacological and behavioral profile of N-(4-fluorophenylmethyl)-N-(1-methylpiperidin-4-yl)-N'-(4-(2-methyl propyloxy) phenylmethyl) carbamide (2R,3R)-dihydroxybutanedioate (2: 1) (ACP-103), a novel 5-hydroxytryptamine$_{2A}$ receptor inverse agonist. J Pharmacol Exp Ther 2006; 317: 910–18.
121. ACADIA Pharmaceuticals. Treating Parkinson's disease—clinical trial Pimavanserin ACADIA. [Available from: http://www.acadiapharm.com/pipeline/pimavanserin.htm]

122. Meltzer HY, Mills R, Ravell S, et al. Pimavanserin, a serotonin(2A) receptor inverse agonist, for the treatment of Parkinson's disease psychosis. Neuropsychopharmacology 2010; 35: 881–92.
123. Weintraub D, Chen P, Ignacio RV, et al. Patterns and trends in antipsychotic prescribing for Parkinson disease psychosis. Arch Neurol 2011; 68: 899–904.
124. Miyasaki JM, Shannon K, Voon V, et al. Practice Parameter: Evaluation and treatment of depression, psychosis, and dementia in Parkinson disease (an evidence-based review): Report of the Quality Standards Subcommittee of the American Academy of Neurology. Neurology 2006; 66: 996.
125. Ozer F, Meral H, Aydin B, et al. Electroconvulsive therapy in drug-induced psychiatric states and neuroleptic malignant syndrome. J Ect 2005; 21: 125–7.
126. Hurwitz TA, Calne DB, Waterman K. Treatment of dopaminomimetic psychosis in Parkinson's disease with electroconvulsive therapy. Can J Neurol Sci 1988; 15: 32–4.
127. Factor SA, Molho ES, Brown DL. Combined clozapine and electroconvulsive therapy for the treatment of drug-induced psychosis in Parkinson's disease. J Neuropsychiatry Clin Neurosci 1995; 7: 304–7.
128. Fernandez HH, Donnelly EM, Friedman JH. Long-term outcome of clozapine use for psychosis in parkinsonian patients. Mov Disord 2004; 19: 831–3.
129. Fernandez HH, Trieschmann ME, Okun MS. Rebound psychosis: Effect of discontinuation of antipsychotics in Parkinson's disease. Mov Disord 2005; 20: 104–5.
130. Emre M, Aarsland D, Brown R, et al. Clinical diagnostic criteria for dementia associated with Parkinson's disease. Mov Disord 2007; 22: 1689–707.
131. Hughes AJ, Daniel SE, Blankson S, et al. A clinicopathologic study of 100 cases of Parkinson's disease. Arch Neurol 1993; 50: 140–8.
132. Hughes AJ, Ben-Shlomo Y, Daniel SE, et al. What feature improve the accuracy of clinical diagnosis in Parkinson's disease: a clinicopathologic study. Neurology 1992; 42: 1142–6.
133. Dubois B, Burn D, Goetz C, et al. Diagnostic procedures for Parkinson's disease dementia: Recommendations form the movement disorder society task force. Mov Disord 2007; 22: 2314–24.
134. Emre M, Aarsland D, Brown R, et al. Clinical diagnostic criteria for dementia associated with Parkinson's disease. Mov Disord 2007; 22: 1689–707.
135. Dubois B, Burn D, Goetz C, et al. Diagnostic procedures for Parkinson's disease dementia: recommendations form the movement disorder society task force. Mov Disord 2007; 22: 2314–24.
136. McKeith IG, Galasko D, Kosaka K, et al. Consensus guidelines for the clinical and pathologic diagnosis of dementia with Lewy bodies (DLB): report of the consortium on DLB international workshop. Neurology 1996; 47: 1113–24.
137. Cummings JL. Third International Workshop on Dementia with Lewy Bodies and Parkinson's Disease Dementia. Newcastle upon Tyne, United Kingdom: MedReviews, LLC, 2003: 31–4.
138. Aarsland D, Ballard CG, Halliday G. Are Parkinson's disease with dementia and dementia with Lewy bodies the same entity? J Geriatr Psychiatry Neurol 2004; 17: 137–45.
139. Troster AI. Neuropsychological characteristics of dementia with Lewy bodies and Parkinson's disease with dementia: differentiation, early detection, and implications for "mild cognitive impairment" and biomarkers. Neuropsychol Rev 2008; 18: 103–19.
140. McKeith IG, Perry EK, Perry RH. Report of the second dementia with Lewy body international workshop: diagnosis and treatment. Consortium on dementia with lewy bodies. Neurology 1999; 53: 902–5.
141. Girotti F, Soliveri P, Carella F, et al. Dementia and cognitive impairment in Parkinson's disease. J Neurol Neurosurg Psychiatry 1988; 51: 1498–502.
142. Mayeux R, Stern Y, Rosenstein R, et al. An estimate of the prevalence of dementia in idiopathic Parkinson's disease. Arch Neurol 1988; 45: 260–2.
143. Friedman A, Barcikowska M. Dementia in Parkinson's disease. Dementia 1994; 5: 12–16.
144. Aarsland D, Andersen K, Larsen JP, et al. Prevalence and characteristics of dementia in Parkinson disease: an 8-year prospective study. Arch Neurol 2003; 60: 387–92.

145. Tison F, Dartigues JF, Auriacombe S, et al. Dementia in Parkinson's disease: a population-based study in ambulatory and institutionalized individuals. Neurology 1995; 45: 705–8.
146. Hobson P, Meara J. The detection of dementia and cognitive impairment in a community population of elderly people with Parkinson's disease by use of the CAMCOG neuropsychological test. Age Ageing 1999; 28: 39–43.
147. Hobson P, Meara J. Risk and incidence of dementia in a cohort of older subjects with Parkinson's disease in the United Kingdom. Mov Disord 2004; 19: 1043–9.
148. Aarsland D, Zaccai J, Brayne C. A systematic review of prevalence studies of dementia in Parkinson's disease. Mov Disord 2005; 20: 1255–63.
149. Hughes TA, Ross HF, Musa S, et al. A 10-year study of the incidence of and factors predicting dementia in Parkinson's disease. Neurology 2000; 54: 1596–602.
150. Aarsland D, Andersen K, Larsen JP, et al. Risk of dementia in Parkinson's disease: a community-based, prospective study. Neurology 2001; 56: 730–6.
151. Marder K, Tang MX, Cote L, et al. The frequency and associated risk factors for dementia in patients with Parkinson's disease. Arch Neurol 1995; 52: 695–701.
152. Levy G, Schupf N, Tang MX, et al. Combined effect of age and severity on the risk of dementia in Parkinson's disease. Ann Neurol 2002; 51: 722–9.
153. Levy G, Tang MX, Cote LJ, et al. Do risk factors for Alzheimer's disease predict dementia in Parkinson's disease? An exploratory study. Mov Disord 2002; 17: 250–7.
154. Weisskopf MG, Grodstein F, Ascherio A. Smoking and cognitive function in Parkinson's disease. Mov Disord 2007; 22: 660–5.
155. Alves G, Kurz M, Lie SA, et al. Cigarette smoking in Parkinson's disease: influence on disease progression. Mov Disord 2004; 19: 1087–92.
156. Gilberto L, Tang MX, Cote LJ, et al. Do risk factors for Alzheimer's disease predict dementia in Parkinson's disease? An exploratory study. Mov Disord 2002; 17: 250–7.
157. Inzelberg R, Bonuccelli U, Schechtman E, et al. Association between amantadine and the onset of dementia in Parkinson's disease. Mov Disord 2006; 21: 1375–9.
158. Harhangi BS, de Rijk MC, van Duijn CM, et al. APOE and the risk of PD with or without dementia in a population-based study. Neurology 2000; 54: 1272–6.
159. Parsian A, Racette B, Goldsmith LJ, et al. Parkinson's disease and apolipoprotein E: possible association with dementia but not age at onset. Genomics 2002; 79: 458–61.
160. Lane R, He Y, Morris C, et al. BuChE and APOE e4 allele frequencies in Lewy body dementias, and influence of genotype and hyperhomocysteinemia on cognitive decline. Mov Disord 2009; 24: 392–400.
161. Kehagia AA, Barker RA, Robbins TW. Neuropsychological and clinical heterogeneity of cognitive impairment and dementia in patients with Parkinson's disease. Lancet Neurol 2010; 9: 1200–13.
162. Foltynie T, Goldberg TE, Lewis SG, et al. Planning ability in Parkinson's disease is influenced by the COMT val158met polymorphism. Mov Disord 2004; 19: 885–91.
163. Williams-Gray CH, Hampshire A, Barker RA, et al. Attentional control in Parkinson's disease is dependent on COMT val 158 met genotype. Brain 2008; 131: 397–408.
164. Williams-Gray CH, Hampshire A, Robbins TW, et al. Catechol O-methyltransferase Val158Met genotype influences frontoparietal activity during planning in patient's with Parkinoson's disease. J Neurosci 2007; 27: 4832–8.
165. Camicioli R, Rajput A, Rajput M, et al. Apolipoprotein E-ε4 and catechol-O-methyltransferase alleles in autopsy-proven Parkinson's disease: relationship to dementia and hallucinations. Mov Disord 2005; 20: 989–94.
166. Neumann J, Bras J, Deas E, et al. Glucocerebrosidase mutations in clinical and pathological proven Parkinson's disease. Brain 2009; 132: 1783–94.
167. Goker-Alpan O, Lopez G, Vithayathil J, et al. The spectrum of parkinsonian manifestations associated with glucocerebrosidase mutations. Arch Neurol 2008; 65: 1353–7.
168. Spira PJ, Sharpe DM, Halliday G, et al. Clinical and pathological features of a Parkinsonian syndrome in a family with an Ala53Thr alpha-synuclein mutation. Ann Neurol 2001; 49: 313–19.
169. Zarranz JJ, Alegre J, Gomez-Esteban JC, et al. The new mutation, E46K, of alpha-synuclein causes Parkinson's and Lewy body dementia. Ann Neurol 2004; 55: 164–73.

170. Foltynie T, Brayne CEG, Robbins TW, et al. The cognitive ability of an incident cohort of Parkinson's patients in the UK. The CamPaIGN study. Brain 2004; 127: 550–60.
171. Uc EY, McDermott MP, Marder KS, et al. Incidence of and risk factors for cognitive impairment in an early Parkinson disease clinical trial cohort. Neurology 2009; 73: 1469–77.
172. Dubois B, Pillon B. Cognitive deficits in Parkinson's disease. J Neurol 1997; 244: 2–8.
173. Aarsland D, Bronnick K, Williams-Gray C, et al. Mild cognitive impairment in Parkinson disease. A multicenter pooled analysis. Neurology 2010; 75: 1062–9.
174. Petersen RC, Smith GE, Waring SC, et al. Mild cognitive impairment: clinical characterization and outcome. Arch Neurol 1999; 56: 303–8.
175. Williams-Gray CH, Foltynie T, Brayne CE, et al. Evolution of cognitive dysfunction in an incident Parkinson's disease cohort. Brain 2007; 130: 1787–98.
176. Janvin CC, Larsen JP, Aarsland D, et al. Subtypes of mild cognitive impairment in Parkinson's diseasee: progression to dementia. Mov Disord 2006; 21: 1343–9.
177. Cahn-Weiner DA, Grace J, Ott BR, et al. Cognitive and behavioral features discriminate between Alzheimer's and Parkinson's disease. Neuropsychiatry Neuropsychol Behav Neurol 2002; 15: 79–87.
178. Ballard CG, Aarsland D, McKeith I, et al. Fluctuations in attention: PD dementia vs DLB with parkinsonism. Neurology 2002; 59: 1714–20.
179. Aarsland D, Andersen K, Larsen JP, et al. The rate of cognitive decline in Parkinson disease. Arch Neurol 2004; 61: 1906–11.
180. Hely MA, Reid WGJ, Adena MA, et al. The Sydney multicenter study of Parkinson's disease: the inevitable of dementia at 20 years. Mov Disord 2008; 23: 837–44.
181. Brooks DJ, Ibanez V, Sawle GV, et al. Differing patterns of striatal 18F-dopa uptake in Parkinson's disease, multiple system atrophy, and progressive supranuclear palsy. Ann Neurol 1990; 28: 547–55.
182. Chou KL, Hurtig HI, Stern MB, et al. Diagnostic accuracy of [(99m)Tc]TRODAT-1 SPECT imaging in early Parkinson's disease. Parkinsonism Relat Disord 2004; 10: 375–9.
183. Seibyl JP, Marek KL, Quinlan D, et al. Decreased single-photon emission computed tomographic [123I]beta-CIT striatal uptake correlates with symptom severity in Parkinson's disease. Ann Neurol 1995; 38: 589–98.
184. Rinne JO, Rummukainen J, Paljarvi L, et al. Dementia in Parkinson's disease is related to neuronal loss in the medial substantia nigra. Ann Neurol 1989; 26: 47–50.
185. Growdon JH, Kieburtz K, McDermott MP, et al. Levodopa improves motor function without impairing cognition in mild non-demented Parkinson's disease patients. Parkinson Study Group. Neurology 1998; 50: 1327–31.
186. Perry EK, Curtis M, Dick DJ, et al. Cholinergic correlates of cognitive impairment in Parkinson's disease: comparisons with Alzheimer's disease. J Neurol Neurosurg Psychiatry 1985; 48: 413–21.
187. Whitehouse PJ, Hedreen JC, White CL 3rd, et al. Basal forebrain neurons in the dementia of Parkinson disease. Ann Neurol 1983; 13: 243–8.
188. Mattila PM, Roytta M, Lonnberg P, et al. Choline acetytransferase activity and striatal dopamine receptors in Parkinson's disease in relation to cognitive impairment. Acta Neuropathol 2001; 102: 160–6.
189. Perry EK, Irving D, Kerwin JM, et al. Cholinergic transmitter and neurotrophic activities in Lewy body dementia: similarity to Parkinson's and distinction from Alzheimer disease. Alzheimer Dis Assoc Disord 1993; 7: 69–79.
190. Ruberg M, Ploska A, Javoy-Agid F, et al. Muscarinic binding and choline acetyltransferase activity in Parkinsonian subjects with reference to dementia. Brain Res 1982; 232: 129–39.
191. Cash R, Dennis T, L'Heureux R, et al. Parkinson's disease and dementia: norepinephrine and dopamine in locus ceruleus. Neurology 1987; 37: 42–6.
192. Paulus W, Jellinger K. The neuropathologic basis of different clinical subgroups of Parkinson's disease. J Neuropathol Exp Neurol 1991; 50: 743–55.
193. Klein JC, Eggers C, Kalbe E, et al. Neurotransmitter changes in dementia with Lewy bodies and Parkinson disease dementia in vivo. Neurology 2010; 74: 885–92.

194. Brown DF, Dababo MA, Bigio EH, et al. Neuropathologic evidence that the Lewy body variant of Alzheimer disease represents coexistence of Alzheimer disease and idiopathic Parkinson disease. J Neuropathol Exp Neurol 1998; 57: 39–46.
195. Jellinger KA. Morphological substrates of dementia in parkinsonism. A critical update. J Neural Transm Suppl 1997; 51: 57–82.
196. Hurtig HI, Trojanowski JQ, Galvin J, et al. Alpha-synuclein cortical Lewy bodies correlate with dementia in Parkinson's disease. Neurology 2000; 54: 1916–21.
197. Ince P, Irving D, MacArthur F, et al. Quantitative neuropathological study of Alzheimer-type pathology in the hippocampus: comparison of senile dementia of Alzheimer type, senile dementia of Lewy body type, Parkinson's disease and non-demented elderly control patients. J Neurol Sci 1991; 106: 142–52.
198. Apaydin H, Ahlskog JE, Parisi JE, et al. Parkinson disease neuropathology: later-developing dementia and loss of the levodopa response. Arch Neurol 2002; 59: 102–12.
199. Parnetti L, Tiraboschi P, Lanari A, et al. Cerebrospinal fluid biomarkers in Parkinson's disease with dementia and dementia of Lewy bodies. Biol Psychiatry 2008; 64: 850–5.
200. Kanemaru K, Kameda N, Yamanouchi H, et al. Decreased CSF amyloid β42 and normal tau levels in dementia with Lewy bodies. Neurology 2000; 54: 1875–6.
201. Mollenhauer B, Trenkwalder C, von Ahsen N, et al. Beta-amlyoid 1-42 and tau-protein in cerebrospinal fluid of patients with Parkinson's disease dementia. Dement Geriatr Cogn Disord 2006; 22: 200–8.
202. Physicians Desk Reference, 56th edn. Montvale, NJ: Medical Economics Company, Inc, 2002.
203. Whitehouse PJ. Clinical and neurochemical consequences of neuronal loss in the nucleus basalis of Meynert in Parkinson's disease and Alzheimer's disease. Adv Neurol 1987; 45: 393–7.
204. Grace J, Daniel S, Stevens T, et al. Long-term use of rivastigmine in patients with dementia with Lewy bodies: an open-label trial. Int Psychogeriatr 2001; 13: 199–205.
205. McKeith I, Del Ser T, Spano P, et al. Efficacy of rivastigmine in dementia with Lewy bodies: a randomised, double-blind, placebo-controlled international study. Lancet 2000; 356: 2031–6.
206. Aarsland D, Bronnick K, Karlsen K. Donepezil for dementia with Lewy bodies: a case study. Int J Geriatr Psychiatry 1999; 14: 69–72.
207. Kaufer DI, Catt KE, Lopez OL, et al. Dementia with Lewy bodies: response of delirium-like features to donepezil. Neurology 1998; 51: 1512.
208. Lanctot KL, Herrmann N. Donepezil for behavioural disorders associated with Lewy bodies: a case series. Int J Geriatr Psychiatry 2000; 15: 338–45.
209. Giladi N, Shabtai H, Gurevich T, et al. Rivastigmine (Exelon) for dementia in patients with Parkinson's disease. Acta Neurol Scand 2003; 108: 368–73.
210. Minett TS, Thomas A, Wilkinson LM, et al. What happens when donepezil is suddenly withdrawn? An open label trial in dementia with Lewy bodies and Parkinson's disease with dementia. Int J Geriatr Psychiatry 2003; 18: 988–93.
211. Werber EA, Rabey JM. The beneficial effect of cholinesterase inhibitors on patients suffering from Parkinson's disease and dementia. J Neural Transm 2001; 108: 1319–25.
212. Aarsland D, Laake K, Larsen JP, et al. Donepezil for cognitive impairment in Parkinson's disease: a randomised controlled study. J Neurol Neurosurg Psychiatry 2002; 72: 708–12.
213. Leroi I, Brandt J, Reich SG, et al. Randomized placebo-controlled trial of donepezil in cognitive impairment in Parkinson's disease. Int J Geriatr Psychiatry 2004; 19: 1–8.
214. Poewe W, Wolters E, Emre M, et al. Long-term benefits of rivastigmine in dementia associated with Parkinson's disease: An active treatment extension study. Mov Disord 2006; 21: 456–61.
215. Aarsland D, Ballard Walker Z, et al. Memantine in patients with Parkinson's disease dementia or dementia with Lewy bodies: a double-blind, placebo-controlled, multicentre trial. Lancet Neurol 2009; 8: 613–18.

216. Emre M, Tsolaki M, Bonuccelli U, et al. Memantine for patients with Parkinson's disease dementia or dementia with Lewy bodies: a randomised, double-blind, placebo-controlled trial. Lancet Neurol 2010; 9: 969–77.
217. Bedard MA, el Massioui F, Malapani C, et al. Attentional deficits in Parkinson's disease: partial reversibility with naphtoxazine (SDZ NVI-085), a selective noradrenergic alpha 1 agonist. Clin Neuropharmacol 1998; 21: 108–17.
218. Marder K, Tang MX, Alfaro B, et al. Postmenopausal estrogen use and Parkinson's disease with and without dementia. Neurology 1998; 50: 1141–3.
219. Fernandez HH, Lapane KL. Estrogen use among nursing home residents with a diagnosis of Parkinson's disease. Mov Disord 2000; 15: 1119–24.
220. Wolozin B, Wang SW, Li NC, et al. Simvastatin is associated with a reduced incidence of dementia and Parkinson's disease. BMC Med 2007; 5: 20.

11 Neuroimaging

David J. Brooks

INTRODUCTION

The value of structural and functional imaging for diagnosing, understanding, and managing parkinsonian disorders and their complications is discussed in this chapter. It is argued that magnetic resonance imaging (MRI), transcranial sonography (TCS), positron emission tomography (PET), and single photon emission computed tomography (SPECT) all can play a valuable role in supporting clinical diagnoses of parkinsonian disorders when there is question and providing a rationale for the use of dopaminergic medications. Imaging can also detect subclinical disease activity in at-risk subjects and potentially monitor the functional effects of putative neuroprotective and restorative therapies.

STRUCTURAL IMAGING

Parkinsonism involves bradykinesia, rigidity, and tremor and it can result either from lesions of the nigrostriatal dopaminergic projections or when striatal and pallidal outflow tracts are damaged. Parkinson's disease (PD) is characterized by Lewy body inclusions targeting the dopaminergic neurons of the substantia nigra pars compacta (SNc). Multiple system atrophy (MSA) is an atypical form of degenerative parkinsonism associated with autonomic failure and ataxia. Here, argyrophilic alpha-synuclein containing inclusions are found in the neurons and glia of the white matter, SNc, and striatum. In progressive supranuclear palsy (PSP), another form of parkinsonism, neurofibrillary tangles target the SNc, basal ganglia, and oculomotor nuclei.

Magnetic Resonance Imaging

Conventional MRI sequences weighted to detect T1- and T2-relaxation times of water protons can detect brain atrophy and hydrocephalus, and sensitively exclude structural causes of parkinsonism, such as basal ganglia tumors, necrosis due to toxins, such as manganese and methcathinone (ephedrone), small vessel basal ganglia ischemic disease, and calcification (1). Volumetric MRI has so far failed to consistently demonstrate SNc atrophy in PD—probably because of the difficulty in defining the borders of this structure due to the high iron content of the neighboring substantia nigra reticulata (SNr). It has been recently reported, however, that MRI performed at 7 tesla can detect scalloping of the nigral signal in PD, which was not seen in healthy normal subjects (Fig. 11.1A) (2).

Diffusion tensor imaging (DTI) uses field gradient sequences, which allows MRI to detect the directionality (anisotropy) and amplitude (diffusion coefficient) of water movement along fiber tracts. In a recent series, DTI has been reported to detect reduced anisotropy of SNc water diffusion in 100% of de novo PD cases (3).

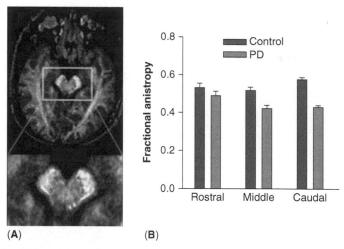

(A)   **(B)**

FIGURE 11.1   (A) FA of the midbrain. (B) Nigral FA is reduced in a rostral caudal gradient in PD. *Abbreviation*: FA, fractional anisotorpy. *Source*: From Ref. 3.

Signal changes were small but consistently evident in the lateral SNC where Lewy body pathology is known to be most severe (Fig. 11.1B).

The striatum does not degenerate in PD, but in MSA the putamen is targeted and can show reduced signal on T_2-weighted MRI due to the iron deposition that accumulates (Fig. 11.2A) (4). On occasion, this is accompanied by a lateral rim of increased signal, due to gliosis. At conventional field strengths, however, these findings tend to only be evident in the more established cases. Additionally, at 3 tesla field strengths reduced putamen T2 signal with a lateral rim of raised signal can also be seen in some normal subjects. If degeneration of the pons is present, the lateral as well as longitudinal pontine fibers become evident as high signal and produce the "hot cross bun" sign (4) (Fig. 11.2B) (5). Advanced MSA cases show cerebellar and pontine atrophy and increased T2 signal can also be detected in the middle cerebellar peduncles.

PSP patients do not show the putamen signal changes that characterize MSA but instead develop third ventricular widening and midbrain atrophy (4). This has been termed the "humming bird sign" on sagittal views. In PSP the superior cerebellar peduncle degenerates in contrast to MSA where the middle cerebellar peduncle is targeted (6). Again, these MRI changes lack sensitivity only being seen in well-established cases of PSP.

The conventional MRI lacks sensitivity for discriminating neurodegenerative causes of parkinsonism, whereas the diffusion-weighted MRI has been reported to reliably discriminate atypical from typical PD. A majority of cases of clinically probable MSA and PSP based on consensus criteria show increased putamen water diffusivity, whereas this is normal in typical PD (7). Although MSA and PSP cannot be readily distinguished by putamen water diffusivity, they can be discriminated from one another by the presence of altered water diffusion in the cerebellar peduncles—MSA targeting the middle and PSP the superior cerebellar peduncles (8,9).

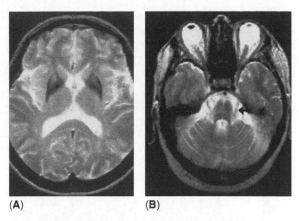

(A)   (B)

FIGURE 11.2   (A) T2-weighted MRI showing low lateral putamen signal at the same level as the pallidum in MSA. (B) T2-weighted MRI showing the pontine hot cross bun sign in MSA. *Abbreviations*: MRI, magnetic resonance imaging; MSA, multiple system atrophy.

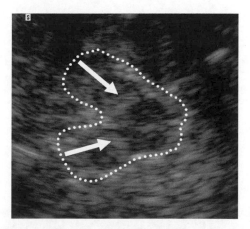

FIGURE 11.3   Transcranial sonography showing hyperechogenicity from the lateral midbrain (substantia nigra) in Parkinson's disease. *Source*: From Ref. 10.

Transcranial Sonography

Transcranial sonography (TCS) emits an ultrasound signal and detects structural midbrain and striatal changes in parkinsonian disorders as hyperechogenic signals (Fig. 11.3). Over 90% of cases with clinically established PD have been reported to show increased midbrain echogenicity with TCS but this is not a highly specific finding as it can also be seen in 10% of elderly normals and 15% of elderly essential tremor cases (10). The extent of SNc hyperechogenicity detected with TCS does not correlate well with motor disability in PD and appears to remain static over five years of follow up despite clinical progression (11). It has been suggested that its presence is a trait marker of susceptibility to PD rather than a state marker of the disorder and may be reflecting the presence of midbrain iron deposition and gliosis rather than dopamine neuron loss (12). In support of this, abnormal nigral hyper-echogenicity can be detected in high-risk subjects for PD, such as carriers of alpha-synuclein, LRRK2, parkin, and DJ1 gene mutations (13) or subjects with late-onset hyposmia (14). Nigral hyperechogenicity is not seen in atypical parkinsonian disorders despite the presence of postmortem dopamine cell loss. In MSA, however, the lentiform nucleus can be hyperechogenic and this, combined with an absence of midbrain hyperechogenicity is a highly specific finding, although it discriminates MSA from PD with a sensitivity of 59% only (15,16).

FUNCTIONAL IMAGING

The changes in regional cerebral function that characterize different parkinsonian disorders can be examined in two main ways: (*i*) Changes in resting levels or patterns of regional cerebral metabolism, blood flow, and neuroreceptor binding can be measured. (*ii*) Abnormal brain activation manifested as changes in regional blood flow or levels of neurotransmitter release can be detected when parkinsonian patients perform motor and cognitive tasks or are exposed to drug challenges.

Parkinson's Disease
The Presynaptic Dopaminergic System
There are a now a large number of PET and SPECT markers of dopamine terminal function (Fig. 11.4) (17). Striatal ^{18}F-dopa uptake reflects terminal dopa decarboxylase activity and dopamine storage capacity. Vesicle monoamine transporter (VMAT2) availability, the protein that takes up dopamine from the cytosol into vesicles, can be studied with PET using [11]C- or ^{18}F-dihydrotetrabenazine (DTBZ). Dopamine transporter (DAT) function can be assessed with tropane-based PET and SPECT markers, such as ^{11}C-CFT, ^{18}F-FP-CIT, ^{123}I-altropane, ^{123}I-IPT, ^{123}I-beta-CIT, and ^{123}I-FP-CIT and with the PET tracers ^{11}C-methylphenidate (MP) and ^{11}C-nomifensine.

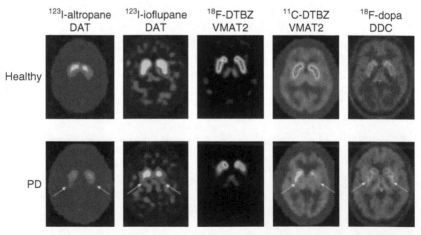

FIGURE 11.4 SPECT and PET images of dopamine terminal function in normal subjects and early PD patients. *Abbreviations*: PD, Parkinson's disease; PET, photon emission tomography; SPECT, single photon emission computed tomography.

In early, clinically unilateral PD, the reduction in putamen dopamine terminal function is invariably bilateral, tracer uptake being more depressed in the putamen contralateral to the clinically affected limbs (18). Head of caudate dopamine terminal function remains relatively preserved until late in the condition. It has been estimated that onset of symptoms occurs after a 30–50% loss of putamen dopamine terminal function (19). Severity of limb rigidity and bradykinesia correlate inversely with levels of putamen dopamine terminal function although severity of tremor does not, suggesting that loss of nigro-striatal projections are not directly responsible for this aspect of PD (20,21).

Striatal DAT imaging has been reported to differentiate clinically probable PD from normal healthy subjects and essential or dystonic tremor patients with a sensitivity and specificity around 90% (22). Reduced DAT binding supports a diagnosis of a dopamine-deficient parkinsonian syndrome and provides a rationale for a therapeutic trial of dopaminergic agents, whereas a normal scan effectively excludes this diagnosis.

Several studies have examined the impact of using DAT imaging to determine whether parkinsonian cases of uncertain etiology are associated with striatal dopamine deficiency (SDD). In the Query PD study, clinicians referred uncertain cases for assessment by two movement disorder experts and ^{123}I-beta-CIT SPECT (23). The standard of truth (SOT) was the clinical impression of the two movement disorder experts after six months of clinical follow up. The referring clinicians showed 92% sensitivity for diagnosing dopamine-deficient parkinsonism but their baseline clinical specificity was poor (30%) compared with the SOT. In contrast, the baseline specificity for detecting dopamine-deficient parkinsonism with ^{123}I-beta-CIT SPECT was 100%. These findings suggest that clinicians tend to overdiagnose PD when uncertain.

The Clinically Uncertain Parkinsonian Syndromes (CUPS) trial was done to determine whether a knowledge of baseline striatal DAT binding would influence the diagnosis and management plan of patients with uncertain PD (24). When FP-CIT SPECT findings were revealed to participating clinicians, the diagnosis of dopamine-deficient parkinsonian syndrome was revised in 52% and the management strategy changed in 72% of the 118 cases. After two years, a clinical review found that 90% of subjects still retained the diagnosis assigned after a knowledge of baseline FP-CIT SPECT findings (25).

Although the CUPS consortium concluded that including a measure of striatal dopaminergic function in the work-up of uncertain parkinsonian cases influenced subsequent management, no non-imaged control group was included in their study as a comparator. Given this, the prevalence of change in management plan without availability of SPECT was not determined. To address this drawback the PDT409 study was designed similar to the CUPS protocol but included a non-imaged control arm (26). Around 130 cases in each arm with possible PD were clinically assessed at baseline and assigned a diagnosis and management plan. Twelve weeks after either FP-CIT SPECT or no DAT imaging they were re-assessed and their diagnosis and management reviewed. Forty-four percent of those who had SPECT had a change in their diagnosis after 12 weeks of follow-up compared with 12% of those who were not imaged. Forty-nine percent of those imaged versus 31% in the nonimaged arm had a change in their management plan. While the CUPS and PDT409 trials clearly show the influence of DAT imaging on patient management in cases of uncertain PD, the utility of imaging in terms of improving quality of life still remains to be determined.

A common cause of confusion with PD is adult-onset dystonic tremor that can present as an asymmetric resting arm tremor with impaired arm swing and cogwheel rigidity but without latency of onset or evidence of true akinesia (27). In these cases, normal DAT imaging can be helpful as inappropriate medication with dopaminergic agents can be avoided. Normal DAT imaging can also help discriminate drug-associated and psychogenic parkinsonism from idiopathic PD. A question that arises is whether it is safe to withdraw dopaminergic agents from cases that have been mistakenly diagnosed as having a dopamine-deficient parkinsonian syndrome and treated for some years. Eleven such patients who initially fulfilled diagnostic criteria for PD and were treated with dopaminergic agents but in whom emerging diagnostic doubts led to DAT imaging with FP-CIT SPECT have been reported (28). Striatal DAT binding was found to be normal and subsequent antiparkinsonian therapy withdrawal was achieved without clinical deterioration suggesting that dopaminergic imaging can be valuable where inappropriate use of antiparkinsonian medication is suspected.

Measuring Striatal Dopamine in PD

The striatum contains mainly dopamine D1 and D2 receptor subtypes and these both play a role in modulating motor function. In untreated PD, D1 site binding measured with ^{11}C-SCH23390 PET is normal, whereas D2 availability measured with ^{123}I-IBZM SPECT or ^{11}C-raclopride PET is normal or mildly raised (Fig. 11.6) (29,30). As ^{11}C-raclopride competes with endogenous dopamine for D2 binding, rises in receptor availability probably reflect synaptic dopamine depletion rather than an adaptive rise in receptor numbers. In chronically levodopa-exposed PD cases, levels of putamen D1 become mildly reduced and D2 binding normalizes as synaptic levels of dopamine are restored.

As ^{11}C-raclopride competes with synaptic dopamine for D2-binding sites, its uptake is sensitive to changes in synaptic levels of striatal dopamine. ^{11}C-raclopride PET can, therefore, be used as a marker of changes in brain dopamine levels induced by drugs or behavioral tasks. Microdialysis studies in animals suggest that a 10% reduction in striatal ^{11}C-raclopride binding reflects a fivefold increase in synaptic dopamine levels (31). Oral L-dopa leads to transient rises in synaptic dopamine levels in PD and the resultant improvements in disability correlate with estimated rises in putamen dopamine estimated from the induced reductions in striatal ^{11}C-raclopride uptake (32). Some PD patients compulsively take far larger doses of levodopa than are clinically required—this has been termed the dopamine dysregulation syndrome. Compared with PD patients matched for disability who are not compulsively taking excess medication, DDS patients show enhanced levodopa-induced dopamine release in ventral striatum (33). PD cases who develop impulse control disorders such as compulsive gambling when administered dopamine agonist therapy have been shown to release higher levels of ventral striatal dopamine when exposed to the relevant stimuli, such as games of chance (34).

Detection of Preclinical PD

It has been estimated from postmortem studies that there are 10 subclinical cases with incidental brainstem Lewy body disease in the community for every patient who develops clinical symptoms of PD (35). The greatest risk factors for PD are age and a family history, but late onset idiopathic hyposmia and rapid eye movement behavior sleep disorder (RBD) are both associated with subsequent development of

Lewy body disorders. Subclinically reduced levels of dopamine terminal function have been detected in asymptomatic identical twins and relatives of idiopathic PD cases with ^{18}F-dopa PET and also in mutation carriers of the susceptibility genes parkin and LRRK2 (36–39). Reduced striatal DAT binding has been detected in 10–25% of late-onset hyposmic subjects (14,40) and also in patients with idiopathic RBD (41).

Mechanisms Underlying Motor Complications
As loss of dopamine terminals in PD becomes severe, the striatum fails to store dopamine and buffer synaptic levels when exogenous L-dopa is taken. This is magnified by the relatively greater loss of dopamine transporters from terminals, the route for dopamine re-uptake, compared with dopa decarboxylase activity (42). PD patients with a sustained therapeutic response to L-dopa show a reduction in striatal ^{11}C-raclopride binding after an oral levodopa challenge that is maintained for 4 hours implying a stable increase in synaptic dopamine levels and intact dopamine buffering (43). In contrast, patients with fluctuating motor responses to levodopa show larger amplitude, but shorter lived, falls in ^{11}C-raclopride uptake compatible with pulsatile swings in synaptic dopamine levels. Pulsatile swings in synaptic dopamine levels will promote internalization of dopamine receptors, which are then unavailable and fluctuating treatment responses result.

Peak dose dyskinesia are likely to involve overstimulation of dopamine receptors by excessive levels of synaptic dopamine generated from exogenous levodopa when striatal buffering fails. In line with this, the severity of peak dose dyskinesia following oral L-dopa administration to PD patients has been shown to correlate with induced reductions in putaminal ^{11}C-raclopride binding, which reflect rises in synaptic dopamine (32).

The striatum contains high densities of adenosine A2A sites, which are expressed by striatal neurons of the indirect pathway projecting to the external pallidum. Uptake of ^{11}C-SCH442416, a marker of A2A binding, is normal in the striatum of nondyskinetic, but raised in dyskinetic cases (44). This could result in underactivity of the indirect pathway, which normally acts to inhibit unwanted motor programs.

N-methyl-D-aspartate (NMDA) receptors are a subclass of glutamate receptors that contain a voltage-gated ion channel, which is opened during learning and memory tasks. ^{11}C-CNS5161 PET is a marker of NMDA ion channel activity and recently striatal signals have been shown to be increased while PD patients are experiencing L-dopa-induced dyskinesia (45). This finding may help explain the beneficial mode of action of amantadine, an NMDA channel blocker.

Monitoring PD Progression with Molecular Imaging
As functional imaging can objectively follow loss of dopamine terminal function in PD, it provides a potential approach for monitoring the efficacy of putative neuroprotective agents. Early PD patients were reported to lose dopamine terminal function around one third more slowly if treated with a dopamine agonist compared with L-dopa with ^{18}F-dopa PET in the REAL PET trial and with beta-CIT SPECT in the CALM PD study (46,47). Despite this, the improvements in disability were greater in the levodopa cohorts. The interpretation of these data has remained unclear—it is possible that levodopa directly acts to downregulate beta-CIT and ^{18}F-dopa uptake, confounding the utility of these imaging biomarkers for assessing neuroprotective efficacy in the presence of this agent. ^{18}F-dopa PET has also been

used as an imaging biomarker to examine the possible neuroprotective efficacy of riluzole and beta-CIT SPECT, the neuroprotective efficacy of TCH346, and CEP1347 in PD—these trials were all negative and CEP1347 treatment was shown to directly depress striatal beta-CIT uptake in untreated cases (48).

Two double-blind controlled trials on the efficacy of striatal implantation of human fetal midbrain cells in PD have shown both histologic and ^{18}F-dopa PET evidence of graft function (49,50). Despite this, neither of these controlled trials demonstrated consistent clinical efficacy of transplantation although younger, more severely affected patients showed a trend toward benefit. An issue raised by both these trials was the occurrence of problematic "off" period dyskinesia after grafting in a significant minority of the implanted patients.

Glial-derived neurotrophic factor (GDNF) is known to prevent the degeneration of dopamine neurons in rodents and nonhuman primates exposed to the nigral toxins 6-OHDA or MPTP. A small, open pilot trial showed efficacy of intraputaminal infusions of GDNF in all the five treated PD patients along with 16–26% increases in ^{18}F-dopa storage at the site of the catheter tip (51). A randomized placebo-controlled study of 36 cases, however, failed to show a clinical benefit of this procedure despite consistent focal increases in ^{18}F-dopa storage at the catheter tip being detected in patients receiving the active agent (52). These restorative trials suggest that increasing dopamine storage capacity by implanting fetal cells, or by inducing terminal sprouting with trophic factors, is not enough to guarantee a therapeutic response unless appropriate connectivity to postsynaptic receptors is also established.

Nonmotor Complications of PD

A majority of PD patients will experience nonmotor complications and, in later disease, these can significantly impact the quality of life. Depression, dementia, sleep disorders, fatigue, and autonomic problems are all commonly reported problems. It has been widely assumed that loss of serotonergic function due to Lewy body involvement of the median raphe contributes to depression in PD, however, results from neuroimaging studies have not supported this viewpoint. Equally disabled PD patients with and without significant depression have shown similar median raphe uptake of ^{11}C-WAY 100635 binding, a marker of HT1A sites on the serotonergic cell bodies reflecting integrity of the neurons (53,54). Additionally, midbrain uptake of ^{123}I-β-CIT, which reflects serotonin transporter availability did not differ between PD patients with and without depression or correlate with Hamilton Depression Rating Scale scores (55). The PET tracer ^{11}C-RTI32 binds with similar affinity to dopamine and noradrenaline transporters. Remy and co-workers have scanned PD patients with and without depression with ^{11}C-RTI32 PET (56). The depressed PD patients had lower ^{11}C-RTI32 binding in locus coeruleus and areas of the limbic system than the nondepressed PD patients. This finding suggests that loss of limbic dopamine and noradrenaline rather than serotonin may be more relevant to the pathogenesis of depression in patients with PD.

It is now known that 80% of PD patients will develop dementia if they survive for 20 years or longer with their illness. The mechanisms underlying dementia are multiple including involvement of the cortical association areas by Lewy body disease, amyloid deposition, and the degeneration of dopaminergic and cholinergic projections to these cortical regions. Resting levels of ^{18}F-2-fluoro-2-deoxyglucose (FDG) uptake reflect basal neuronal synaptic activity. In nondemented PD patients cortical FDG uptake is usually normal but covariance analysis reveals an abnormal profile of relatively increased lentiform nucleus and reduced frontoparietal metabolism, which has been termed the PD-related profile (PDRP) (57). The degree of expression of the PDRP correlates with degree of motor disability in patients withdrawn from medication and the profile normalizes after successful treatment with either dopaminergic drugs or deep brain stimulation (58,59). PD patients with overt dementia show an Alzheimer's disease (AD) pattern of impaired brain glucose utilization, posterior cingulate, parietal and temporal association areas being most affected (60). This pattern of glucose hypometabolism could reflect either cortical Lewy body disease or coincidental AD. It has been reported that cases later proved to have cortical Lewy body disease show greater occipital cortex hypometabolism than AD patients but this finding has relatively low discriminatory power (61).

[11]C-PIB is a neutral thioflavin-T analogue developed to allow detection of β-amyloid plaques with PET. It has been employed to assess both dementia with Lewy body (DLB) patients and PD patients with later dementia. Although a majority of DLB cases show cortical amyloid this is evident in a minority of PD cases with late dementia (62,63). This suggests that amyloid pathology is not a major contributor toward late-onset dementia in PD and that their cognitive problems are more related to Lewy body pathology.

Cholinergic terminal function can be assessed with ^{11}C-NMP4A or ^{11}C-PMP PET, markers of acetylcholinesterase activity. Nondemented PD patients show reduced cholinergic function in parietal and occipital cortex while this becomes global and more severe when dementia is present (64). Levels of PD cortical acetylcholinesterase activity correlated with Mini-Mental State Examination scores and performance on executive tests, such as card sorting and trail making (65). These results suggest progressive cognitive impairment in PD arises in part as a consequence of a cholinergic deficit.

Cardiac Sympathetic Function
^{123}I-MIBG (metaiodobenzylguanidine) SPECT is a marker of adrenergic terminal function and can be used to study functional integrity of cardiac sympathetic innervation in PD. Mediastinal ^{123}I-MIBG signal is reduced in a majority of PD cases, even when no clinical evidence of autonomic failure is present. However, in early PD, 50% of cases have been reported to show normal cardiac MIBG uptake, so this approach is not as sensitive a marker for PD as striatal DAT imaging (66).

Atypical Parkinsonian Syndromes
Multiple System Atrophy
Patients with MSA show reduced resting levels of striatal, brainstem, and cerebellar glucose metabolism with [18]FDG PET studies in contrast to PD where these are preserved (67,68). In both MSA and PD, the nigral dopaminergic projections to the posterior putamen are targeted and while ^{18}F-dopa PET, VMAT2, and DAT imaging can all reliably separate PD and MSA from healthy controls, they are unable to discriminate between these two parkinsonian conditions.

Putamen dopamine D2 binding is preserved in PD, whereas it is reduced by around 20% in MSA (Fig. 11.5). There is, however, a significant overlap in the PD and MSA ranges and striatal D2 measurements do not provide a sensitive discriminator of these conditions (17). In one series, ^{123}I-IBZM SPECT detected reduced striatal D2 binding in only two-thirds of de novo parkinsonian patients who had a negative apomorphine response and were thought to have early MSA-P (69).

^{123}I-MIBG SPECT, a marker of myocardial adrenergic terminal function, is normal in MSA as autonomic dysfunction results from loss of pre- rather than postsynaptic innervation (70). This differentiates MSA from PD where the sympathetic loss is postsynaptic and potentially provides a means of discriminating these two conditions (Fig. 11.6).

Progressive Supranuclear Palsy

PSP is characterized pathologically by neuronal loss in the substantia nigra, pallidum, superior colliculi, brainstem nuclei, and the periaqueductal gray matter with intraneuronal neurofibrillary tangle formation. FDG PET reveals depressed frontal cortex, basal ganglia, cerebellar, and thalamic glucose metabolism in PSP, which correlates with disease duration and performance on psychometric tests of frontal function (17,71). The presence of reduced striatal metabolism sensitively discriminates 90% of PSP cases from PD, however, as striatal hypometabolism is also a feature of MSA, FDG PET cannot reliably discriminate these atypical conditions.

The pathology of PSP uniformly targets nigrostriatal dopaminergic projections and so, in contrast to PD and MSA, putamen and caudate ^{18}F-dopa uptake and

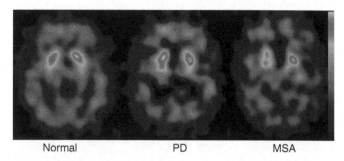

Normal   PD   MSA

FIGURE 11.5   ^{123}I-IBZM SPECT images of dopamine D2 receptor binding in a normal subject, PD, and MSA cases. Striatal D2 binding is reduced in the MSA case. *Abbreviations*: MSA, multiple system atrophy; PD, Parkinson's disease; SPECT, single photon emission computed tomography. *Source*: Courtesy of Dr G Wenning.

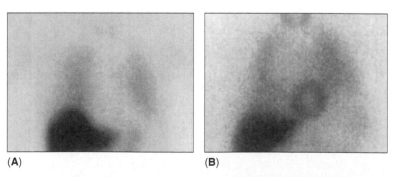

(A)   **(B)**

FIGURE 11.6   ^{123}I-MIBG images of cardiac sympathetic function in PD (**A**) and MSA (**B**). *Abbreviations*: MIBG, metaiodobenzylguanidine; MSA, multiple system atrophy; PD, Parkinson's disease. *Source*: From Ref. 73.

DAT binding are equivalently reduced resulting in a uniform and often symmetrical loss of striatal signal (72). Striatal D2 binding is reduced in a majority of PSP cases and this can be detected with ^{11}C-raclopride PET or IBZM SPECT (17).

CONCLUSIONS

- Structural changes in PD nigra can now be detected with 7 tesla MRI, diffusion tensor imaging, and transcranial sonography.
- Midbrain hyperechogenicity detects susceptibility to PD but does not correlate with severity of disease.
- PET and SPECT can sensitively detect dopamine terminal dysfunction when present in parkinsonian disorders and provide a rationale for a trial of dopaminergic medication. Dopamine transporter imaging, however, cannot discriminate typical from atypical PD.
- MSA cases give abnormal putamen signal on T2-weighted MRI, diffusion-weighted imaging, and transcranial sonography and show striatal hypometabolism with FDG PET, discriminating them from PD.
- PET and SPECT can detect subclinical dopamine terminal dysfunction in subjects at risk for PD when present. This could help identify cases for neuroprotective approaches if a successful therapy is identified.
- Imaging potentially enables PD progression to be objectively monitored and the efficacy of putative neuroprotective and restorative approaches to be evaluated. However, direct effects of any intervention on the imaging modality can be a confound.

REFERENCES

1. Brooks DJ. Technology insight: imaging neurodegeneration in Parkinson's disease. Nat Clin Pract Neurol 2008; 4: 267–77.
2. Cho ZH, Oh SH, Kim JM, et al. Direct visualization of Parkinson's disease by in vivo human brain imaging using 7.0T magnetic resonance imaging. Mov Disord 2011; 26: 713–18.
3. Vaillancourt DE, Spraker MB, Prodoehl J, et al. High-resolution diffusion tensor imaging in the substantia nigra of de novo Parkinson's disease. Neurology 2009; 72: 1378–84.
4. Schrag A, Good CD, Miszkiel K, et al. Differentiation of atypical parkinsonian syndromes with routine MRI. Neurology 2000; 54: 697–702.
5. Brooks DJ, Seppi K. Proposed neuroimaging criteria for the diagnosis of multiple system atrophy. Mov Disord 2009; 24: 949–64.
6. Paviour DC, Price SL, Jahanshahi M, Lees AJ, Fox NC. Regional brain volumes distinguish PSP, MSA-P, and PD: MRI-based clinico-radiological correlations. Mov Disord 2006; 21: 989–96.
7. Seppi K, Schocke MF, Esterhammer R, et al. Diffusion-weighted imaging discriminates progressive supranuclear palsy from PD, but not from the Parkinson variant of multiple system atrophy. Neurology 2003; 60: 922–7.
8. Nicoletti G, Lodi R, Condino F, et al. Apparent diffusion coefficient measurements of the middle cerebellar peduncle differentiate the Parkinson variant of MSA from Parkinson's disease and progressive supranuclear palsy. Brain 2006; 129: 2679–87.
9. Paviour DC, Thornton JS, Lees AJ, Jager HR. Diffusion-weighted magnetic resonance imaging differentiates Parkinsonian variant of multiple-system atrophy from progressive supranuclear palsy. Mov Disord 2007; 22: 68–74.
10. Berg D, Siefker C, Becker G. Echogenicity of the substantia nigra in Parkinson's disease and its relation to clinical findings. J Neurol 2001; 248: 684–9.

11. Berg D, Merz B, Reiners K, Naumann M, Becker G. Five-year follow-up study of hyper-echogenicity of the substantia nigra in Parkinson's disease. Mov Disord 2005; 20: 383–5.
12. Berg D, Roggendorf W, Schroder U, et al. Echogenicity of the substantia nigra: association with increased iron content and marker for susceptibility to nigrostriatal injury. Arch Neurol 2002; 59: 999–1005.
13. Walter U, Klein C, Hilker R, et al. Brain parenchyma sonography detects preclinical parkinsonism. Mov Disord 2004; 19: 1445–9.
14. Sommer U, Hummel T, Cormann K, et al. Detection of presymptomatic Parkinson's disease: combining smell tests, transcranial sonography, and SPECT. Mov Disord 2004; 19: 1196–202.
15. Behnke S, Berg D, Naumann M, Becker G. Differentiation of Parkinson's disease and atypical parkinsonian syndromes by transcranial ultrasound. J Neurol Neurosurg Psychiatry 2005; 76: 423–5.
16. Walter U, Dressler D, Probst T, et al. Transcranial brain sonography findings in discriminating between parkinsonism and idiopathic Parkinson's disease. Arch Neurol 2007; 64: 1635–40.
17. Brooks DJ. Imaging approaches to Parkinson's disease. J Nucl Med 2010; 51: 596–609.
18. Morrish PK, Sawle GV, Brooks DJ. Clinical and [18F]dopa PET findings in early Parkinson's disease. J Neurol Neurosurg Psychiat 1995; 59: 597–600.
19. Morrish PK, Rakshi JS, Sawle GV, Brooks DJ. Measuring the rate of progression and estimating the preclinical period of Parkinson's disease with [18F]dopa PET. J Neurol Neurosurg Psychiat 1998; 64: 314–19.
20. Vingerhoets FJG, Schulzer M, Calne DB, Snow BJ. Which clinical sign of Parkinson's disease best reflects the nigrostriatal lesion? Ann Neurol 1997; 41: 58–64.
21. Benamer HTS, Patterson J, Wyper DJ, et al. Correlation of Parkinson's disease severity and duration with I-123-FP-CIT SPECT striatal uptake. Mov Disord 2000; 15: 692–8.
22. Benamer TS, Patterson J, Grosset DG, et al. Accurate differentiation of parkinsonism and essential tremor using visual assessment of [123I]-FP-CIT imaging: The [123I]-FP-CIT study group. Mov Disord 2000; 15: 503–10.
23. Jennings DL, Seibyl JP, Oakes D, et al. (123I) beta-CIT and single-photon emission computed tomographic imaging vs clinical evaluation in Parkinsonian syndrome: unmasking an early diagnosis. Arch Neurol 2004; 61: 1224–9.
24. Catafau AM, Tolosa E. Impact of dopamine transporter SPECT using 123I-Ioflupane on diagnosis and management of patients with clinically uncertain Parkinsonian syndromes. Mov Disord 2004; 19: 1175–82.
25. Tolosa E, Borght TV, Moreno E. Accuracy of DaTSCAN ((123)I-ioflupane) SPECT in diagnosis of patients with clinically uncertain parkinsonism: 2-Year follow-up of an open-label study. Mov Disord 2007; 22: 2346–51.
26. Kupsch A, Bajaj N, Weiland F, et al. Changes in clinical management following DaTscan (TM) (ioflupane) imaging in patients with a clinically uncertain parkinsonian syndrome: interim report. Neurology 2011; 76: A276.
27. Schwingenschuh P, Ruge D, Edwards MJ, et al. Distinguishing SWEDDs patients with asymmetric resting tremor from Parkinson's disease: a clinical and electrophysiological study. Mov Disord 2010; 25: 560–9.
28. Marshall VL, Patterson J, Hadley DM, Grosset KA, Grosset DG. Successful antiparkinsonian medication withdrawal in patients with Parkinsonism and normal FP-CIT SPECT. Mov Disord 2006; 21: 2247–50.
29. Turjanski N, Lees AJ, Brooks DJ. PET studies on striatal dopaminergic receptor binding in drug naive and L-dopa treated Parkinson's disease patients with and without dyskinesia. Neurology 1997; 49: 717–23.
30. Antonini A, Schwarz J, Oertel WH, et al. [11C]raclopride and positron emission tomography in previously untreated patients with Parkinson's disease: influence of L-dopa and lisuride therapy on striatal dopamine D2-receptors. Neurology 1994; 44: 1325–9.
31. Laruelle M, Abi-Dargham A, van Dyck CH, et al. Single photon emission computerized tomography imaging of amphetamine-induced dopamine release in drug-free schizophrenic subjects. Proc Natl Acad Sci U S A 1996; 93: 9235–40.

32. Pavese N, Evans AH, Tai YF, et al. Clinical correlates of levodopa-induced dopamine release in Parkinson's disease: a PET study. Neurology 2006; 67: 1612–17.
33. Evans AH, Pavese N, Lawrence AD, et al. Compulsive drug use linked to sensitized ventral striatal dopamine transmission. Ann Neurol 2006; 59: 852–8.
34. Steeves TD, Miyasaki J, Zurowski M, et al. Increased striatal dopamine release in Parkinsonian patients with pathological gambling: a [11C] raclopride PET study. Brain 2009; 132: 1376–85.
35. Golbe LI. The genetics of Parkinson's disease: A reconsideration. Neurology 1990; 40: 7–16.
36. Piccini P, Morrish PK, Turjanski N, et al. Dopaminergic function in familial Parkinson's disease: A clinical and 18F-dopa PET study. Ann Neurol 1997; 41: 222–9.
37. Piccini P, Burn DJ, Ceravalo R, Maraganore DM, Brooks DJ. The role of inheritance in sporadic Parkinson's disease: evidence from a longitudinal study of dopaminergic function in twins. Ann Neurol 1999; 45: 577–82.
38. Khan NL, Brooks DJ, Pavese N, et al. Progression of nigrostriatal dysfunction in a parkin kindred: an [18F]dopa PET and clinical study. Brain 2002; 125: 2248–56.
39. Adams JR, van Netten H, Schulzer M, et al. PET in LRRK2 mutations: comparison to sporadic Parkinson's disease and evidence for presymptomatic compensation. Brain 2005; 128: 2777–85.
40. Ponsen MM, Stoffers D, Booij J, et al. Idiopathic hyposmia as a preclinical sign of Parkinson's disease. Ann Neurol 2004; 56: 173–81.
41. Stiasny-Kolster K, Doerr Y, Moller JC, et al. Combination of 'idiopathic' REM sleep behaviour disorder and olfactory dysfunction as possible indicator for alpha-synucleinopathy demonstrated by dopamine transporter FP-CIT-SPECT. Brain 2005; 128: 126–37.
42. Troiano AR, de la Fuente-Fernandez R, Sossi V, et al. PET demonstrates reduced dopamine transporter expression in PD with dyskinesias. Neurology 2009; 72: 1211–16.
43. de la Fuente-Fernandez R, Sossi V, Huang Z, et al. Levodopa-induced changes in synaptic dopamine levels increase with progression of Parkinson's disease: implications for dyskinesias. Brain 2004; 127: 2747–54.
44. Ramlackhansingh AF, Bose SK, Ahmed I, et al. Adenosine 2A receptor availability in dyskinetic and nondyskinetic patients with Parkinson's disease. Neurology 2011; 76: 1811–16.
45. Ahmed I, Bose SK, Pavese N, et al. Glutamate NMDA receptor dysregulation in Parkinson's disease with dyskinesias. Brain 2011; 134: 979–86.
46. Whone AL, Watts RL, Stoess IJ, et al. Slower progression of PD with ropinirol versus L-dopa: the REAL-PET study. Ann Neurol 2003; 54: 93–101.
47. Parkinson Study Group. Dopamine transporter brain imaging to assess the effects of Pramipexole vs levodopa Parkinson's disease progression. JAMA 2002; 287: 1653–61.
48. Parkinson Study Group. Mixed lineage kinase inhibitor CEP-1347 fails to delay disability in early Parkinson's disease. Neurology 2007; 69: 1480–90.
49. Freed CR, Greene PE, Breeze RE, et al. Transplantation of embryonic dopamine neurons for severe Parkinson's disease. N Engl J Med 2001; 344: 710–19.
50. Olanow CW, Goetz CG, Kordower JH, et al. A double-blind controlled trial of bilateral fetal nigral transplantation in Parkinson's disease. Ann Neurol 2003; 54: 403–14.
51. Gill SS, Patel NK, Hotton GR, et al. Direct brain infusion of glial cell line-derived neurotrophic factor in Parkinson's disease. Nat Med 2003; 9: 589–95.
52. Lang AE, Gill S, Patel NK, et al. Randomized controlled trial of intraputamenal glial cell line-derived neurotrophic factor infusion in Parkinson's disease. Ann Neurol 2006; 59: 459–66.
53. Doder M, Rabiner EA, Turjanski N, Lees AJ, Brooks DJ. Brain serotonin HT1A receptors in Parkinson's disease with and without depression measured by positron emission tomography and 11C-WAY100635. Mov Disord 2000; 15: 213.
54. Brooks DJ. Imaging non-dopaminergic function in Parkinson's disease. Mol Imaging Biol 2007; 9: 217–22.
55. Kim SE, Choi JY, Choe YS, Choi Y, Lee WY. Serotonin transporters in the midbrain of Parkinson's disease patients: a study with 123I-beta-CIT SPECT. J Nucl Med 2003; 44: 870–6.

56. Remy P, Doder M, Lees AJ, Turjanski N, Brooks DJ. Depression in Parkinson's disease: loss of dopamine and noradrenaline innervation in the limbic system. Brain 2005; 128: 1314–22.
57. Eidelberg D, Moeller JR, Dhawan V, et al. The metabolic topography of parkinsonism. J Cereb Blood Flow Metab 1994; 14: 783–801.
58. Trost M, Su S, Su P, et al. Network modulation by the subthalamic nucleus in the treatment of Parkinson's disease. Neuroimage 2006; 31: 301–7.
59. Feigin A, Fukuda M, Dhawan V, et al. Metabolic correlates of levodopa response in Parkinson's disease. Neurology 2001; 57: 2083–8.
60. Kuhl DE, Metter EJ, Benson DF. Similarities of cerebral glucose metabolism in Alzheimer's and Parkinsonian dementia. J Cereb Blood Flow Metab 1985; 5: S169–S70.
61. Bohnen NI, Koeppe RA, Minoshima S, et al. Cerebral glucose metabolic features of Parkinson's disease and incident dementia: longitudinal study. J Nucl Med 2011; 52: 848–55.
62. Edison P, Rowe CC, Rinne JO, et al. Amyloid load in Parkinson's disease dementia and Lewy body dementia measured with [11C]PIB positron emission tomography. J Neurol Neurosurg Psychiatry 2008; 79: 1331–8.
63. Gomperts SN, Rentz DM, Moran E, et al. Imaging amyloid deposition in Lewy body diseases. Neurology 2008; 71: 903–10.
64. Hilker R, Thomas AV, Klein JC, et al. Dementia in Parkinson's disease: functional imaging of cholinergic and dopaminergic pathways. Neurology 2005; 65: 1716–22.
65. Bohnen NI, Kaufer DI, Hendrickson R, et al. Cognitive correlates of cortical cholinergic denervation in Parkinson's disease and parkinsonian dementia. J Neurol 2006; 253: 242–7.
66. Nagayama H, Hamamoto M, Ueda M, Nagashima J, Katayama Y. Reliability of MIBG myocardial scintigraphy in the diagnosis of Parkinson's disease. J Neurol Neurosurg Psychiatry 2005; 76: 249–51.
67. Antonini A, Kazumata K, Feigin A, et al. Differential diagnosis of parkinsonism with [18F]Fluorodeoxyglucose and PET. Mov Disord 1998; 13: 268–74.
68. Spetsieris PG, Ma Y, Dhawan V, Eidelberg D. Differential diagnosis of parkinsonian syndromes using PCA-based functional imaging features. Neuroimage 2009; 45: 1241–52.
69. Schwarz J, Tatsch K, Arnold G, et al. 123I-iodobenzamide-SPECT predicts dopaminergic responsiveness in patients with de-novo parkinsonism. Neurology 1992; 42: 556–61.
70. Druschky A, Hilz MJ, Platsch G, et al. Differentiation of Parkinson's disease and multiple system atrophy in early disease stages by means of I-123-MIBG-SPECT. J Neurol Sci 2000; 175: 3–12.
71. Eckert T, Tang C, Ma Y, et al. Abnormal metabolic networks in atypical parkinsonism. Mov Disord 2008; 23: 727–33.
72. Messa C, Volonte MA, Fazio F, et al. Differential distribution of striatal [123I]b-CIT in Parkinson's disease and progressive supranuclear palsy, evaluated with single-photon emission tomography. Eur J Nucl Med 1998; 25: 1270–6.
73. Braune S, Reinhardt M, Schnitzer R, et al. Cardiac uptake of [123-I])-MIBG separates Parkinson's disease from multiple system atrophy. Neurology 1999; 53: 1020–5.

12 Neuropathology of parkinsonism

Dennis W. Dickson

INTRODUCTION

The common denominator of virtually all disorders associated with clinical parkinsonism is neuronal loss in the substantia nigra, particularly the dopaminergic neurons in the *pars compacta* that project to the striatum (Fig. 12.1). The ventrolateral group of neurons (A9) appears to be the most vulnerable in many parkinsonian disorders (1), and these tend to project heavily to the putamen (2). The more medial group of neurons send projections to limbic forebrain and medial temporal lobe and are less affected, but may be preferentially affected in individuals with cognitive impairment (3). The dorsal tier of neurons may be vulnerable to neuronal loss associated with aging (2).

PARKINSON'S DISEASE

The clinical features of Parkinson's disease (PD) are bradykinesia, rigidity, tremor, postural instability, autonomic dysfunction, and bradyphrenia. The most frequent pathologic substrate for this clinical syndrome is Lewy body disease. The diagnostic accuracy rate can approach as high as 90% in some series (4). In the brain bank for neurodegenerative disorders at Mayo Clinic, more than 80% of cases with a clinical diagnosis of PD made by a referring movement disorder specialist had Lewy bodies (Table 12.1). Lewy body disease is also the most common finding at autopsy in cases with a broader clinical diagnosis of parkinsonism, which includes patients with dementia or focal cortical syndromes in addition to parkinsonism. Disorders most likely to present clinically as PD with underlying pathologic diagnoses other than Lewy body disease are progressive supranuclear palsy (PSP), multiple system atrophy (MSA), and vascular disease. Non-Lewy body disorders are less uncommon when the clinical diagnosis is made after several years of clinical follow-up (5,6).

Macroscopic Findings in PD

The brain in patients with PD is usually grossly normal when viewed from the outer surface. There may be mild frontal atrophy in some cases, but this is variable. The most obvious visible change in PD is seen after the brainstem is sectioned. The loss of neuromelanin pigmentation in the substantia nigra and locus coeruleus is usually grossly apparent and may be associated with a rust color in the *pars reticulata* of the substantia nigra, which correlates with increased iron deposition in the tissue.

Microscopic Findings in PD

Histologically, there is neuronal loss in the substantia nigra *pars compacta* along with compensatory astrocytic and microglial proliferation. While biochemically there is

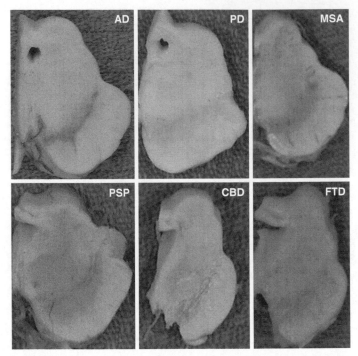

FIGURE 12.1   Midbrain sections from a variety of disorders associated with parkinsonism, including PD, MSA, PSP, CBD, FTD and AD, a disorder not associated with parkinsonism. Note loss of pigment in the substantia nigra in all disorders except AD. *Abbreviations*: PD, Parkinson's disease; MSA, multiple system atrophy; PSP, progressive supranuclear palsy; CBD, corticobasal degeneration; FTD, frontotemporal dementia; AD, Alzheimer's disease.

TABLE 12.1   Neuropathology of PD and Parkinsonism

Clinical Diagnosis	PD N (%)	Parkinsonism N (%)
Pathologic Diagnosis:		
Lewy body disease	75 (84%)	164 (73%)
Progressive supranuclear palsy	5 (6%)	30 (13%)
Vascular disease	4 (4%)	10 (4%)
Corticobasal degeneration	0 (0%)	7 (3%)
Multiple system atrophy	3 (3%)	5 (2%)
"Nonspecific" SN degeneration	2 (2%)	3 (1%)
Lewy Body Disease Subtype		
Brainstem predominant	21 (28%)	34 (21%)
Limbic/transitional	37 (49%)	67 (41%)
Diffuse cortical	17 (23%)	63 (38%)

Pathology of cases from the brain bank for neurodegenerative disorders at Mayo Clinic who had been referred by a movement disorder specialist with diagnosis of PD (N = 89) or Parkinsonism – which included PD cases as well as cases with parkinsonism with dementia or focal cortical syndromes (N = 219). For cases with Lewy body pathology as the primary diagnosis, the distribution of Lewy bodies is provided in the lower table.

loss of dopaminergic termini in the striatum, the striatum is histologically unremarkable on routine stains, but with α-synuclein immunohistochemistry, Lewy neurites can be detected in many cases. In the substantia nigra and locus coeruleus, neuromelanin pigment may be found in the cytoplasm of macrophages. Less common are neurons undergoing neuronophagia (i.e., phagocytosis by macrophages). Hyaline cytoplasmic inclusions, so-called Lewy bodies and less well-defined "pale bodies" are found in some of the residual neurons in the substantia nigra (Fig. 12.2). Similar pathology is found in the locus coeruleus, the dorsal motor nucleus of the vagus, as well as the basal forebrain (especially the basal nucleus of Meynert). The convexity neocortex usually does not have Lewy bodies, but the limbic cortex and the amygdala may be affected. Depending on the age of the individual, varying degrees of Alzheimer-type pathology may be detected, but if the person is not demented, this usually falls within the limits for that age. Some cases may have abundant senile plaques, but few or no neurofibrillary tangles.

The Lewy bodies are proteinaceous neuronal cytoplasmic inclusions [reviewed in Refs. (7–9)]. In some regions of the brain, such as the dorsal motor nucleus of the vagus, Lewy bodies tend to form within neuronal processes and are sometimes referred to as intraneuritic Lewy bodies. In most cases, Lewy bodies are accompanied by a variable number of abnormal neuritic profiles, referred to as Lewy neurites. Lewy neurites were first described in the hippocampus (10), but are also found in other regions of the brain, including the amygdala, cingulate gyrus, and temporal cortex. At the electron microscopic level, Lewy bodies are composed of densely aggregated filaments (11) and Lewy neurites also are filamentous, but they are usually not as densely packed (10).

The chemical composition of Lewy bodies has been inferred from immunohistochemical studies. While antibodies to neurofilament were first shown to label Lewy bodies (12), ubiquitin (13) and α-synuclein (14) antibodies are better markers for Lewy bodies, and α-synuclein is the most specific marker currently available for Lewy bodies (Fig. 12.2). Lewy neurites have the same immunoreactivity profile as

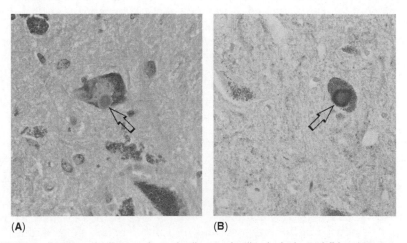

(A)   (B)

FIGURE 12.2 Parkinson's disease: Lewy bodies are hyaline inclusions visible with routine histologic methods in pigmented neurons of the substantia nigra (arrow in **A**). They are strongly immunoreactive with α-synuclein immunohistochemistry (arrow in **B**).

Lewy bodies (15). Biochemical studies of purified Lewy bodies have not been accomplished, but evidence suggests that they may contain a mixture of proteins, including neurofilament and α-synuclein (16–18).

Distribution of α-Synuclein Pathology in PD

Neurons that are most vulnerable to Lewy bodies include the monoaminergic neurons of the substantia nigra, locus coeruleus, and dorsal motor nucleus of the vagus, as well as cholinergic neurons in the basal forebrain. Lewy bodies are uncommon in the basal ganglia or thalamus, but are frequent in the hypothalamus, especially the posterior and lateral hypothalamus, and the brainstem reticular formation. The oculomotor nuclear complex is also vulnerable. In the pons, the dorsal raphe and pedunculopontine nuclei are often affected, but neurons of the pontine base are not. Lewy bodies have not been described in the cerebellar cortex. In the spinal cord, the neurons of the intermediolateral cell column are most vulnerable. Lewy bodies can be found in the autonomic ganglia, including submucosal ganglia of the esophagus (19). Increasingly, they have been detected in the peripheral autonomic nervous system (20).

While not usually numerous in typical PD, Lewy bodies can be found in cortical neurons, especially in the limbic lobe. Cortical Lewy bodies can be difficult to detect with routine histology, but are visible with α-synuclein immunohistochemistry and are usually most numerous in small nonpyramidal neurons in lower cortical layers. Similar lesions in the substantia nigra are referred to as "pale bodies" or as "pre-Lewy bodies." Ultrastructural studies of cortical Lewy bodies demonstrate poorly organized filamentous structures.

Braak and co-workers have proposed a staging scheme for progression of α-synuclein pathology in PD, with six stages and the earliest changes are in the lower brainstem and the olfactory bulb, with "spread" of the disease process to progressively higher levels of the neuraxis (21). In this scheme, locus coeruleus is involved at stage 2, substantia nigra is involved at stage 3, basal forebrain and limbic lobe at stage 4, multimodal association neocortex at stage 5, and primary neocortex at stage 6. The hypothesis predicts that preclinical manifestations of PD would be nonmotor (e.g., autonomic dysfunction and anosmia) and that the late stage would be associated with cortical Lewy body dementia. The scheme remains to be confirmed, but there is intriguing evidence that would suggest that sleep disorders, constipation, and anosmia may precede overt parkinsonism in some cases by many years (22–24). There is increasing interest in the cell-to-cell spread or transmission of abnormal conformers of α-synuclein (25), and detection of Lewy bodies and Lewy neurites in fetal grafts placed in the striatum of PD patients after nine or more years seems to support this hypothesis (26,27).

Neuropathology of Dementia in PD

Pathologic findings considered to account for dementia in PD include severe pathology in monoaminergic and cholinergic nuclei that project to the cortex producing a "subcortical dementia" (39%), coexistent Alzheimer's disease (29%), and diffuse cortical Lewy bodies (26%) (28). A subset of cases, particularly those with diffuse cortical Lewy bodies and concurrent Alzheimer type pathology, have neuronal inclusions composed of the protein found in frontotemporal lobar degeneration, namely, TDP-43 (29,30). The basal forebrain cholinergic system is the subcortical region most often implicated in dementia, and neurons in this region are damaged in both Alzheimer's and Lewy body disease. Neuronal loss in the basal nucleus is consistently found in PD, especially PD with dementia (31). Cholinergic deficits are common in PD (32), and they may contribute to dementia in PD in those cases that do not have concurrent Alzheimer's disease or cortical Lewy bodies.

Although virtually all PD brains have a few cortical Lewy bodies (28), they are usually neither widespread nor numerous in PD patients who were not demented [reviewed in Ref. (33)]. Several recent studies have shown, however, that cortical Lewy bodies are numerous and widespread in PD with dementia (34–36) and that the density of cortical Lewy bodies and Lewy neurites, especially in the medial temporal lobe (37), correlates with the severity of dementia (38). There are exceptions to this rule with occasional reports of patients with many Lewy bodies who were clinically normal (39).

MULTIPLE SYSTEM ATROPHY

The term multiple system atrophy (MSA) is used for a neurodegenerative disease characterized by parkinsonism, cerebellar ataxia, and autonomic dysfunction (40). MSA has an average age of onset between 30 and 50 years and a disease duration of approximately a decade. It is classified into MSA-C for cases with predominant cerebellar ataxia and MSA-P for cases with predominant atypical parkinsonism (41). There are ethnic differences in the frequency of MSA subtypes, with MSA-C more common in Japanese and MSA-P more common in western countries (42,43). Most cases of MSA have no family history of similar disease, and there are no known genetic risk factors for MSA, but variants in the synuclein gene have been suggested to be a risk factor for MSA (44).

Macroscopic Findings in MSA

The MSA brain shows varying degrees of atrophy of cerebellum, cerebellar peduncles, pontine base, and inferior olive, as well as atrophy and discoloration of the posterolateral putamen and pigment loss in the substantia nigra. For MSA-C, the findings are those of an olivopontocerebellar degeneration, whereas for MSA-P, the findings are those of a striatonigral degeneration.

Microscopic Findings in MSA

The histopathologic findings include neuronal loss, gliosis, and microvacuolation, involving the putamen, substantia nigra, cerebellum, olivary nucleus, pontine base, and intermediolateral cell column of the spinal cord. White matter inevitably shows demyelination, with the brunt of the changes affecting white matter tracts in cerebellum and pons (Fig. 12.3).

Lantos and co-workers first described oligodendroglial inclusions in MSA and named them glial cytoplasmic inclusions (GCI) (45). GCI can be detected with silver stains, such as the Gallyas silver stain, but are best seen with α-synuclein immunohistochemistry, where they appear as flame- or sickle-shaped inclusions in oligodendrocytes (Fig. 12.3). Like Lewy bodies, GCI are also immunostained with antibodies to ubiquitin (45). At the ultrastructural level, GCI are non–membrane-bound cytoplasmic inclusions composed of filaments (7–10 nm) and granular material that often coats the filaments making precise measurements difficult (46). GCI are specific for MSA and have not been found in other neurodegenerative diseases. In addition to GCI, synuclein immunoreactive inclusions are also detected in some neurons in MSA, particularly in the putamen, pontine base, and inferior olivary nucleus. Biochemical studies of synuclein in MSA have shown changes in its solubility (47).

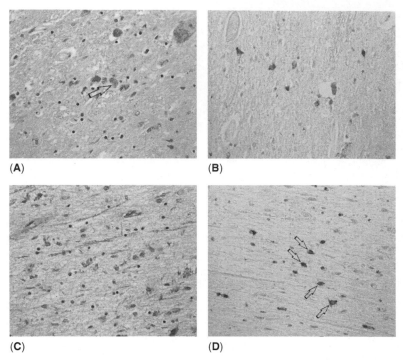

(A)   (B)

(C)   (D)

FIGURE 12.3 MSA: Substantia nigra neuronal loss in MSA is obvious in the cluster of pigment-laden macrophages (arrow in **A**), but neuronal inclusions are not present. Immunohistochemistry for α-synuclein shows many small glial inclusions in oligodendroglial cells, so-called GCI (**B**). The white matter in the cerebellum shows marked myelin loss (Luxol fast blue stain for myelin) (**C**) and in the affected areas there are many synuclein-immunoreactive GCI (arrows) (**D**). *Abbreviations*: MSA, multiple system atrophy; GCI, glial cytoplasmic inclusion.

PROGRESSIVE SUPRANUCLEAR PALSY

Progressive supranuclear palsy is an atypical parkinsonian disorder associated with progressive axial rigidity, vertical gaze palsy, dysarthria, and dysphagia first described by Steele–Richardson–Olszewski (48). Some cases present with a clinical syndrome similar to PD, including asymmetry and response to dopamine replacement therapy, before developing more characteristic signs of PSP at a later stage (49). Others present with pure akinesia with gait failure and freezing of gait (50). Focal cortical syndrome presentations, such as frontal lobe dementia or corticobasal syndrome, are rare (51).

Macroscopic Findings in PSP

In contrast to PD, gross examination of the brain often has distinctive findings in PSP. Most cases have varying degrees of frontal atrophy that may involve the precentral gyrus. The midbrain, especially the midbrain tectum, and to a lesser extent the pons shows atrophy. The third ventricle and aqueduct of Sylvius is often dilated. The substantia nigra shows loss of pigment, whereas the locus coeruleus is often better preserved. The subthalamic nucleus is smaller than expected and may

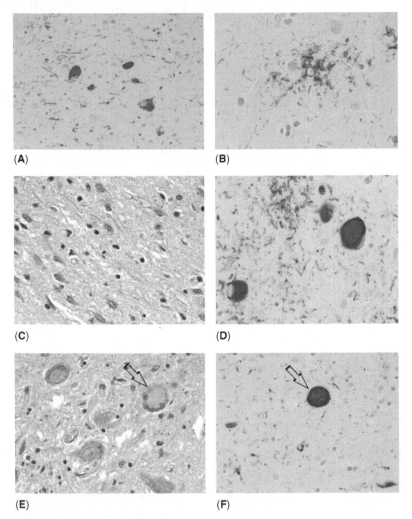

FIGURE 12.4   Progressive supranuclear palsy: The basal ganglia have neurofibrillary tangles and threads (**A**) and tufted astrocytes (**B**) with tau immunohistochemistry. There is severe neuronal loss and gliosis in the subthalamic nucleus (**C**) and many neurofibrillary tangles and glial lesions in the subthalamic nucleus (**D**). The substantia nigra has neuronal loss and neurofibrillary tangles visible in a pigmented neuron with hematoxylin and eosin histologic stain (arrow in **E**) or with tau immunohistochemistry (arrow in **F**).

have discoloration. The superior cerebellar peduncle and the hilus of the cerebellar dentate nucleus are usually atrophic and have discoloration due to myelinated fiber loss (52).

Microscopic Findings in PSP

Microscopic findings include neuronal loss, gliosis, and tau immunoreactive neurofibrillary tangles affecting basal ganglia, diencephalon, and brainstem (Fig. 12.4). The nuclei most affected are the globus pallidus, subthalamic nucleus, and substantia nigra. The cerebellar dentate nucleus is also affected. The cerebral cortex is relatively spared, but lesions are common in the premotor and motor cortices. Recent studies suggest that cortical pathology may be more widespread in cases of PSP with atypical features, such as dementia (53). The limbic lobe is preserved in PSP.

The striatum and thalamus often have some degree of neuronal loss and gliosis, especially ventral anterior and lateral thalamic nuclei. The basal nucleus of Meynert usually has mild cell loss. The brainstem regions that are affected include the superior colliculus, periaqueductal gray matter, oculomotor nuclei, locus coeruleus, pontine nuclei, pontine tegmentum, vestibular nuclei, medullary tegmentum, and inferior olives. The cerebellar dentate nucleus may show grumose degeneration, a type of neuronal degeneration associated with clusters of degenerating presynaptic terminals around dentate neurons (54). The dentato-rubro-thalamic pathway consistently shows fiber loss. The cerebellar cortex is preserved, but there may be mild Purkinje loss with scattered axonal torpedoes. The spinal cord is often affected, where neuronal inclusions can be found in anterior horn and intermediolateral cells.

Silver stains (e.g., Gallyas stain) or immunohistochemistry for tau reveal neurofibrillary tangles in residual neurons in the basal ganglia, diencephalon, brainstem, and spinal cord. In addition to neurofibrillary tangles, special stains demonstrate argyrophilic, tau-positive inclusions in both astrocytes and oligodendrocytes. Tufted astrocytes are increasingly recognized as a characteristic feature of PSP (55) and are commonly found in motor cortex and striatum (Fig. 12.4) (56). They are fibrillary lesions within astrocytes based on double immunolabeling of tau and glial fibrillary acidic protein. Oligodendroglial lesions appear as argyrophilic and tau-positive perinuclear fibers, so-called coiled bodies, which are often accompanied by thread-like processes in the white matter, especially in the diencephalon, brainstem, and cerebellar white matter.

Neurofibrillary tangles in PSP are composed of 15-nm straight filaments (57). The abnormal filaments in glial cells in PSP also contain straight filaments. Biochemical studies also show differences between tau in AD and PSP. In AD the abnormal insoluble tau migrates as three major bands (68, 64, and 60 kDa) on Western blots, whereas in PSP it migrates as two bands (68 and 64 kDa) (58). This reflects the preferential involvement of specific splice forms of tau, so-called 4-repeat tau, which is tau containing alternatively spliced exon 10 that has four ~32 amino acid repeats in the microtubule-binding domain (59).

CORTICOBASAL DEGENERATION

Corticobasal degeneration (CBD) is only rarely mistaken for PD due to characteristic focal cortical signs that are the clinical hallmark of this disorder (Table 12.1). On the other hand, most cases of CBD have some degree of bradykinesia and rigidity, with dystonia and myoclonus more common than parkinsonian rest tremor. CBD often presents with focal cortical syndromes, including progressive asymmetrical rigidity and apraxia, progressive aphasia and progressive frontal lobe dementia (60). The ability to correctly diagnose CBD is very poor at present (61), and the corticobasal clinical syndrome can have a range of different underlying pathologies, including AD (62).

Macroscopic Findings in CBD

Given the prominent cortical findings on clinical evaluations, it is not surprising that gross examination of the brain often reveals focal cortical atrophy. The atrophy may be severe and "knife-edge" in some cases or subtle and hardly noticeable in others. It may be asymmetrical. Atrophy is often most marked in the medial superior frontal gyrus, parasagittal pre- and postcentral gyri and the superior parietal lobule. The temporal and occipital lobes are usually preserved. The brainstem does not have gross atrophy as in PSP, but pigment loss is common in the substantia nigra. In contrast to PSP, the superior cerebellar peduncle and the subthalamic nucleus are grossly normal.

The cerebral white matter in affected areas is often attenuated and may have a gray discoloration. The corpus callosum is sometimes thinned and the frontal horn of the lateral ventricle is frequently dilated. The caudate head may have flattening. The thalamus may be smaller than usual.

Microscopic Findings in CBD

Microscopic examination of atrophic cortical sections shows neuronal loss with superficial spongiosis, gliosis, and usually many achromatic or ballooned neurons (63). Ballooned neurons are swollen and vacuolated neurons found in middle and lower cortical layers, which are variably positive with silver stains and tau immunohistochemistry, but intensely stained with immunohistochemistry for alpha-B-crystallin, a small heat shock protein, and for neurofilament (Fig. 12.5).

Cortical neurons in atrophic areas also have tau-immunoreactive lesions. In some neurons, tau is densely packed into a small inclusion body somewhat reminiscent of a Pick body or a small neurofibrillary tangle. In other neurons, the filamentous inclusions are more dispersed and diffuse consistent with so-called pretangles. As in PSP, neurofibrillary lesions in CBD are not detected well with most diagnostic silver stains and thioflavin fluorescent microscopy. Neurofibrillary lesions in brainstem monoaminergic nuclei, such as the locus coeruleus and substantia nigra, sometimes resemble globose neurofibrillary tangles.

In addition to fibrillary lesions in perikarya of neurons, the neuropil of CBD invariably contains a large number of thread-like tau-immunoreactive processes. They are usually profuse in both gray and white matter, and this latter feature is an important attribute of CBD and a useful feature in differentiating it from other disorders (63).

The most characteristic tau-immunoreactive lesion in the cortex in CBD is an annular cluster of short, stubby processes with fuzzy outlines that may be highly suggestive of a neuritic plaque of AD (64). In contrast to Alzheimer plaques, they do not contain amyloid, but rather tau-positive astrocytes and have been referred to as "astrocytic plaques" (Fig. 12.5). Astrocytic plaques differ from the tufted astrocytes seen in PSP, and the two lesions do not co-exist in the same brain (55). The astrocytic plaque may be the most specific histopathologic lesion of CBD (65).

In addition to cortical pathology, deep gray matter is consistently affected in CBD. The globus pallidus and putamen show mild neuronal loss with gliosis. Thalamic nuclei may also be affected. In the basal ganglia, thread-like processes are often extensive, often in the pencil fibers of the striatum. Tau-positive neurons, but not neurofibrillary tangles, are common in the striatum and globus pallidus. The internal capsule and thalamic fasciculus often have many thread-like processes. The subthalamic nucleus usually has a normal neuronal population, but neurons may have

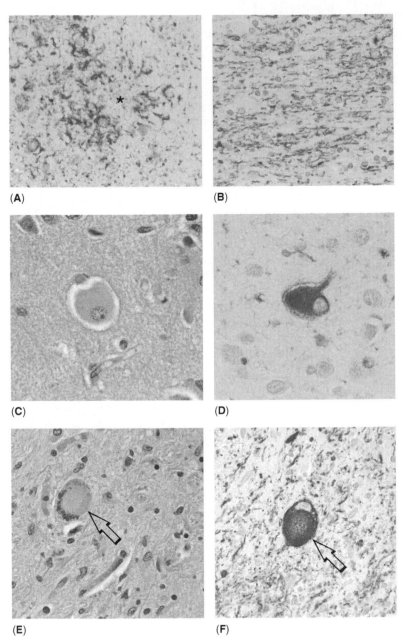

(A)   (B)

(C)   (D)

(E)   (F)

FIGURE 12.5   CBD: The hallmark lesion in CBD is the astrocytic plaque (asterisk in A), which is a cluster of irregular tau processes around a central astrocyte. Both white matter and gray matter in CBD have numerous tau-immunoreactive thread-like processes (**B**). Cortical neurons have swelling characteristic of ballooning degeneration (**C**) and the ballooned neurons have intense immunoreactivity with the stress protein alpha-B-crystallin (**D**). Neurons in the substantia nigra have round inclusions called corticobasal bodies (arrow in **E**) that are positive with tau immunohistochemistry (arrow in **F**). Note also the many thread-like processes in (**F**). *Abbreviation*: CBD, corticobasal degeneration.

tau inclusions, and there may be many thread-like lesions in the subthalamic nucleus. Fibrillary gliosis typical of PSP is not seen in the subthalamic nucleus in CBD.

The substantia nigra usually shows moderate-to-severe neuronal loss with extraneuronal neuromelanin and gliosis. Many of the remaining neurons contain neurofibrillary tangles, which have also been termed "corticobasal bodies" (Fig. 12.5) (66). The locus coeruleus and raphe nuclei have similar inclusions. In contrast to PSP where neurons in the pontine base usually have at least a few neurofibrillary tangles, the pontine base is largely free of neurofibrillary tangles in CBD. On the other hand, tau inclusions in glia and thread-like lesions are frequent in the pontine base. The cerebellum has mild Purkinje cell loss and axonal torpedoes. There is also mild neuronal loss in the dentate nucleus, but grumose degeneration is much less common than in PSP.

In CBD the filaments have a paired helical appearance at the electron microscopic level, but the diameter is wider and the periodicity is longer than the paired helical filaments of AD (64). These structures have been referred to as twisted ribbons. Similar to PSP, abnormal insoluble tau in CBD migrates as two prominent bands (68 and 64 kDa) on western blots (58).

GUAM PARKINSON–DEMENTIA COMPLEX
A characteristic parkinsonism with dementia [Parkinson–dementia complex (PDC)] with a number of features that overlap with PSP (67) has been reported in the native Chamorro population of Guam since the 1950s (68). The frequency of PDC is declining in recent years for unknown reasons, and the etiology is unknown.

Macroscopic Findings in PDC
The gross findings in PDC are notable for cortical atrophy affecting frontal and temporal lobes, as well as atrophy of the hippocampus and the tegmentum of the rostral brainstem (69). The substantia nigra often has severe loss of neuromelanin pigment.

Microscopic Findings in PDC
The cortex and hippocampus have neuronal loss and gliosis with many neurofibrillary tangles in residual neurons. In the cortex, neurofibrillary tangles show a different laminar distribution from AD, with more neurofibrillary tangles in superficial cortical layers in Guam PDC and in lower cortical layers in AD (70). The hippocampus has numerous neurofibrillary tangles, with many extracellular neurofibrillary tangles. The substantia nigra and locus coeruleus also have marked neuronal loss and many neurofibrillary tangles (Fig. 12.6). The basal nucleus and large neurons in the striatum are also vulnerable to neurofibrillary tangles. Astrocytic tau pathology has also been reported in PDC (Fig. 12.6) (71). In addition to tau pathology, most cases of Guam PDC have neuronal and glial lesions that contain TDP-43 (72). Biochemically and morphologically, neurofibrillary tangles in Guam PDC are indistinguishable from those in AD (73).

CHRONIC TRAUMATIC ENCEPHALOPATHY
Chronic traumatic encephalopathy (CTE) is an akinetic-rigid syndrome with dysarthria and dementia that is sometimes a long-term outcome of repeated closed-head trauma, as seen in professional athletes. The clinical syndrome is characterized by

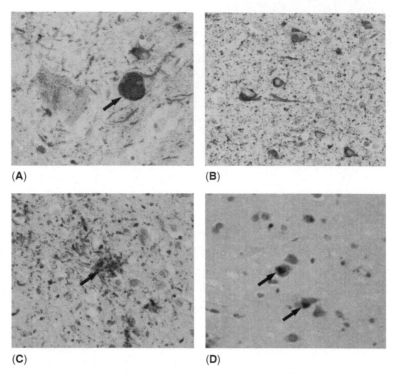

(A)   (B)

(C)   (D)

FIGURE 12.6 PDC: Many neurofibrillary tangles are the hallmark of PDC, with neurofibrillary tangles readily apparent with tau immunohistochemistry in the substantia nigra (arrow in **A**) and in the superficial cortical layers (**B**). Astrocytic inclusions are also noted in subcortical areas (**C**). There are also neurons with cytoplasmic inclusions (arrows) composed of TDP-43 (**D**). *Abbreviation*: PDC, Guam Parkinson–dementia complex.

memory disturbances, behavioral and personality changes, parkinsonism, and speech and gait abnormalities (74).

Macroscopic Findings in CTE
The pathology on gross examination, other than lesions that can be attributed to trauma, (e.g., subdural membranes and cortical contusions), is nonspecific, but may be associated with cerebral atrophy and ventricular dilation. The substantia nigra may also show pigment loss.

Microscopic Findings in CTE
Microscopically, there are neurofibrillary tangles similar to those in AD in brainstem monoaminergic nuclei, cortex, and hippocampus and some cases also have amyloid plaques (75,76). At the electron microscopic level, neurofibrillary tangles in CTE are composed of paired helical filaments and biochemically composed 68, 64, and 60 kDa forms (77). Most characteristic are patchy foci of neuronal and glial tau pathology in the frontal and temporal cortices with a propensity for sulcal depths (Fig. 12.7) (78). Tau pathology in astrocytes, similar to so-called thorn-shaped astrocytes that

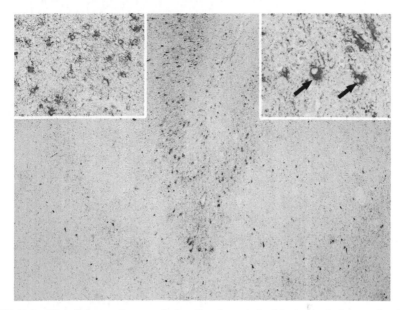

FIGURE 12.7 Chronic traumatic encephalopathy characterized by tau pathology at the depth of sulci that includes both cortical and white matter astrocytic lesions (left inset) and cortical neurofibrillary tangles (right inset).

occur in aging (79), is prominent in perivascular, periventricular, and subpial distribution (Fig. 12.7). Some cases have TDP-43 pathology, as well (80).

FAMILIAL PARKINSONISM

While most parkinsonian disorders are sporadic, rare familial forms have been described and mutations have been found or genetic linkage analyses have suggested a strong genetic factor in their etiology (81). Perhaps the most common cause of early-onset familial PD is autosomal recessive juvenile PD (ARJP) due to mutations in the gene for Parkin (PRKN) (82). The clinical features are somewhat atypical in that dystonia is common in ARJP (83). The pathology of ARJP is based on only a few autopsy reports. Initial studies emphasized severe neuronal loss in the substantia nigra with no Lewy bodies, but a more recent report of an individual who died prematurely of an automobile accident had Lewy bodies in the substantia nigra and other vulnerable regions (84,85). Even in sporadic PD, there is an inverse relationship between the disease duration and the number of Lewy bodies in the substantia nigra. When the disease is very severe, there are very few residual neurons. Since Lewy bodies are intraneuronal inclusions that are phagocytosed after the neuron dies, it is not surprising that there are few Lewy bodies in cases of very long duration.

Less common than ARJP are autosomal dominant forms of early-onset PD. The best characterized is the Contursi kindred, a familial PD due to a mutation in the α-synuclein gene (86). The pathology of the Contursi kindred is typical Lewy body PD; however, given the young age of onset, by the time the individual dies, Lewy body pathology is typically widespread in the brain. Lewy neurites are also prominent in many cortical areas. Some cases have TDP-43 pathology (87). Some young-onset autosomal dominant PD kindreds, such as the Iowa kindred, have atypical clinical presentations and include family members with dementia and psychosis. The Iowa kindred has been shown to have a multiplication of the α-synuclein gene (88). Families with duplications have a milder phenotype than those with a triplication of the α-synuclein gene, suggesting a role for over expression of α-synuclein in the pathogenesis of even sporadic PD (89). The pathology in cases with gene triplication is associated with severe Lewy body-related pathology in the cortex, hippocampus, and amygdala in addition to the substantia nigra and other brainstem nuclei, and in some cases glial inclusions similar to those found in MSA are present (Fig. 12.8) (90).

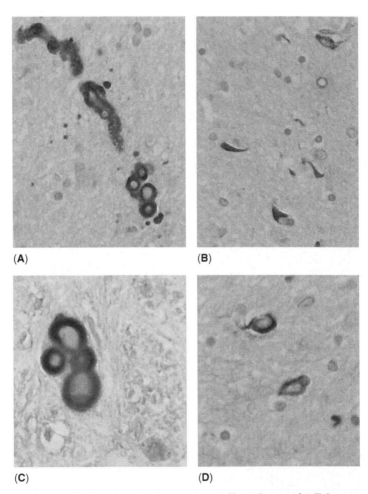

(A)   (B)

(C)   (D)

FIGURE 12.8 Familial PD: Many Lewy bodies are detected in early-onset familial cases and some of the inclusions have unusual morphologies (**A, B**). Like multiple system atrophy, synuclein-immunoreactive glial inclusions are also detected in some cases of familial early-onset PD. *Abbreviation*: PD, Parkinson's disease.

The most common cause of autosomal dominant late-onset PD is mutation in the *LRRK2* gene on chromosome 12 (91,92). The pathology in most cases, is characterized by Lewy bodies (93), but in some individuals other types of pathology, including neurofibrillary pathology or ubiquitin immunoreactive inclusions, are detected (91,94). In some cases, the neuronal inclusions are immunoreactive for TDP-43 (95). The genetic influence of *LRRK2* to seemingly sporadic PD continues to expand (96–98), with problems in interpretation of genetic results related to the incomplete penetrance of the mutations, reaching more than 80% only after 70 years of age (99).

ACKNOWLEDGMENTS
Supported by NIH P50-AG16574, P01-AG03949, P50-NS20187, Mangurian Foundation, Mayo Foundation, State of Florida Alzheimer Disease Initiative and CurePSP/Society for Progressive Supranuclear Palsy.

REFERENCES
1. Dickson DW, Braak H, Duda JE, et al. Neuropathological assessment of Parkinson's disease: refining the diagnostic criteria. Lancet Neurol 2009; 8: 1150–7.
2. Gibb WR, Lees AJ. Anatomy, pigmentation, ventral and dorsal subpopulations of the substantia nigra, and differential cell death in Parkinson's disease. J Neurol Neurosurg Psychiatry 1991; 54: 388–96.
3. Rinne JO, Rummukainen J, Paljarvi L, et al. Dementia in Parkinson's disease is related to neuronal loss in the medial substantia nigra. Ann Neurol 1989; 26: 47–50.
4. Hughes AJ, Daniel SE, Lees AJ. Improved accuracy of clinical diagnosis of Lewy body Parkinson's disease. Neurology 2001; 57: 1497–9.
5. Rajput AH, Rozdilsky B, Rajput A. Accuracy of clinical diagnosis in parkinsonism–a prospective study. Can J Neurol Sci 1991; 18: 275–8.
6. Hughes AJ, Daniel SE, Kilford L, et al. Accuracy of clinical diagnosis of idiopathic Parkinson's disease: a clinico-pathological study of 100 cases. J Neurol Neurosurg Psychiatry 1992; 55: 181–4.
7. Pollanen MS, Dickson DW, Bergeron C. Pathology and biology of the Lewy body. J Neuropathol Exp Neurol 1993; 52: 183–91.
8. Shults CW. Lewy bodies. Proc Natl Acad Sci USA 2006; 103: 1661–8.
9. Wakabayashi K, Tanji K, Odagiri S, et al. The Lewy body in Parkinson's disease and related neurodegenerative disorders. Mol Neurobiol 2012.
10. Dickson DW, Ruan D, Crystal H, et al. Hippocampal degeneration differentiates diffuse Lewy body disease (DLBD) from Alzheimer's disease: light and electron microscopic immunocytochemistry of CA2-3 neurites specific to DLBD. Neurology 1991; 41: 1402–9.
11. Galloway PG, Mulvihill P, Perry G. Filaments of Lewy bodies contain insoluble cytoskeletal elements. Am J Pathol 1992; 140: 809–22.
12. Goldman JE, Yen SH, Chiu FC, et al. Lewy bodies of Parkinson's disease contain neurofilament antigens. Science 1983; 221: 1082–4.
13. Kuzuhara S, Mori H, Izumiyama N, et al. Lewy bodies are ubiquitinated. A light and electron microscopic immunocytochemical study. Acta Neuropathol (Berl) 1988; 75: 345–53.
14. Spillantini MG, Schmidt ML, Lee VM, et al. Alpha-synuclein in Lewy bodies. Nature 1997; 388: 839–40.
15. Irizarry MC, Growdon W, Gomez-Isla T, et al. Nigral and cortical Lewy bodies and dystrophic nigral neurites in Parkinson's disease and cortical Lewy body disease contain alpha-synuclein immunoreactivity. J Neuropathol Exp Neurol 1998; 57: 334–7.
16. Pollanen MS, Bergeron C, Weyer L. Detergent-insoluble cortical Lewy body fibrils share epitopes with neurofilament and tau. J Neurochem 1992; 58: 1953–6.

17. Iwatsubo T, Yamaguchi H, Fujimuro M, et al. Lewy bodies: purification from diffuse Lewy body disease brains. Ann NY Acad Sci 1996; 786: 195–205.
18. Baba M, Nakajo S, Tu PH, et al. Aggregation of alpha-synuclein in Lewy bodies of sporadic Parkinson's disease and dementia with Lewy bodies. Am J Pathol 1998; 152: 879–84.
19. Wakabayashi K, Takahashi H, Ohama E, et al. Lewy bodies in the visceral autonomic nervous system in Parkinson's disease. Adv Neurol 1993; 60: 609–12.
20. Beach TG, Adler CH, Sue LI, et al. Multi-organ distribution of phosphorylated alpha-synuclein histopathology in subjects with Lewy body disorders. Acta Neuropathol 2010; 119: 689–702.
21. Braak H, Ghebremedhin E, Rub U, et al. Stages in the development of Parkinson's disease-related pathology. Cell Tissue Res 2004; 318: 121–34.
22. Abbott RD, Petrovitch H, White LR, et al. Frequency of bowel movements and the future risk of Parkinson's disease. Neurology 2001; 57: 456–62.
23. Schenck CH, Bundlie SR, Mahowald MW. Delayed emergence of a parkinsonian disorder in 38% of 29 older men initially diagnosed with idiopathic rapid eye movement sleep behaviour disorder. Neurology 1996; 46: 388–93.
24. Berendse HW, Booij J, Francot CM, et al. Subclinical dopaminergic dysfunction in asymptomatic Parkinson's disease patients' relatives with a decreased sense of smell. Ann Neurol 2001; 50: 34–41.
25. Danzer KM, Ruf WP, Putcha P, et al. Heat-shock protein 70 modulates toxic extracellular alpha-synuclein oligomers and rescues trans-synaptic toxicity. FASEB J 2011; 25: 326–36.
26. Kordower JH, Chu Y, Hauser RA, et al. Lewy body-like pathology in long-term embryonic nigral transplants in Parkinson's disease. Nat Med 2008; 14: 504–6.
27. Li JY, Englund E, Holton JL, et al. Lewy bodies in grafted neurons in subjects with Parkinson's disease suggest host-to-graft disease propagation. Nat Med 2008; 14: 501–3.
28. Hughes AJ, Daniel SE, Blankson S, et al. A clinicopathologic study of 100 cases of Parkinson's disease. Arch Neurol 1993; 50: 140–8.
29. Higashi S, Iseki E, Yamamoto R, et al. Concurrence of TDP-43, tau and alpha-synuclein pathology in brains of Alzheimer's disease and dementia with Lewy bodies. Brain Res 2007; 1184C: 284–94.
30. Nakashima-Yasuda H, Uryu K, Robinson J, et al. Co-morbidity of TDP-43 proteinopathy in Lewy body related diseases. Acta Neuropathol 2007; 114: 221–9.
31. Whitehouse PJ, Hedreen JC, White CL 3rd, et al. Basal forebrain neurons in the dementia of Parkinson disease. Ann Neurol 1983; 13: 243–8.
32. Perry EK, McKeith I, Thompson P, et al. Topography, extent, and clinical relevance of neurochemical deficits in dementia of Lewy body type, Parkinson's disease, and Alzheimer's disease. Ann NY Acad Sci 1991; 640: 197–202.
33. Emre M, Aarsland D, Brown R, et al. Clinical diagnostic criteria for dementia associated with Parkinson's disease. Mov Disord 2007; 22: 1689–707.
34. Mattila PM, Roytta M, Torikka H, et al. Cortical Lewy bodies and Alzheimer-type changes in patients with Parkinson's disease. Acta Neuropathol (Berl) 1998; 95: 576–82.
35. Apaydin H, Ahlskog JE, Parisi JE, et al. Parkinson disease neuropathology: later-developing dementia and loss of the levodopa response. Arch Neurol 2002; 59: 102–12.
36. Hurtig HI, Trojanowski JQ, Galvin J, et al. Alpha-synuclein cortical Lewy bodies correlate with dementia in Parkinson's disease. Neurology 2000; 54: 1916–21.
37. Churchyard A, Lees AJ. The relationship between dementia and direct involvement of the hippocampus and amygdala in Parkinson's disease. Neurology 1997; 49: 1570–6.
38. Lennox G, Lowe J, Landon M, et al. Diffuse Lewy body disease: correlative neuropathology using anti-ubiquitin immunocytochemistry. J Neurol Neurosurg Psychiatry 1989; 52: 1236–47.
39. Parkkinen L, Kauppinen T, Pirttila T, et al. Alpha-synuclein pathology does not predict extrapyramidal symptoms or dementia. Ann Neurol 2005; 57: 82–91.
40. Wenning GK, Tison F, Ben Shlomo Y, et al. Multiple system atrophy: a review of 203 pathologically proven cases. Mov Disord 1997; 12: 133–47.
41. Gilman S, Wenning GK, Low PA, et al. Second consensus statement on the diagnosis of multiple system atrophy. Neurology 2008; 71: 670–6.

42. Ozawa T, Paviour D, Quinn NP, et al. The spectrum of pathological involvement of the striatonigral and olivopontocerebellar systems in multiple system atrophy: clinicopathological correlations. Brain 2004; 127: 2657–71.
43. Ozawa T, Tada M, Kakita A, et al. The phenotype spectrum of Japanese multiple system atrophy. J Neurol Neurosurg Psychiatry 2010; 81: 1253–5.
44. Scholz SW, Houlden H, Schulte C, et al. SNCA variants are associated with increased risk for multiple system atrophy. Ann Neurol 2009; 65: 610–14.
45. Lantos PL. The definition of multiple system atrophy: a review of recent developments. J Neuropathol Exp Neurol 1998; 57: 1099–111.
46. Dickson DW, Lin W, Liu WK, et al. Multiple system atrophy: a sporadic synucleinopathy. Brain Pathol 1999; 9: 721–32.
47. Dickson DW, Liu W, Hardy J, et al. Widespread alterations of alpha-synuclein in multiple system atrophy. Am J Pathol 1999; 155: 1241–51.
48. Steele JC, Richardson JC, Olszewski J. Progressive supranuclear palsy. A heterogeneous degeneration involving the brain stem, basal ganglia and cerebellum with vertical gaze and pseudobulbar palsy, nuchal dystonia and dementia. Arch Neurol 1964; 10: 333–59.
49. Williams DR, de Silva R, Paviour DC, et al. Characteristics of two distinct clinical phenotypes in pathologically proven progressive supranuclear palsy: richardson's syndrome and PSP-parkinsonism. Brain 2005; 128: 1247–58.
50. Williams DR, Holton JL, Strand K, et al. Pure akinesia with gait freezing: a third clinical phenotype of progressive supranuclear palsy. Mov Disord 2007; 22: 2235–41.
51. Dickson DW, Ahmed Z, Algom AA, et al. Neuropathology of variants of progressive supranuclear palsy. Curr Opin Neurol 2010; 23: 394–400.
52. Tsuboi Y, Slowinski J, Josephs KA, et al. Atrophy of superior cerebellar peduncle in progressive supranuclear palsy. Neurology 2003; 60: 1766–9.
53. Bigio EH, Brown DF, White CL 3rd. Progressive supranuclear palsy with dementia: cortical pathology. J Neuropathol Exp Neurol 1999; 58: 359–64.
54. Ishizawa K, Lin WL, Tiseo P, et al. A qualitative and quantitative study of grumose degeneration in progressive supranuclear palsy. J Neuropathol Exp Neurol 2000; 59: 513–24.
55. Komori T. Tau-positive glial inclusions in progressive supranuclear palsy, corticobasal degeneration and Pick's disease. Brain Pathol 1999; 9: 663–79.
56. Dickson DW. In: Esiri MM, Lee VM-Y, Trojanowski JQ, eds. Sporadic Tauopathies: Pick's Disease, Corticobasal Degeneration, Progressive Supranuclear Palsy and Argyrophilic Grain Disease. New York: Cambridge University Press, 2004: 227–56.
57. Tellez-Nagel I, Wisniewski HM. Ultrastructure of neurofibrillary tangles in Steele-Richardson-Olszewski syndrome. Arch Neurol 1973; 29: 324–7.
58. Buee L, Delacourte A. Comparative biochemistry of tau in progressive supranuclear palsy, corticobasal degeneration, FTDP-17 and Pick's disease. Brain Pathol 1999; 9: 681–93.
59. Lee VM, Goedert M, Trojanowski JQ. Neurodegenerative tauopathies. Annu Rev Neurosci 2001; 24: 1121–59.
60. Litvan I, Grimes DA, Lang AE, et al. Clinical features differentiating patients with postmortem confirmed progressive supranuclear palsy and corticobasal degeneration. J Neurol 1999; 246: II1–5.
61. Ling H, O'Sullivan SS, Holton JL, et al. Does corticobasal degeneration exist? A clinicopathological re-evaluation. Brain 2010; 133: 2045–57.
62. Boeve BF, Maraganore DM, Parisi JE, et al. Pathologic heterogeneity in clinically diagnosed corticobasal degeneration. Neurology 1999; 53: 795–800.
63. Dickson DW, Bergeron C, Chin SS, et al. Office of rare diseases neuropathologic criteria for corticobasal degeneration. J Neuropathol Exp Neurol 2002; 61: 935–46.
64. Dickson DW, Liu WK, Ksiezak-Reding H, et al. Neuropathologic and molecular considerations. Adv Neurol 2000; 82: 9–27.
65. Feany MB, Dickson DW. Widespread cytoskeletal pathology characterizes corticobasal degeneration. Am J Pathol 1995; 146: 1388–96.
66. Gibb WR, Luthert PJ, Marsden CD. Corticobasal degeneration. Brain 1989; 112: 1171–92.

67. Steele JC. Parkinsonism-dementia complex of Guam. Mov Disord 2005; 20: S99–S107.
68. Hirano A, Kurland LT, Krooth RS, et al. Parkinsonism-dementia complex, an endemic disease on the island of Guam. I. Clinical features. Brain 1961; 84: 642–61.
69. Oyanagi K, Makifuchi T, Ohtoh T, et al. Amyotrophic lateral sclerosis of Guam: the nature of the neuropathological findings. Acta Neuropathol (Berl) 1994; 88: 405–12.
70. Hof PR, Perl DP, Loerzel AJ, et al. Neurofibrillary tangle distribution in the cerebral cortex of parkinsonism-dementia cases from Guam: differences with Alzheimer's disease. Brain Res 1991; 564: 306–13.
71. Oyanagi K, Makifuchi T, Ohtoh T, et al. Distinct pathological features of the gallyas- and tau-positive glia in the Parkinsonism-dementia complex and amyotrophic lateral sclerosis of Guam. J Neuropathol Exp Neurol 1997; 56: 308–16.
72. Hasegawa M, Arai T, Akiyama H, et al. TDP-43 is deposited in the Guam parkinsonism-dementia complex brains. Brain 2007; 130: 1386–94.
73. Buee-Scherrer V, Buee L, Hof PR, et al. Neurofibrillary degeneration in amyotrophic lateral sclerosis/parkinsonism-dementia complex of Guam. Immunochemical characterization of tau proteins. Am J Pathol 1995; 146: 924–32.
74. Stern RA, Riley DO, Daneshvar DH, et al. Long-term consequences of repetitive brain trauma: chronic traumatic encephalopathy. PMR 2011; 3: S460–7.
75. Roberts GW, Allsop D, Bruton C. The occult aftermath of boxing. J Neurol Neurosurg Psychiatry 1990; 53: 373–8.
76. Graham DI, Gentleman SM, Nicoll JA, et al. Altered beta-APP metabolism after head injury and its relationship to the aetiology of Alzheimer's disease. Acta Neurochir Suppl 1996; 66: 96–102.
77. Schmidt ML, Zhukareva V, Newell KL, et al. Tau isoform profile and phosphorylation state in dementia pugilistica recapitulate Alzheimer's disease. Acta Neuropathol (Berl) 2001; 101: 518–24.
78. McKee AC, Cantu RC, Nowinski CJ, et al. Chronic traumatic encephalopathy in athletes: progressive tauopathy after repetitive head injury. J Neuropathol Exp Neurol 2009; 68: 709–35.
79. Schultz C, Ghebremedhin E, Del Tredici K, et al. High prevalence of thorn-shaped astrocytes in the aged human medial temporal lobe. Neurobiol Aging 2004; 25: 397–405.
80. McKee AC, Gavett BE, Stern RA, et al. TDP-43 proteinopathy and motor neuron disease in chronic traumatic encephalopathy. J Neuropathol Exp Neurol 2010; 69: 918–29.
81. Gasser T. Genetics of Parkinson's disease. J Neurol 2001; 248: 833–40.
82. Hattori N, Kitada T, Matsumine H, et al. Molecular genetic analysis of a novel Parkin gene in Japanese families with autosomal recessive juvenile parkinsonism: evidence for variable homozygous deletions in the Parkin gene in affected individuals. Ann Neurol 1998; 44: 935–41.
83. Hattori N, Shimura H, Kubo S, et al. Autosomal recessive juvenile parkinsonism: a key to understanding nigral degeneration in sporadic Parkinson's disease. Neuropathology 2000; 20(Suppl): S85–90.
84. Farrer M, Chan P, Chen R, et al. Lewy bodies and parkinsonism in families with parkin mutations. Ann Neurol 2001; 50: 293–300.
85. Pramstaller PP, Schlossmacher MG, Jacques TS, et al. Lewy body Parkinson's disease in a large pedigree with 77 Parkin mutation carriers. Ann Neurol 2005; 58: 411–22.
86. Polymeropoulos MH, Lavedan C, Leroy E, et al. Mutation in the alpha-synuclein gene identified in families with Parkinson's disease. Science 1997; 276: 2045–7.
87. Markopoulou K, Dickson DW, McComb RD, et al. Clinical, neuropathological and genotypic variability in SNCA A53T familial Parkinson's disease. Variability in familial Parkinson's disease. Acta Neuropathol 2008; 116: 25–35.
88. Singleton AB, Farrer M, Johnson J, et al. Alpha-Synuclein locus triplication causes Parkinson's disease. Science 2003; 302: 841.
89. Farrer M, Kachergus J, Forno L, et al. Comparison of kindreds with parkinsonism and alpha-synuclein genomic multiplications. Ann Neurol 2004; 55: 174–9.
90. Gwinn-Hardy K, Mehta ND, Farrer M, et al. Distinctive neuropathology revealed by alpha-synuclein antibodies in hereditary parkinsonism and dementia linked to chromosome 4p. Acta Neuropathol (Berl) 2000; 99: 663–72.

91. Zimprich A, Biskup S, Leitner P, et al. Mutations in LRRK2 cause autosomal-dominant parkinsonism with pleomorphic pathology. Neuron 2004; 44: 601–7.
92. Paisan-Ruiz C, Jain S, Evans EW, et al. Cloning of the gene containing mutations that cause PARK8-linked Parkinson's disease. Neuron 2004; 44: 595–600.
93. Ross OA, Toft M, Whittle AJ, et al. Lrrk2 and Lewy body disease. Ann Neurol 2006; 59: 388–93.
94. Wszolek ZK, Pfeiffer RF, Tsuboi Y, et al. Autosomal dominant parkinsonism associated with variable synuclein and tau pathology. Neurology 2004; 62: 1619–22.
95. Wider C, Dickson DW, Wszolek ZK. Leucine-rich repeat kinase 2 gene-associated disease: redefining genotype-phenotype correlation. Neurodegener Dis 2010; 7: 175–9.
96. Gilks WP, Abou-Sleiman PM, Gandhi S, et al. A common LRRK2 mutation in idiopathic Parkinson's disease. Lancet 2005; 365: 415–16.
97. Di Fonzo A, Rohe CF, Ferreira J, et al. A frequent LRRK2 gene mutation associated with autosomal dominant Parkinson's disease. Lancet 2005; 365: 412–15.
98. Nichols WC, Pankratz N, Hernandez D, et al. Genetic screening for a single common LRRK2 mutation in familial Parkinson's disease. Lancet 2005; 365: 410–12.
99. Kachergus J, Mata IF, Hulihan M, et al. Identification of a novel LRRK2 mutation linked to autosomal dominant parkinsonism: evidence of a common founder across European populations. Am J Hum Genet 2005; 76: 672–80.

Neurophysiology

Erwin B. Montgomery Jr.

OVERVIEW

The basal ganglia comprise a set of subcortical nuclei that include the putamen (PT), globus pallidus interna (GPi), globus pallidus externa (GPe), subthalamic nucleus (STN), substantia nigra pars compacta, and substantia nigra pars reticularlis. However, the basal ganglia are integral parts of a larger system, which includes at the minimum, the supplementary motor area, motor cortex (MC), and ventorlateral and ventroanterior thalamus, as these structures are interdigitated among the nuclei traditionally associated with the basal ganglia. When viewed physiologically, in terms of propagation of information, the functional systems are far more extensive. Hence, there is little sense in discussing the physiology or pathophysiology of the basal ganglia alone. Rather, the physiology and pathophysiology of the basal ganglia–thalamic–cortical system (and beyond) should be discussed.

This chapter proceeds from the notion that current concepts of motor physiology have suffered because they are inherently anatomical rather than physiological. Furthermore, the anatomical presuppositions are very much a top–down approach where the physiology is extrapolated from the anatomy (1) with relatively little regard for what the physiology must actually accomplish particularly in terms of the dynamics necessary for normal movement. Further, the anatomical approaches have been dominated by a long tradition known as the Neuron Doctrine (2) and an approach to motor physiology that is hierarchical and sequential (3). Neither of these approaches is valid. Consequently, this chapter will take the opposite approach by first carefully analyzing what the motor system has to accomplish and then work backward to how the basal ganglia–thalamic–cortical system might achieve these requirements as informed by the abnormalities of movement associated with disorders of the basal ganglia.

The basal ganglia–thalamic–cortical system is a network of innumerable and interconnected oscillators. Each oscillator has nodes, which are local collections of individual neurons within the classic anatomical structures of the basal ganglia–thalamic–cortical system. Individual nodes can be components of multiple oscillators. Each oscillator is formed as physiologically closed reentrant loops. The activities of the neurons are highly nonlinear conferring onto the oscillator properties of discrete, as compared with continuous oscillators. These oscillators interact by a variety of means, including phase and frequency changes, synchronizations, positive and negative resonance, and beat interactions. These interactions provide a rich set of dynamics over multiple time scales that are necessary to produce the variety and complexity of movements available to humans.

The rich dynamics over multiple time scales matches well with the dynamics of the peripheral motor system comprising the lower motor neurons (LMN) in the brainstem and spinal cord and the muscle fibers innervated by the individual motor neurons collectively known as the motor unit. As Binder et al noted, "Sherrington referred to the motoneuron as the 'the final common pathway' to emphasize the axiom that every part of the nervous system involved in the control of movement must do so by acting either directly or indirectly on motoneurons" (4). Consequently, any full theory of the physiology and pathophysiology of the basal ganglia–thalamic–cortical system must match the dynamics of the peripheral motor system. The different but integrated time scales in behavior range from milliseconds, in terms of the timing of discharges of the LMN to seconds in terms of the orchestration of multiple muscles over multiple joints.

Ultimately, any motor physiology must modulate the activities of individual motor units at the most fundamental level and simultaneously be orchestrated with the activities of all the other motor units involved. Furthermore, the modulation and orchestration evolves over multiple time frames with separate but linked dynamics on different time scales. Modulation of individual motor units requires the recruitment into activity followed by changes in the rate of maintained discharge followed by de-recruitment. Each of these is abnormal in Parkinson's disease (PD), thus arguing for a role of the basal ganglia–thalamic–cortical system at the level of modulation of individual motor units. Further, each aspect of control for the individual motor units also is true of the orchestration between the motor units, again occurring over multiple time frames, thereby suggesting independent but linked dynamics. These dynamics for the orchestration of multiple muscles are altered in PD. Furthermore, these dynamics operating within large networks of loosely coupled nonlinear oscillators are capable of self-organization that drives different behaviors. Abnormalities in these dynamics of the basal ganglia–thalamic–cortical system then disrupt the dynamics of the peripheral motor system to produce the symptoms, signs, and disabilities of movement disorders such as PD.

INTRODUCTION

A full accounting of the physiology and pathophysiology of the basal ganglia has yet to be achieved. Indeed, one requirement for advancing the state of knowledge is the necessity to discard previous theories and to begin to offer radical new alternatives. Current theories include the Globus Pallidus Interna Rate theory and its derivative for normal physiology, the Action Selection/Focused Attention theory. The Globus Pallidus Interna Rate theory posits abnormal increased activity in the GPi that inhibits activity within the ventrolateral thalamic–cortical system. Also, there is the Beta Oscillations theory, which posits increased power in the beta frequency band of neuronal activities as somehow causal to parkinsonism. Consequently, the Beta Oscillations theory is kin to the Globus Pallidus Interna Rate theory and shares the same limitations due to the one-dimensional push–pull nature of the dynamics. The weaknesses of these theories have been reviewed elsewhere (5). Another theory parses movements on a spectrum of automatic versus explicit or consciously intentioned movements (6). The problem with these theories is that they fail to recognize and consequently, fail to explain abnormalities at the level of the motor units.

The failure to include any explanation at the level of the motor unit probably resulted from a number of factors. First and perhaps foremost, is the dichotomization of the symptoms and signs of movement disorders into hypokinetic disorders (absent and slowed movements) such as PD, and hyperkinetic disorders (involuntary movements) such as Huntington's disease. However, such dichotomization is not true as patients with Huntington's disease have bradykinesia (7,8) and patients with PD simultaneously can have hypokinesia and hyperkinesia, the latter in the form of levodopa-induced dyskinesia (9). Unfortunately, such false dichotomizations have a very long history in neurology and neuroscience, indeed in explanation of nature dating back to Aristotle. Any heuristic value of such dichotomizations, from the standpoint of a convenient simplification for the instruction of nonexperts, is counterproductive, as experts evolve from novices who still carry the false dichotomization. Thus, the current theories, such as the Globus Pallidus Interna Rate, the Action Selection/Focused Attention, and the Beta Oscillations theories, posit the pathophysiology of the basal ganglia as simply the production of too little or too much movement.

A second reason for the failure of theories of basal ganglia physiology and pathophysiology to include accounts for control of motor units relates to the notion that such control was unnecessary. The motor unit recruitment patterns were thought to be controlled by the LMN based on their biophysical properties or local circuitry (10). Small lower neurons innervating a small number of muscle fibers were recruited into activity early at the lowest force requirements. As force requirements increased, progressively larger LMN, with their large number of muscle fibers, were recruited to generate larger forces. Roger Enoka writes, "The great advantage of a spinally based control scheme [*recruitment order determined by motor neuron biophysics—author*], such as orderly recruitment, is that it relieves higher centers [*e.g., the basal ganglia—author*] of the responsibility to select the motor neurons that must be activated for a specific task" (11). It is no wonder that theories of basal ganglia physiology and pathophysiology did not include notions of how motor units were recruited.

THE DYNAMICS OF LOWER MOTOR NEURON CONTROL
Recruitment of Motor Unit Activity to Threshold for Movement

In order to generate a rotation about a joint, which is the basis for movement of the limbs and other body parts, there has to be sufficient tension developed by the muscles. The tension is a function of the kinds of muscle fibers activated, the frequency at which they are activated, and the number of muscle fibers activated. The latter two are directly controlled by the LMN. Each LMN synapses on a specific number of muscle fibers to constitute the motor unit.

Motor units vary in their size, although the definition of "size" is somewhat problematic, but generally relates to the force each motor unit is able to contribute. Small motor units provide fine precise force control, whereas large motor units provide for greater force. This correlates well with the phenomena that distal muscles, such as those that control finger dexterity, primarily comprise small motor units, whereas proximal muscles that have to support the weight of the limb or body, primarily have large motor units. One can appreciate that if large motor units were recruited prematurely in a fine dexterous task, the forces would be abnormal or excessive. This is exactly what is seen in PD (Fig. 13.1).

Muscular forces to generate movement must overcome a number of resistances. First, the muscular forces must overcome the inertia of the limb (inertial loads) to be moved, following Newton's second law of motion, which states that the force necessary to accelerate an object is directly proportional to its mass. As can be

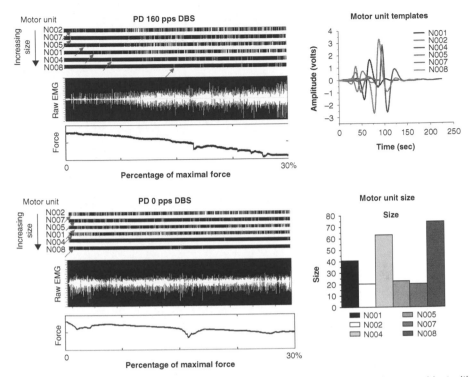

FIGURE 13.1 Example of the EMG recordings from an intramuscular electrode as a subject with PD made a wrist flexion force from rest to 30% of maximum voluntary force under STN DBS at therapeutic frequencies (in this case 160 pps) and 0 pps. The rows show the discharge from 6 individual motor units ordered from smallest (*top*) to largest (*bottom*). The waveforms of the EMG associated with each motor unit and the sizes, measured as the area under the waveform, are shown. As can be seen under therapeutic DBS, the smaller units begin to discharge (indicated by the red arrow) at lower forces compared with larger motor units. As the force is increased, progressively larger motor units are engaged. This is the same as seen in normal subjects. However, under ineffective DBS, the order of recruitment is abnormal. The force tracings show a regular pattern of force production under therapeutic DBS but abnormal force production with excessive early force generation under ineffective DBS. *Abbreviations*: EMG, electromyograph; DBS, deep brain stimulation; PD, Parkinson's disease; STN, subthalamic nucleus; pps, pulses per second.

appreciated, to achieve different velocities of movement different accelerations will be required and consequently, different forces will be required, and thereby requiring different patterns of activations of the LMN. As will be discussed latter, normal individuals dynamically control the velocities of their movements depending on target conditions, which means they engage different patterns of LMN activities. Patients with PD tend to adopt the same velocities irrespective of the target conditions (12,13). Thus, one cause of bradykinesia may be engaging suboptimal patterns of LMN recruitment for the given target conditions. This is very different from the one-dimensional dynamics of the Globus Pallidus Interna Rate, the Action Selection/Focused Attention (1), and the Beta Oscillations theories that result from a dichotomization of the phenomenology of basal ganglia disorders. These theories posit a paucity or excess of movements based on the notion that the basal ganglia acts as a gate to allow intended movement while suppressing undesired movements. In hypokinetic disorders, such as PD, the gait is presumed to be "too closed" and therefore, desired movements are prevented. There is little accounting for how disorders of the basal ganglia would result in suboptimal movements.

Muscular forces also must overcome resistance consequent to stretching the opposing muscles (elastic loads). The elastic loads have passive and active components. The passive elastic loads relate to the elasticity of the joint ligaments, tendons, and muscles that must be stretched. The resistance of the opposing muscle to stretch also can be increased by ongoing active contraction of the opposing muscle. Consider a wrist flexion movement that must start from a position in extension. The extensor muscles must actively contract to hold the wrist in the initial position in extension. With the onset of movement, the extensor muscles, which would oppose (antagonist) the movement, stop contracting (relax) before the wrist flexor muscles (agonist) contract. This is what occurs normally, but in patients with PD the extensor muscles continue to contract requiring greater flexor muscle force to stretch the extensor muscle in order to generate movement and consequently slows movement onset (14).

There is evidence that the rate of build-up to motor unit activity to reach the threshold for movement is slower resulting in the prolonged reaction times seen as bradykinesia in patients with PD. Performing a wrist flexion task to a target is slower in patients with PD compared with normal controls when starting from rest. However, if the patient already is engaged in a wrist flexion movement and receives a signal to move to a further target, the reaction time to initiate this movement is the same as normal controls (15). One interpretation is that the LMN already were activated above the threshold necessary for movement as the wrist flexion movement was already underway. All that was necessary was to further increase the motor unit recruitments and discharge frequencies to continue the movement to the new target.

The slower rate of motor unit recruitment in PD is consistent with the slower rate of recruitment of upper motor neurons in the MC of nonhuman primates rendered parkinsonian using the neurotoxin, 1-methyl-4-phenyl-1, 2, 3, 6-tetrahydropyridine (MPTP) (Fig. 13.2) (16). As discussed later, the appropriate rate of recruitment of upper motor neurons is dependent on resonance within the oscillators of the basal ganglia–thalamic–cortical system.

Given that reaction times for behaviors such as rapid wrist flexion in response to a "go" signal are on the order of 100–200 msec, the initial evolution of motor unit recruitment must be very fast. Thus, the dynamics involved in recruiting motor units are operating on a short time scale. As will be discussed latter, the short time scale dynamics must be associated with similarly rapid dynamics within the basal ganglia–thalamic–cortical system, and therefore engage oscillators with high intrinsic frequencies.

Motor Unit Recruitment Order and Rate of Change

Normally as one generates a progressively increasing muscle force the small motor units are engaged or recruited first. As larger forces are required, increasingly larger motor units are recruited. This order of recruitment from small to progressively larger motor units is called the Henneman Size Principle and has been a fundamental concept of motor control. However, the order of motor unit recruitment is abnormal and even reversed in PD, but normalized with therapeutic high-frequency deep brain stimulation (DBS) supporting the concept that the basal ganglia–thalamic–cortical

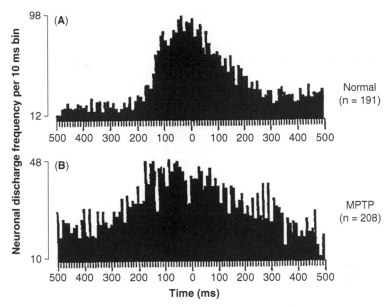

FIGURE 13.2 Time interval histograms of neuronal activities recorded from the motor cortex in two nonhuman primates performing a wrist flexion and extension task. Movement onset occurred at time 0. As can be seen in the recordings in the normal animals, there is a sharp rise in neuronal activity approximately 200 msec before the onset of movement and a rapid fall to a new steady-state at approximately 300 msec after movement onset. Following parkinsonism induced by 1-methyl-4-phenyl-1, 2, 3, 6-tetrahydropyridine, the neuronal activities raise and fall more slowly. The slower rise correlates with the greater time required to generate sufficient force for movement onset. *Source*: Adapted from Ref. 16.

system is important in controlling which motor units, small or large, are recruited for a behavior (Fig. 13.1).

In addition to the time when a motor unit is recruited into activity, the rate at which the activity within a motor unit increases also is important for controlling the time course of the force generated. Normally, small motor units increase their discharge rate faster than large motor units, thereby allowing maintained precision as the force requirements increase. The control of motor unit discharge rate is abnormal in PD causing further imprecision in movements (unpublished observations).

The fact that PD can disrupt and even reverse the motor unit recruitment order argues that each motor unit is under relatively independent control. Thus the suprasegmental oscillators involved in driving the lower motor neuron of a small motor unit are relatively independent of those suprasegmental oscillators that drive the lower motor neuron of the large motor units. The fact that Size Principle of the motor unit recruitment order is ubiquitous in normal conditions argues that there is considerable coordination between these oscillators. However, PD disrupts this coordination.

PARALLEL AND DISTRIBUTED CONTROL OF MOTOR UNIT RECRUITMENT

There is an important conceptual advance here; that is suprasegmental structures, particularly the basal ganglia–thalamic–cortical system, are involved in the most fundamental level of motor control. Clearly, the local biophysical properties of the LMN and local or segmental circuitry is not a sufficient condition for normal motor unit recruitment, otherwise PD would not disrupt normal motor unit recruitment. This means that the function of controlling motor unit recruitment is not localized in the segmental structures but is distributed throughout the networks that connect the basal ganglia–thalamic–cortical–LMN system (and quite probably the cerebellum and brainstem). Furthermore, given the fast time scales involved, this distributed system, for practical purposes, is occurring simultaneously, which means that the different components are acting in a parallel and distributed manner, which is a very different approach than the Globus Pallidus Interna Rate and the Action Selection/Focused Attention theories which, fundamentally, are hierarchical and sequential (1,17).

These observations impose a greater and more complex role for the basal ganglia–thalamic–cortical system, which is to orchestrate the recruitment of different motor units. The complexity of this orchestration is enormous given the range of possible patterns of motor unit recruitment and discharge frequency control. For example, consider the not uncommon experience of lifting an object that appears to be much heavier than it is. The result often is that the object is excessively accelerated resulting in a movement that is difficult to control. Clearly, there are suprasegmental controls that estimate the mass of the object to be lifted and adjust the patterns of motor unit recruitment and discharge frequencies that are the best match. If there is potentially a very large (potentially infinite) number of objects of different masses, then there a very large number (potentially infinite) of control schemes. The question is how can a physically limited brain control for a very large (potentially infinite) number of motor unit control schemes to accommodate a very large (potentially infinite) number of objects? The Systems Oscillators theory posits that a limited number of interconnected reentrant nonlinear oscillators can self-organize into a very large (potentially infinite) number of states or transitions between states to meet the very large number of potential motor unit control schemes that would be necessary for movement.

HIGHER LEVELS OF MOTOR UNIT CONTROL

The concept of motor unit control schemes is seen in Fitt's Law of the speed/accuracy trade off, which states that movements to small or close targets are slower than movements to large or further targets. Thus, there is a specific and reciprocal relationship between the speed of the movement and the accuracy required. The quantitative relationship can be considered as the gain and offset of that relationship. For example, if the movement velocity is doubled when the size of the target is doubled (or halving the accuracy requirement), then the system can be considered as operating with a gain of one. Although the movement speed/accuracy tradeoff of Fitt's Law holds in patients with untreated PD, the gain is abnormal. Thus, the mechanisms, presumably within the basal ganglia–thalamic–cortical system, that organize the suprasegmental mechanisms to control the gain of the movement speed/accuracy relationship are abnormal. Patients with PD can increase the speed of their movements in response to lower accuracy requirements but are slower than normal subjects for the same accuracy requirement (18). The impairment of self-organization within the networks of oscillators within the basal ganglia–thalamic–motor cortical system resulting in abnormal control of the movement speed/accuracy trade off may be a mechanism that produces the bradykinesia of PD.

Modulation of Ongoing Motor Unit Activity

Inertial loads are particularly significant in rapid movements. Not only does the inertia while at rest resist attempts to move the limb, the inertia once the limb is moving, may continue the movement past the target. Consequently, in rapid movements a large initial burst of the agonist muscle occurs to overcome the inertia at rest but then the agonist muscle is rapidly de-recruited (reduced) to lessen the tendency of now increased inertia to move the limb past the target. Indeed, the de-recruitment of the agonist muscle is associated with recruitment of the antagonist muscle to "brake" to slow the movement. Often, the de-recruitment of the agonist muscles and/or the recruitment of the antagonist muscles result in the limb segment failing short of the target (13). In this case, a second agonist muscle recruitment is necessary to bring the limb to the final target. If the final position is past the neutral point, the point where the elastic loads in the opposing directions, such as flexion and extension are balanced, then the agonist muscle recruitment must be maintained to hold the limb at the target. If the movement begins on the opposite side of the neutral position, such as in wrist extension preceding a wrist flexion task, then the muscle antagonistic to the intended movement must be maintained in recruitment so as to hold the limb in the initial position against the elastic loads (Fig. 13.3).

In the scenario described above, there is modulation of the muscle antagonistic to the intended movement that is first a de-recruitment to allow the limb to begin

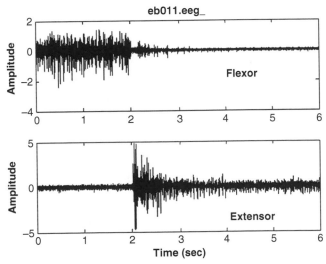

FIGURE 13.3 An example of a variation of the triphasic patterns in a ballistic wrist flexion movement; in this case the isometric analogue in a normal subject. The "go" signal occurred at 2 sec. The variation begins with activity in the flexor muscles to hold the wrist in the initial flexor position. This is followed by relaxation of the flexor and burst in the extensor to accelerate the hand. This is followed by an antagonist (flexor) burst to brake the movement to control the termination to a target that is not limited by mechanical stops. Finally, there is a burst in the extensor to bring the wrist to final position and sustained extensor activity to hold at the target until the subject relaxed at the 3-sec time mark.

to move followed by a recruitment, then, de-recruitment burst to brake the moving inertia so that the limb does not overshoot. For the motor units agonistic to the intended movement, there is an initial recruitment—de-recruitment constituting the initial agonist burst to overcome the inertia at rest. This is followed by recruitment and then maintained recruitment of motor unit activity to bring the limb to the target and hold at the target. These patterns of recruitment and de-recruitment constitute the modulation of motor unit activity and occur at a slower time scale than the activation of the motor units during the individual recruitments. Patients with PD are abnormal in these dynamics. Often the initial and subsequent agonist activations are insufficient to bring the limb to the target. Repeated activations are required which consequently require more time resulting in slowing of the movement and the symptoms and signs of bradykinesia.

Orchestration Among Muscles for Simple Single Joint Rotations

The example above demonstrates another level of dynamics necessary for normal movement. That is the precise relationships between recruitments and de-recruitments of muscle agonistic and antagonistic to the intended movement. In the scenario described above, the initial activity of the muscle antagonistic to the intended movement maintaining the limb in the initial start position normally de-recruits prior to the initial recruitment of muscles agonistic to the intended movement. However, in patients with PD, there is a slower de-recruitment of the muscle antagonistic to the intended movement such that it persists even as the muscles agonistic to the intended movement are recruited and thus, the persistent activity in the antagonist muscle impedes the onset of movement and contributes to the prolonged reaction times and bradykinesia.

The abnormally slow de-recruitment of the motor units antagonistic to the intended movement at the onset of the task is consistent with the slower abnormal de-recruitment of neurons in the MC at the completion of the task in nonhuman primates with MPTP-induced parkinsonism (Fig. 13.2) (16). The Systems Oscillators theory posits that the abnormal persistent activity in the motor cortical neurons reflects the difficulty of the networks of oscillators to self-organize to bifurcate or transition to new states, which may be due to a number of mechanisms such as increased coupling between oscillators or a failure of negative resonance.

Orchestration Among Muscles for Complex Multijoint Rotations

The complexities associated with the control of motor units for a simple single-joint rotation are vastly increased as more complex movements involve more complex rotations around individual joints as well as integration of rotations about multiple joints. The complexity is both spatial, in terms of specific muscles engaged, and temporal, in terms of timing of their engagement. Consider the relatively simple act of grasping a glass and bringing it to one's lips. It is generally not possible, or typical, to make such a movement as a single virtually straight-line trajectory to the lips using a single joint or through a series of independent sequential single-joint rotations. There are simultaneous rotations about the interphalange joints, wrist, supination/pronation of the forearm, rotations about the elbow and shoulder, each with all the complexities associated with the single joint rotations as described above. To be sure, there are physical limitations to the range of complex-joint rotations and there probably are a number of physically possible, although seldom used, sets of joint rotations, but nevertheless the range of sets of relevant complex multijoint rotations are very large if not effectively infinite.

PD affects the patient's ability to orchestrate over large spatially and temporally complex movements that require complex control over complex multijoint rotations (19). One patient stated that he found reaching for his wallet in his back pocket, opening the wallet, reaching for a dollar bill and handing it to the clerk was very difficult. He noted that he had no trouble doing each of these movements independently but it was orchestrating them into a whole and integrated behavior that was most difficult.

Whole Body Orchestration

Limb movements are superimposed on a flexible support frame, that being the trunk and legs, which also must be integrated with the control of limb movements. Consider the scenario where one initially has their arms at their side and then quickly raises the arms extended in front of them. The weight of the arm acting through the lever of the limb produces a torque that tends to rotate the body forward. The body compensates by rotating backward at the hips and/or ankles in order to maintain the center of gravity, which has shifted forward, over the center of support, which is the feet. This trunk rotation is not just a reflex following the shift in the center of gravity, but occurs either just preceding or simultaneous with the actual movement. Thus, the orchestration of motor unit activities occurs throughout the limb as well as the trunk and legs simultaneously (20). Such anticipatory postural adjustments are abnormal in PD (21).

The rapidity of limb movements also has an effect on anticipatory postural adjustments. For rapid limb movements, the inertia of the trunk provides stabilization, and active control by proximal muscles is not needed. However, in slow movements the proximal muscles are activated to provide the stabilizing force.

Integration of Multiple and Independent Dynamics

The time course of the various motor unit recruitments and de-recruitments for the sequence of individual joint rotations and the orchestration of these over multiple joints, operate at larger or slower time scales. The Systems Oscillators theory posits that the longer, hence slower or lower frequencies within the basal ganglia side loops, provides the control of the faster thalamic–motor cortical loop, to modulate the recruitment of individual motor units. Self-organization of the networks of oscillators, through mechanisms such as positive resonance, frequency locking, and/or phase locking among the different oscillators allows for the simultaneous control of multiple motor units across multiple joints (22).

PD affects every dynamic of motor unit control. It affects the initial activations to threshold for movement, the motor unit recruitment order and motor unit discharge frequencies over the early and temporally brief period requiring dynamics on a short time scale. The Systems Oscillators theory relates these rapid dynamics to components of the basal ganglia–thalamic–cortical system that operate at high frequencies, such as the ventrolateral thalamic–motor cortical oscillator. The Systems Oscillators theory posits other oscillators operating at somewhat slower frequencies as primarily related to the temporal dynamics of antagonist and agonist control in single-joint rotations. Similarly, the timing of motor unit activations for various synergistic muscles for more complex multijoint rotations operate over a larger time frame, thereby requiring oscillators of lower frequencies to control these dynamics.

Similarly, other slower time scale dynamics may be involved in the anticipatory postural adjustments. To some degree, the different dynamics are independently controlled in order to allow for the very large (if not infinite) numbers of different movements, but at the same time they are integrated so as to allow coordination.

The integration means that the self-organizations for the different dynamics are occurring simultaneously. Thus, later actions operating over long time scales still influence the early actions operating over shorter time scales. An analogy comes from speech. How a phoneme (roughly equivalent to a syllable) is pronounced is affected by the nature of the phoneme as much as nine phonemes later. Another example of the long time scale dynamics are seen in anticipatory paraphasic errors, such as Spoonerisms, where instead of saying "beef noodle" one says "neef boodle" clearly whatever mechanisms that would be engaged to produce the "n" in "noodles" was operating when the "b" in "beef" was being organized. Analogous studies in typing demonstrate similar typographical errors.

ROLE OF THE BASAL GANGLIA–THALAMIC–CORTICAL SYSTEM IN DYNAMICS OF MOTOR UNIT CONTROL

The physiology of the basal ganglia–thalamic–cortical system is comprised of many reentrant closed loops of differing lengths that result in continuous although shifting oscillations over a wide range of frequencies. These oscillators interact, for example, by having groups of neurons in common between oscillators. These interactions allow for a variety of mechanisms such as frequency and phase interactions and positive and negative resonance [for an introduction to these concepts see Ref. (22)]. Information is contained in the different frequency bands such that the same oscillators can encode multiple functions simultaneously and operate independently but still interact. The self-organizing interactions among these oscillators drive behaviors. PD alters the physiology of these interacting oscillators to produce the symptoms, signs, and disability of the disease.

Evidence of Oscillatory Activity within the Basal Ganglia–Thalamic–Cortical System

Gale, Huang, and Montgomery (23) recorded neuronal activity from 279 neurons in different anatomical structures in three nonhuman primates at rest. A variation of the Schuster periodogram (24) was used to detect oscillatory activity in the neuronal spike train. The periodogram is mathematically equivalent to the Fourier Transform (25,26), but is easier to implement (25,26). The periodogram was applied over a 2-second window that was moved in 0.2 msec steps to demonstrate the frequency content over time.

Figure 13.4 shows a representative periodogram over time for a GPe neuron. As can be seen, the neuronal spike train contains several frequencies over time. Table 13.1 shows the number of neurons recorded in each structure, the mean and standard deviation of the number of frequencies present in the periodogram, and the mean and standard deviation of the frequencies in the periodogram. In a limited study, similar findings were demonstrated in the neuronal spike train of human STN neurons. From these observations, it is clear that the neuronal spike train can entrain multiple oscillations simultaneously. An analogy is a cable television cable can simultaneously carry many channels over a single wire. Thus, activities of electrons within the single wire can simultaneously entrain many separate streams of

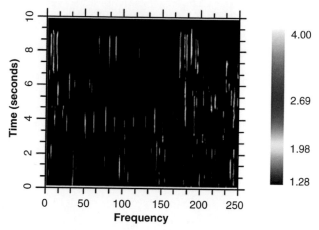

FIGURE 13.4 The appearance and disappearance of operationally defined significant frequencies in the discharge of a neuron recorded in the globus pallidus externa in a nonhuman primate at rest. The circular statistics method is applied repeatedly over 10- to 2-sec windows, which are then moved through time at 0.2-sec increments. The circular statistics method is applied for periods (the inverse of the frequency) corresponding to frequencies from 1 to 250 Hz. The color scale shows the z-scores above the circular statistic for a random control spike train. At every instant of time, multiple frequencies are represented in the neuronal spike train. Further, it appears as though there are different sets of frequencies at different times and that there are shifts between these different sets of frequencies.

information. The Systems Oscillators theory posits that the basal ganglia–thalamic–cortical system is comprised of a large number of loosely coupled nonlinear oscillators. Such systems have been demonstrated mathematically as capable of entraining multiple frequencies simultaneously (27). Computer simulations of interconnected nonlinear oscillators likewise demonstrate that individual neurons can entrain multiple frequencies simultaneously. Indeed, periodograms over time of simulated neurons are indistinguishable for biologic neurons recorded in nonhuman primates and humans. Neurons can occupy nodes that are common to multiple oscillators, either of the same or different frequencies. Because of the nonlinear nature of the neurons and consequently, the neural oscillators (presence of thresholds to discharge and refractory periods) can entrain multiple frequencies simultaneously by having multiple action potentials traversing the oscillator simultaneously.

The multiple simultaneous frequencies are important to simultaneously convey the multiple time scale dynamics necessary for motor unit control in the same output to the LMN. The potential for individual oscillators operating over a limited but different set of frequencies can be appreciated from Inverse Fourier Transforms [for introduction to Fourier and Inverse Fourier Transforms see chap. 14 Oscillator Basics in Ref. (22)]. The idea is that any complex waveform, such as the patterns of motor unit activity over time, can be represented by a series of individual simple oscillations. Thus, the complex waveform is just a weighted sum of the individual oscillators. The key is that all the oscillators representing different time scales interact simultaneously, thus slow oscillators that determine activity later in the movement still have an effect early in the movement, which explains why in speech, later phonemes influence the production of early phonemes.

TABLE 13.1   Frequency Contents of 279 Spectrograms from 3 Nonhuman Primates

	sCtx	mCtx	Cd/Pt	GPe	GPi	STN
Animal M1 and M4						
Number of neurons analyzed	49	25	16	24	15	9
Mean number of frequencies (standard deviation)	114 (18)	102 (31.5)	108 (26.2)	102 (27.2)	92 (34.4)	97 (28.6)
Mean frequency (Hz)	135	135	135	140	136	138
Mean of the standard deviations around the mean of each spectrogram (Hz)	74.9	73.5	74.1	74.9	70.8	73.2
Animal M3						
Number of neurons analyzed	–	48	21	37	20	–
Mean number of frequencies (standard deviation)	–	108 (37)	103 (13)	111.4 (30)	113.4 (28)	–
Mean frequency (Hz)	–	132.9	138.2	140	136	–
Mean of the standard deviations around the mean of each spectrogram (Hz)	–	72.9	74.7	74.4	76.0	–

Note: Only 15 neurons were recorded in animal M4 and all were from the sCtx. Consequently, data from animal M1 and M4 were pooled.
Abbreviations: Cd/Pt, caudate nucleus and putamen; GPe, globus pallidus externa; GPi, globus pallidus interna; mCtx, motor cortex; sCtx, somatosensory cortex; STN, subthalamic nucleus.

This notion of the Inverse Fourier Transform creating complex waveforms appropriate to complex movements has important implications for skill acquisition. Simulations in holographic memory demonstrate that a bank of oscillators representing multiple frequencies can be trained, by affecting the degree of interaction between the oscillators, to reproduce any complex waveform (28–31). Furthermore, if only a fragment of the complex waveform is introduced to the bank of oscillators, the entire waveform can be reproduced. Thus, skill acquisition may involve shaping the interactions between oscillators to produce the desired complex movement. Furthermore, generating the complex movement no longer requires the amount of information used during the training, but only a fragment. This would give the appearance of an "automatic" or habitual movement as distinguished from an intentional or goal-directed movement (6). The former are thought to be affected in PD and may reflect disruption of holographic memory.

Convergence and Divergence Between Oscillator States

The periodograms over time demonstrate clustering in the distributions of frequencies in the neuronal spike train (Fig. 13.3). It appears that the neurons enter one state represented by a specific set of frequencies in the spike train than bifurcate to another set and then return to the initial set of frequencies. Such transitions may be important in the large-scale orchestration of motor units.

Oscillator Mechanism

The Globus Pallidus Interna Rate, Action Selection/Focused Attention, and Beta Oscillation theories are one-dimensional push–pull systems. The former two are explicitly one-dimensional push–pull systems where putative decreases in activity in one structure of the basal ganglia causes an increase in another that subsequently decreases activity in yet another structure. The Beta Oscillations theory is an implicit one-dimensional system where normalcy or parkinsonism is solely a function of the power in the beta frequencies. In some unspecified way the increased beta oscillations interfere with movement.

The Systems Oscillators theory posits a much richer set of dynamics and interactions. Increasing or decreasing neuronal activity can be accomplished by positive or negative resonance as in the other theories. Resonance effects are familiar to anyone who has pushed a child on a swing (Fig. 13.5). The effect of the push depends on the exact timing of the push and the child's motion on the swing. If the person pushes the child just after the child has reached the top of the swing and is starting to head in the opposite direction, the push will have an additive effect or positive resonance. However, if the person pushes while the child is still ascending the push will have a negative effect or negative resonance. Consider the same situation but now the child is moving in a complete circle (Fig. 13.6). The motion has gone from a pendulum motion to a circular or oscillator motion. Nonetheless, the same dynamics related to the pushing still apply. Now imagine the person pushing is on a wheel in rotation (Fig. 13.6). The person's ability to increase or decrease the child's motion depends on the rate of the person's rotation on the wheel (frequency) and position in the rotation (phase) as well as the child's rate of rotation (frequency) and the child's position in the rotation (phase).

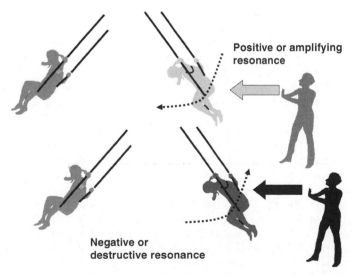

FIGURE 13.5 Example of positive and negative resonance between two periodic functions, one a child swing and the other, a person pushing the child. If the person pushes at the right time, when the child is beginning her descent near the person, the child's swing will be amplified (positive resonance). However, if the person pushes while the child is ascending, the push will work against the swing and reduce the child's swing (negative resonance).

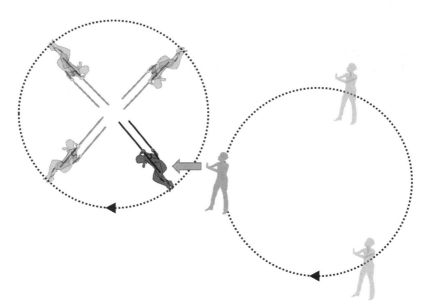

FIGURE 13.6 Consider the extension of the dynamics shown in Figure 13.5 where the child swings completely around and no longer in a pendulum-like fashion. Further, the person pushing the child is on a rotating platform. Again, the most optimal push will be when the person and the child line up just at the child is moving past the person. Thus, the frequencies of the child and the person are important and the phase of each in the rotations for introduction to frequency and phase.

The effects of DBS, which improve the symptoms of PD, cause a frequency-dependent increase in neuronal activities in nuclei of the basal ganglia–thalamic–cortical system. Figure 13.7 shows the time course of neuronal activities following a DBS pulse at time 0. The changes in neuronal activities are measured in z-scores based on the pre-stimulation baseline. For example, a z-score of 1 means that the neuronal activity was 1 standard deviation above the baseline. As can be seen, the patterns of responses were similar across the different frequencies, including 100 and 50 pps, which are considered ineffective. It is the increased magnitude of the response with 130 pps DBS, which is therapeutic, that distinguished between therapeutic and nontherapeutic DBS. Thus, the pattern of responses to DBS of different frequencies is the same, but the magnitude is different and consistent with positive resonance.

The Systems Oscillators theory posits that there is a positive resonance interaction between the high-frequency oscillator in the basal ganglia–thalamic–cortical system, probably the ventrolateral thalamic–motor cortical oscillator, and the high-frequency DBS. The resonance amplification in the ventrolateral thalamic–motor cortical oscillator then drives motor unit recruitment. An example is shown in Figure 13.8. Intramuscular fine-wire electromyographic electrodes were placed in the flexor carpi ulnaris as the patient with PD made a wrist flexion force at 30% of his or her maximum force. Individual motor units were isolated from the recordings before and after onset of 160 pps STN DBS. As can be seen, there is very little motor unit activity before stimulation but much more during DBS. Also, as can be seen there was a progressive build up of activity in addition to the burst of motor unit activity associated with each DBS pulse (Walker, Huang, Guthrie, Watts, and Montgomery unpublished observations).

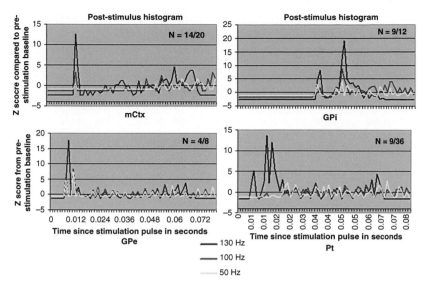

FIGURE 13.7 Graphic representation of the characteristic changes in neuronal activities in various structures of the basal ganglia of nonhuman primates during DBS-like stimulation of the STN. The denominator (following "N") is the number of neurons demonstrating this pattern while the numerator is the total number of neurons studied. As can be seen, the overall pattern of responses are similar across the different stimulation frequencies but the magnitude is greatest with the 130 pps DBS. *Abbreviations*: DBS, deep brain stimulation; mCTX, motor cortex; GPi, globus pallidus interna; GPe, globus pallidus externa; pps, pulses per second; PT, putamen; STN, subthalamic nucleus.

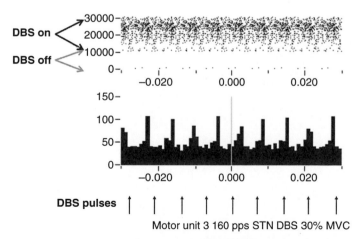

FIGURE 13.8 Activities of a motor unit recording from the flexor carpi ulnaris in a patient with Parkinson's disease performing an isometric wrist flexion force at 30% of her or his maximum before and after the 160 pps STN DBS was turned on. The figure at the top is a raster where each dot represents the discharge of the motor unit. Each row represents the time period between successive DBS pulses. The figure at the bottom is a histogram, which collapses the individual epochs in the raster to better see the trend over time. The time of each DBS pulse is shown relative to the index pulse at time zero. *Abbreviations*: DBS, deep brain stimulation; MVC, Maximum Voluntary Contraction; STN, subthalamic nucleus. *Source*: From Ref. 10.

As can be seen, the increase in motor unit activity over time is typical of resonance effects. The Tacoma Narrows Bridge collapsed because of resonance amplification during a gale. As the winds continued, the bridge began to oscillate with increasing amplitude until it collapsed. Figure 13.9 shows a schematic representation of the possible positive resonance effect in the ventrolateral thalamic–motor cortical oscillator with high frequency DBS. With each successive DBS, greater numbers of neurons are activated within the VL and MC. Similar mechanisms may operate for normal recruitment of muscle activity without DBS and negative resonance may be responsible for de-recruitment.

ANATOMICAL NATURE OF THE BASAL GANGLIA–THALAMIC–CORTICAL OSCILLATORS NETWORK

The Systems Oscillators theory posits that the basal ganglia–thalamic–cortical system is organized into a large number of closed loop reentrant polysynaptic non-linear oscillators (1). Each oscillator contains some number of nodes where each node is some subset of neurons within the specific anatomical structures. A schematic

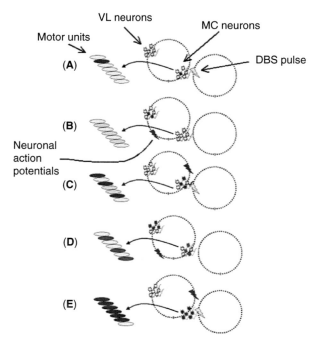

FIGURE 13.9 Schematic representation of positive resonance effects within the VL–MC oscillator in response to STN DBS. As shown in (**A**), the DBS pulse causes activation of MC neurons, presumably by antidromic activation from motor cortical projections to the STN. The MC neuron also causes activations of neurons in VL (**B**) that in turn cause a subsequent increase in neuron activity in MC that occurs and the next DBS pulse activates other MC neurons (**C**). These MC neurons lead to more VL neurons becoming active (**D**) as well as driving more motor units. This process repeats driving more MC neurons and motor units to activity (**E**). *Abbreviations*: DBS, deep brain stimulation; MC, motor cortical; STN, subthalamic nucleus; VL, ventrolateral. *Source*: Adapted from Refs. 41,42.

representation of some of the structures and interconnections are shown in Figure 13.10. This schematic only includes some of the anatomical structures related to the basal ganglia–thalamic–cortical system and excludes, for example, the supplementary motor area, centromedian nucleus of the thalamus, parafascicular nucleus of the thalamus, and pendunculopontine nucleus. However, the limited set of structures and oscillators resulting from the set of structures is used primarily to illustrate the dynamics. The dynamical properties of this subset of oscillators can be applied to any set of oscillators.

Figure 13.10A shows a number of possible oscillators. The figure demonstrates multiple neurons within each node. In this representation, each neuron within all the nodes participates in a separate oscillator. Figure 13.10B shows what has been referred to as the direct pathway by which the cortex (in this case the MC) projects to the PT, which in turn projects to the GPi, which in turn projects to the ventrolateral thalamus (VL) which finally projects back to the cortex, specifically MC. Figure 13.10C shows what has been referred to as the hyperdirect pathway where the cortex projects to the STN which then projects to the GPi, then to the VL and then back to the cortex. Figure 13.10D represents the indirect pathway, which connects the MC to the PT to the GPe to the STN to the GPi to the VL and ultimately back to the MC. These particular pathways are important to the Globus Pallidus Interna Rate theory.

An additional oscillator is the feedback loop between the VL and the MC (Fig. 13.10E). However, one can construct many more oscillators such as seen in Figure 13.10F, which consists of the MC to the PT to the GPe to the STN to the GPi

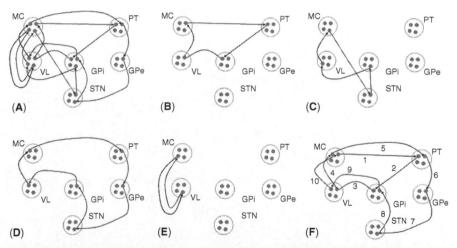

FIGURE 13.10 Schematic of a subset of nuclei in the basal ganglia and the VL and MC that comprise the basal ganglia–thalamic–cortical system. The basal ganglia structures included the PT; GPe; GPi; and STN. (**A**) shows just some of the potential oscillators. (**B**) shows what is referred to as the direct pathway; while **C**, the hyperdirect pathway; and **D**, the indirect pathway. Also shown is the VL–MC oscillator (**E**). (**F**) shows another potential oscillator that is much longer involving at least two "passes" through the basal ganglia–thalamic–cortical system. *Abbreviations*: MC, motor cortex; GPe, globus pallidus externa; GPi, globus pallidus interna; PT, putamen; STN, subthalamic nucleus; VL, ventrolateral thalamus;

to the VL to the MC to the PT (different set of neurons) to the GPi to the VL (different set of neurons) and back to the MC.

The fundamental frequency of each of these oscillators is fixed by the number of nodes and the conduction times and synaptic delays for each of the connections. If one makes the reasonable assumption that information takes approximately 3.5 milliseconds between nodes, then the time it takes to traverse the VL to MC oscillator (Fig. 13.10E) is 7 milliseconds, which corresponds to a fundamental frequency of 143 Hz. The four-node loop would have a fundamental frequency of 71 Hz. A six-node loop (Fig. 13.10D) would have a frequency of 48 Hz. Finally, the very long 10-node loop would have frequency of 29 Hz. Note, because of the nonlinear nature of the neurons in each loop, activities of much higher frequencies are possible within each loop because refractory period, which would limit the maximum frequency is quite small relative to the time it takes for an impulse to traverse the loop (Fig. 13.4 and Table 13.1). The important feature is that all these different frequencies represent the range of oscillators needed to produce the time course of motor unit activations in the manner of holographic memory as described above.

Figure 13.11 shows a hypothetical example of how activities of different frequencies within the basal ganglia–thalamic–cortical system could interact to produce the complex pattern of motor unit activity associated with movement

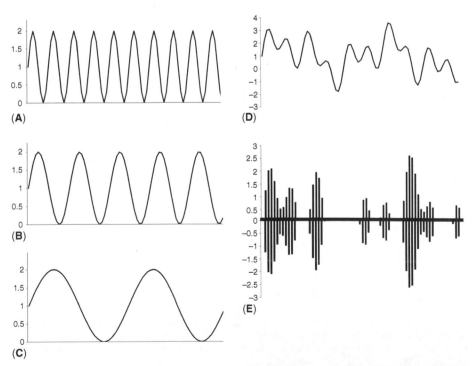

FIGURE 13.11 Hypothetical example of how regular oscillations in three oscillators can combine into a complex waveform and then translated into motor unit activity (see text).

such as shown in Figure 13.3. Figure 13.11A shows activity at 143 Hz within the ventrolateral thalamic–motor cortical oscillator as shown in Figure 13.11E, Figure 13.11B is the 71 Hz oscillator that could reflect the motor cortical–STN–GPi–ventrolateral thalamus–motor cortical oscillator (Fig. 13.11C), whereas Figure 13.11B reflects the long oscillator shown in Figure 13.11F at 29 Hz. Figure 13.11D shows the sum of 143, 71, and 29 Hz, which would reflect the integrated inputs in the ventrolateral thalamus and MC. The complex waveform of the summed oscillations (Fig. 13.11D) can be transformed into a series of motor unit discharges by using the magnitude of the waveform as the relative probability of a motor unit discharge as shown in Figure 13.11E. The appearance of the simulated motor unit activity in Figure 13.11E is very reminiscent of actual motor unit activity as shown in Figure 13.3.

ROLE OF INHIBITION AND POSTINHIBITORY REBOUND EXCITATION

The Systems Oscillators theory posits ongoing oscillations within the various loops within the basal ganglia–thalamic–cortical system. Yet, many of the interconnections are inhibitory so the question is how can oscillations be sustained. The fact of the matter is that inhibition frequently is followed by rebound excitation such that an inhibitory connection actually is delayed excitation (1,32). Indeed, some invertebrate nervous systems are composed entirely if inhibitory interconnections, yet because of postinhibitory rebound excitation, these systems are capable of sustained oscillations (33).

THE GLOBUS PALLIDUS INTERNA RATE THEORY

The Globus Pallidus Interna Rate theory posits that the loss of dopamine input to the striatum (the combination of PT and caudate nucleus) from degeneration of the substantia nigra causes increased activity in the GPi. Because the GPi is inhibitory onto VL neurons, overactivity of the GPi, associated with PD, causes reduction in the ventrolateral thalamic–motor cortical system and consequently, bradykinesia. Loss of dopamine in the PT neurons of the indirect pathway causes decreased inhibition of the PT neurons. As these PT neurons are inhibitory onto the GPe, there is increased inhibition of the GPe neurons. The GPe neurons are inhibitory onto the subthalamic neurons, which increase their activity as a consequence of increased inhibition of the GPe. The increased activity of the STN causes increased activity in the GPi with reduction of activity within the ventrolateral thalamic–motor cortical system as described above.

Similar changes are postulated to occur in the direct pathway. Putamen neurons normally excited by dopaminergic input from the substantia nigra pars compacta, decrease their activity in PD. The decreased PT neuronal activity reduces the inhibition of the GPi with the consequent increased inhibition of the ventrolateral thalamic–motor cortical system.

This theory fails on a number of counts. First, increased neuronal activity in the GPi is not a necessary condition for parkinsonism as several studies have demonstrated parkinsonism in the absence of increased GPi activity (34). Also, several studies have demonstrated no increase in STN neuronal activity in parkinsonism (5). Also, increased STN and GPi activity is not a necessary condition as manipulations that increase STN and GPi neuronal activities are not associated with parkinsonism (32,35–37). As increased activities in the STN and GPi are neither necessary nor sufficient conditions for parkinsonism, those studies demonstrating such changes are describing epiphenomena.

Finally, the Globus Pallidus Interna Rate theory fails as its fundamental tenet that is the GPi inhibits the VL neurons, is not true. Rather, the initial inhibition of the VL neurons by GPi activity is followed by rebound excitation (32).

THE BETA OSCILLATION THEORY

A theory of the pathophysiology of PD is the demonstration of increased activity in the beta frequencies (13–30 Hz), such as local field potentials, in various recordings of neural structures in the basal ganglia (38,39). The precise manner by which increased beta activity causes the types of abnormalities of motor unit recruitment is unknown. However, there is evidence that increased power in the beta frequencies is not a necessary condition as recording of neural activities fail to demonstrate increased beta activity. Furthermore, increased beta activity is not a sufficient condition for parkinsonism reasoning from studies where low-frequency stimulation may improve speech (40) and gait in patients with PD and does not produce parkinsonism in patients with dystonia.

REFERENCES

1. Montgomery EB Jr. Dynamically coupled, high-frequency reentrant, non-linear oscillators embedded in scale-free basal ganglia-thalamic-cortical networks mediating function and deep brain stimulation effects. Nonlinear Stud 2004; 11: 385–421.
2. Guillery RW. Observations of synaptic structures: origins of the Neuron Doctrine and its current status. Philos Trans R Soc Lond B Biol Sci 2005; 360: 1281–307.
3. Sherrington CS. The Integrative Action of the Nervous System. New Haven, CT: Yale University Press, 1920.
4. Binder MC, Heckman CJ, Powers RK. The physiological control of motoneuron activity. Compr Physiol 2011; 3–53.
5. Montgomery EB Jr. Basal ganglia physiology and pathophysiology: a reappraisal. Parkinsonism Relat Disord 2007; 13: 455–65.
6. Redgrave P, Rodriguez M, Smith Y, et al. Goal-directed and habitual control in the basal ganglia: implications for Parkinson's disease. Nat Rev Neurosci 2010; 11: 760–72.
7. Sánchez-Pernaute R, Künig G, del Barrio A, et al. Bradykinesia in early Huntington's disease. Neurology 2000; 54: 119–25.
8. Delval A, Krystkowiak P, Blatt JL, et al. A biomechanical study of gait initiation in Huntington's disease. Gait Posture 2007; 25: 279–88.
9. Nutt JG, Chung KA, Holford NHG. Dyskinesia and the antiparkinson response always temporally coincide: a retrospective study. Neurology 2010; 74: 1191–7.
10. Huang H, Watts RL, Guthrie BL, Walker HC, Montgomery EB. Jr. Role of the basal ganglia in motor unit recruitment: effects of Parkinson's disease (PD) and Deep Brain Stimulation (DBS) of the subthalamic nucleus (STN). International Motoneuron Meeting. Sydney, Australia, 2012.
11. Enoka RM. Morphological features and activation patterns of motor units. J Clin Neurophysiol 1995; 12: 538–59.
12. Montgomery EB Jr, Koller WC, LaMantia TJK, et al. Early detection of probable idiopathic Parkinson's disease: I. Development of a diagnostic test battery. Mov Disord 2000; 15: 467–73.
13. Hallett M, Khoshbin S. A physiological mechanism of bradykinesia. Brain 1980; 103: 301–14.

14. Montgomery EB Jr, Nuessen J, Gorman DS. Reaction time and movement velocity abnormalities in Parkinson's disease under different conditions. Neurology 1991; 41: 1476–81.
15. Montgomery EB Jr, Gorman DS, Nuessen J. Motor initiation versus execution in normal and Parkinson's disease subjects. Neurology 1991; 41: 1469–75.
16. Watts RM, Mandir AS. The role of motor cortex in the pathophysiology of voluntary movement deficits associated with parkinsonism. Neurol Clin 1992; 10: 451–69.
17. Montgomery EB Jr, Buchholz SR. The striatum and motor cortex in motor initiation and execution. Brain Res 1991; 549: 222–9.
18. Montgomery EBJ, Nuessen J. The movement speed/accuracy operator in Parkinson's disease. Neurology 1990; 40: 269–72.
19. Bertram CP, Lemay M, Stelmach GE. The effect of Parkinson's disease on the control of multi-segmental coordination. Brain Cogn 2005; 57: 16–20.
20. Bouisseta S, Zattaraa M. Biomechanical study of the programming of anticipatory postural adjustments associated with voluntary movement J Biomech. 1987; 20: 735–42.
21. Latash ML, Aruin AS, Neyman I, Nicholas JJ. Anticipatory postural adjustments during self inflicted and predictable perturbations in Parkinson's disease. J Neurol Neurosurg Psychiatry 1995; 58: 326–34.
22. Montgomery EB Jr. Deep Brain Stimulation Programming: Principles and Practice. Oxford: Oxford University Press, 2010.
23. Gale JT. Basis of Periodic Activities in the Basal Ganglia -Thalamic-Cortical System of the Rhesus Macaque. Kent: Kent State University, 2004.
24. Schuster A. The periodogram and its optical analogy. Proceedings of the Royal Society of London. 1905. 77: 136–40.
25. Batschelet E. Circular Statistics in Biology. New York: Academic Press, 1981.
26. Takeshita D, Gale JT, Montgomery EB Jr, Bahar S, Moss F. Analyzing spike trains with circular statistics. Am J Phys 2009; 77: 424–9.
27. Hoppensteadt FC, Izhikevich EM. Weakly Connected Neural Networks. In: Marsden JE, Sirovich L, John F, eds. New York: Springer, 1997.
28. Longuet-Higgins HC. Holographic model of temporal recall. Nature 1968; 217: 104.
29. Gabor D. Improved holographic model of temporal recall. Nature 1968; 217: 1288–9.
30. Borsellino A, Poggio T. Holographic aspects of temporal memory and optomotor responses. Kybernetik 1972; 10: 58–60.
31. Yoshioka M, Shiino M. Associative memory storing an extensive number of patterns based on a network of oscillators with distributed natural frequencies in the presence of external white noise. Phys Rev E Stat Phys Plasmas Fluids Relat Interdiscip Topics 2000; 61: 4732–44.
32. Montgomery EB Jr. Effects of GPi stimulation on human thalamic neuronal activity. Clin Neurophysiol 2006; 117: 2691–702.
33. Marder E, Bucher D. Central pattern generators and the control of rhythmic movements. Curr Biol 2001; 11: R986–R96.
34. Wang Z, Jensen A, Baker KB, et al. Neurophysiological changes in the basal ganglia in mild parkinsonism: a study in the non-human primate model of Parkinson's disease. Program No 8289. 2009 Neuroscience Meeting Planner. Chicago, IL: Society for Neuroscience, 2009.
35. Walker HC, Watts RL, Schrandt CJ, et al. Activation of subthalamic neurons by contralateral subthalamic deep brain stimulation in Parkinson Disease. J Neurophysiol 2011; 105: 1112–21.
36. Anderson ME, Postupna N, Ruffo M. Effects of high-frequency stimulation in the internal globus pallidus on the activity of thalamic neurons in the awake monkey. J Neurophysiol 2003; 89: 1150–60.
37. Hashimoto T, Elder CM, Okun MS, Patrick SK, Vitek JL. Stimulation of the subthalamic nucleus changes the firing pattern of pallidal neurons. J Neurosci 2003; 23: 1916–23.
38. Brown P. Bad oscillations in Parkinson's disease. J Neural Transmission 2006: 27–30.

39. Hutchison WD, Dostrovsky JO, Walters JR, et al. Neuronal oscillations in the basal gan-
    glia and movement disorders: evidence from whole animal and human recordings.
    J Neuroscience 2004; 24: 9240–3.
40. Wojtecki L, Timmermann L, Jorgens S, et al. Frequency-dependent reciprocal modula-
    tion of verbal fluency and motor functions in subthalamic deep brain stimulation. Arch
    Neurol 2006; 63: 1273–6.
41. Baker K, Montgomery EB Jr, Rezai AR, Burgess R, Lüders HO. Subthalamic nucleus
    deep brain stimulus evoked potentials: physiology and therapeutic implications. Mov
    Disord 2002; 17: 969–83.
42. Montgomery EB Jr, Gale JT. Mechanisms of action of Deep Brain Stimulation (DBS).
    Neurosci Biobehav Rev 2008; 32: 388–407.

14 Animal models of Parkinson's disease and related disorders

Giselle M. Petzinger and Michael W. Jakowec

INTRODUCTION

Although the cause of Parkinson's disease (PD) remains unknown, in the last several decades the understanding of the role of the environment along with the role of familial and genetic risk factors has contributed to an expansive knowledge base regarding potential mechanisms. Specifically, animal models have contributed to our understanding of PD by allowing researchers to test specific hypothesis generated from these various known contributors of disease. Through the years, animal models have also provided an important and necessary tool for screening and validating new therapeutic modalities. This review highlights the wide spectrum of animal models, generated through chemical or neurotoxin lesioning or genetic manipulation (transgenic rodents, vector targeting), as well as delineating some of their strengths and limitations.

When designing animal models for human neurological disorders, a researcher's goal is to recapitulate many of the primary pathological, neurochemical and behavioral aspects of the disorder. Although this has been achieved for several metabolic disorders, such as diabetes, it can be a challenging objective in the setting of a neurological disorder, such as PD, because it may in fact represent a spectrum of disease with diverse etiology and clinical symptomology. Another challenge for researchers pursuing animal model research in PD is the aspect of aged animals. PD is generally considered a disorder of aging, yet practically speaking there are prohibitory challenges with working in aged animals that include, but are not limited to, costs and availability. A common approach in the research field is to choose an animal model of PD that can address a specific hypothesis regarding a mechanism, or a therapeutic question. Given the wide variety of animal models in PD, this is a useful and realistic approach that has yielded a vast body of knowledge and therapeutics. In essence the utility of an animal model often depends on the specific scientific question. As mentioned, animal models of PD exist in a wide variety of species (i.e., pig, nonhuman primate, rodent, cat, Drosophila, Zebra fish, worms), and are generated using a variety of approaches that include (*i*) pharmacological manipulation; (*ii*) administration of neurotoxicants; (*iii*) genetic manipulations; and (*iv*) surgical lesioning. Although not providing all the answers, these models have yielded significant advancements in our understanding of the underlying mechanisms and treatment of PD and serve as excellent templates for research and drug development.

PD is characterized by bradykinesia, rigidity, postural instability, and resting tremor. The primary pathological and biochemical features of PD are the loss of nigrostriatal dopaminergic neurons in the substantia nigra pars compacta, the appearance of intracellular inclusions called Lewy bodies, and the depletion of striatal dopamine. Clinical features are apparent when striatal dopamine depletion reaches 80%, and when 40% of nigrostriatal dopaminergic neurons have degenerated (1). While other regions of the brain, including nondopaminergic areas, are also affected in PD, the focus of the majority of the animal models is on the primary deficits of the nigrostriatal system and consequent depletion of striatal dopamine. In this chapter, each model, when applicable, is discussed with respect to its development, behavioral profile, biochemical and neuropathological alterations, and contribution to the field. While highlighting some of the more common animal models of PD, this review does not cover surgical lesion-based models, such as that used to investigate basal ganglia circuitry.

PHARMACOLOGICAL/NEUROTOXIN-INDUCED MODELS OF PARKINSON'S DISEASE

Pharmacological/neurotoxin-induced manipulation of the dopaminergic system can take on two basic approaches, that is, either through the selective targeting of dopamine biosynthesis and/or storage, or the loss of nigrostriatal dopaminergic neurons and its respective terminals. Both reserpine and alpha-methyl-para-tyrosine (AMPT) interfere with dopamine production/storage and result in a temporary dopamine depletion lasting hours to days, while neurotoxicants such as 6-hydroxy-dopamine (6-OHDA) and 1-methyl-4-phenyl-1,2,3,6-tetrahydropyridine (MPTP) result in permanent midbrain dopaminergic neuronal cell death. Methamphetamine is a class of compound that selectively destroys axonal terminals of nigrostriatal dopaminergic neurons usually without significant cell death to midbrain dopaminergic neurons. Other compounds, particularly pesticides, such as rotenone and proteasome inhibitors, have been utilized as selective toxins targeting the dopaminergic system since the mitochondria of these cells display enhanced vulnerability during chronic exposure. The utility of compounds to generate animal models of parkinsonism are discussed in the following sections.

Reserpine

In the 1950s, scientists were interested in better understanding catecholamine biosynthesis in the mammalian brain. Arvid Carlsson used reserpine, a catecholamine-depleting agent that blocks vesicular storage of monoamines to deplete dopamine in rabbits (2). Several interesting historical accounts written by Carlsson have been published (3,4). The akinetic state, resulting from reserpine-induced dopamine depletion in the caudate nucleus and putamen, led Carlsson to speculate that PD was due to loss of dopamine neurotransmission. This speculation was supported by the discovery of reduced striatal dopamine in postmortem brain tissue of PD patients and led to the subsequent use of levodopa (in conjunction with a peripheral dopa-decarboxylase inhibitor) for symptomatic treatment of PD (5,6). Thus, the initial observations derived from an animal model led to an important clinical therapy that still remains the "gold standard." Another entertaining account of this historical clinical period can be found in Oliver Sacks' book *Awakenings* and its theatrical version starring Robin Williams.

Alpha-Methyl-Para-Tyrosine

Although less commonly used, AMPT, similar to reserpine, serves as an effective biosynthetic catecholamine-depleting agent (7). By directly inhibiting tyrosine hydroxylase (TH) (the rate-limiting enzyme in dopamine biosynthesis), the nascent synthesis of dopamine in neurons of the substantia nigra pars compacta and ventral tegmental area is prevented.

Both reserpine and AMPT have been used to discover new dopaminomimetics for the treatment of PD, but because their effects are transient (hours to days) these models are primarily useful for acute studies. In addition, neither agent can duplicate the extensive biochemical nor pathological changes seen in PD. Consequently, other models with long-lasting neurochemical and behavioral alterations have been sought using site-specific neurotoxicant injury.

NEUROTOXIN-INDUCED MODELS OF PARKINSON'S DISEASE
6-Hydroxydopmine

6-Hydroxydopamine (6-OHDA or 2,4,5-trihydroxyphenylethylamine) is a specific catecholaminergic neurotoxin structurally analogous to both dopamine and noradrenalin. Acting as a "false-substrate," 6-OHDA is rapidly accumulated in catecholaminergic neurons. The mechanism of 6-OHDA toxicity is complex and involves (*i*) alkylation, (*ii*) rapid auto-oxidization (leading to the generation of hydrogen peroxide, superoxide, and hydroxyl radicals), and (*iii*) impairment of mitochondrial energy production (8,9). The 6-OHDA-induced rat model of PD was initially carried out by Ungerstedt in 1968, using stereotaxic bilateral intracerebral injections into the substantia nigra or lateral hypothalamus (targeting the medial forebrain bundle) (10). An unfortunate limitation of the model was that bilateral administration of 6-OHDA resulted in catalepsy, generalized inactivity, aphagia, adipsia, and a high degree of animal morbidity and mortality. Consequently, the administration of 6-OHDA was modified to a unilateral intracerebral lesion (targeting the substantia nigra and/or medial forebrain bundle). A unilateral lesioning approach led to a model characterized by (*i*) minimal postoperative morbidity, (*ii*) behavioral asymmetry, and (*iii*) a nonlesioned side to serve as a control (11,12). An additional modification of 6-OHDA delivery was the development of a chronic low-dose striatal injection approach. This approach was demonstrated to lead to progressive dopaminergic cell death and to more closely resemble the human condition (13). Thus, an important caveat of 6-OHDA-lesioning to consider when examining intervention or therapeutic strategies in this model is the prolonged time course of cell death, which may be on the order of one to three weeks (13,14).

A distinctive behavioral feature of the unilateral lesioned model is rotation (15,16). This motor feature is due to asymmetry in dopaminergic neurotransmission between the lesioned and intact sides. Specifically, animals rotate away from the side of greater dopaminergic activity. Nomenclature describes the direction of rotation as either ipsilateral (toward) or contralateral (away) with respect to the lesioned side. Initial reports of rotation examined both spontaneous and pharmacologically induced rotation. Spontaneous rotation consists of ipsilateral rotation (toward the lesioned side), whereas pharmacologically induced rotation may be either contra- or ipsilateral rotation. For example, apomorphine and other dopamine agonists induce contralateral rotation (away from the lesioned side). This is due to their direct action on supersensitized dopaminergic receptors on the lesioned side. Conversely, D-amphetamine phenylisopropylamine (AMPH) induces ipsilateral rotation by blocking dopamine re-uptake and increasing dopamine receptor activity on the nonlesioned side. In general, a greater than 80% depletion of dopamine is necessary to manifest rotation in this model (7,17). Circling behavior can be measured either by observation or by special devices called rotameters. The rate of rotation correlates with the severity of the lesion, and animals with more extensive striatal dopamine depletions are less likely to show behavioral recovery. This simple model of rotation away from the side with the most dopamine receptor occupancy has proved to be more complex and less predictable than previously thought, especially in the context of various pharmacological treatments and neuronal transplantation (18,19). In addition to rotation other behavioral assessments in the 6-OHDA model may include tests of (*i*) forelimb use, (*ii*) bilateral tactile stimulation, and (*iii*) single-limb akinesia [for review see Ref. (20)]. A study on the behavioral and electromyographic analysis of the 6-OHDA-lesioned rat demonstrated extensive gait impairment, including alterations in limb movement and use, as well as evidence of myoclonus (21).

The 6-OHDA-lesioned rat model has proved to be a valuable tool in evaluating (*i*) the pharmacological action of new drugs on the dopaminergic system, (*ii*) the mechanisms of motor complications, (*iii*) the neuroplasticity of the basal ganglia in response to nigrostriatal injury, and (*iv*) the safety and efficacy of neuronal transplantation in PD. Extensive pharmacological studies have utilized the 6-OHDA-lesioned rat to investigate the role of various dopamine receptor (D1–D5) agonists and antagonists, and other neurotransmitter systems (including glutamate, adenosine, nicotine, or opioids) on modulating dopamine neurotransmission. These studies elucidate the role of these compounds on electrophysiological, behavioral, and molecular (signal transduction) properties of the basal ganglia. A review of this vast amount of pharmacological literature in this model is beyond the scope of this chapter (16).

The 6-OHDA-lesioned rat model has also been an important tool in elucidating the mechanism(s) underlying motor complications, including wearing off phenomenon and dyskinesia (22,23). The chronic administration of levodopa (over a period of weeks) in the 6-OHDA rat has been demonstrated to lead to a shortening response similar to the wearing off complication in idiopathic PD, as well as to choreiform and dystonic movements observed with long-term levodopa use in humans (24). This altered motor response occurs when greater than 95% of nigrostriatal dopaminergic neurons are lost. Studies using glutamate antagonists have demonstrated improvement in the wearing off response and dyskinesia and have implicated the role of glutamate receptor subtypes in the development of motor complications (25–27). These findings have been supported by molecular studies that demonstrate alterations in the phosphorylation state of glutamate receptor subunits of the NMDA subtype (28). Unlike the nonhuman primate model, 6-OHDA-lesioned rats do not typically develop severe limb and truncal dyskinesia as seen in PD but rather a form localized primarily to the jaw (23,29).

In the context of neuroplasticity, the 6-OHDA-lesioned rat model demonstrates behavioral recovery and has been instrumental in characterizing the neurochemical, molecular, and morphological alterations related to compensatory mechanisms within the basal ganglia and its circuitry in response to nigrostriatal dopamine depletion (30). These mechanisms of neuroplasticity in surviving dopaminergic neurons and their striatal terminals include (*i*) increased turnover of dopamine and its metabolites, (*ii*) alterations in the expression of TH, the rate-limiting step in dopamine biosynthesis, (*iii*) decreased dopamine uptake through altered dopamine transporter expression, (*iv*) alterations in the electrophysiological phenotype (both pattern and rate of neuronal firing) of striatal and substantia nigra neurons, and (*v*) sprouting of new striatal dopaminergic terminals. These molecular mechanisms may provide new targets for novel therapeutic interventions, such as growth factors, to enhance the function of surviving dopaminergic neurons and their targets.

The 6-OHDA-lesioned rat model has also been useful for determining important parameters for successful transplantation. These parameters include (*i*) target site (striatum versus substantia nigra); (*ii*) volume of innervation at the target site; (*iii*) number of cells transplanted; (*iv*) type and species of cells transplanted, including fetal mesencephalon, engineered cell lines, and stem cells; (*v*) age of host and donor tissues; (*vi*) pretreatment of transplant tissue or host with neurotrophic factors, antioxidants, immunosuppressive therapy, or neuroprotective pharmacological agents; and (*vii*) surgical techniques, including needle design, cell suspension media, and transplant cell delivery methods (31,32). The near absence of dopaminergic neurons and terminals within the striatum due to 6-OHDA lesioning provides a template for the assessment of sprouting axons and terminals originating from the transplant. Measures of transplant success in this model include reduction in the rotational behavior and the survival, sprouting, and innervation (synapse formation) of dopaminergic fibers within the denervated striatum. The reduction of rotational behavior suggests increased striatal dopamine production originating from the transplanted tissue. Interestingly, not all behavioral measures appear to respond to transplant. The advancements made in the 6-OHDA-lesioned rat provide a framework for the further testing of transplantation in nonhuman primates and future human clinical trials.

Although the 6-OHDA-lesioned rat model has many advantages, it serves primarily as a model of dopamine dysfunction. Lesioning with 6-OHDA is highly specific for catecholaminergic neurons and does not replicate all of the behavioral, neurochemical, and pathological features of human PD. For example, the 6-OHDA-lesioned rat does not manifest alterations in the cholinergic and serotonergic neurotransmitter systems, which are commonly affected in PD. Stereotaxic injections of 6-OHDA to precise targets does not replicate the extensive pathology of PD where other anatomical regions of the brain (including the locus coeruleus, nucleus basalis of Meynert, and raphe nuclei) are affected. In addition, Lewy body formation, a pathological hallmark of PD, has not been reported in this model. Interestingly, a report using a regimen of chronic administration of 6-OHDA into the third ventricle did show a more extensive lesioning pattern reminiscent of human PD (33). In addition to the rat, other species including the nonhuman primate (specifically the marmoset) have served as models for 6-OHDA lesioning (34,35). Lesioning in nonhuman primates provides for the analysis of behaviors not observed in the rat, such as targeting and retrieval tasks of the arm and hand. In addition, lesioning in the nematode *Caenorhabditis elegans* provides a potential genetic tool to investigate mechanisms involved in cell death with this toxin and to provide large-scale screenings (36,37).

Overall, lesioning with 6-OHDA has provided a rich source of information regarding the consequences of precise dopamine depletion and its effects on rotational behavior, dopamine biosynthesis, biochemical and morphological aspects of recovery, and serves as an excellent template to study both pharmacological and transplantation treatment modalities for PD. While the vast majority of studies utilizing 6-OHDA have been in the rat owing to its larger size for anatomical targeting, the 6-OHDA mouse has re-emerged as a legitimate model. Improved stereotactic targeting, behavioral analysis, and the emergence of scientific questions that can be specifically addressed in unique transgenic mouse models have supported the utility of the 6-OHDA mouse in the PD research field including the onset of levodopa-induced dyskinesia (38–41).

1-Methyl-4-Phenyl-1,2,3,6-Tetrahydropyridine

The inadvertent self-administration of MPTP by heroin addicts in the early 1980s induced an acute form of parkinsonism with clinical and biochemical features indistinguishable from idiopathic PD (42,43). Similar to PD, this MPTP cohort demonstrated an excellent response to levodopa and dopamine agonist treatment but developed motor complications within a short period of time (over weeks). The rapidity with which these motor complications appeared reflected the severity of substantia nigra pars compacta neuronal degeneration induced by MPTP. Given the clinical similarities between the human model of MPTP-induced parkinsonism and PD, MPTP was quickly administered to nonhuman primates and mice to evaluate its efficacy for generating an animal model of PD.

The subsequent administration of MPTP to a wide range of animal species demonstrates a spectrum of sensitivity to its toxic effects. These differences were shown to be species, strain, and age dependent. For example, the nonhuman primate is exquisitely sensitive to the toxic effects of MPTP. The mouse, cat, dog, and guinea pig are less sensitive and the rat is the least sensitive, displaying near resistance. Even within species there are strain differences. For example, the C57BL/6 mouse is the most sensitive of all mouse strains tested, whereas strains such as CD-1 appear almost resistant (44,45). Some differences among strains may also be supplier dependent as seen with variability in the Swiss Webster strain (46). In addition to strain type, sensitivity may be influenced by the animal's age with old mice being more sensitive than young mice (47,48). Studies suggest that age-dependent differences may be due to differences in MPTP metabolism (49). To bypass potential confounders involved in MPTP delivery to the brain and its conversion to the MPP^+ toxin form some investigators have utilized stereotaxic delivery via cannulae into the striatum (50). Similar to 6-OHDA lesioning this approach still has technical issues regarding targeting and diffusion, and has yet to be tested in a wide range of species.

The mechanism of MPTP toxicity has been thoroughly investigated. The meperidine analog MPTP is converted to 1-methyl-4-pyridinium (MPP^+) by monoamine oxidase B. MPP^+ acts as a substrate of the dopamine transporter (DAT) leading to the inhibition of mitochondrial complex I, the depletion of ATP, and cell death of dopaminergic neurons. MPTP administration to mice and nonhuman primates selectively destroys dopaminergic neurons of the substantia nigra pars compacta (SNpc), the same neurons affected in PD (51). Similar to PD other catecholaminergic neurons, such as those in the ventral tegmental area and locus coeruleus, may be affected to a lesser degree. In addition, dopamine depletion occurs in both the putamen and the caudate nucleus. The preferential lesioning of either the putamen or the caudate nucleus may depend on animal species and regimen of MPTP administration (52–54). Unlike PD, Lewy bodies have not been reported, however, eosinophilic inclusions (reminiscent of Lewy bodies) have been described in aged nonhuman primates (55). The time course of MPTP-induced neurodegeneration is rapid, and therefore represents a major difference with idiopathic PD, which is a chronic progressive disease. Interestingly, data from humans exposed to MPTP indicate that the toxic effects of MPTP may be more protracted than initially believed (56). Details of MPTP toxicity, safety, and utility are described in several excellent reviews (57).

The MPTP-Lesioned Mouse Model

The administration of MPTP to mice results in behavioral alterations that may resemble human parkinsonism. For example, hypokinesia, bradykinesia, and akinesia can be observed through various behavioral analyses including open field activity monitoring, swim test, pole test, inverted grip, and rotarod. Whole body tremor and postural abnormalities have also been reported but primarily in the acute phase (58). Cognitive changes have been reported with respect to spatial learning (59). In general these behavioral alterations tend to be highly variable with some mice showing severe deficits while others show little or no behavioral change [for review see Ref. (58). This behavioral variability may be due to a number of factors, including the degree of lesioning, mouse strain, time course after lesioning, and the reliability and validity of the behavioral analysis (60–64).

The MPTP-lesioned mouse model has proved to be valuable to investigate potential mechanisms of neurotoxic-induced dopaminergic cell death. For example, mechanisms under investigation have included mitochondrial dysfunction, energy (ATP) depletion, free-radical production, apoptosis, and glutamate excitotoxicity (65–70). In addition to its utility in studying acute cell death, the MPTP-lesioned model also provides an opportunity to study injury-induced neuroplasticity. The MPTP-lesioned mouse displays the return of striatal dopamine several weeks to months after lesioning (52,54,71,72). The molecular mechanism of this neuroplasticity of the injured basal ganglia is an area of investigation, and appears to encompass both neurochemical and morphological components. In addition, this plasticity may be facilitated through activity-dependent processes using treadmill training (73,74).

MPTP-Lesioned Nonhuman Primate

Administration of MPTP to nonhuman primates results in parkinsonian symptoms, including bradykinesia, postural instability, and rigidity. In some species resting or action/postural tremor has been observed (75). The nonhuman primate model is one of the most extensively used research models in PD for examining novel pharmacological treatments, transplantation, mechanisms of motor complications, deep brain stimulation, behavioral recovery, cognitive impairment, and the development of novel neuroprotective and restorative therapies. The strongest asset of this model is its close behavioral and anatomical proximity to the human condition. Similar to PD, the MPTP-lesioned nonhuman primate responds to traditional antiparkinsonian therapies, such as levodopa and dopamine receptor agonists. After the administration of MPTP, the nonhuman primate progresses through acute (hours), subacute (days), and chronic (weeks) behavioral phases of toxicity that are due to the peripheral and central effects of MPTP. The acute phase is characterized by sedation, and a hyperadrenergic state, the subacute phase by the development of varying degrees of parkinsonian features, and the chronic phase by initial recovery (by some, but not all animals) followed by the stabilization of motor deficits (76). In general the behavioral response to MPTP lesioning may vary at both the inter- and intraspecies levels. Variability may be due to age and species phylogeny. For example, older animals and Old World monkeys (such as rhesus, *Macaca mulatta or*

African Green, *Cercopithecus aethiops*) tend to be more sensitive than young and New World monkeys (such as the squirrel monkey, *Saimiri sciureus* or marmoset, *Callithrix jacchus*) (77–79).

Behavioral recovery after MPTP-induced parkinsonism has been reported in most species of nonhuman primate. The degree and time course of behavioral recovery is dependent on age, species, and mode of MPTP administration (76). In general the more severely affected animal is less likely to recover (75). The molecular mechanisms underlying behavioral recovery of the nonhuman primate is a major focus of our laboratory. Results of our work and others have identified that the mechanisms underlying recovery may include (*i*) alterations in dopamine biosynthesis (increased TH protein and mRNA expression) and turnover; (*ii*) downregulation of DAT; (*iii*) increased dopamine metabolism; (*iv*) sprouting and branching of TH fibers; (*iv*) alterations of other neurotransmitter systems, including glutamate and serotonin; and (*v*) alterations of signal transduction pathways in both the direct (D1) and indirect (D2) pathways (80,81).

The administration of MPTP through a number of different dosing regimens has led to the development of several distinct models of parkinsonism in the nonhuman primate, which are characterized by distinct behavioral and neurochemical parameters as well as unique advantages and limitations. For example, in some models there is profound striatal dopamine depletion and denervation with little or no dopaminergic axons or terminals remaining. This model provides an optimal setting to test fetal tissue grafting since the presence of any TH positive axons or sprouting cells would be due to transplanted tissue survival. Other models have less extensive dopamine depletion and only partial denervation with a modest-to-moderate degree of dopaminergic axons and terminals remaining. This partially denervated model best resembles mild to moderately affected PD patients. Therefore, sufficient dopaminergic neurons and axons as well as compensatory mechanisms are likely to be present. The effects of growth factors (inducing sprouting) or neuroprotective factors (promoting cell survival) are best evaluated in this situation. The following section reviews the most commonly used MPTP-lesioned nonhuman primate models.

In the *systemic lesioned* model, MPTP may be administered via intramuscular, intravenous, intraperitoneal, or subcutaneous injection (82–85). This leads to bilateral depletion of striatal dopamine and nigrostriatal cell death. A feature of this model is that the degree of lesioning can be titrated resulting in a range (mild to severe) of parkinsonian symptoms. The presence of clinical asymmetry is common with one side more severely affected. Levodopa administration leads to the reversal of all behavioral signs of parkinsonism in a dose-dependent fashion. After several days to weeks of levodopa administration, animals develop reproducible motor complications, both wearing-off and dyskinesia. Animal behavior in this model and others may be assessed using (*i*) cage-side or video-based observation; (*ii*) automated activity measurements in the cage through infrared-based motion detectors or accelerometers; and (*iii*) examination of hand reaching movements tasks. The principal advantage of this model is that the behavioral syndrome closely resembles the clinical features of idiopathic PD. The systemic model has partial dopaminergic denervation bilaterally and probably best represents the degree of loss seen in all stages of PD including the end-stage disease where some dopaminergic neurons are still present. This model is well suited for therapeutics that interact with remaining dopaminergic neurons including growth factors, neuroprotective agents, and dopamine modulation. The easily reproducible dyskinesia in this model allows for extensive investigation of its underlying mechanism and treatment. Disadvantages of this model include spontaneous recovery in mildly affected animals. Alternatively, bilaterally severely affected animals may require extensive veterinary care and dopamine supplementation.

Administration of MPTP via unilateral intracarotid infusion has been used to induce a hemiparkinsonian state in the primate, called the *hemiparkinsonian* model (86). The rapid metabolism of MPTP to MPP+ in the brain may account for the localized toxicity to the hemisphere ipsilateral to the infusion. Motor impairments appear primarily on the contralateral side. Hemi-neglect, manifested by a delayed motor reaction time, also develops on the contralateral side. In addition, spontaneous ipsilateral rotation may develop. Levodopa administration reverses the parkinsonian symptoms and induces contralateral rotation. Substantia nigra neurodegeneration and striatal dopamine depletion (greater than 99%) on the ipsilateral side to the injection is more extensive than seen in the systemic model. The degree of unilateral lesioning in this model is dose dependent.

Major advantages of the *hemi-lesioned* model include: (*i*) the ability for animals to feed and maintain themselves without supportive care, (*ii*) the availability of the unaffected limb on the ipsilateral side to serve as a control, and (*iii*) the utility of the dopamine-induced rotation for pharmacological testing. In addition, due to the absence of dopaminergic innervation in the striatum, *the hemi-lesioned* model is well suited for examining neuronal sprouting of transplanted tissue. A disadvantage of this model is that only a subset of parkinsonian features are evident and are restricted to one side of the body, a situation never seen in idiopathic PD.

The *bilateral intracarotid* model employs an intracarotid injection of MPTP followed several months later by another intracarotid injection on the opposite side (87). This model combines the less debilitating features of the carotid model as well as creating bilateral clinical features, a situation more closely resembling idiopathic PD. The advantage of this model is its prolonged stability and limited interanimal variability. Similar to the hemi-lesioned model, where there is extensive striatal dopamine depletion and denervation, the bilateral intracarotid model is well suited for evaluation of transplanted tissue. However, levodopa administration may result in only partial improvement of parkinsonian motor features and food retrieval tasks. This can be a disadvantage since high doses of test drug may be needed to demonstrate efficacy, increasing the risk for medication-related adverse effects.

A novel approach to MPTP lesioning is the administration of MPTP via intracarotid infusion followed by a systemic injection. This *overlesioned* model is characterized by severe dopamine depletion ipsilateral to the MPTP–carotid infusion and a partial depletion on the contralateral side due to the systemic MPTP injection. Consequently, animals are still able to maintain themselves due to a relatively intact side. The behavioral deficits consist of asymmetric parkinsonian features. The more severely affected side is contralateral to the intracarotid injection (88). Levodopa produces a dose-dependent improvement in behavioral features, however, the complications of levodopa therapy such as dyskinesia have not been as consistently observed. This model combines some of the advantages of both the systemic and intracarotid MPTP models including stability. This model is suitable for both transplant studies, utilizing the more depleted side, and neuro-regeneration with growth factors, utilizing the partially depleted side where dopaminergic neurons still remain.

Finally, the *chronic low-dose* model consists of intravenous injections of a low dose of MPTP administration over a 5- to 13-month period (89). This model is characterized by cognitive deficits consistent with frontal lobe dysfunction reminiscent of PD or normal-aged monkeys. These animals have impaired attention and short-term memory processes and perform poorly in tasks of delayed response or delayed alternation. Since gross parkinsonian motor symptoms are essentially absent at least in early stages, this model is well adapted for studying cognitive deficits analogous to those that accompany idiopathic PD.

The MPTP-lesioned nonhuman primate has provided a valuable tool for investigating potential mechanisms underlying motor complications related to long-term levodopa use in human idiopathic PD. The MPTP-lesioned nonhuman primate has been shown to demonstrate both wearing-off and dyskinesia. Although the etiology of dyskinesia is unknown, electrophysiological, neurochemical, molecular, and neuroimaging studies in the nonhuman primate models suggest that the pulsatile delivery of levodopa may lead to (i) changes in the neuronal firing rate and pattern of the globus pallidus and subthalamic nucleus, (ii) enhancement of D1- and/or D2-receptor–mediated signal transduction pathways, (iii) supersensitivity of the D2 receptor, (iv) alterations in the phosphorylation state and subcellular localization of glutamate (NMDA subtype) receptors, (v) modifications in the functional links between dopamine receptor subtypes (D1 and D2, and D1 and D3), (vi) changes in glutamate receptors (AMPA and NMDA receptor subtypes), and (vii) enhancement of opioid-peptide–mediated neurotransmission (90–94).

While the presence of a nigral lesion has long been considered an important prerequisite for the development of dyskinesia in the MPTP model, studies demonstrate that even normal nonlesioned nonhuman primates when given sufficiently large doses of levodopa (with a peripheral decarboxylase inhibitor) over two to eight weeks may develop peak-dose dyskinesia (95). The high levels of plasma levodopa in this dosing regimen may serve to exhaust the buffering capacity within the striatum of the normal animal and therefore lead to pulsatile delivery of levodopa and priming of postsynaptic dopaminergic sites for dyskinesia.

In addition to its central effects, the administration of MPTP may lead to systemic effects, which may prove detrimental to any animal during the induction of a parkinsonian state. For example, the peripheral conversion of MPTP to MPP+ in the liver could lead to toxic injury of the liver and heart. To address these potential peripheral effects of MPTP, squirrel monkeys were administered MPTP (a series of six subcutaneous injections of 2 mg/kg, free-base, two weeks apart) and were given a comprehensive exam 1, 4, and 10 days after each injection. This exam included measurements of body weight, core body temperature, heart rate, blood pressure, liver and kidney function, and white blood cell count. Biochemical markers of hepatocellular toxicity were evident within days of MPTP lesioning and persisted for several weeks after the last injection. In addition, animals had significant hypothermia within 48 hours after lesioning that persisted for up to 10 days after the last MPTP injection (Petzinger et al., Manuscript in preparation). The pathophysiology of these effects may be directly related to MPTP itself and/or its metabolites. The systemic effects of MPTP on animal models should be taken into consideration during the design of any pharmacological study.

MPTP Lesioning in Other Species
Although mice and nonhuman primates continue to remain the primary species in the majority of studies with MPTP, researchers have reported the effects of MPTP in a wide range of other species. These include the leech (*Hirudo medicinakis*),

planarian flatworm (*Dugesia japonica*), rainbow trout (*Oncorhynchus mykiss*), goldfish (*Carassius auratus*), zebrafish (*Brachydanio rerio*), frog (*Rana pipiens* and *R. clamitans*), salamander (*Taricha torosa*), snake (*Elaphe obsolete* and *Nerodia fasciata*), lizard (*Anolis carolinensis*), chicken (*Gallus gallus*), rat (*Rattus rattus* and *R. norvegicus*), guinea pig (*Cavia porcellus*), rabbit (*Oryctolagus cuniculus*), dog (*Canis familiaris*), and pig (*Susscrofa domestica*). Some of these species may have some advantages, such as the zebra fish where powerful genetic tools involved in large scale screening can be applied (96). Despite the novel application of MPTP to these species there are limitations that restrict their popularity including animal availability, biosafety exposure and disposal, genetic background, and standardization of lesioning regimen and its efficacy.

METHAMPHETAMINE

Amphetamine and its derivatives [including methamphetamine (METH)] causes long-lasting depletion of both dopamine and serotonin when administered to rodents and nonhuman primates (97,98). METH, one of the most potent of these derivatives, causes terminal degeneration of dopaminergic neurons in the caudate–putamen, nucleus accumbens, and neocortex. In contrast to MPTP, the axonal trunks and soma of SNpc and VTA neurons are spared (99). However, there have been occasional reports of METH-induced cell death in the substantia nigra (100). In general the effects of severe METH lesioning are long lasting. There is evidence of recovery of dopaminergic innervation depending on the METH regimen and species used (101). Despite the severe depletion of striatal dopamine, the motor behavioral alterations seen in rodents and nonhuman primates are subtle (102).

The neurotoxic effects of METH are dependent on the efflux of dopamine since agents that deplete dopamine or block its uptake are neuroprotective (103,104). The metabolic mechanisms underlying METH-induced neurotoxicity involve the perturbation of antioxidant enzymes, such as glutathione peroxidase or catalase, leading to the formation of reactive oxygen/nitrogen species, including H_2O_2, superoxide, and hydroxyl radicals (105–109). The administration of antioxidant therapies or over-expression of superoxide dismutase (SOD) in transgenic mice models is neuroprotective against METH toxicity (110,111). In addition, both glutamate receptors and nitric oxide synthase (NOS) are important to METH-induced neurotoxicity since the administration of either NMDA receptor antagonists or NOS inhibitors are also neuroprotective (112). Other factors important to METH-induced neurotoxicity include the inhibition of both TH and DAT activity and METH induced hyperthermia (108).

The administration of METH to adult animals has played an important role in testing the molecular and biochemical mechanisms underlying dopaminergic and serotonergic neuronal axonal degeneration especially the role of free radicals and glutamate neurotransmission. Understanding these mechanisms has led to testing different neuroprotective therapeutic modalities. An advantage of the METH model over MPTP is that the serotonergic and dopaminergic systems can be lesioned *in utero* during the early stages of the development of these neurotransmitter systems. Such studies have indicated that there is a tremendous degree of architectural rearrangement that occurs within the dopaminergic and serotonergic systems of injured animals as they develop. These changes may lead to altered behavior in the adult animal (113).

In light of the toxic nature of these compounds in animals, studies in humans have suggested that abusers of METH and substituted amphetamines (including MDMA "ecstasy") may suffer from the long-lasting effects of these drugs (114,115). Specifically these individuals may be prone to develop parkinsonism (116).

ROTENONE

Epidemiological studies have suggested that environmental factors such as pesticides may increase the risk for PD (117,118). The demonstration of specific neurochemical and pathological damage to dopaminergic neurons by the application of various pesticides such as rotenone (an inhibitor of mitochondrial complex I due to impaired oxidative phosphorylation through inhibition of NADH-ubiquitin reductase), have been consistent with these epidemiological findings. For example, using a chronic rotenone infusion paradigm (2 or 3 mg/kg/day for three weeks) through either jugular vein cannulation or systemic delivery with an osmotic pump, Greenamyre and colleagues reported degeneration of a subset of nigrostriatal dopaminergic neurons, the formation of cytoplasmic inclusions, and the development of parkinsonian motor behavior (including hunched posture, rigidity, unsteady movement, and paw tremor) in the rat (119,120). Researchers have used a number of different delivery modalities to evaluate the effects of rotenone on features overlapping with those seen in PD (120–123). Limitations to the rotenone model include (*i*) long administration period of weeks to months, (*ii*) variability due to dose, (*iii*) low animal survival, (*iv*) variable pathological outcomes and specificity, and (*v*) species and strain differences (122,124–130). Despite these potential confounders this model provides valuable insight into one potential mechanism relevant to the etiology of parkinsonism (131). Studies examining the different parameters of this and other pesticides in animal models may lead to insights into the mechanisms of neuronal death in PD (132–134).

PARAQUAT

Paraquat (*N, N'*-dimethyl-4, 4'bipyridium dichloride) is a pesticide analog of MPP+ and etiologically linked to parkinsonism through epidemiological studies (132,135,136). Paraquat acts to induce oxidative stress by interfering with mitochondria electron transport, especially in the more vulnerable nigrostriatal dopaminergic neurons with a mechanism different from rotenone and MPP+ (137–139). Acute exposure can result in extensive brain damage and death in humans without specific parkinsonian-like pathology (140,141). However, more chronic exposures in rodents (over 24 weeks) can manifest with many features due to dopaminergic dysfunction including selective loss of nigrostriatal dopaminergic neurons and motor deficits (142,143). Therefore, paraquat, as well as a number of other related reagents, including other pesticides, may replicate features of human parkinsonism when administered in chronic but not acute delivery regimens most likely due to specific uptake and poisoning of nigrostriatal dopaminergic neurons. Paraquat-induced models have similar limitations as rotenone models but due to issues of specificity and technical issues, this model has not achieved wide usage beyond studies in cell culture and limited animal studies. However, studies are beginning to examine the effects of paraquat and other pesticides on dopamine systems including those of Drosophila and other lower animals (144–148). Recent identification of familial forms of PD and their genes has promoted studies examining the effects of paraquat and pesticides as potential risk factors in the context of genetic background, including DJ-1, α-synuclein, and parkin (149–152).

PROTEASOME INHIBITORS

An important regulatory system within cells is the ubiquitin proteasome system (UPS), a large enzymatic complex involved in detoxification and degradation of ubiquitin-tagged proteins (153,154). Inhibition of the UPS can lead to the inability to remove toxic protein moieties, accumulation of protein aggregates, neuronal dysfunction, and cell death (155,156). The identification of genes involved in familial forms of parkinsonism, especially parkin (an E3 ligase of UPS) and UCH-L1 (ubiquitin carboxy terminal hydrolase L1) have implicated a role of the UPS in PD (155–158). Therefore, targeting the UPS through elevated oxidative stress, introduction of various gene mutants, or pharmacological targeting have been tested for developing parkinsonian features in animal models. The infusion of inhibitors of the UPS, such as lactacystin and epoxymycin, to the basal ganglia has been reported to result in the loss of TH and DAT immunoreactivity, dopamine depletion, and the occurrence of protein inclusions in midbrain dopaminergic neurons spared from cell death (159,160). The potential impact of using proteasome inhibitors to generate models of PD is in its early phase where the reproducibility of different regimens is being evaluated, including differences in species (rats vs. mice) and strain susceptibility, efficacy of different chemical agents, and mode of delivery. It is interesting to note that there has been a shift in the role of some genes involved in familial PD such as parkin originally identified as playing a role in the UPS may also be involved in mitochondria integrity as well.

GENETIC MODELS OF PARKINSON'S DISEASE

In addition to pharmacological and neurotoxicant models of PD, which can be induced in a variety of different species, there are also rodent models derived from either spontaneous or directed genetic manipulation. Spontaneous rodent models of movement disorders (such as the founder mutations seen in the *weaver* mouse and *AS/AGU* rat) tend to arise fortuitously and depend on their recognition by researchers followed by successful breeding. Another approach for establishing genetic rodent models is through targeting specific genes of interest to create a transgenic mouse line. The recent identification of genes implicated in the etiology of familial forms of PD, including α-synuclein (PARK1/4), parkin (PARK2), UCH-L1 (PARK5), PINK1 (PARK6), DJ-1 (PARK7), and LRRK2 (PARK8), have provided a starting point in the development of specific transgenic mouse lines (161). The goal of these transgenic lines is to replicate in the rodent some of the neurochemical, pathological, or behavioral features of the human condition. The generation of transgenic mouse models can be rather complex, as illustrated by the wide range of outcomes observed through the characterization of existing α-synuclein transgenic lines. Although many different laboratories have generated α-synuclein transgenic mice the importance of transgene sequence (wild-type or different mutant alleles), promoter strength and cell-type specificity, copy number, insertion site, and background strain all influence features of this model. The following sections highlight both spontaneous and transgenic rodent models of PD, many of which are still in their early stages of development and characterization.

SPONTANEOUS RODENT MODELS FOR PARKINSON'S DISEASE

There are several naturally occurring spontaneous mutations in rodents that are of particular interest in PD. Spontaneous rodent models include the *weaver, lurcher, reeler, Tshr*[hyt]*, tottering, coloboma* mice and the *AS/AGU* and *circling* (*ci*) rat. These models possess unique characteristics that may provide insight into neurodegenerative processes of PD and related disorders. Several of these spontaneous rodent models display altered dopaminergic function or neurodegeneration, and have deficits in motor behavior (162). For example, the *weaver* mouse displays cell death of dopaminergic neurons, whereas the *tottering* mouse displays TH hyperinnervation. The *AS/AGU* rat is a spontaneous model characterized by progressive rigidity, staggering gait, tremor, and difficulty in initiating movements (163). This strain arises from a recessive mutation within the gene encoding protein kinase C-gamma suggesting another interesting gene implicated in neurodegeneration (164,165) affecting both the dopaminergic and serotonergic systems (164). Microdialysis in the *AS/AGU* rat model has revealed that even prior to dopaminergic neuronal cell death, there is dysfunction in dopaminergic neurotransmission that correlates with behavioral deficits. Another potentially interesting rodent model is the *circling* (*ci*) rat (166). This animal model displays spontaneous rotational behavior as a result of an imbalance in dopaminergic neurotransmission despite the absence of asymmetric nigral cell death.

Another interesting, naturally occurring mutation is the aphakia mouse. This mutation affects a gene called Pitx3, which is a developmentally regulated homeobox containing transcription factor necessary for the establishment of midbrain dopaminergic neurons (167). Mice carrying mutations in Pitx3 display behavioral and neurochemical characteristics similar to the anatomical and functional deficits seen in PD, including cell loss in the substantia nigra dopaminergic neurons, a feature not seen in most transgenic mouse lines (168). The deficits in motor behavior can be rescued with levodopa replacement therapy. These mice demonstrate the importance of developmental factors for midbrain dopaminergic neurons and could reveal key therapeutic targets for treating PD (169).

TRANSGENIC MOUSE MODELS

The development of transgenic animal models is dependent on identifying the potential role of genes of interest to the etiology of PD. A transgenic mouse is an animal in which a specific gene of interest has been altered through one of several techniques including (*i*) the excision of the host gene (knockout), (*ii*) the introduction of a mutant gene (knock-in), and (*iii*) the alteration of gene expression (knockdown, null, or overexpression). In PD, one source of transgenic targeting is derived from genes identified through epidemiological and linkage analysis studies. Examples of genes that have been identified through linkage analysis in familial forms of parkinsonism are α-synuclein and parkin. Once the transgene has been constructed, the degree of its expression and its impact on the phenotype of the animal depends on many factors including the selection of sequence (mutant vs wild-type), site of genomic integration, number of copies recombined, selection of transcription promoter, and upstream controlling elements (enhancers). Other important factors may include the background strain and age of the animal. These different features may account for some of the biochemical and pathological variations observed among transgenic mouse lines.

α-Synuclein

Rare cases of autosomal dominant familial forms of PD (the Contursi, German, and Iowa kindreds) have been linked to A30P and A53T substitution mutations in the gene encoding α-synuclein or triplicate of the gene (170–172). The normal function of α-synuclein is unknown but its localization and developmental expression suggests a role in neuroplasticity, neurotransmission, and vesicular function (173–175). The disruption of normal neuronal function may lead to the loss of synaptic maintenance and subsequent degeneration. It is interesting that mice with knockout of α-synuclein are viable, suggesting that a "gain-in-function" phenotype or other protein–protein interactions may contribute to neurodegeneration. Although no mutant forms of α-synuclein have been identified in idiopathic PD, its localization to Lewy bodies (including PD and related disorders) has suggested a pathophysiological link between α-synuclein aggregation and neurodegenerative disease (176,177). An interesting caveat is that the mutant allele of α-synuclein in the Contursi kindred is identical to the wild-type mouse suggesting that protein expression and/or protein–protein interactions leading to a yet unidentified gain of function may be more important than loss of function due to missense mutation. Since the identification of α-synuclein in familial PD, many groups have developed transgenic mouse models (178–192). A review of the transgene construction parameters (species and/or mutant forms), promoter selection (neuron or glia specific), and gene and protein expression patterns or levels demonstrate a high degree of variability in the resulting transgenic strains. Some transgenic mouse lines show neurochemical or pathological changes in dopaminergic neurons (including inclusions, decreased striatal dopamine, and loss of striatal TH immunoreactivity), behavioral deficits (rotarod and attenuation of dopamine-dependent locomotor response to amphetamine), whereas other lines show no deficits. No group has reported the specific loss of substantia nigra dopaminergic neurons despite inclusion pathology or cell death in other areas of the brain. This range of results with different α-synuclein constructs from different laboratories underscores the important link between protein expression (mutant vs wild-type alleles) and pathological and behavioral outcome. Important applications of α-synuclein transgenic mice are occurring at the level of understanding the role of this protein in basal ganglia function. For example, the response of α-synuclein expression to neurotoxic injury as well as interactions with other proteins, including parkin, will provide valuable insights into mechanisms important to neurodegeneration (193). Interestingly, some groups report evidence of neuronal dysfunction (either physiological or motor behavioral changes) without cell death. This suggests that cell death may in fact be a component of the late phase in the progression of basal ganglia degeneration, whereas neuronal dysfunction may occur at the level of the synapse and connectivity.

Parkin

An autosomal recessive form of juvenile parkinsonism (AR-JP) led to the identification of a gene on chromosome 6q27 called parkin (194,195). Mutations in parkin may account for the majority of autosomal recessive familial cases of PD. Parkin protein has a large N-terminal ubiquitin-like domain and C-terminal cysteine ring structure and is expressed in the brain (196–198). Biochemical studies indicate that parkin protein may play a critical role in mediating interactions with a number of different proteins involved in the proteasome-mediated degradation pathway including α-synuclein (193,199). Null mutations in mice appear normal with respect to motor behavior with no evidence of cell loss; however, striatal dopamine levels are elevated with enhanced synaptic excitability in striatal neurons (200). Mutations of the parkin gene have been introduced into transgenic mice. At present there is very little known about pathological or behavioral alterations due to mutations in parkin protein. However, parkin transgenic models enable investigation of the ubiquitin-mediated protein degradation pathways and the relationship to neurodegenerative disease.

DJ-1

Mutations in the DJ-1 gene (PARK7) are associated with rare forms of autosomal recessive early-onset PD (201). Mice with knockout of DJ-1 appear hypoactive, show no apparent loss of midbrain dopaminergic neurons, but do display altered electrophysiological properties in striatal neurons that can be rescued by targeting dopamine receptor D1 (202). Analysis of the structure, function, and pattern of expression of DJ-1 in mice, Drosophila, and in cell culture indicate that DJ-1 protein interacts with mitochondria playing a role in oxidative stress and apoptosis (203,204). Interestingly, DJ-1 has been shown to interact with a number of other proteins implicated in familial parkinsonism (205).

UCH-L1

Ubiquitin carboxyl-terminal hydrolase L1 (UCH-L1) is a member of the family of de-ubiquitinating enzymes responsible for mediating monomeric subunits from poly-ubiquitin chains (206). Mutations in UCH-L1 result in impaired clearance of ubiquitin and ubiquitinated proteins, therefore leading to elevated cell toxicity, protein accumulation, and cell death. At present, transgenic mice with altered UCH-L1 expression have been examined in the context of spermatogenesis and not extensively on alterations in basal ganglia function (207,208). Some studies have reported increased α-synuclein accumulation and neuropathology in UCH-L1 transgenic mice supporting interactions between α-synuclein and the UPS (209).

LRRK2

The leucine-rich repeat kinase 2 gene (LRRK2 termed PARK8) also called Dardarin encodes a large polymer of 2527-amino acid protein with multiple structural motifs and has recently been implicated in the etiology of PD based on genetic studies (210,211). Mutations in this gene have been identified in familial forms of PD that result in autosomal dominant late-onset PD (212–214). The precise function of LRRK2 is currently unknown but studies have suggested that this cytoplasmic protein can associate with other PD proteins including Parkin and possesses a wide range of biochemical features including multiple kinase activities and various structural motifs (215,216). Ongoing structural/function analysis of this large complex protein will reveal more precisely its role in neurodegenerative disorders and will guide the development of transgenic animals for study. LRRK2 presents multiple challenges in generating transgenic mice not only because of its size but the lack of precise knowledge of its pattern of expression and protein interactions. This challenge is not unlike those faced early in the generation of α-synuclein transgenic mice. Currently, transgenic mice and other species are being generated in a wide spectrum of configurations and the effects of LRRK2 mutations on PD features are being evaluated (217–223).

PINK1

A locus for a rare familial form of PD maps to chromosome 1p36 (PARK6) and is termed PINK1 (phosphatase and tensin homolog-induced kinase-1) (224). The function of PINK1 is thought to be in the protection of mitochondria from the ravages of oxidative stress (225,226). In addition, PINK1 may serve to control interactions with regulatory factors involved in mitochondrial function, morphology, and apoptosis (226). A number of PINK1 transgenic mice have been used to investigate its role in mitochondria function and its interactions with other familial PD genes, including Parkin, LRRK2, and DJ-1 (221,227–232). These interactions with DJ-1, and Parkin have been important in supporting the critical role of mitochondria health in neurodegenerative disorders such as PD.

NURR1

Nurr1 is a transcription factor that is highly expressed in early development, and disruption of this gene results in the failure to develop nigrostriatal dopaminergic neurons in postnatal life (233,234). Nurr1 expression decreases with age and in patients with PD suggesting that this protein may play a role in maintaining dopamine cell function and integrity (235). Transgenic mice disrupting Nurr1 expression show lack of development of nigrostriatal dopaminergic neurons based on TH immunoreactivity (236–240). While the time course of midbrain dopaminergic cell death in PD is unclear, the Nurr1 transgenic strains may provide insight into understanding dopamine cell development, potential susceptibility to PD in the context of dopamine dysfunction, and elucidation of the role of Nurr1 may act to guide stem cells as a therapeutic replacement for lost neurons.

Multiple Transgenic Mouse Models

The technological advancements in developing transgenic mouse models and facilities that assist the researcher to genetically manipulate genes of interest has also led to the establishment of models with multiple transgenics and multiple gene knockouts. For example, triple knockout transgenic mice have been reported in which genes for the three related synuclein proteins, α, β, and γ-synuclein have been removed (241). Other multiple transgenic models targeting Parkin, Pink, and DJ-1 in combination with α-synuclein or LRRK2 have been used to reveal potential interactions between these proteins (231). Transgenic rodents can also serve as templates for additional gene manipulation through the use of viral delivery approaches. This is especially highlighted in how pathway-specific mechanisms have been revealed for many PD-related genes in the structure and function of mitochondria. Such findings support the important role of mitochondria in disease etiology and identify novel therapeutic targets for treatment.

Other Transgenic Mice

The function of the basal ganglia is dependent on a wide range of proteins involved in dopamine biosynthesis, metabolism, uptake, and neurotransmission. To elucidate the role of numerous proteins in basal ganglia development, function, dysfunction, and their potential role in PD and its treatments, a wide spectrum of transgenic animals have been developed. These include transgenic mice and rats targeting TH, DAT, monoamine oxidase A and B, catechol-O-methyl-transferase, dopamine receptors, and vesicular monoamine transporter-2 as examples. These rodents are instrumental in elucidating the regulation of dopamine neurotransmission and its link to motor behavior. In addition, transgenics targeting proteins involved in basal ganglia neurotransmission or susceptibility to toxicity have also been developed including those for neurotrophic factors such as brain-derived neurotrophic factor (BDNF), glia-derived neurotrophic factor (GDNF) and their receptors, immune response components (cytokines and chemokines), and other neurotransmitter systems including glutamate, adenosine, and acetylcholine. Many of these distinctive transgenic animals have been developed to investigate the modulatory role of other neurotransmitter systems and signaling pathways within the basal ganglia in order to better understand function and behavior (both motor and nonmotor).

Novel transgenic mouse lines from the Gene Expression Nervous System Atlas (GENSAT) program, and ascertained through the Mutant Mouse Regional Resource Centers (MMRRC), have become available to better understand the circuitry of the basal ganglia. This library of mice employs BAC technology to selectively express the green fluorescent protein (GFP) under the control of a promoter in a small subset of neurons within a specific circuit. For example, GFP under the control of the dopamine D1 promoter expresses GFP within striatonigral projection medium spiny neurons (the direct pathway), whereas GFP under the control of the dopamine D2 promoter expresses GFP exclusively within striatopallidal neurons of the indirect pathway (242,243). These and other BAC-GFP transgenic mice allow studies that can begin to discern the involvement of specific circuits and their role in the pathophysiology of PD.

Transgenic Rat Models

Advances in the development of transgenic technologies have allowed the generation of transgenic rats. While some may consider a transgenic rat simply a larger version of a transgenic mouse there are some unique advantages. These include a long history of sensitive behavioral tests, a larger brain thus providing more tissues for analysis, and a relatively low cost. At this point a number of rat transgenic models have been developed, including those for LRRK2, α-synuclein, parkin, and others (223,244). As this technological approach gains popularity it is expected that many more genes will be manipulated in the rat genome and soon may rival in numbers to those available in mice.

Conditional Knockout and Vector Targeting

A major concern for all transgenic rodents is the possibility of developmental compensatory mechanisms as a consequence of a genetic knockout or transgenic. For example, other genes may be expressed or redundancies revealed in offspring from such manipulations. This challenge is clearly displayed when first developing any transgenic or knockout when researchers must evaluate issues of embryonic or early postnatal lethality, differential expression, gene silencing, and developmental disorders when establishing a founder line. Although researchers attempt to control all parameters it is not uncommon for screening to involve dozens of founders before a successful transgenic is developed. This challenge highlights the amount of work and validation required to establish the utility of a transgenic mouse model.

Now many of the potential confounders of transgenic approaches can be avoided by new genetic approaches. Specifically, the advent of new vector technologies based on infectious viruses, including the lentivirus and adeno-associated virus and others, allows genes of interest to be introduced directly into the brain with a high degree of anatomical targeting through a stereotaxic approach. Genes can be introduced to adult animals at any age thus avoiding the potential confounders observed in the development of a transgenic line including problems with embryonic lethality and developmental disruptions, especially with compensatory mechanisms. For example, induction of neurodegeneration can be achieved by direct targeting of α-synuclein or tau into the midbrain dopaminergic neurons (245–248). These engineered vectors have been constructed to introduce almost any gene of interest within the central nervous system, with the goal of increasing expression through the use of a wide variety of promoters. Genes beneficial to neuron protection and repair, including GDNF, BDNF, or neurotrophic factors, can be delivered directly to their site of action in the brain, such as the substantia nigra, striatum, or cortex (249–253). This technology also permits genes to be either overexpressed or silenced, depending on the research question. For example, viral vectors carrying short hairpin or small interfering RNA sequences (termed shRNA and siRNA), used to suppress mRNA transcripts in a gene-specific fashion, can also be delivered through this technology. The obvious advantage is that viral targeting can occur at any age of the animal with a high degree of anatomical specificity. In addition, this approach is fast and gene expression occurs within days and persists for months. Manipulations can be done in any transgenic line and is not limited to rodents but is available to other species including nonhuman primates. These approaches have advanced rather quickly and have a high degree of safety as demonstrated by current clinical trials in patients with PD. For example, targeting to specific brain regions (subthalamic nucleus) to regulate basal ganglia circuitry and improve motor function is currently being evaluated as a therapeutic modality (254). Studies are underway to evaluate different parameters of delivery, stability, toxicity, and long-term efficacy, which include research in nonhuman primate and rodent models of PD, prior to clinical applications.

Another approach to avoid developmental compensatory issues in transgenic rodents is the development of conditional knockout mouse models. For example, a gene of interest can be introduced via traditional transgenic methods, and expressed under the control of an inducible promoter, such as the tetracycline operator (255). The addition of doxycycline in the water of these transgenic animals leads to the induction of the gene construct in a dose-dependent manner. Thus a gene of interest can be turned on or off as desired. Another more approach is the development of transgenic mice in which a gene of interest is flanked by sequences of the cre-lox system, a construct termed flox. In this design the gene or a key sequence of a gene is flanked by a short inverted repeat sequences called loxP sites derived from the bacteriophage P1. In the presence of the enzyme recombinase, termed cre-recombinase, these flanking *loxP* sites are used to excise any intervening sequences they flank. As a consequence of this excision by the cre-recombinase, a floxed gene of interest can be removed at any developmental stage, including postnatal or adult stages. For example, cre-recombinase can be carried on a viral vector under the control of a promoter of interest that can be stereotaxically targeted to any brain region and lead to selective expression in specific subsets of cells. Similar target-specific expression can also be achieved through crossing of transgenic mice having floxed genes with another transgenic having either an inducible cre-recombinase or cre-recombinase under control of a promoter having tissue-specific expression. Examination of the literature demonstrates the increasing popularity of these approaches (256).

INVERTEBRATE GENETIC MODELS

Although the anatomical differences between *Homo sapiens* and *Drosophila melanogaster* are somewhat dramatic, invertebrates such as *D. melanogaster* are now providing an important avenue for understanding neurodegenerative disorders (257). Similar to studies in rodents, flies have served as a template for exposure to toxins implicated in PD, including rotenone and paraquat (258). A number of identified genes involved in familial forms of PD, including α-synuclein, parkin, LRRK2, PINK1, and DJ-1, in conjunction with the molecular tools available for gene transfer, have resulted in the establishment of transgenic fly lines expressing these genes of interest (150,219,221,259–264). These new models are significant because they can be used to elucidate the biochemical function of these proteins, and identify other interacting proteins, modifiers, and regulatory genes. In addition, their potential for high volume screening of large chemical libraries may lead to new therapeutic agents (265). One of the first examples of fly models of human neurodegenerative disorders was the introduction of both wild-type and mutant forms of human α-synuclein that resulted in loss of TH dopaminergic neurons, the formation of intracytoplasmic and neurite protein aggregates, and progressive motor behavior impairment (259). The availability of powerful transposon-based screens can be used to find compensatory mutants and proteins that interact with α-synuclein, such as the chaperone protein Hsp-70, thus providing insights into structure and function relationships (266).

The success of α-synuclein transgenic flies has provided a strong foundation for the development of other transgenic *D. melanogaster* models. For example, targeting of the parkin gene, despite showing little evidence of specific dopaminergic neuron cell death (267) has revealed the important role of mitochondrial pathology and neuromuscular dysfunction (268). In addition, the parkin Drosophila transgenic demonstrate increased sensitivity to oxidative stress and wide scale degeneration, which may provide insight into the relationship between vulnerability of cell types having a high energy demand to injury and degeneration (269). Another example of the impact of *D. melanogaster* models in neurodegenerative disorders is the demonstration of the development of DJ-1 transgenic flies. *D. melanogaster* possesses two alleles of DJ-1, but P-element-based gene disruption leads to impaired climbing ability that is progressive with age and localized to mitochondria, but with no apparent loss of dopaminergic neurons (270). Studies in *D. melanogaster* suggest that DJ-1 may function as a redox-sensitive molecular chaperone that can protect against oxidative stress, underlying the susceptibility of mitochondria (271). Hence, flies with disruption of DJ-1 show increased sensitivity to induction of oxidative stress by hydrogen peroxide, rotenone, and paraquat (272). These studies highlight insights into the function of DJ-1 in *D. melanogaster* and provide a better understanding of its potential role in PD (273).

MODELS OF PD VARIANTS

While the models discussed in the above sections provide insights into PD there have been additional animal models developed to begin to understand clinical variants of PD, including multiple system atrophy (MSA) and progressive supranuclear palsy (PSP).

MULTIPLE SYSTEM ATROPHY AND STRIATONIGRAL DEGENERATION

MSA is a variant of PD characterized by a combination of clinical symptoms involving cerebellar, extrapyramidal, and autonomic systems. The predominant subtype of MSA is striatonigral degeneration (SND), a form of levodopa unresponsive parkinsonism. Neuropathological changes of SND include degeneration of the nigrostriatal pathway, medium spiny striatal GABAergic projection pathways (putamen greater than caudate), as well as other regions of the brain stem, cerebellum, and spinal cord. Inclusion-like aggregates that immuno-stain for ubiquitin and α-synuclein are seen in oligodendrocytes and neurons.

The basis for developing an animal model for SND emerged from established animal models for both parkinsonism (having SNpc pathology) and Huntington's disease (HD) (having striatal pathology). For example, rodent models for SND have been generated through sequential stereotaxic injections of 6-OHDA and quinolinic acid (QA) into the medial forebrain bundle and striatum, respectively, or striatal injections of MPP[+] and 3-nitropropionic acid (3-NP) (274–276). These double-lesioning models are characterized morphologically by neuronal degeneration in the SNpc and ipsilateral striatum. The order of neurotoxic lesioning may influence the degree of nigral or striatal pathology. For example, animals receiving 6-OHDA prior to QA exhibit predominantly nigral pathology while animals receiving QA prior to 6-OHDA show predominantly striatal pathology. This may be due to QA-induced terminal damage or other complex interactions after lesioning that reduce terminal uptake of 6-OHDA. Glial inclusions have not been reported in any of these models indicating a significant difference compared with the human condition.

Motor deficits in models for MSA and SND are assessed by ipsilateral and contralateral motor tasks (including stepping response, impaired paw reaching, and balance) and drug-induced circling behavior. As described earlier, characteristic drug-induced circling behavior occurs after 6-OHDA lesioning resulting in ipsilateral rotation in response to amphetamine and contralateral rotation in response to apomorphine. The subsequent striatal lesioning with QA diminishes (or has no affect on) amphetamine-induced ipsilateral rotation and reduces (or abolishes) apomorphine-induced contralateral rotation. This observation may be mediated by dopamine release on the intact side (in response to amphetamine) and/or the loss of dopamine receptor activation on the lesioned side (in response to apomorphine). The lack of response to apomorphine has been shown to correlate with the volume of the striatal lesion and is analogous to the diminished efficacy of levodopa therapy observed in the majority of SND patients.

A nonhuman primate (*Macaca fasicularis*) model of SND has been generated through the sequential systemic administration of MPTP and 3-NP (274,277). The parkinsonian features after MPTP-lesioning are levodopa responsive, however, subsequent administration of 3-NP worsen motor symptoms and nearly eliminate the levodopa response. Levodopa occasionally induces facial dyskinesia as sometimes seen in human MSA. Similar to SND, morphological changes include cell loss in the SNpc (typical of MPTP-lesioning) and severe circumscribed degeneration of striatal GABAergic projection neurons (typical of 3-NP lesioning). Despite the similarities with the human condition, the MSA model is characterized by an equal degree of lesioning in the putamen and caudate nucleus, whereas in human SND the putamen is more affected. In addition, inclusion bodies that may underlie the pathogenesis of SND have not been reported in this nonhuman primate model.

THE TAUOPATHIES INCLUDING PROGRESSIVE SUPRANUCLEAR PALSY AND OTHER TAU-RELATED DISORDERS

The low molecular weight microtubule–associated protein tau has been implicated in a number of neurodegenerative diseases, including Alzheimer's disease, PSP, Pick's disease, frontotemporal dementia with parkinsonism, and amyotrophic lateral sclerosis/parkinsonism–dementia complex (ALS/PDC) of Guam. Together these neurodegenerative diseases comprise what is referred to as tauopathies since they share common neuropathological features, including abnormal hyperphosphorylation and filamentous accumulation of aggregated tau proteins (278). Reports in the literature have implicated either alternative RNA splicing (generating different isoforms) or missense mutations as mechanisms underlying many of the tauopathies. Therefore, transgenic mice have been generated that overexpress specific splice variants or missense mutations of tau (279). One such transgenic line has been developed to overexpress the shortest human tau isoform (280). These mice showed progressive motor weakness, intraneuronal and intra-axonal inclusions (detectable by one-month postnatal), and reduced axonal transport. Fibrillary tau inclusions developed in the neocortical neurons after 18 months of age implicating age-specific processes in the pathogenesis of fibrous tau inclusions. An interesting tau transgenic has been developed in *D. melanogaster* where expression of a tau missense mutation showed no evidence of large filamentous aggregates (neurofibrillary tangles). However, aged flies showed evidence of vacuolization and degeneration of cortical neurons (281). These observations suggest that tau-mediated neurodegeneration is age dependent and may take place independent of protein aggregation.

CONCLUSIONS

Our understanding of PD and related disorders has been advanced through animal models using genetic, pharmacological, and neurotoxicant manipulation. Each animal model has its own unique strengths and limitations. There is no "best model" for PD. Rather investigators must select the most appropriate model for the specific research question under investigation. Therefore, justification of nonhuman primates, the 6-OHDA rat, or the MPTP-mouse can be made in different cases and the most appropriate model selected. The nonhuman primate, rodent, and Drosophila models have contributed to the development of symptomatic (dopamine modulation), neuroprotective (antioxidants, free-radical scavengers), and restorative (growth factors, transplantation) therapies. In addition, these animal models have furthered our understanding of important aspects in the human condition shedding light on critical aspects of PD, including motor complications (wearing off and dyskinesia), neuronal cell death, nondopaminergic systems, and neuroplasticity of the basal ganglia. Future direction in PD research is through the continued development of animal models with altered genes and proteins of interest. In conjunction with existing models, these genetic-based models will help researchers better understand PD and will lead to improved treatments and the eventual cure of PD and related disorders.

ACKNOWLEDGMENTS

We would like to thank our colleagues at the University of Southern California for their support. Studies in our laboratory were made possible through the generous support of the Parkinson's Disease Foundation, Parkinson Alliance, The Baxter

Foundation, The Zumberge Foundation, the NIH (1RO1NS44327), and US Army NETRP. Special thanks to the friends of the USC Parkinson's Disease Research Group for their generous support. Thank you to Nicolaus, Pascal, and Dominique for their patience and encouragement.

REFERENCES

1. Jellinger K. Pathology of Parkinson's syndrome. In: Calne DB, ed. Handbook of Experimental Pharmacology. Berlin: Springer, 1988: 47–112.
2. Carlsson A, Lindqvist M, Magnusson T. 3,4-Dihydroxyphenylalanine and 5-hydroxytryptophan as reserpine antagonists. Nature 1957; 180: 1200.
3. Carlsson A. A half-century of neurotransmitter research: impact on neurology and psychiatry. Nobel lecture. Biosci Rep 2001; 21: 691–710.
4. Carlsson A. Treatment of Parkinson's with L-DOPA. The early discovery phase, and a comment on current problems. J Neural Transm 2002; 109: 777–87.
5. Birkmayer W, Hornykiewicz O. Der 1-3,4-dioxy-phenylanin (l-DOPA)-effek bei der Parkinson-akinesia. Klin Wochenschr 1961; 73: 787.
6. Ehringer H, Hornykiewicz O. Verteilung von noradrenalin und dopamin (3-hydroxytyramin) in gehrindes menschen und ihr verhalten bei erkrankungen des extrapyramidalen systems. Klin Wochenschr 1960; 38: 1238–9.
7. Schultz W. Depletion of dopamine in the striatum as an experimental model of Parkinsonism: direct effects and adaptive mechanisms. Prog Neurobiol 1982; 18: 121–66.
8. Glinka Y, Youdim MBH. Mechanisms of 6-hydroxydopamine neurotoxicity. J Neural Transm 1997; 50: 55–66.
9. Blum D, Torch S, Lambeng N, et al. Molecular pathways involved in the neurotoxicity of 6-OHDA, dopamine and MPTP: contribution to the apoptotic theory in Parkinson's disease. Prog Neurobiol 2001; 6+5: 135–72.
10. Ungerstedt U. 6-Hydroxy-dopamine induced degeneration of central monoamine neurons. Eur J Pharmacol 1968; 5: 107–10.
11. Ungerstedt U, Arbuthnott GW. Quantitative recording of rotational behavior in rats after 6-hydroxydopamine lesions of the nigrostriatal dopamine system. Brain Res 1970; 24: 485–93.
12. Ungerstedt U. Postsynaptic supersensitivity after 6-hydroxydopamine induced degeneration of the nigro-striatal dopamine system. Acta Physiol Scand 1971; 367(Suppl): 69–93.
13. Sauer H, Oertel W. Progressive degeneration of nigrostriatal dopamine neurons following intrastriatal terminal lesions with 6-hydroxydopamine: a combined retrograde tracing and immunocytochemical study in the rat. Neuroscience 1994; 59: 401–15.
14. Przedborski S, Levivier M, Jiang H, et al. Dose-dependent lesions of the dopaminergic nigrostriatal pathway induced by intranigrostriatal injection of 6-hydroxydopamine. Neuroscience 1995; 67: 631–47.
15. Yuan H, Sarre S, Ebinger G, et al. Histological, behavioural and neurochemical evaluation of medial forebrain bundle and striatal 6-OHDA lesions as rat models of Parkinson's disease. J Neurosci Methods 2005; 144: 35–45.
16. Schwarting RK, Huston JP. Unilateral 6-hydroxydopamine lesions of meso-striatal dopamine neurons and their physiological sequelae. Prog Neurobiol 1996; 49: 215–66.
17. Schwarting RK, Huston JP. The unilateral 6-hydroxydopamine lesion model in behavioral brain research. Analysis of functional deficits, recovery and treatments. Prog Neurobiol 1996; 20: 275–331.
18. Metz GA, Whishaw IQ. Drug-induced rotation intensity in unilateral dopamine-depleted rats is not correlated with end point or qualitative measures of forelimb or hindlimb motor performance. Neuroscience 2002; 111: 325–36.
19. Olds ME, Jacques DB, Kopyov O. Relation between rotation in the 6-OHDA lesioned rat and dopamine loss in striatal and substantia nigra subregions. Synapse 2006; 59: 532–44.

20. Schallert T, Tillerson J. Interventive strategies for degeneration of dopamine neurons in parkinsonism: optimizing behavioral assessment of outcome. In: Emerich D, Dean R, Sanberg P, eds. Central Nervous System Diseases. Totawa, NJ: Humana Press, 2000: 131–51.

21. Metz GA, Tse A, Ballermann M, Smith LK, Fouad K. The unilateral 6-OHDA rat model of Parkinson's disease revisited: an electromyographic and behavioural analysis. Eur J Neurosci 2005; 22: 735–44.

22. Cenci MA, Whishaw IQ, Schallert T. Animal models of neurological deficits: how relevant is the rat? Nat Rev Neurosci 2002; 3: 574–9.

23. Monville C, Torres EM, Dunnett SB. Validation of the l-dopa-induced dyskinesia in the 6-OHDA model and evaluation of the effects of selective dopamine receptor agonists and antagonists. Brain Res Bull 2005; 68: 16–23.

24. Papa SM, Engber TM, Kask AM, et al. Motor fluctuations in levodopa treated parkinsonian rats: relation to lesion extent and treatment duration. Brain Res 1994; 662: 69–74.

25. Papa SM, Boldry RC, Engber TM, Kask AM, Chase TN. Reversal of levodopa-induced motor fluctuations in experimental parkinsonism by NMDA receptor blockade. Brain Res 1995; 701: 13–18.

26. Chase TN, Engber TM, Mouradian MM. Contribution of dopaminergic and glutamatergic mechanisms to the pathogenesis of motor response complications in Parkinson's disease. Adv Neurol 1996; 69: 497–501.

27. Chase TN, Konitsiotis S, Oh JD. Striatal molecular mechanisms and motor dysfunction in Parkinson's disease. Adv Neurol 2001; 86: 355–60.

28. Oh JD, Russell DS, Vaughan CL, et al. Enhanced tyrosine phosphorylation of striatal NMDA receptor subunits: effect of dopaminergic denervation and L-DOPA administration. Brain Res 1998; 813: 150–9.

29. Henry B, Crossman AR, Brotchie JM. Characterization of enhanced behavioral responses to L-DOPA following repeated administration in the 6-hydroxydopamine-lesioned rat model of Parkinson's disease. Exp Neurol 1998; 151: 334–42.

30. Zigmond MJ, Abercrombie ED, Berger TW, et al. Compensations after lesions of central dopaminergic neurons: some clinical and basic implications. Trends Neurosci 1990; 13: 290–5.

31. Winkler C, Kirik D, Bjorklund A, et al. Transplantation in the rat model of Parkinson's disease: ectopic versus homotopic graft placement. Prog Brain Res 2000; 127: 233–65.

32. Nikkhah G, Olsson M, Eberhard J, et al. A microtransplantation approach for cell suspension grafting in the rat Parkinson model: a detailed account of the methodology. Neuroscience 1994; 63: 57–72.

33. Rodriguez M, Barroso-Chinea P, Abdala P, et al. Dopamine cell degeneration induced by intraventricular administration of 6-hydroxydopamine in the rat: similarities with cell loss in Parkinson's disease. Exp Neurol 2001; 169: 163–81.

34. Eslamboli A. Marmoset monkey models of Parkinson's disease: which model, when and why? Brain Res Bull 2005; 68: 140–9.

35. Annett LE, Rogers DC, Hernandez TD, et al. Behavioral analysis of unilateral monoamine depletion in the marmoset. Brain 1992; 115: 825–56.

36. Nass R, Hall DH, Miller DM, et al. Neurotoxin-induced degeneration of dopamine neurons in Caenorhabditis elegans. Proc Natl Acad Sci USA 2002; 99: 3264–9.

37. Nass R, Hahn MK, Jessen T, et al. A genetic screen in Caenorhabditis elegans for dopamine neuron insensitivity to 6-hydroxydopamine identifies dopamine transporter mutants impacting transporter biosynthesis and trafficking. J Neurochem 2005; 94: 774–85.

38. Lundblad M, Usiello A, Carta M, et al. Pharmacological validation of a mouse model of l-DOPA-induced dyskinesia. Exp Neurol 2005; 194: 66–75.

39. Lundblad M, Picconi B, Lindgren H, et al. A model of L-DOPA-induced dyskinesia in 6-hydroxydopamine lesioned mice: relation to motor and cellular parameters of nigrostriatal function. Neurobiol Dis 2004; 16: 110–23.

40. Branchi I, D'Andrea I, Armida M, et al. Striatal 6-OHDA lesion in mice: Investigating early neurochemical changes underlying Parkinson's disease. Behav Brain Res 2010; 208: 137–43.

41. Mandel RJ, Randall PK. Quantification of lesion-induced dopaminergic supersensitivity using the rotational model in the mouse. Brain Res 1985; 330: 358–63.
42. Davis GC, Williams AC, Markey SP, et al. Chronic parkinsonism secondary to intravenous injection of meperidine analogues. Psychiatry Res 1979; 1: 249–54.
43. Langston JW, Ballard P, Tetrud JW, et al. Chronic parkinsonism in humans due to a product of meperidine-analog synthesis. Science 1983; 219: 979–80.
44. Muthane U, Ramsay KA, Jiang H, et al. Differences in nigral neuron number and sensitivity to 1-methyl-4-phenyl-1,2,3,6-tetrahydropyridinium in C57/bl and CD-1 mice. Exp Neurol 1994; 126: 195–204.
45. Hamre K, Tharp R, Poon K, et al. Differential strain susceptibility following 1-methyl-4-phenyl-1,2,3,6-tetrahydropyridine (MPTP) administration acts in an autosomal dominant fashion: quantitative analysis in seven strains of Mus musculus. Brain Res 1999; 828: 91–103.
46. Heikkila RE. Differential neurotoxicity of 1-methyl-4-phenyl-1,2,3,6-tetrahydropyridine (MPTP) in Swiss-Webster mice from different sources. Eur J Pharmacol 1985; 117: 131–3.
47. Jarvis MF, Wagner GC. Age-dependent effects of 1-methyl-4-phenyl-1,2,3,6-tetrahydropyridine (MPTP). Neuropharmacology 1985; 24: 581–3.
48. Ali S, David SN, Newport GD, Cadet JL, Slikker W Jr. MPTP-induced oxidative stress and neurotoxicity are age-dependent: evidence from measures of reactive oxygen species and striatal dopamine levels. Synapse 1994; 18: 27–34.
49. Saura J, Richards J, Mahy N. Age-related changes on MAO in Bl/C57 mouse tissues: a quantitative radioautographic study. J Neural Transm 1994; 41: 89–94.
50. Yazdani U, German DC, Liang CL, et al. Rat model of Parkinson's disease: chronic central delivery of 1-methyl-4-phenylpyridinium (MPP(+)). Exp Neurol 2006; 200: 172–83.
51. Jackson-Lewis V, Jakowec M, Burke RE, Przedborski S. Time course and morphology of dopaminergic neuronal death caused by the neurotoxin 1-methyl-4-phenyl-1,2,3,6-tetrahydropyridine. Neurodegen 1995; 4: 257–69.
52. Ricaurte GA, Langston JW, Delanney LE, et al. Fate of nigrostriatal neurons in young mature mice given 1-methyl-4-phenyl-1,2,3,6-tetrahydropyridine: a neurochemical and morphological reassessment. Brain Res 1986; 376: 117–24.
53. Kalivas PW, Duffy P, Barrow J. Regulation of the mesocortocolimbic dopamine system by glutamic acid receptor subtypes. J Pharmacol Exp Ther 1989; 251: 378–87.
54. Bezard E, Dovero S, Imbert C, et al. Spontaneous long-term compensatory dopaminergic sprouting in MPTP-treated mice. Synapse 2000; 38: 363–8.
55. Forno LS, Langston JW, DeLanney LE, et al. Locus ceruleus lesions and eosinophilic inclusions in MPTP-treated monkeys. Ann Neurol 1986; 20: 449–55.
56. Langston JW, Forno LS, Tetrud J, et al. Evidence of active nerve cell degeneration in the substantia nigra of humans years after 1-methyl-4-phenyl-1,2,3,6-tetrahydropyridine exposure. Ann Neurol 1999; 46: 598–605.
57. Przedborski S, Jackson-Lewis V, Naini AB, et al. The parkinsonian toxin 1-methyl-4-phenyl-1,2,3,6-tetrahydropyridine (MPTP): a technical review of its utility and safety. J Neurochem 2001; 76: 1265–74.
58. Sedelis M, Schwarting RK, Huston JP. Behavioral phenotyping of the MPTP mouse model of Parkinson's disease. Behav Brain Res 2001; 125: 109–25.
59. Tanila H, Bjorklund M, Riekkinen P Jr. Cognitive changes in mice following moderate MPTP exposure. Brain Res Bull 1998; 45: 577–82.
60. Sedelis M, Hofele K, Auburger GW, et al. MPTP susceptibility in the mouse: behavioral, neurochemical, and histological analysis of gender and strain differences. Behav Genet 2000; 30: 171–82.
61. Tillerson JL, Miller GW. Grid performance test to measure behavioral impairment in the MPTP-treated-mouse model of parkinsonism. J Neurosci Methods 2003; 123: 189–200.
62. Kurosaki R, Muramatsu Y, Kato H, et al. Biochemical, behavioral and immunohistochemical alterations in MPTP-treated mouse model of Parkinson's disease. Pharmacol Biochem Behav 2004; 78: 143–53.

63. Rousselet E, Joubert C, Callebert J, et al. Behavioral changes are not directly related to striatal monoamine levels, number of nigral neurons, or dose of parkinsonian toxin MPTP in mice. Neurobiol Dis 2003; 14: 218–28.
64. Tillerson JL, Caudle WM, Reveron ME, et al. Detection of behavioral impairments correlated to neurochemical deficits in mice treated with moderate doses of 1-methyl-4-phenyl-1,2,3,6-tetrahydropyridine. Exp Neurol 2002; 178: 80–90.
65. Meredith GE, Totterdell S, Beales M, Meshul CK. Impaired glutamate homeostasis and programmed cell death in a chronic MPTP mouse model of Parkinson's disease. Exp Neurol 2009; 219: 334–40.
66. Chin MH, Qian WJ, Wang H, et al. Mitochondrial dysfunction, oxidative stress, and apoptosis revealed by proteomic and transcriptomic analyses of the striata in two mouse models of Parkinson's disease. J Proteome Res 2008; 7: 666–77.
67. Przedborski S, Tieu K, Perier C, et al. MPTP as a mitochondrial neurotoxic model of Parkinson's disease. J Bioenerg Biomembr 2004; 36: 375–9.
68. Royland JE, Langston JW. MPTP: a dopamine neurotoxin. In: Kostrzewa RM, ed. Highly Selective Neurotoxins. Totawa, NJ: Humana Press, 1998: 141–94.
69. Smith TS, Trimmer PA, Khan SM, et al. Mitochondrial toxins in models of neurodegenerative diseases. II: elevated zif268 transcription and independent temporal regulation of striatal D1 and D2 receptors mRNAs and D1 and D2 receptor-binding sites in C57BL/6 mice during MPTP treatment. Brain Res 1997; 765: 189–97.
70. Smith TS, Bennett JP Jr. Mitochondrial toxins in models of neurodegenerative diseases. I: in vivo brain hydroxyl radical production during systemic MPTP treatment or following microdialysis infusion of methylpyridinium or azide ions. Brain Res 1997; 765: 183–8.
71. Jakowec MW, Nixon K, Hogg E, et al. Tyrosine hydroxylase and dopamine transporter expression following 1-methyl-4-phenyl-1,2,3,6-tetrahydropyridine-induced neurodegeneration in the mouse nigrostriatal pathway. J Neurosci Res 2004; 76: 539–50.
72. Ho A, Blum M. Induction of interleukin-1 associated with compensatory dopaminergic sprouting in the denervated striatum of young mice: model of aging and neurodegenerative disease. J Neurosci 1998; 18: 5614–29.
73. Tillerson JL, Caudle WM, Reveron ME, et al. Exercise induces behavioral recovery and attenuates neurochemical deficits in rodent models of Parkinson's disease. Neuroscience 2003; 119: 899–911.
74. Fisher BE, Petzinger GM, Nixon K, et al. Exercise-induced behavioral recovery and neuroplasticity in the 1-methyl-4-phenyl-1,2,3,6-tetrahydropyridine-lesioned mouse basal ganglia. J Neurosci Res 2004; 77: 378–90.
75. Taylor JR, Elsworth JD, Roth RH, et al. Severe long-term 1-methyl-4-phenyl-1,2,3,6-tetrahydropyridine-induced parkinsonism in the vervet monkey (Cercopithecus aethiops sabaeus). Neuroscience 1997; 81: 745–55.
76. Petzinger GM, Langston JW. The MPTP-lesioned non-human primate: a model for Parkinson's disease. In: Marwah J, Teitelbbaum H, eds. Advances in Neurodegenerative Disease. Volume I: Parkinson's Disease. Scottsdale, AZ: Prominent Press, 1998: 113–48.
77. Rose S, Nomoto M, Jackson EA, et al. Age-related effects of 1-methyl-4-phenyl-,2,3,6-tetrahydropyridine treatment of common marmosets. Eur J Pharmacol 1993; 230: 177–85.
78. Gerlach M, Reiderer P. Animal models of Parkinson's disease: an empiracal comparison with the phenomenology of the disease in man. J Neural Transm 1996; 103: 987–1041.
79. Ovadia A, Zhang Z, Gash DM. Increased susceptibility to MPTP toxicity in middle-aged rhesus monkeys. Neurobiol Aging 1995; 16: 931–7.
80. Petzinger GM, Fisher B, Hogg E, et al. Behavioral recovery in the MPTP (1-methyl-4-phenyl-1,2,3,6-tetrahydropyridine)-lesioned Squirrel Monkey (Saimiri sciureus): Analysis of Striatal Dopamine and the expression of tyrosine hydroxylase and Dopamine transporter proteins. J Neuorsci Res 2005; 83: 332–47.
81. Bezard E, Gross C. Compensatory mechanisms in experimental and human parkinsonism: towards a dynamic approach. Progr Neurobiol 1998; 55: 96–116.

82. Tetrud JW, Langston JW. MPTP-induced parkinsonism as a model for Parkinson's disease. Acta Neurol Scand 1989; 126: 35–40.
83. Elsworth JD, Deutch AY, Redmond DE, et al. MPTP-induced parkinsonism: relative changes in dopamine concentration in subregions of substantia nigra, ventral tegmental area and retrorubral field of symptomatic and asymptomatic vervet monkeys. Brain Res 1990; 513: 320–4.
84. Waters CM, Hunt SP, Jenner P, et al. An immunohistochemical study of the acute and long-term effects of 1-methyl-4-phenyl-1,2,3,6-tetrahydropyridine in the marmoset. Neuroscience 1987; 23: 1025–39.
85. Eidelberg E, Brooks BA, Morgan WW, et al. Variability and functional recovery in the N-methyl-4-phenyl-1,2,3,6-tetrahydropyridine model of parkinsonism in monkeys. Neuroscience 1986; 18: 817–22.
86. Bankiewicz KS, Oldfield EH, Chiueh CC, et al. Hemiparkinsonism in monkeys after unilateral internal carotid infusion of 1-methyl-4-phenyl-1,2,3,6-tetrahydropyridine. Life Sci 1986; 39: 7–16.
87. Smith R, Zhang Z, Kurlan R, et al. Developing a stable bilateral model of parkinsonism in rhesus monkeys. Neuroscience 1993; 52: 7–16.
88. Eberling JL, Jagust WJ, Taylor S, et al. A novel MPTP primate model of Parkinson's disease: neurochemical and clinical changes. Brain Res 1998; 805: 259–62.
89. Bezard E, Imbert C, Deloire X, et al. A chronic MPTP model reproducing the slow evolution of Parkinson's disease: evolution of motor symptoms in the monkey. Brain Res 1997; 766: 107–12.
90. Bezard E, Brotchie JM, Gross CE. Pathophysiology of levodopa-induced dyskinesia: potential for new therapies. Nat Rev Neurosci 2001; 2: 577–88.
91. Hurley MJ, Mash DC, Jenner P. Dopamine D1 receptor expression in human basal ganglia and changes in Parkinson's disease. Brain Res Mol Brain Res 2001; 87: 271–9.
92. Papa SM, Chase TN. Levodopa-induced dyskinesias improved by a glutamate antagonist in parkinsonian monkeys. Ann Neurol 1996; 39: 574–8.
93. Bedard PJ, Mancilla BG, Blanchette P, Gagnon C, Di Paolo T. Levodopa-induced dyskinesia: facts and fancy. What does the MPTP monkey model tell us? Can J Neurol Sci 1992; 19: 134–7.
94. Calon F, Morissette M, Ghribi O, et al. Alteration of glutamate receptors in the striatum of dyskinetic 1-methyl-4-phenyl-1,2,3,6-tetrahydropyridine-treated monkeys following dopamine agonist treatment. Prog Neuropsychopharmacol Biol Psychiatry 2002; 26: 127–38.
95. Pearce RK, Heikkila M, Linden IB, et al. L-Dopa induces dyskinesia in normal monkeys: behavioural and pharmacokinetic observations. Psychopharmacology (Berl) 2001; 156: 402–9.
96. McKinley ET, Baranowski TC, Blavo DO, et al. Neuroprotection of MPTP-induced toxicity in zebrafish dopaminergic neurons. Brain Res Mol Brain Res 2005; 141: 128–37.
97. Ricaurte GA, Schuster CR, Seiden LS. Long-term effects of repeated methylamphetamine administration on dopamine and serotonin neurons in the rat brain: a regional study. Brain Res 1980; 193: 153–63.
98. Ricaurte GA, Guillery RW, Seiden LS, et al. Dopamine nerve terminal degeneration produced by high doses of methylamphetamine in the rat brain. Brain Res 1982; 235: 93–103.
99. Kim BG, Shin DH, Jeon GS, et al. Relative sparing of calretinin containing neurons in the substantia nigra of 6-OHDA treated rat Parkinsonian model. Brain Res 2000; 855: 162–5.
100. Sonsalla PK, Jochnowitz ND, Zeevalk GD, et al. Treatment of mice with methamphetamine produces cell loss in the substantia nigra. Brain Res 1996; 738: 172–5.
101. Harvey DC, Lacan G, Melega WP. Regional heterogeneity of dopaminerigc deficits in vervet monkey striatum and substantia nigra after methamphetamine exposure. Exp Brain Res 2000; 133: 349–58.
102. Walsh SL, Wagner GC. Motor impairments after methamphetamine-induced neurotoxicity in the rat. J Pharmacol Exp Ther 1992; 263: 617–26.

103. Westphale RI, Stadlin A. Dopamine uptake blockers nullify methamphetamine-induced decrease in dopamine uptake and plasma membrane potential in rat striatal synaptosomes. Ann NY Acad Sci 2000; 914: 187–93.

104. Fumagalli F, Gainetdinov RR, Valenzano KJ, et al. Role of dopamine transporter in methamphetamine-induced neurotoxicity: evidence from mice lacking the transporter. J Neurosci 1998; 18: 4861–9.

105. Cubells JF, Rayport S, Rajendran G, et al. Methamphetamine neurotoxicity involves vacuolation of endocytic organelles and dopamine-dependent intracellular oxidative stress. J Neurosci 1994; 14: 2260–71.

106. Gluck MR, Moy LY, Jayatilleke E, et al. Parallel increases in lipid and protein oxidative markers in several mouse brain regions after methamphetamine treatment. J Neurochem 2001; 79: 152–60.

107. Yamamoto BK, Zhu W. The effects of methamphetamine on the production of free radicals and oxidative stress. J Pharmacol Exp Ther 1998; 287: 107–14.

108. Imam SZ, el-Yazal J, Newport GD, et al. Methamphetamine-induced dopaminergic neurotoxicity: role of peroxynitrite and neuroprotective role of antioxidants and peroxynitrite decomposition catalysts. Ann NY Acad Sci 2001; 939: 366–80.

109. Davidson C, Gow AJ, Lee TH, et al. Methamphetamine neurotoxicity: necrotic and apoptotic mechanisms and relevance to human abuse and treatment. Brain Res Brain Res Rev 2001; 36: 1–22.

110. Cadet JL, Ladenheim B, Baum I, et al. CuZn-superoxide dismutase (CuZnSOD) transgenic mice show resistance to the lethal effects of methylenedioxyamphetamine (MDA) and of methylenedioxymethamphetamine (MDMA). Brain Research, 1994; 655: 259–62.

111. Hirata H, Ladenheim B, Carlson E, et al. Autoradiographic evidence for methamphetamine-induced striatal dopaminergic loss in mouse brain: attenuation in CuZn-superoxide dismutase transgenic mice. Brain Res 1996; 714: 95–103.

112. Sonsalla PK, Riordan DE, Heikkila RE. Competitive and noncompetitive antagonists at N-methyl-D-asparate receptors protect against methamphetamine-induced dopaminergic damage in mice. J Pharmacol Exp Ther 1991; 256: 506–12.

113. Frost DO, Cadet JL. Effects of methamphetamine-induced neurotoxicity on the development of neural circuitry: a hypothesis. Brain Res Brain Res Rev 2000; 34: 103–18.

114. McCann UD, Wong DF, Yokoi F, et al. Reduced striatal dopamine transporter density in abstinent methamphetamine and methcathinone users: evidence from positron emission tomography studies with [11C]WIN-35,428. J Neurosci 1998; 18: 8417–22.

115. Paulus MP, Hozack NE, Zauscher BE, et al. Behavioral and functional neuroimaging evidence for prefrontal dysfunction in methamphetamine-dependent subjects. Neuropsychopharmacology 2002; 26: 53–65.

116. Guilarte TR. Is methamphetamine abuse a risk factor in parkinsonism? Neurotoxicology 2001; 22: 725–31.

117. Tanner CM, Ottman R, Goldman SM, et al. Parkinson disease in twins: an etiologic study. JAMA 1999; 281: 341–6.

118. Brown TP, Rumsby PC, Capleton AC, et al. Pesticides and Parkinson's disease–is there a link? Environ Health Perspect 2006; 114: 156–64.

119. Betarbet R, Sherer TB, MacKenzie G, et al. Chronic systemic pesticide exposure reproduces features of Parkinson's disease. Nat Neurosci 2000; 3: 1301–6.

120. Sherer TB, Kim JH, Betarbet R, et al. Subcutaneous rotenone exposure causes highly selective dopaminergic degeneration and alpha-synuclein aggregation. Exp Neurol 2003; 179: 6–18.

121. Pan-Montojo F, Anichtchik O, Dening Y, et al. Progression of Parkinson's disease pathology is reproduced by intragastric administration of rotenone in mice. PLoS One 2010; 5: e8762.

122. Testa CM, Sherer TB, Greenamyre JT. Rotenone induces oxidative stress and dopaminergic neuron damage in organotypic substantia nigra cultures. Brain Res Mol Brain Res 2005; 134: 109–18.

123. Xiong N, Huang J, Zhang Z, et al. Stereotaxical infusion of rotenone: a reliable rodent model for Parkinson's disease. PLoS One 2009; 4: e7878.

124. Hoglinger GU, Feger J, Prigent A, et al. Chronic systemic complex I inhibition induces a hypokinetic multisystem degeneration in rats. J Neurochem 2003; 84: 491–502.
125. Huang J, Liu H, Gu W, et al. A delivery strategy for rotenone microspheres in an animal model of Parkinson's disease. Biomaterials 2006; 27: 937–46.
126. Sherer TB, Betarbet R, Testa CM, et al. Mechanism of toxicity in rotenone models of Parkinson's disease. J Neurosci 2003; 23: 10756–64.
127. Greenamyre JT, Betarbet R, Sherer TB. The rotenone model of Parkinson's disease: genes, environment and mitochondria. Parkinsonism Relat Disord 2003; 9: S59–64.
128. Panov A, Dikalov S, Shalbuyeva N, et al. Rotenone model of Parkinson's disease: multiple brain mitochondria dysfunctions after short-term systemic rotenone intoxication. J Biol Chem 2005; 280: 42026–35.
129. Fleming SM, Zhu C, Fernagut PO, et al. Behavioral and immunohistochemical effects of chronic intravenous and subcutaneous infusions of varying doses of rotenone. Exp Neurol 2004; 187: 418–29.
130. Cicchetti F, Drouin-Ouellet J, Gross RE. Viability of the rotenone model in question. Trends Pharmacol Sci 2010; 31: 142–3.
131. Cannon JR, Tapias V, Na HM, et al. A highly reproducible rotenone model of Parkinson's disease. Neurobiol Dis 2009; 34: 279–90.
132. Thiruchelvam M, Richfield EK, Baggs RB, et al. The nigrostriatal dopaminergic system as a preferential target of repeated exposures to combined paraquat and maneb: implications for Parkinson's disease. J Neurosci 2000; 20: 9207–14.
133. Freestone PS, Chung KK, Guatteo E, et al. Acute action of rotenone on nigral dopaminergic neurons: involvement of reactive oxygen species and disruption of Ca2+ homeostasis. Eur J Neurosci 2009; 30: 1849–59.
134. Mirzaei H, Schieler JL, Rochet JC, et al. Identification of rotenone-induced modifications in alpha-synuclein using affinity pull-down and tandem mass spectrometry. Anal Chem 2006; 78: 2422–31.
135. McCormack AL, Thiruchelvam M, Manning-Bog AB, et al. Environmental risk factors and Parkinson's disease: selective degeneration of nigral dopaminergic neurons caused by the herbicide paraquat. Neurobiol Dis 2002; 10: 119–27.
136. Uversky VN. Neurotoxicant-induced animal models of Parkinson's disease: understanding the role of rotenone, maneb and paraquat in neurodegeneration. Cell Tissue Res 2004; 318: 225–41.
137. Richardson JR, Quan Y, Sherer TB, et al. Paraquat neurotoxicity is distinct from that of MPTP and rotenone. Toxicol Sci 2005; 88: 193–201.
138. Tawara T, Fukushima T, Hojo N, et al. Effects of paraquat on mitochondrial electron transport system and catecholamine contents in rat brain. Arch Toxicol 1996; 70: 585–9.
139. Fukushima T, Yamada K, Hojo N, et al. Mechanism of cytotoxicity of paraquat. III. The effects of acute paraquat exposure on the electron transport system in rat mitochondria. Exp Toxicol Pathol 1994; 46: 437–41.
140. Grant H, Lantos PL, Parkinson C. Cerebral damage in paraquat poisoning. Histopathology 1980; 4: 185–95.
141. Hughes JT. Brain damage due to paraquat poisoning: a fatal case with neuropathological examination of the brain. Neurotoxicology 1988; 9: 243–8.
142. Ossowska K, Wardas J, Smiałowska M, et al. A slowly developing dysfunction of dopaminergic nigrostriatal neurons induced by long-term paraquat administration in rats: an animal model of preclinical stages of Parkinson's disease? Eur J Neurosci 2005; 22: 1294–304.
143. Brooks AI, Chadwick CA, Gelbard HA, et al. Paraquat elicited neurobehavioral syndrome caused by dopaminergic neuron loss. Brain Res 1999; 823: 1–10.
144. Bonilla E, Medina-Leendertz S, Villalobos V, et al. Paraquat-induced oxidative stress in drosophila melanogaster: effects of melatonin, glutathione, serotonin, minocycline, lipoic acid and ascorbic acid. Neurochem Res 2006; 31: 1425–32.
145. Bretaud S, Lee S, Guo S. Sensitivity of zebrafish to environmental toxins implicated in Parkinson's disease. Neurotoxicol Teratol 2004; 26: 857–64.

146. Cicchetti F, Drouin-Ouellet J, Gross RE. Environmental toxins and Parkinson's disease: what have we learned from pesticide-induced animal models? Trends Pharmacol Sci 2009; 30: 475–83.
147. Gomez C, Bandez MJ, Navarro A. Pesticides and impairment of mitochondrial function in relation with the parkinsonian syndrome. Front Biosci 2007; 12: 1079–93.
148. Miller RL, Sun GY, Sun AY. Cytotoxicity of paraquat in microglial cells: Involvement of PKCdelta- and ERK1/2-dependent NADPH oxidase. Brain Res 2007; 1167: 129–39.
149. Kwon HJ, Heo JY, Shim JH, et al. DJ-1 mediates paraquat-induced dopaminergic neuronal cell death. Toxicol Lett 2011; 202: 85–92.
150. Lavara-Culebras E, Paricio N. Drosophila DJ-1 mutants are sensitive to oxidative stress and show reduced lifespan and motor deficits. Gene 2007; 400: 158–65.
151. Fernagut PO, Hutson CB, Fleming SM, et al. Behavioral and histopathological consequences of paraquat intoxication in mice: effects of alpha-synuclein over-expression. Synapse 2007; 61: 991–1001.
152. Gatto NM, Rhodes SL, Manthripragada AD, et al. Alpha-Synuclein gene may interact with environmental factors in increasing risk of Parkinson's disease. Neuroepidemiology 2010; 35: 191–5.
153. Betarbet R, Sherer TB, Greenamyre JT. Ubiquitin-proteasome system and Parkinson's diseases. Exp Neurol 2005; 191:S17–27.
154. Ross CA, Pickart CM. The ubiquitin-proteasome pathway in Parkinson's disease and other neurodegenerative diseases. Trends Cell Biol 2004; 14: 703–11.
155. Tanaka K, Suzuki T, Hattori N, et al. Ubiquitin, proteasome and parkin. Biochim Biophys Acta 2004; 1695: 235–47.
156. Petrucelli L, Dawson TM. Mechanism of neurodegenerative disease: role of the ubiquitin proteasome system. Ann Med 2004; 36: 315–20.
157. McNaught KS, Belizaire R, Isacson O, et al. Altered proteasomal function in sporadic Parkinson's disease. Exp Neurol 2003; 179: 38–46.
158. Healy DG, Abou-Sleiman PM, Wood NW. Genetic causes of Parkinson's disease: UCHL-1. Cell Tissue Res 2004; 318: 189–94.
159. McNaught KS, Perl DP, Brownell AL, et al. Systemic exposure to proteasome inhibitors causes a progressive model of Parkinson's disease. Ann Neurol 2004; 56: 149–62.
160. Fornai F, Lenzi P, Gesi M, et al. Fine structure and biochemical mechanisms underlying nigrostriatal inclusions and cell death after proteasome inhibition. J Neurosci 2003; 23: 8955–66.
161. Dawson TM, Ko HS, Dawson VL. Genetic animal models of Parkinson's disease. Neuron 2010; 66: 646–61.
162. Heintz N, Zoghbi HY. Insights from mouse models into the molecular basis of neurodegeneration. Annu Rev Physiol 2000; 62: 779–802.
163. Payne AP, Campbell JM, Russell D, et al. The AS/AGU rat: a spontaneous model of disruption and degeneration in the nigrostriatal dopaminergic system. J Anat 2000; 196: 629–33.
164. Al-Fayez M, Russell D, Wayne Davies R, et al. Deficits in the mid-brain raphe nuclei and striatum of the AS/AGU rat, a protein kinase C-gamma mutant. Eur J Neurosci 2005; 22: 2792–8.
165. Craig NJ, Duran Alonso MB, Hawker KL, et al. A candidate gene for human neurodegenerative disorders: a rat PKC gamma mutation causes a Parkinsonian syndrome. Nat Neurosci 2001; 4: 1061–2.
166. Richter A, Ebert U, Nobrega JN, et al. Immunohistochemical and neurochemical studies on nigral and striatal functions in the circling (ci) rat, a genetic animal model with spontaneous rotational behavior. Neuroscience 1999; 89: 461–71.
167. Nunes I, Tovmasian LT, Silva RM, et al. Pitx3 is required for development of substantia nigra dopaminergic neurons. Proc Natl Acad Sci USA 2003; 100: 4245–50.
168. van den Munckhof P, Gilbert F, Chamberland M, et al. Striatal neuroadaptation and rescue of locomotor deficit by L-dopa in aphakia mice, a model of Parkinson's disease. J Neurochem 2006; 96: 160–70.

169. Smidt MP, Smits SM, Burbach JP. Molecular mechanisms underlying midbrain dopamine neuron development and function. Eur J Pharmacol 2003; 480: 75–88.
170. Polymeropoulos M, Lavedan C, Leroy E, et al. Mutation in the α-synuclein gene identified in families with Parkinson's disease. Science 1997; 276: 2045–7.
171. Kruger R, Kuhn W, Muller T, et al. Ala30Pro mutation in the gene encoding α-synuclein in parkinson's disease. Nat Genet 1998; 18: 106–8.
172. Singleton AB, Farrer M, Johnson J, et al. Alpha-synuclein locus triplication causes Parkinson's disease. Science 2003; 302: 841.
173. George JM, Jin H, Woods WS, Clayton DF. Characterization of a novel protein regulated during the critical period for song learning in the zebra finch. Neuron, 1995; 15: 361–72.
174. Jakowec MW, Donaldson DM, Barba J, et al. The postnatal expression of α-synuclein in the substantia nigra and striatum of the rodent. Dev Neurosci 2001; 23: 91–9.
175. Lykkebo S, Jensen PH. Alpha-synuclein and presynaptic function: implications for Parkinson's disease. Neuromolecular Med 2002; 2: 115–29.
176. Fornai F, Soldani P, Lazzeri G, et al. Neuronal inclusions in degenerative disorders Do they represent static features or a key to understand the dynamics of the disease? Brain Res Bull 2005; 65: 275–90.
177. Lundvig D, Lindersson E, Jensen PH. Pathogenic effects of alpha-synuclein aggregation. Brain Res Mol Brain Res 2005; 134: 3–17.
178. Abeliovich A, Schmitz Y, Farinas I, et al. Mice lacking alpha-synuclein display functional deficits in the nigrostriatal dopamine system. Neuron 2000; 25: 239–52.
179. Masliah E, Rockenstein E, Veinbergs I, et al. Dopaminergic loss and inclusion body formation in alpha-synuclein mice: implications for neurodegenerative disorders. Science 2000; 289: 1265–9.
180. van der Putten H, Wiederhold KH, Probst A, et al. Neuropathology in mice expressing human alpha-synuclein. J Neurosci 2000; 20: 6021–9.
181. Kahle PJ, Neumann M, Ozmen L, et al. Physiology and pathophysiology of alpha-synuclein. Cell culture and transgenic animal models based on a Parkinson's disease-associated protein. Ann NY Acad Sci 2000; 920: 33–41.
182. Richfield EK, Thiruchelvam MJ, Cory-Slechta DA, et al. Behavioral and neurochemical effects of wild-type and mutated human alpha-synuclein in transgenic mice. Exp Neurol 2002; 175: 35–48.
183. Gispert S, Del Turco D, Garrett L, et al. Transgenic mice expressing mutant A53T human alpha-synuclein show neuronal dysfunction in the absence of aggregate formation. Mol Cell Neurosci 2003; 24: 419–29.
184. Giasson BI, Duda JE, Quinn SM, et al. Neuronal alpha-synucleinopathy with severe movement disorder in mice expressing A53T human alpha-synuclein. Neuron 2002; 34: 521–33.
185. Shults CW, Rockenstein E, Crews L, et al. Neurological and neurodegenerative alterations in a transgenic mouse model expressing human alpha-synuclein under oligodendrocyte promoter: implications for multiple system atrophy. J Neurosci 2005; 25: 10689–99.
186. Unger EL, Eve DJ, Perez XA, et al. Locomotor hyperactivity and alterations in dopamine neurotransmission are associated with overexpression of A53T mutant human alpha-synuclein in mice. Neurobiol Dis 2005; 21: 431–43.
187. Lee MK, Stirling W, Xu Y, et al. Human alpha-synuclein-harboring familial Parkinson's disease-linked Ala-53 –> Thr mutation causes neurodegenerative disease with alpha-synuclein aggregation in transgenic mice. Proc Natl Acad Sci USA 2002; 99: 8968–73.
188. Gomez-Isla T, Irizarry MC, Mariash A, et al. Motor dysfunction and gliosis with preserved dopaminergic markers in human alpha-synuclein A30P transgenic mice. Neurobiol Aging 2003; 24: 245–58.
189. Yavich L, Oksman M, Tanila H, et al. Locomotor activity and evoked dopamine release are reduced in mice overexpressing A30P-mutated human alpha-synuclein. Neurobiol Dis 2005; 20: 303–13.

190. Matsuoka Y, Vila M, Lincoln S, et al. Lack of nigral pathology in transgenic mice expressing human alpha-synuclein driven by the tyrosine hydroxylase promoter. Neurobiol Dis 2001; 8: 535–9.

191. Martin LJ, Pan Y, Price AC, et al. Parkinson's disease alpha-synuclein transgenic mice develop neuronal mitochondrial degeneration and cell death. J Neurosci 2006; 26: 41–50.

192. Yazawa I, Giasson BI, Sasaki R, et al. Mouse model of multiple system atrophy alpha-synuclein expression in oligodendrocytes causes glial and neuronal degeneration. Neuron 2005; 45: 847–59.

193. Shimura H, Schlossmacher MG, Hattori N, et al. Ubiquitination of a new form of {alpha}-synuclein by parkin from human brain: Implications for Parkinson's disease. Science 2001; 293: 263–9.

194. Kitada T, Asakawa S, Hattori N, et al. Mutations in the parkin gene cause autosomal recessive juvenile parkinsonism. Nature 1998; 392: 605–8.

195. Hattori N, Kitada T, Matsumine H, et al. Molecular genetic analysis of a novel Parkin gene in Japanese families with autosomal recessive juvenile parkinsonism: evidence for variable homozygous deletions in the Parkin gene in affected individuals. Ann Neurol 1998; 44: 935–41.

196. Fallon L, Moreau F, Croft BG, et al. Parkin and CASK/LIN-2 associate via a PDZ-mediated interaction and are co-localized in lipid rafts and postsynaptic densities in brain. J Biol Chem 2002; 277: 486–91.

197. Huynh DP, Dy M, Nguyen D, et al. Differential expression and tissue distribution of parkin isoforms during mouse development. Brain Res Dev Brain Res 2001; 130: 173–81.

198. Solano SM, Miller DW, Augood SJ, et al. Expression of alpha-synuclein, parkin, and ubiquitin carboxy-terminal hydrolase L1 mRNA in human brain: genes associated with familial Parkinson's disease. Ann Neurol 2000; 47: 201–10.

199. Tanaka K, Suzuki T, Chiba T, et al. Parkin is linked to the ubiquitin pathway. J Mol Med 2001; 79: 482–94.

200. Goldberg MS, Fleming SM, Palacino JJ, et al. Parkin-deficient mice exhibit nigrostriatal deficits but not loss of dopaminergic neurons. J Biol Chem 2003; 278: 43628–35.

201. Bonifati V, Rizzu P, Squitieri F, et al. DJ-1(PARK7), a novel gene for autosomal recessive, early onset parkinsonism. Neurol Sci 2003; 24: 159–60.

202. Goldberg MS, Pisani A, Haburcak M, et al. Nigrostriatal dopaminergic deficits and hypokinesia caused by inactivation of the familial Parkinsonism-linked gene DJ-1. Neuron 2005; 45: 489–96.

203. Junn E, Taniguchi H, Jeong BS, et al. Interaction of DJ-1 with Daxx inhibits apoptosis signal-regulating kinase 1 activity and cell death. Proc Natl Acad Sci USA 2005; 102: 9691–6.

204. Martinat C, Shendelman S, Jonason A, et al. Sensitivity to oxidative stress in DJ-1-deficient dopamine neurons: an ES- derived cell model of primary Parkinsonism. PLoS Biol 2004; 2: e327.

205. Shendelman S, Jonason A, Martinat C, et al. DJ-1 is a redox-dependent molecular chaperone that inhibits alpha-synuclein aggregate formation. PLoS Biol 2004; 2: e362.

206. Leroy E, Boyer R, Auburger G, et al. The ubiquitin pathway in Parkinson's disease. Nature 1998; 395: 451–2.

207. Kwon J, Wang YL, Setsuie R, et al. Developmental regulation of ubiquitin C-terminal hydrolase isozyme expression during spermatogenesis in mice. Biol Reprod 2004; 71: 515–21.

208. Wang YL, Liu W, Sun YJ, et al. Overexpression of ubiquitin carboxyl-terminal hydrolase L1 arrests spermatogenesis in transgenic mice. Mol Reprod Dev 2006; 73: 40–9.

209. Wang YL, Takeda A, Osaka H, et al. Accumulation of beta- and gamma-synucleins in the ubiquitin carboxyl-terminal hydrolase L1-deficient gad mouse. Brain Res 2004; 1019: 1–9.

210. Paisan-Ruiz C, Jain S, Evans EW, et al. Cloning of the gene containing mutations that cause PARK8-linked Parkinson's disease. Neuron 2004; 44: 595–600.

211. Cookson MR. The role of leucine-rich repeat kinase 2 (LRRK2) in Parkinson's disease. Nat Rev Neurosci 2010; 11: 791–7.

212. Mata IF, Kachergus JM, Taylor JP, et al. Lrrk2 pathogenic substitutions in Parkinson's disease. Neurogenetics 2005; 6: 171–7.

213. Skipper L, Shen H, Chua E, et al. Analysis of LRRK2 functional domains in nondominant Parkinson's disease. Neurology 2005; 65: 1319–21.

214. Ozelius LJ, Senthil G, Saunders-Pullman R, et al. LRRK2 G2019S as a cause of Parkinson's disease in Ashkenazi Jews. N Engl J Med 2006; 354: 424–5.

215. West AB, Moore DJ, Biskup S, et al. Parkinson's disease-associated mutations in leucine-rich repeat kinase 2 augment kinase activity. Proc Natl Acad Sci USA 2005; 102: 16842–7.

216. Smith WW, Pei Z, Jiang H, et al. Leucine-rich repeat kinase 2 (LRRK2) interacts with parkin and mutant LRRK2 induces neuronal degeneration. Proc Natl Acad Sci USA 2005; 102: 18676–81.

217. Lee SB, Kim W, Lee S, et al. Loss of LRRK2/PARK8 induces degeneration of dopaminergic neurons in Drosophila. Biochem Biophys Res Commun 2007; 358: 534–9.

218. Lin X, Parisiadou L, Gu XL, et al. Leucine-rich repeat kinase 2 regulates the progression of neuropathology induced by Parkinson's-disease-related mutant alpha-synuclein. Neuron 2009; 64: 807–27.

219. Liu Z, Wang X, Yu Y, et al. A Drosophila model for LRRK2-linked parkinsonism. Proc Natl Acad Sci USA 2008; 105: 2693–8.

220. Ramonet D, Daher JP, Lin BM, et al. Dopaminergic neuronal loss, reduced neurite complexity and autophagic abnormalities in transgenic mice expressing G2019S mutant LRRK2. PLoS One 2011; 6: e18568.

221. Venderova K, Kabbach G, Abdel-Messih E, et al. Leucine-Rich Repeat Kinase 2 interacts with Parkin, DJ-1 and PINK-1 in a Drosophila melanogaster model of Parkinson's disease. Hum Mol Genet 2009; 18: 4390–404.

222. Yao C, El Khoury R, Wang W, et al. LRRK2-mediated neurodegeneration and dysfunction of dopaminergic neurons in a Caenorhabditis elegans model of Parkinson's disease. Neurobiol Dis 2010; 40: 73–81.

223. Zhou H, Huang C, Tong J, et al. Temporal expression of mutant LRRK2 in adult rats impairs dopamine reuptake. Int J Biol Sci 2011; 7: 753–61.

224. Valente EM, Abou-Sleiman PM, Caputo V, et al. Hereditary early-onset Parkinson's disease caused by mutations in PINK1. Science 2004; 304: 1158–60.

225. Shen J, Cookson MR. Mitochondria and dopamine: new insights into recessive parkinsonism. Neuron 2004; 43: 301–4.

226. Petit A, Kawarai T, Paitel E, et al. Wild-type PINK1 prevents basal and induced neuronal apoptosis, a protective effect abrogated by Parkinson disease-related mutations. J Biol Chem 2005; 280: 34025–32.

227. Kim KH, Son JH. PINK1 gene knockdown leads to increased binding of parkin with actin filament. Neurosci Lett 2010; 468: 272–6.

228. Matsuda N, Sato S, Shiba K, et al. PINK1 stabilized by mitochondrial depolarization recruits Parkin to damaged mitochondria and activates latent Parkin for mitophagy. J Cell Biol 2010; 189: 211–21.

229. Murphy AN. In a flurry of PINK, mitochondrial bioenergetics takes a leading role in Parkinson's disease. EMBO Mol Med 2009; 1: 81–4.

230. Wood-Kaczmar A, Gandhi S, Yao Z, et al. PINK1 is necessary for long term survival and mitochondrial function in human dopaminergic neurons. PLoS One 2008; 3: e2455.

231. Kitada T, Tong Y, Gautier CA, et al. Absence of Nigral Degeneration in aged Parkin/DJ-1/PINK1 triple knockout mice. J Neurochem 2009; 111: 692–702.

232. Liu W, Acin-Perez R, Geghman KD, et al. Pink1 regulates the oxidative phosphorylation machinery via mitochondrial fission. Proc Natl Acad Sci USA 2011; 108: 12920–4.

233. Law SW, Conneely OM, DeMayo FJ, O'Malley BW. Identification of a new brain-specific transcription factor, NURR1. Mol Endocrinol 1992; 6: 2129–35.

234. Zetterstrom RH, Solomin L, Jansson L, et al. Dopamine neuron agenesis in Nurr1-deficient mice. Science 1997; 276: 248–50.

235. Chu Y, Le W, Kompoliti K, et al. Nurr1 in Parkinson's disease and related disorders. J Comp Neurol 2006; 494: 495–514.
236. Tornqvist N, Hermanson E, Perlmann T, et al. Generation of tyrosine hydroxylase-immunoreactive neurons in ventral mesencephalic tissue of Nurr1 deficient mice. Brain Res Dev Brain Res 2002; 133: 37–47.
237. Jankovic J, Chen S, Le WD. The role of Nurr1 in the development of dopaminergic neurons and Parkinson's disease. Prog Neurobiol 2005; 77: 128–38.
238. Eells JB. The control of dopamine neuron development, function and survival: insights from transgenic mice and the relevance to human disease. Curr Med Chem 2003; 10: 857–70.
239. Eells JB, Lipska BK, Yeung SK, et al. Nurr1-null heterozygous mice have reduced meso-limbic and mesocortical dopamine levels and increased stress-induced locomotor activity. Behav Brain Res 2002; 136: 267–75.
240. Witta J, Baffi JS, Palkovits M, et al. Nigrostriatal innervation is preserved in Nurr1-null mice, although dopaminergic neuron precursors are arrested from terminal differentiation. Brain Res Mol Brain Res 2000; 84: 67–78.
241. Greten-Harrison B, Polydoro M, Morimoto-Tomita M, et al. αβγ-Synuclein triple knock-out mice reveal age-dependent neuronal dysfunction. Proc Natl Acad Sci USA 2010; 107: 19573–8.
242. Ade KK, Wan Y, Chen M, et al. An improved BAC Transgenic fluorescent reporter line for sensitive and specific identification of striatonigral medium spiny neurons. Front Syst Neurosci 2011; 5: 32.
243. Gong S, Zheng C, Doughty ML, et al. A gene expression atlas of the central nervous system based on bacterial artificial chromosomes. Nature 2003; 425: 917–25.
244. Sato H, Arawaka S, Hara S, et al. Authentically phosphorylated alpha-synuclein at Ser129 accelerates neurodegeneration in a rat model of familial Parkinson's disease. J Neurosci 2011; 31: 16884–94.
245. Klein RL, Dayton RD, Lin WL, et al. Tau gene transfer, but not alpha-synuclein, induces both progressive dopamine neuron degeneration and rotational behavior in the rat. Neurobiol Dis 2005; 20: 64–73.
246. Kirik D, Georgievska B, Bjorklund A. Localized striatal delivery of GDNF as a treatment for Parkinson disease. Nat Neurosci 2004; 7: 105–10.
247. Kirik D, Annett LE, Burger C, et al. Nigrostriatal alpha-synucleinopathy induced by viral vector-mediated overexpression of human alpha-synuclein: a new primate model of Parkinson's disease. Proc Natl Acad Sci USA 2003; 100: 2884–9.
248. Klein RL, King MA, Hamby ME, et al. Dopaminergic cell loss induced by human A30P alpha-synuclein gene transfer to the rat substantia nigra. Hum Gene Ther 2002; 13: 605–12.
249. Bankiewicz KS, Eberling JL, Kohutnicka M, et al. Convection-enhanced delivery of AAV vector in parkinsonian monkeys; in vivo detection of gene expression and restoration of dopaminergic function using pro-drug approach. Exp Neurol 2000; 164: 2–14.
250. Azzouz M, Martin-Rendon E, Barber RD, et al. Multicistronic lentiviral vector-mediated striatal gene transfer of aromatic L-amino acid decarboxylase, tyrosine hydroxylase, and GTP cyclohydrolase I induces sustained transgene expression, dopamine production, and functional improvement in a rat model of Parkinson's disease. J Neurosci 2002; 22: 10302–12.
251. Bjorklund A, Kirik D, Rosenblad C, et al. Towards a neuroprotective gene therapy for Parkinson's disease: use of adenovirus, AAV and lentivirus vectors for gene transfer of GDNF to the nigrostriatal system in the rat Parkinson model. Brain Res 2000; 886: 82–98.
252. Kordower JH, Emborg ME, Bloch J, et al. Neurodegeneration prevented by lentiviral vector delivery of GDNF in primate models of Parkinson's disease. Science 2000; 290: 767–73.
253. Torres EM, Monville C, Lowenstein PR, et al. Delivery of sonic hedgehog or glial derived neurotrophic factor to dopamine-rich grafts in a rat model of Parkinson's disease using adenoviral vectors Increased yield of dopamine cells is dependent on embryonic donor age. Brain Res Bull 2005; 68: 31–41.

254. During MJ, Kaplitt MG, Stern MB, et al. Subthalamic GAD gene transfer in Parkinson disease patients who are candidates for deep brain stimulation. Hum Gene Ther 2001; 12: 1589–91.
255. Backman CM, Zhang Y, Hoffer BJ, et al. Tetracycline-inducible expression systems for the generation of transgenic animals: a comparison of various inducible systems carried in a single vector. J Neurosci Methods 2004; 139: 257–62.
256. Hnasko TS, Perez FA, Scouras AD, et al. Cre recombinase-mediated restoration of nigrostriatal dopamine in dopamine-deficient mice reverses hypophagia and bradykinesia. Proc Natl Acad Sci USA 2006; 103: 8858–63.
257. Bilen J, Bonini NM. Drosophia as a model for human neurodegenerative disease. Annu Rev Genet 2005; 39: 153–71.
258. Coulom H, Birman S. Chronic exposure to rotenone models sporadic Parkinson's disease in Drosophila melanogaster. J Neurosci 2004; 24: 10993–8.
259. Feany MB, Bender WW. A Drosophila model of Parkinson's disease. Nature 2000; 404: 394–8.
260. Botella JA, Bayersdorfer F, Gmeiner F, et al. Modelling Parkinson's disease in Drosophila. Neuromolecular Med 2009; 11: 268–80.
261. Chaudhuri A, Bowling K, Funderburk C, et al. Interaction of genetic and environmental factors in a Drosophila parkinsonism model. J Neurosci 2007; 27: 2457–67.
262. Hirth F. Drosophila melanogaster in the study of human neurodegeneration. CNS Neurol Disord Drug Targets 2010; 9: 504–23.
263. Sang TK, Chang HY, Lawless GM, et al. A Drosophila model of mutant human parkin-induced toxicity demonstrates selective loss of dopaminergic neurons and dependence on cellular dopamine. J Neurosci 2007; 27: 981–92.
264. Whitworth AJ. Drosophila models of Parkinson's disease. Adv Genet 2011; 73: 1–50.
265. Pendleton RG, Parvez F, Sayed M, et al. Effects of pharmacological agents upon a transgenic model of Parkinson's disease in Drosophila melanogaster. J Pharmacol Exp Ther 2002; 300: 91–6.
266. Auluck PK, Chan HY, Trojanowski JQ, et al. Chaperone suppression of alpha-synuclein toxicity in a Drosophila model for Parkinson's disease. Science 2002; 295: 865–8.
267. Pesah Y, Burgess H, Middlebrooks B, et al. Whole-mount analysis reveals normal numbers of dopaminergic neurons following misexpression of alpha-Synuclein in Drosophila. Genesis 2005; 41: 154–9.
268. Greene JC, Whitworth AJ, Kuo I, et al. Mitochondrial pathology and apoptotic muscle degeneration in Drosophila parkin mutants. Proc Natl Acad Sci USA 2003; 100: 4078–83.
269. Pesah Y, Pham T, Burgess H, et al. Drosophila parkin mutants have decreased mass and cell size and increased sensitivity to oxygen radical stress. Development 2004; 131: 2183–94.
270. Park J, Kim SY, Cha GH, et al. Drosophila DJ-1 mutants show oxidative stress-sensitive locomotive dysfunction. Gene 2005; 361: 133–9.
271. Menzies FM, Yenisetti SC, Min KT. Roles of Drosophila DJ-1 in survival of dopaminergic neurons and oxidative stress. Curr Biol 2005; 15: 1578–82.
272. Meulener M, Whitworth AJ, Armstrong-Gold CE, et al. Drosophila DJ-1 mutants are selectively sensitive to environmental toxins associated with Parkinson's disease. Curr Biol 2005; 15: 1572–7.
273. Moore DJ, Dawson VL, Dawson TM. Lessons from Drosophila models of DJ-1 deficiency. Sci Aging Knowledge Environ 2006; 2006: pe2.
274. Ghorayeb I, Puschban Z, Fernagut PO, et al. Simultaneous intrastriatal 6-hydroxydopamine and quinolinic acid injection: a model of early-stage striatonigral degeneration. Exp Neurol 2001; 167: 133–47.
275. Wenning GK, Granata R, Puschban Z, et al. Neural transplantation in animal models of multiple system atrophy: a review. J Neural Transm Suppl 1999; 55: 103–13.
276. Scherfler C, Puschban Z, Ghorayeb I, et al. Complex motor disturbances in a sequential double lesion rat model of striatonigral degeneration (multiple system atrophy). Neuroscience 2000; 99: 42–54.

277. Ghorayeb I, Fernagut PO, Aubert I, et al. Toward a primate model of L-dopa-unresponsive parkinsonism mimicking striatonigral degeneration. Mov Disord 2000; 15: 531–6.
278. Neumann M, Muller V, Gorner K, et al. Pathological properties of the Parkinson's disease-associated protein DJ-1 in alpha-synucleinopathies and tauopathies: relevance for multiple system atrophy and Pick's disease. Acta Neuropathol (Berl) 2004; 107: 489–96.
279. Barbieri S, Hofele K, Wiederhold KH, et al. Mouse models of alpha-synucleinopathy and Lewy pathology. Alpha-synuclein expression in transgenic mice. Adv Exp Med Biol 2001; 487: 147–67.
280. Ishihara T, Hong M, Zhang B, et al. Age-dependent emergence and progression of a tauopathy in transgenic mice overexpressing the shortest human tau isoform. Neuron 1999; 24: 751–62.
281. Wittmann CW, Wszolek MF, Shulman JM, et al. Tauopathy in Drosophila: neurodegeneration without neurofibrillary tangles. Science 2001; 293: 711–14.

15

Genetics

Shinsuke Fujioka, Christina Sundal, Owen A. Ross,
and Zbigniew K. Wszolek

INTRODUCTION

Despite considerable progress in understanding the clinical and pathologic features of Parkinson's disease (PD), the etiology of this condition is still unknown, and the medical and surgical therapies provide only symptomatic relief (1,2). Current working hypotheses are based on two major plausible explanations, the environmental and the genetic hypotheses (3). The scope of environmental factors on causation of PD is discussed in chapter 16. The genetic hypothesis, which gained popularity in the 1990s, stemmed from considerable progress in the development of new molecular genetic techniques and from the description of several large families with a parkinsonian phenotype in many cases closely resembling that of sporadic PD (4–6). However, genetic factors still do not explain the etiology of all cases of PD (7). Thus, a combination of environmental and inherited risk factors may play a crucial role in the development of disease in most cases of parkinsonism.

Understanding the etiology of PD is further complicated by a lack of *in vivo* biologic markers for diagnosis, which requires reliance on clinical or pathologic criteria (8,9). In addition, rather than being a uniform clinical and pathologic entity, PD represents a cluster of heterogeneous syndromes (10). In this chapter, we discuss the contributions of epidemiologic, twin, kindred, and genome-wide association studies in support of the genetic hypothesis of PD. We will also address some basic issues related to the clinical genetic testing for determination of carrier status.

EPIDEMIOLOGIC STUDIES

Epidemiologic studies indicate a genetic contribution to the pathogenesis of PD. Lazzarini and colleagues (11) found that the likelihood of persons in New Jersey having PD at age 80 years was about 2% for the general population and about 5–6% if a parent or sibling was affected. However, if both a parent and a sibling were affected, the probability of having PD increased up to 20–40%. Marder and colleagues (12) assessed the risk of PD among first-degree relatives living in the same geographic region. They found a 2% cumulative incidence of PD at age 75 years among first-degree relatives of patients with PD compared with a 1% incidence among first-degree relatives of control subjects. The risk of PD was greater in male than in female first-degree relatives [relative risk (RR): 2.0; 95% confidence interval (CI): 1.1–3.4]. The risk of PD in any first-degree relative was also higher for whites than for African-Americans or Hispanics (RR: 2.4; 95% CI: 1.4–4.1). However, Shino and colleagues (13) found the opposite, that the risk of PD in first-degree relatives was higher for Hispanics than for non-Hipanic Caucasian cases and controls (RR: 3.7%; 95% CI: 1.0–68.9). Rocca and colleagues (14) reported that relatives of probands who were younger (<66 years) at onset of PD had a significantly increased risk (RR: 2.62; 95% CI: 1.66–4.15), whereas relatives of probands with later onset had no increased risk.

In an Italian case–control study (15), history of familial PD was the most relevant risk factor [odds ratio (OR): 14.6; 95% CI: 7.2–29.6]. In a Canadian study of PD patients (16), the prevalence rate in first- and second-degree relatives was more than five times higher than that of the general population. Even patients who reported a negative family history of PD actually had a prevalence rate in relatives more than three times higher than that of the general population. A study of the Icelandic population (17) revealed the presence of genetic as well as environmental components in the etiology of late-onset PD (onset at >50 years of age). The risk ratio for PD in relatives of patients with late-onset PD was 6.7 (95% CI: 1.2–9.6) for siblings, 3.2 (95% CI: 1.2–7.8) for offspring, and 2.7 (95% CI: 1.6–3.9) for nephews and nieces. The findings of Maher and colleagues (18) for 203 sibling pairs with PD also supported a genetic contribution to the etiology of PD. Sibling pairs with PD were found to have greater similarity for age at symptomatic disease onset than for year of symptomatic disease onset. The frequency of PD in parents (7%) and siblings (5.1%) was greater than that in spouses (2%). Tracker and colleagues (19) conducted a literature-based meta-analysis and found that RR of PD for having a first-degree relative with PD was 2.9 (95% CI: 2.2–3.8). The RR for sibling pairs was 4.4 (95% CI: 3.1–6.1) and for child–parent pairs it was 2.7 (95% CI: 2.0–3.7).

Therefore, based on these studies, it is reasonable to assume that the siblings and/or children of patients affected with PD are at a higher risk of developing PD, but how significant such a risk is, cannot be easily determined particularly for a single case or family situation, and may also be dependent on the race and ethnicity.

STUDIES OF TWINS

Studies of twins may be used to estimate the genetic contribution to the etiology of a neurodegenerative condition. If a genetic component is present, concordance will be greater in monozygotic twins than in dizygotic twins. If a disorder is exclusively genetic in origin and the diagnosis is not compounded by age-associated penetrance, stochastic or environmental factors, monozygotic concordance may be close to 100%. However, PD is a heterogeneous, age-associated disease with reduced penetrance. Even within families in whom parkinsonism is caused by a single gene defect, the age at onset and the progression and severity of symptoms in affected carriers may vary widely. Thus, even large studies of hundreds of twin pairs are likely to be underpowered to exclude a genetic etiology (20).

Although earlier twin studies in PD were inconclusive (21–23), Tanner and colleagues (24) demonstrated the presence of genetic factors in the etiology of PD when disease begins at or before age 50 years. They studied twins enrolled in the twin registry of the National Academy of Science and the National Research Council World War II Veteran Twin Registry. No genetic component was evident when the onset of symptoms occurred after age 50 years. Wirdefeldt and colleagues (25) demonstrated low concordance rates in twins whether monozygotic or dizygotic, using the Swedish Twin Registry. However, both of these studies were largely based on limited, cross-sectional clinical observations (26). A more recent study by the same group with longitudinal and cross-sectional clinical analysis (27) demonstrated that PD and parkinsonism are moderately heritable.

Positron emission tomography (PET) studies with [18F] 6-fluorodopa (6-FD) may in part circumvent the need for extended follow-up. Indeed, reduced striatal uptake of 6-FD has been demonstrated in some clinically asymptomatic co-twins (28). Using longitudinal evaluation with measurement of 6-FD, Piccini and colleagues (29) demonstrated a 75% concordance rate in monozygotic twins versus 22% in dizygotic twins. These results must also be interpreted cautiously. At best, 6-FD uptake is only a surrogate marker of PD and the number of twins studied was relatively small.

EVALUATION OF KINDREDS

Kindreds with a parkinsonian phenotype have been reported in the world medical literature since the 19th century (30). In a 1926 literature review, Bell and Clark (31) described 10 families with "shaking palsy" believed to be hereditary. They also provided 20 references of earlier accounts of familial paralysis agitans. In 1937, Allen (32) detailed an additional 25 families with inherited parkinsonism and speculated that the inheritance was autosomal dominant and probably the result of a single autosomal gene in about two-thirds of these kindreds. In 1949, Mjönes (33) detailed 8 pedigrees with inherited parkinsonism, some with atypical features such as myoclonic epilepsy. In the levodopa era, numerous reports described families with PD and parkinsonism-plus syndrome (34), including two large multigenerational kindreds known as the Contursi and Family C (German-American) families (35,36). As molecular genetic techniques have improved, the importance of collecting data from parkinsonian families with PD has grown exponentially. With the newest molecular genetic techniques of exome and whole genome sequencing advancement and cost reduction, the need for finding large families with multiple members affected is less important as these new techniques allow finding the pathogenic gene mutations based on a smaller number of affected family members (37).

Eighteen genetic PARK loci have been identified (Table 15.1). At the present time, nine pathogenic PD/parkinsonism genes have been confirmed: *PARK1 alpha-synuclein (SNCA)* in 1997 (38), *PARK2 (parkin)* in 1998 (39), *PARK7 (DJ-1)* in 2003 (40), *PARK6 [PTEN-induced putative kinase 1 (PINK1)]* (41) and *PARK8 [leucine-rich repeat kinase 2 (LRRK2)]* in 2004 (42), *PARK9 [ATPase type 13A2 (ATP13A2)]* in 2006 (43), *PARK15 [F-Box only protein 7 (FBX07)]* in 2009 (44), and *PARK17 [vacuolar protein sorting 35 (VPS35)]* and (45,46) *PARK18 [eukaryotic translation initiation factor 4-gamma (eIF4G1)]* in 2011 (47). *PARK5 (UCHL1)* is associated with typical PD, but pathogenecity has not yet been fully established.

PD/Parkinsonism Genes/Loci with Autosomal Dominant Inheritance
PARK1: Alpha-Synuclein
In 1996, linkage analysis in a large family of Italian descent (Contursi), with a parkinsonian phenotype, mapped the *PARK1* locus on chromosome 4q21-q23 (48). In the next year, the first point mutation in the *SNCA* gene, p.A53T, was identified in this family and in three unrelated Greek families (38). Later, two additional rare point mutations were discovered, p.A30P in a German family (49) and p.E46K in Spanish families (50). As of November 2011, three pathogenic point mutations, p.A53T, p.A30P, and p.E46K, have been identified as associated with the *SNCA* gene (51). Besides point mutations, multiplication of the entire *SNCA* gene can also cause parkinsonism through a hypothesized mechanism of overexpression. Several families

TABLE 15.1 Familial Parkinson's Disease with Reported Mutations or Loci

Gene	Locus	MI	AAO	Phenotype	Progression	Pathology	LR
SNCA (PARK1, PARK4)	4q22.1	AD	PM: 20–85, DU: 38–77, TR: 20–48	PM: PD, De, Da[a]; DU: PD, De, Hu, Da[a], My[a]; TR: PD, De, Da, De, Hu, My[a]	PM, DU: C; TR: Rapid	PM, DU: LBs, PND; TR: LBs	Good
Parkin (PARK2)	6q26	AR	16–72	PD, Dy, Hy	Slow	PND, LBs, tau	Good
PARK3	2p13	AD	36–89	PD, De[a]	Unclear	LBs, AD-Path	Good
UCHL1 (PARK5)	4p13	AD	49–58	PD	Slow	NA	Good
PINK1 (PARK6)	1p36.12	AR	20–40	PD	Slow	LBs[b]	Good
DJ-1 (PARK7)	1p36.23	AR	20–40	PD	Slow	NA	Good
LRRK2 (PARK8)	12q12	AD	32–79	PD	C	LBs, NFTs, PND	Good
ATP13A2 (PARK9)	1p36.13	AR	11–40	PD, De, SGP	Rapid	NA	Good
PARK10	1p32	UD	Unclear	Unclear	Unclear	NA	Good
PARK11	2q37.1	AD	49–75	PD, De[a]	Unclear	NA	Good
PARK12	Xq21–q25	X	Unclear	Unclear	Unclear	NA	Unclear
PARK13	2p13.1	AD	44–81	PD	Unclear	NA	Unclear
PLA2G6 (PARK14)	22q13.1	AR	1–30	PD, De, Dy, E, Py, Ps	Unclear	LBs, tau, NFTs, NASs	Good
FBXO7 (PARK15)	22q12.3	AR	10–19	PD, Py, SGP, Dy	Unclear	NA	Good
PARK16	1q32	UD	Unclear	PD	Unclear	NA	Unclear
VPS35 (PARK17)	16q11.2	AD	46–64	PD	Slow	NA[c]	Good
eIF4G1 (PARK18)	3q27.1	AD	40–64	PD, De, PDD	Slow	LBs	Good

[a]Symptom which sometimes occurs.

[b]Only one case available.

[c]Only a limited brain tissue from one patient available from necropsy.

Abbreviations: AAO, age at onset; AD, autosomal dominant; AD-Path, Alzheimer-type pathology; AR, autosomal recessive; ATP13A2, ATPase type 13A2; C, consistence with sporadic PD; Da, dysautonomia; De, dementia; Du, duplication; Dy, dystonia; E, epilepsy; eIF4G1, eukaryotic translation initiation factor 4-gamma; FBXO7, F-box only protein 7; Hy, hyperreflexia; Hu, hallucination; LBs, Lewy bodies; LR, levodopa-responsiveness; LRRK2, leucine-rich repeat kinase 2; MI, mode of inheritance; My, myoclonus; NA, not available; NASs, neuroaxonal spheroids; NFTs, neurofibrillary tangles; PD, Parkinson's disease; PDD, Parkinson's disease with dementia; PINK1, PTEN-induced putative kinase 1; PLA2G6, phospholipase A2, group 6; PM, point mutation; PND, pure nigral degeneration; Ps, psychiatric symptoms; Py, pyramidal sign; SGP, supranuclear gaze palsy; SNCA, alpha-synuclein; TR, triplication; UCHL1, ubiquitin carboxy-terminal hydrolase L1; UD, undetermined; VPS35, vacuolar protein sorting 35; X, X-linked.

have been described with *SNCA* gene triplications and duplications (52–55). Tripli-cation of the *SNCA* gene was first discovered in a family clinically characterized by early-onset parkinsonism and dementia initially referred to as *PARK4* (55). Duplica-tion of the *SNCA* gene was first observed in a French family (53). PD with the *SNCA* triplication presents earlier and with a faster clinical course compared with PD with known point mutations or duplication of the *SNCA* gene. This suggests that disease severity is dependent on alpha-synuclein expression level.

Alpha-synuclein is abundant in the brain and is a highly soluble neuronal cytoplasmic protein. Alpha-synuclein is mainly localized to presynaptic terminals in the central nervous system (56). Aggregated alpha-synuclein is the major compo-nent of Lewy bodies, the pathologic hallmark of PD. Potentially, aggregation of alpha-synuclein plays a role in the pathogenesis of PD, inducing cell death and affecting various mitochondrial pathways (57). However, the precise mechanisms by which the *SNCA* gene point mutations lead to aggregation of the toxic mutant protein are still largely unknown.

PARK3: Gene Unknown
In 1998, linkage analysis in six families of German-American and Danish-American origin (including the previously mentioned Family C) with a typical parkinsonian phenotype and some cases with dementia (58), mapped the *PARK3* locus on chro-mosome 2p13. Linkage to the *PARK3* locus was also confirmed in several other families (59,60); however, the *PARK3* gene has not yet been identified. Among a number of candidate genes, the *sepiapterin reductase* gene is thought to be a candi-date gene for *PARK3* (61,62).

PARK5: Ubiquitin Carboxy-Terminal Hydrolase L1
In 1998, a point mutation, p.I93M, in the *ubiquitin carboxy-terminal hydrolase L1* (*UCHL1*) gene was identified in a single German sib-pair with a clinical phenotype resembling typical PD (63). Lincoln and colleagues (64) identified the new polymor-phic variant p.S18Y in an English PD family and four unrelated PD cases. Since then, several reports (65) failed to confirm the evidence of *UCHL1* as a susceptibility gene for PD. However, the meta-analysis of the PD population of European ances-try (66) showed moderate evidence of the *UCHL1* gene as a susceptibility gene for PD. UCHL1 is one of the most abundant proteins in the brain (67), and also found in Lewy bodies. It plays a pivotal role in the ubiquitin-proteasomal system (67). UCHL1 functions as the dimerization-dependent E3 ubiquitin ligase, which pro-motes alpha-synuclein aggregation (68).

PARK8: Leucine-Rich Repeat Kinase 2
Linkage analysis revealed *PARK8* locus on chromosome 12p11.2-q13.1 in a large Japanese family in 2002 (5). The LRRK2 mutations, p.R1441C, p.R1441G, p.Y1699C, and p.I2020T were then identified by two different groups in 2004 (42,69). Subse-quently, the most common LRRK2 mutation, p.G2019S, was discovered in 2005 (70–73), and p.N1437H was found in a large Norwegian family in 2010 (74). A num-ber of other genetic variants have been reported; however, the established patho-genic mutations include p.R1441C, p.R1441G, p.R1441H, p.Y1699C, p.G2019S, p.I2020T, and p.N1437H (51). Nonetheless, the LRRK2 p.G2019S mutation is the most common form of genetic parkinsonism identified to date (75) accounting for 1–2 % of sporadic and 5–10% of autosomal dominant PD cases in Caucasians in

North America (75). The variety of the *LRRK2* gene mutation depends on ethnicity. For example, the LRRK2 p.G2019S mutation has been found in up to approximately 40% of PD cases in North-African Arabs and Ashkenazi Jews (76), whereas it is rare in Asian populations (77). On the other hand, the p.R1441G mutation can be observed frequently in individuals of Basque ancestry (78), and the p.R1441C mutation is frequent in Belgian ancestry (79). The affected patients present with levodopa-responsive parkinsonism. Subclinical manifestations in apparently healthy *LRRK2* gene mutation carriers have been described (80). Pathologic examination revealed nigral neuronal loss and Lewy body pathology in most of the cases (81,82); however, some cases were associated with tau pathology (83) or did not present with Lewy body pathology (84). Several LRRK2 variants, p.G2385R, p.R1628P, p.M1646T, and p.A419V are thought to be risk factors for PD.

LRRK2 is a protein kinase widely expressed in many organs and tissues, including the brain (69). The *LRRK2* gene encodes a large multidomain protein and the amino acid changes are concentrated in the central region of the protein. The region includes the Ras of complex protein (Roc) domain, C-terminal of Roc (COR), and kinase domain. The Roc domain contains p.R1441C, p.R1441G, p.R1441H, and p.N1437H mutations; COR domain p.Y1699C mutation; and the kinase domain p.G2019S and p.I2020T mutations (85). LRRK2 is thought to act upstream of alpha-synuclein depositions; however, the pathogenic impact of mutant LRRK2 is still unclear.

PARK11: Grb10-Interacting GYF Protein 2
A genome-wide screen performed on 150 families with typical late-onset PD (86) revealed *PARK11* locus on 2q36-37 in 2003. Seven heterozygous mutations were identified in the *Grb10-interacting GYF protein 2 (GIGYF2)* gene in French and Italian familial cases with a typical PD phenotype, but not in controls (87); however, no *GIGYF2* gene mutations have been identified in other populations (88). GIGYF2 interacts with Grb10 adaptor protein, which is involved in insulin signaling (89). The insulin pathway is thought to be implicated in the pathogenesis of PD (90). However, pathogenicity of the *GIGYF2* gene mutations for PD has not been confirmed and does not account for the *PARK11* linkage in the original families (91).

PARK13: Omi/High Temperature Requirement Protein A2
By mutation screening of the *Omi/high temperature requirement protein A2 (Omi/HtrA2)* gene, one heterozygous mutation, p.G399S, was identified in four patients from 512 German PD collections in 2005 (92). However, pathogenicity of the *Omi/HtrA2* gene mutations has not been confirmed in other populations (93–95). Omi/HtrA2 is a protease that localizes to the mitochondrial intermembrane space (96). *In vivo*, loss of Omi/HtrA2 function is related to the phenotype mimicking parkinsonism (97).

PARK17: Vacuolar Protein Sorting 35
Wider and colleagues (98) initially reported a Swiss family with a typical PD phenotype in 2008. The mean age at disease onset was approximately 51 years. The clinical phenotype was slowly progressive, tremor-predominant, levodopa-responsive parkinsonism. Fluorodopa PET presented a marked asymmetric striatal tracer uptake deficiency as in idiopathic PD. By exome sequencing (45), a heterozygous mutation, p.D620N in the *VPS35* gene was identified on chromosome 16p11.2.

Zimprich and colleagues (46) discovered the VPS35 p.D620N and p.R524W mutations in three Austrian families with a typical parkinsonian phenotype. Sheerin and colleagues (99) investigated 160 familial PD cases, 175 young-onset PD cases, and 262 sporadic, neuropathologically confirmed PD cases for the *VPS35* gene mutations. They found one individual harboring the p.D620N mutation with an autosomal dominant family history of PD. VPS35 is a critical component of retromer cargo-recognition complex (45). Thus, the discovery of *VPS35* mutations suggests dysfunction of retromer in neurodegenerative processes in PD.

PARK18: Eukaryotic Translation Initiation Factor 4-Gamma

Five missense mutations, p.R1205H, p.A502V, p.G686C, p.R1197W, and p.S1164R in the *eIF4G1* gene on chromosome 3q27.1 were identified by genome-wide linkage analysis (47). Chartier-Harlin and colleagues investigated 4708 individuals with idiopathic PD and 4050 controls for the eIF4G1 p.R1205H mutation and found nine affected PD patients from seven families. They also screened 4483 individuals with idiopathic PD and 3865 controls for the other eIF4G1 variants and identified two PD cases with the p.A502V mutation from two families and two PD cases with the p.G686C mutation from one family. The majority of the affected patients manifested levodopa-responsive parkinsonism with asymmetric resting tremor and rigidity, and the minority presented with dementia or parkinsonism and dementia (47). eIF4G1 complex helps regulate translation of mRNA and eIF4G1 depletion causes impairment of mitochondrial function leading to the inability of cells to respond to the stress.

PD/Parkinsonism Genes/Loci with Autosomal Recessive Inheritance

PARK2: Parkin

PARK2 locus was mapped to chromosome 6q25.2-q27 in juvenile Japanese PD patients with early-onset parkinsonism with other neurologic symptoms such as dystonia and hyperreflexia in 1997 (100). The next year, deletions in the *parkin* gene were discovered in one of the original Japanese PD families (39). Since then, a number of the *parkin* gene mutations have been reported. *Parkin* gene mutations are the most common autosomal recessive PD gene mutations, accounting for about 50% of early-onset autosomal recessive PD and 10–20% of early-onset sporadic PD (27). As of November 2011, more than 120 pathogenic allelic variants have been identified that are associated with the *parkin* gene (51). Parkin is an E3 ubiquitin ligase and is abundant in the brain, including the substantia nigra (39). Mutant parkin causes a loss of normal E3 ubiqutin ligase activity leading to the accumulation of its substrates. One of the substrates is the glycosylated form of alpha-synuclein (101).

PARK6: PTEN-Induced Putative Kinase 1

PARK6 locus was mapped on chromosome 1p35-p36 in a large Italian family with a slowly progressive PD phenotype in 2001 (102). In 2004, two homozygous point mutations, p.G309A and p.W437OPA, in the *PINK1* gene were identified in an Italian family and a Spanish family with early-onset and slowly progressive PD (41). As of November 2011, more than 25 pathogenic mutations have been identified (51). Frequency of the *PINK1* gene mutations in PD patients has been estimated to be between 0.5% and 9% (27). PINK1 is mitochondrial kinase, which protects cells against oxidative stress–induced apoptosis (41). Mutant PINK1 can lead to apoptosis of dopaminergic cells. PINK1 is thought to interact with parkin to modulate mitochondrial degradation, termed mitophagy (103,104).

PARK7: DJ-1

PARK7 locus was mapped on chromosome 1p36 in a Dutch family with early-onset PD in 2001 (40). In 2003, two homozygous mutations in the DJ-1 gene were identified in Dutch and Italian families (105). Several other DJ-1 mutations have been discovered; however, the DJ-1 mutations seem to be more rare than the par-kin and PINK1 mutations (106). As of November 2011, six pathogenic mutations have been identified as associated with the DJ-1 gene (51). DJ-1 is a ubiquitous protein highly expressed in both neurons and astrocytes in the brain including the basal ganglia, substantia nigra, and many other lesions (59). The function of DJ-1 is still unknown; however, DJ-1 may play an important role in the modulation of transcription, chaperone-like functions, and antioxidant properties (107). Several studies (108) suggest that DJ-1 may directly act to prevent alpha-synuclein aggregation.

PARK9: ATPase Type 13A2

The PARK9 locus was mapped on chromosome 1p36 in the Kufor–Rakeb kindred, with affected family members having atypical parkinsonism associated with dementia, spasticity, and supranuclear gaze palsy (109). Homozygous and compound heterozygous mutations were identified in the ATPase type 13A2 (ATP13A2) gene in a Jordanian family and Chilean family in 2006 (43). Genetic screening of early onset of PD observed several other mutations (110–113).

The ATP13A2 gene is widely expressed in the brain, including the substantia nigra (43). Several studies suggested that ATP13A2 might be involved in protecting cells against alpha-synuclein toxicity (114). Lysosome has been recognized to play an important role in the etiology of PD, and ATP13A2 is localized in lysosome, which indicates the association of this protein with the pathogenesis of PD (115).

PARK14: Phospholipase A2, Group 6

Phospholipase A2, group 6 (PLA2G6) gene mutations were initially identified by Morgan and colleagues (116) in 31 cases of infantile neuroaxonal dystrophy (IND) and neurodegeneration with brain iron accumulation (NBIA). Later, two homozygous mutations in the PLA2G6 gene were also discovered in two unrelated Pakistani families with dystonia-parkinsonism (117). The phenotype of these cases was different from that of the cases of IND and NBIA clinically and radiologically. Since then, some other mutations have been discovered associated with the dystonia-parkinsonism phenotype (118,119). According to a report (120), the PLA2G6 gene mutation can also present with the phenotype of frontotemporal dementia. PLA2G6 is an enzyme that catalyzes the release of fatty acids from phospholipids. At the present time, little is known about the association between mutant PLA2G6 and the phenotype of dystonia-parkinsonism. However, PLA2G6 gene mutations carriers have been shown to present both with Lewy body and tau aggregates (110), which indicates shared pathologic pathways.

PARK15: F-Box Only Protein 7

Davison (121) reported parkinsonism accompanied with spasticity in 1954. Genome-wide linkage analyses (44) identified a homozygous mutation in the FBXO7 gene in an Iranian family with parkinsonian-pyramidal syndrome in 2008. Another homozygous mutation and a compound heterozygous mutation in the FBXO7 gene were found in Italian and Dutch families (122). FBXO7 codes for a member of the F-box family of proteins. FBXO7 immunoreactivity was observed in the nuclei of neurons of the cerebral cortex, globus pallidum, and substantia nigra (123). FBXO7 is thought to play a role in the ubiquitin-proteosome protein-degradation pathway (44).

PD Gene Associated with X-Linked Inheritance
PARK12: Gene Unknown
Pankratz and colleagues (86) performed a multipoint nonparametric linkage analysis on 160 PD families and identified the *PARK12* locus on chromosome Xq21-25 in 2002. Other studies (124,125) also detected this locus; however, the *PARK12* gene has not yet been discovered.

PD Loci with Undetermined Mode of Inheritance
PARK10: Gene Unknown
In 2002, genome-wide linkage analysis on 117 late-onset PD patients from 51 Icelandic families with a typical PD phenotype (124) revealed the *PARK10* locus on chromosome 1p32. The *PARK10* locus was also linked to PD in patients in the United States (126), however, not in other populations. Several genes were reported as candidate genes for the *PARK10* (127–130); however, the pathogenic gene mutation or mutations have not yet been identified.

PARK16: Gene Unknown
PARK16 locus on chromosome 1q32 was discovered by a large association study in the Japanese population in 2009 (131). Another genome-wide linkage analysis from Germany, the United Kingdom, and the United States (132,133) confirmed the same location as a susceptibility locus, however, two other studies (134,135) failed to replicate this locus. Additional PARK loci and contributing genes are likely to be identified through family studies, ultimately facilitating a molecular rather than a clinicopathologic diagnosis. Mutations in the genes implicated in parkinsonism have already been used to create *in vivo* models. These can recapitulate the etiology as well as the symptoms of disease, and they may provide powerful insight into neuronal degeneration. They facilitate validation of biomarkers of disease progression and neuroprotection strategies (102,136). These new tools bring the hope of novel therapies for PD designed to address the causes rather than merely the symptoms of the disease.

Table 15.1 summarizes the status of the current knowledge about the mendelian genetics of PD. It shows genes, the location of known chromosomal loci, the types of inheritance, and clinical and pathologic data for each gene and locus.

Genetic Variants/Susceptibility PD Genes in Mendelian Genes
LRRK2 Variants
The LRRK2 p.R1628P and p.G2385R mutations increase PD risk in East Asian populations (137–140). Tan and colleagues (141) reported that the heterogeneous p.R1628P genotype was associated with an increased risk of PD compared with the controls (OR: 3.3; 95% CI: 1.4–7.9). Kim and colleagues (142) indicated the highest frequency of p.G2385R variants in PD compared with the controls. Ross and colleagues (143) identified new independent risk associations with p.M1646T (OR: 1.43; 95% CI: 1.15–1.78) in Caucasian individuals and p.A419V (OR: 2.27; 95% CI: 1.35–3.83) in Asian individuals.

SNCA Variants
Haplotypic analysis showed that genetic availability in the promoter and toward the 3' end of the gene was associated with PD (144,145). According to the PDGene Database (146), allele length variability in a dinucleotide repeat sequence in the *SNCA* gene (*SNCA* Rep1) has been associated with an increased risk of PD (147).

MAPT: Microtubule-Associated Protein Tau
The *MAPT* gene mutations were initially identified as causative for frontotemporal dementia with parkinsonism linked to chromosome 17 (148). Pastor and colleagues (149) reported a significant association between the *MAPT* A0/A0 genotype and PD. Several other studies supported the significant association between the *MAPT* H1 haplotype and PD (150–152). Elbaz and colleagues investigated the independent effects and joint effects of the *MAPT* H1 haplotype and *SNCA* single nucleotide polymorphisms (SNPs) (153). They found a strong association between *SNCA* SNPs and PD as well as the *MAPT* H1 haplotype and PD; however, there was no evidence of interaction between any *SNCA* SNPs and the *MAPT* H1 haplotype.

GBA: Glucocerebrosidase
Gaucher's disease is a recessive lysosomal storage disorder caused by loss of function of the enzyme GBA (154). Three phenotypes have been reported: Absence (type 1), presence of neurologic involvement during childhood (type 2), and adolescence (type 3) (154). Homozygous mutations in the *GBA* gene cause Gaucher's disease (154). According to a worldwide, multicenter analysis, a strong association between heterozygous *GBA* gene mutations and PD (155) is present. The OR for the *GBA* gene mutations in PD patients compared with that in controls was 5.43, and the symptomatic age at onset of the *GBA* gene mutation carriers was earlier than that of noncarriers. Heterozygous *GBA* gene mutations also increase the risk for dementia with Lewy bodies (156). Nishioka and colleagues (157) investigated 59 pathologically confirmed diffuse Lewy body disease cases and identified four cases with *GBA* gene mutations.

Hereditary Parkinsonism with Non-PARK Genes/Loci
Besides parkinsonism with PARK genes or loci, there are some disorders with known gene mutations that can present with parkinsonian phenotypes. Table 15.2 summarizes the status of the current knowledge of genetics of familial parkinsonism with non-PARK genes or loci. The table includes genes, the location of known chromosomal loci, the types of inheritance, and clinical data.

ASSOCIATION STUDIES AND GENOME-WIDE ASSOCIATION STUDIES
Despite substantial progress in identification, there are still only few known large pedigrees with PD. Furthermore, genetic linkage studies that use "identity-by-descent" mapping have been hampered because of the limited amount of DNA available from affected pedigree members, because of death, lack of consent, or geographic dispersion. Association or "identity-by-state" mapping is an alternative approach using groups of unrelated persons. Association studies measure differences in genetic variability between a group with the disease in question and a group of age, gender, and ethnically matched normal individuals. This method is most powerful in implicating common genetic risk factors for multigenic traits in homogeneous population isolates. Many studies have been confounded by

TABLE 15.2 Examples of Hereditary Parkinsonism with Non-PARK Genes

Disease/Syndrome	Gene	Locus	MI	AAO (average)	Neurologic Phenotype	LR for PD
SCA2	SCA 2	12q24.12	AD	2–65 (30)	C, PD, SS, O, Ch, PD, A	Good
SCA3	SCA 3	14q32.12	AD	Type 1: 10–30 Type 2: 20–50 Type 3: 40–75 Type 4: variable	Type 1: O, Py, Dy, C Type 2: C, Py Type 3: C, PN Type 4: PD, PN	Good*
SCA8	SCA8	13q21	AD	0–73 (38)	C, D, Py, PN, Dysp, PD	May be good
SCA12	PPP2R2B	5q32	AD	8–62 (40)	C, T, Py, D, PD	Unclear
SCA17	TBP	6q27	AD	3–55 (30)	C, D, Ps, PD, Dys, Py, E	Good
DYT5	GCH1	14q22.2	AD	1–12 (5)	Dyst, PD, DF	Good
DYT12	ATP1A3	19q13.2	AD	4–55	Dyst, P[b], Ps	Poor
FTDP-17T	MAPT	17q21.31	AD	25–76 (49)	Pe, B, PD, SGP, Dyst	Maybe good
FTDP-17U	PGRN	17q21.31	AD	48–83 (59)	B, L, PD, MND	Maybe good
FTD-3	CHMP2B	3p11.2	AD	46–65 (57)	Pe, B, PD, Py	Unclear
FTD	FUS	16p11.2	AD	35–74 (42)	Pe, B, PD, Ch	Unclear
FTD	C9ORF72	9p21.2	AD	31–65 (44)	Pe, B, C, MND, PD	Unclear
PS	DCTN1	2p13.1	AD	30–61 (46)	P, Hypov, W, Ps	Good[a]
NF	FTL	19q13.33	AD	10–63 (40)	Dyst, Ch, PD, Py, D, C	Poor
HD	HTT, IT15	4p16.3	AD	2–80 (40)	Ch, D, PD, De	Unclear
HDLS	CSF1R	5q32	AD	18–78 (39)	D, Ps, PD, Py, CBS	Poor
Prion disease	PRNP	20p13	AD	fCJD: 20th–80th GSS: 40th–60th FFI: 40th–50th	fCJD: D, C, My, PD, CBS, E, Ch GSS: C, D, Py, PD, Ps, B, Dysp FFI: I, A, O, D	Unclear
DYT5	TH	11p15.5	AR	Mild type: childhood Severe type: ~6M	Mild type: Dyst, T Severe type: Dyst, PD, DP, A	Mild form: good Severe form: poor
DYT16	PRKRA	2q31.2	AR	2–18 (9)	Dyst, PD, Dysp, Ps, Py	Poor
SPG11	Spatacsin	15q21.1	AR	1–31 (10th–20th)	Py[b], W[c], D, MR, PN, PD, Dyst, Dysp	Maybe initially
WD	ATP7B	13q14.3	AR	3–50th (21)	PD, Ch, Ps, B, D	May be poor

(Continued)

TABLE 15.2 Examples of Hereditary Parkinsonism with Non-PARK Genes (*Continued*)

Disease/Syndrome	Gene	Locus	MI	AAO (average)	Neurologic Phenotype	LR for P
NPC	NPC1	18q11.2	AR	Neonatal-adult	Neonatal/infantile: Hypot, DPD; Childhood: C, O, D, Dyst, E, Dysp; Adolescent/adults: D, Ps, PD	May be poor
PKAN	PANK2	20p13	AR	Classic type: 3–30 (185); Atypical type: ~30th (14)	Classic type: Dyst, PD, Py, PR; Atypical type: Ps, Pe, D, L, Dyst, Py, PD	May be partially
CHAC	VPS13A	9q21.2	AR	10th–70th (30)	Cho, PD, Dyst, D, B, E, PN, Myoc	Unclear
DYT3	TAF1	Xq13.1	X	Male: 12–64 (39); Female: 26–75 (52)	PD, Dyst, Cho[b], Myoc	May be good in early stage
FXTAS	FMR1	Xq27.3	X	(62)	C, T, PD, PN, A[b]	May be good

[a]With high dose.

[b]Predominantly seen in lower extremities.

Abbreviations: A, autonomic dysfunction; AAO, age at onset; ATP1A3, ATPase, Na+/K+ transporting, alpha-3 polypeptide; ATP7B, ATPase, Cu2+-transporting, beta polypeptide; C, cerebellar sign; CBS, corticobasal syndrome; Ch, chorea; CHAC, Chorea-acanthocytosis; CHMP2B, CHMP family, member 2B; CSF1R, colony-stimulating factor 1 receptor; C9ORF72, chromosome 9 open reading frame 72; D, dementia; DCTN1, dynactin 1; DF, diurnal fluctuation; DPD, delay in psychomotor development; Dyst, dystonia; Dysp, dysphasia; DYT, dystonia; E, epilepsy; fCJD, familial Creutzfeldt-Jakob disease; FTD, frontotemporal dementia; FTDP-17T, frontotemporal dementia and parkinsonism linked to chromosome 17 associated with tau gene mutations; FTDP-17U, frontotemporal dementia and parkinsonism linked to chromosome 17 associated with ubiquitin- and TDP-43-positive inclusions in the frontotemporal cortex, striatum and hippocampus; FFI, fatal familial insomnia; FTL, ferritin light chain; FUS, fused in sarcoma; FXTAS, fragile X-associated tremor/ataxia syndrome; GCH1, GTP cyclohydrolase 1; GSS, Gerstrann–Sträussler–Scheinker syndrome; HD, Huntington disease; HDLS, hereditary diffuse leukoencephalopathy with spheroids; HTT, huntingtin; Hypot, hypotonia; Hypov, hypoventilation; I, insomnia; L, language problem; LB, Lewy bodies; LR, levodopa-responsiveness; M, months; MAPT, microtubule-associated protein tau; MI, mode of inheritance; MND, motor neuron disease; MR, mental retardation; Myoc, myoclonus; Myop, myopathy; NF, neuroferritinopathy; NPC, Niemann–Pick disease, type C; O, ophthalmoparesis; PANK2, pantothenate kinase 2; PD, Parkinson's disease; Pe, personality change; PGRN, progranulin; PIE, progressive infantile encephalopathy; PKAN, pantothenate kinase-associated neurodegeneration; PN, peripheral neuropathy; PPP2R2B, protein phosphatase 2, regulatory subunit B, beta; PR, pigmentary retinopathy; PRKRA, protein kinase, interferon-inducible double-stranded RNA dependent activator; PRNP, prion protein; Ps, psychiatric syndrome; PS, Perry syndrome; Py, pyramidal sign; SCA, spinocerebellar ataxia; SGP, supranuclear gaze palsy; SPG, spastic paraplegia; SS, slow saccade; T, tremor; TAF1, transcription initiation factor TFIID subunit 1; TBP, TATA box-binding protein; TH, tyrosine hydroxylase; VPS13A, vacuolar protein sorting 13, yeast, homolog of; A; W, weakness; WD, Wilson's disease; X, X-linked.

misconceived *a priori* notions about the causes of disease, by the candidate genes or variants chosen for analysis, and by clinical, locus, and allelic heterogeneity. Results must be reproducible, preferably in different ethnic populations, and the genetic variability associated with disease should have some functional consequence (either directly or in disequilibrium) that alters gene expression or the resultant protein.

The genes for *SNCA, parkin, UCHL1, PINK1, DJ-1, LRRK2, ATP13A2, PLA2G6, FBXO7, VPS35, and eIF4G1* harbor mutations that segregate with parkinsonism in affected family members. Although the relevance of these findings for sporadic PD is still unclear, these proteins may mark pathways that are perturbed in both familial and sporadic PD. Understanding the components of the pathway and its regulation is the first step toward elucidating the molecular causes of parkinsonism (158). In some studies, common genetic variability in genes for *SNCA* (159,160), *parkin* (161), *UCHL1* (162,163), *PINK1* (164,165), *DJ-1* (106,166), and *LRRK2* (143,158,167) has been implicated in sporadic PD by association. These genes clearly contribute to risk in at least a subset of patients with idiopathic PD.

Mendelian forms of parkinsonism are rare compared with the far more common typical PD. Genetic and environmental factors are believed to moderate disease risk. Therefore, the traditional association studies are limited to identifying loci detectable by linkage analysis. Advances in genotyping technology have allowed rapid genome-wide screening of common variants in large populations. The first genome-wide association study in PD was performed in 2005 by Maraganore and colleagues (168), although the results did not reach genome-wide significance. Subsequently, several genome-wide association studies (7,131,169–174) have been performed on PD cases (Table 15.3). According to these data, *SNCA* and *MAPT* have consistently shown associations. *LRRK2* and *BST1* have been implicated in some studies but these associations have not been completely replicated. However, there are some limitations to genome-wide association studies. One of the limitations is that all gene association studies can have both false-positive and false-negative errors due to the number of comparisons performed per study. To avoid this problem, future analyses should employ highly stringent statistical correction procedures for data assessments (175). Another limitation is that genome-wide association studies can only identify genes that exhibit significant main effects; genes that require the interacting factor to be included in the study to show their association with disease are missed. Therefore, despite the success of these studies, the heredity of common disorders cannot be completely explained by genetic factors. To solve such a problem, future genome-wide gene–environment studies could potentially address this deficiency. Hamza and colleagues (176) performed the genome-wide association and interaction study, in which they tested each SNP's main effect plus its interaction with coffee. In this study, the most significant signal was identified from rs4998386 in the *GRIN2A* gene and its signal was present in heavy coffee-drinkers (OR: 0.43; $P = 6 \times 10^{-7}$) but not in light coffee-drinkers. Furthermore, among the heavy coffee-drinkers, rs4998386_T carriers had lower PD risk than rs4998386_CC carriers (OR: 0.59; $P = 1 \times 10^{-3}$). Compared with light coffee-drinkers with the rs4998386_CC genotype, heavy coffee-drinkers with this genotype had 18% lower PD risk. On the other hand, heavy coffee-drinkers with this genotype had a 59% lower risk. Future research may require testing of the gene–environment interactions on a whole genome scale and the whole genome scale sequences between gene and environmental factors.

TABLE 15.3   Examples of Association Results From Previous Genome-Wide Association Studies

Country or Population	Number of PD/Controls	Genes with Strong Association with PD	OR	*P* Value	References
Japan	2011/18381	SNCA	1.4	7.3×10^{-17}	Satake et al. (131)
		PARK16	1.3	1.5×10^{-12}	
		BST1	1.2	3.9×10^{-9}	
		LRRK2	1.3	2.7×10^{-8}	
Europe	3361/4573	MAPT	0.8	2.0×10^{-16}	Simón-Sánchez
		SNCA	1.2	2.2×10^{-16}	et al. (169)
United States	2000/1986	SNCA	1.4	3.4×10^{-11}	Hamza et al. (170)
		HLA-DRA	1.3	2.9×10^{-8}	
United States, Europe	7053/9007	SNCA	1.3	4.2×10^{-23}	Nalls et al. (172)
		MAPT	0.8	1.4×10^{-13}	
		BST1	0.9	2.4×10^{-9}	
		LRRK2	1.3	1.1×10^{-8}	
United States	3426/29624	LRRK2	9.6	1.8×10^{-28}	Do et al. (7)
		GBA	4.0	5.2×10^{-21}	
		SNCA	1.3	2.3×10^{-19}	
		MAPT	0.8	2.7×10^{-14}	
		MCCC1/LAMP3	0.8	2.7×10^{-10}	
		SCARB2	0.8	7.6×10^{-10}	
		GAK	1.3	3.9×10^{-8}	
United States, Europe	12386/21026	STX1B		2.7×10^{-12}	Plagnol et al. (174)
		FGF20		7.5×10^{-11}	
		RAB7L1/PARK16		1.0×10^{-10}	
		GPNMB		3.3×10^{-10}	
		STBD1		7.5×10^{-10}	
		MMP16		2.3×10^{-9}	
		NMD3		1.8×10^{-8}	

Abbreviations: BST1, bone marrow stromal cell antigen 1; fibroblast growth factor 20; GAK, cyclin G-associated kinase; GBA, glucosidase, beta, acid; FGF20, GPNMB, glycoprotein NMB; HLA-DRA, major histocompatibility complex, class II, DR alpha; LAMP3, lysosome-associated membrain protein 3; LRRK2, leucine-rich repeat kinase 2; MAPT, microtubule-associated protein tau; MCCC1, methylcrotonyl-CoA carboxylase 1; MMP16, matrix metalloproteinase 16; NMD3, S. cerevisiae, homolog of; OR, odds ratio; PD, Parkinson's disease; RAB7L1, RAB7-like 1; SCARB2, scavenger receptor class B, member 2; SNCA, alpha-synuclein; STBD1, starch-binding domain-containing protein 1; STX1B, syntaxin 1B.

DIGENIC INHERITANCE

It has been proposed in families with an autosomal recessive inheritance pattern, that the interaction of two genes may strengthen the expression of a phenotype, a mechanism referred to as digenic inheritance. PD patients carrying both the heterozygous PINK1 p.A39S mutation and heterozygous DJ-1 p.P399L mutation were reported by Tang and colleagues in 2006 (177). Two individuals harboring both mutations presented with the typical PD phenotype. The average age at disease onset was 26.5 years, which was younger than that of the symptomatic carriers with only one of the heterozygous gene mutations. However, one family member carrying both gene mutations was still an asymptomatic carrier at the age of 42 years. Dächsel and colleagues (178) identified three Spanish PD patients, two sporadic cases harboring compound heterozygotes with the parkin p.M192V mutation and the LRRK2 p.R1441G mutation, and one familial case carrying compound heterozygotes with the parkin p.N52Stop80 mutation and the LRRK2 p.R1441G mutation. The patients harboring digenic mutations did not present with an earlier age of disease onset, a faster progression of disease, or any exhibited clinical differences compared with the patients with either a *parkin* or *LRRK2* gene mutation alone. Funayama and colleagues (179) detected two sibling pairs and one sporadic PD case harboring both the parkin p.T175PfsX2 mutation and PINK1 p.R58_V59insGR mutation in Japan. The patients carrying both the homozygous *parkin* mutation and the heterozygous *PINK1* mutation had an earlier symptomatic disease onset than the patients with only the homozygous *parkin* mutation. These results may indicate an interaction between the *parkin* and *PINK1* gene. Charles and colleagues (180) reported two siblings harboring both the *SCA2* repeat expansion and the LRRK2 p.G2019S mutation. The age at disease onset in both was earlier than their parent, with only the *SCA* repeat expansion, indicating the additive interaction between the *SCA2* and the *LRRK2* genes.

PHENOCOPY

Phenocopy means the nonhereditary phenotype identical to the one of another individual whose phenotype is produced by the genotype (181). Phenocopy also indicates the individuals with mutations different from the main genetic cause in a given family and the individuals with an unknown environmental or genetic cause of the disorder (182). Latourelle and colleagues (183) identified the frequency of over 14% for phenocopies in the pedigrees of PD with the *LRRK2* gene mutations. Klein and colleagues (182) reviewed publications from 1997 to 2009, regarding familial PD with *SNCA, LRRK2, parkin*, and *PINK1* mutations. Of all patients with clinical PD, 5% of affected individuals from approximately 14% of all selected pedigrees represented phenocopies. Among these mutations, the *SNCA* gene was most frequent to have phenocopies (20%), followed by the *LRRK2* gene (18%). An overall phenocopy rate of 3.8% of all blood relatives was reported in the pedigrees containing phenocopies and 1.3% in the entire study sample. This retrospective study has several limitations, so prospective studies may identify an even higher frequency of phenocopies in familial PD.

CLINICAL MOLECULAR GENETIC TESTING

At present, diagnostic molecular genetic testing is commercially available for five PD genes, *SNCA, parkin, PINK1, DJ-1*, and *LRRK2* (184). Diagnostic genetic testing is not essential in the current management of PD patients. However, if genetic testing is performed, it would likely have the greatest yield in the early-onset PD cases, as they most frequently have *parkin* or *PINK1* gene mutations as well as *SNCA* and *LRRK2* gene mutations. From the point of view of prevalence of each gene mutation and cost reduction, *parkin* should be tested first in early-onset PD (<50 years old) and *LRRK2* for the typical later-onset idiopathic PD (>50 years old). After genetic testing, appropriate counseling should be provided either by the treating physician or a clinical geneticist along with psychological support if needed.

Commercial genetic testing for parkinsonian genes for asymptomatic cases should be interpreted with caution. A positive finding contributes only to the probability that the person will become affected because most mutations gain or lose function and are associated with age-dependent penetrance. Indeed, for most genes and mutations, the age-associated risk to carriers has yet to be formally described. Despite the explosive progress in genetic research, not all mutations in PD have been functionally validated and some rare variants could be either benign polymorphisms or indeed represent pathogenic mutations. Moreover, there may be other problems such as phenocopies. For example, affected patients not harboring the same PD gene mutations as the affected members in their own families may carry the causative PD gene mutation in another gene. Technical problems in test–retest reliability may also occur. These issues should be carefully and comprehensively discussed with physicians and their patients who are seeking genetic advice, as well as with asymptomatic family members who are genealogically at risk. Genetic testing should be performed in specialized centers that can provide expertise in neurology, genetics, and genetic counseling (184).

For the familial cases presenting with atypical parkinsonism, sequencing analysis may be recommended. Sequence analysis of *SCA2, SCA3, SCA8, SCA12, SCA17, GCH1, ATP1A3, MAPT, PGRN, DCTN1, IT15, TH, NPC1*, and *FMR* are commercially available. Results of genetic testing for asymptomatic family members are easier to interpret in genes with high penetrance. Given the earlier and rapid nature of disease onset with these gene mutations, the genetic screening is more useful for making life-related decisions, such as having children.

SUMMARY

The genetics of PD and related conditions is complex, even in monogenic parkinsonism. The discovery of mutations in the genes for *SNCA, parkin, UCHL1, PINK1, DJ-1, LRRK2, ATP13A2, PLA2G6, FBXO7, VPS35, and eIF4G1* has created a unique glimpse into the basic mechanisms responsible for this neurodegenerative process. Further genetic studies of already known PD loci will undoubtedly uncover more mutations and more genes. Subsequent clinical and pathologic correlations will aid not only our understanding of the mechanisms involved in cell dysfunction and death, but also our ability to intervene.

The new techniques of genetic sequencing will aid to expand the possibility of genetic association for PD. With this background, an understanding of gene–gene and gene–environment interactions is also emerging, which will promote the discovery of gene therapy for PD and protection from environmental factors. After almost 190 years since the first description of PD in 1817, only symptomatic treatments are presently available, but hope now exists that genetics studies will lead to curative treatments for PD.

ACKNOWLEDGMENTS

The authors thank patients with PD and their families for their cooperation, patience, and continued support for genetic research on parkinsonian conditions.

ZKW is partially supported by the NIH/NINDS R01NS078086, 1RC2NS070276, NS057567, P50 NS072187, Mayo Clinic Florida (MCF) Research Committee CR program, Dystonia Medical Research Foundation, and the gift from Carl Edward Bolch, Jr., and Susan Bass Bolch.

REFERENCES

1. Gardian G, Vecsei L. Medical treatment of Parkinson's disease: today and the future. Int J Clin Pharmacol Ther 2010; 48: 633–42.
2. Bronstein JM, Tagliati M, Alterman RL, et al. Deep brain stimulation for Parkinson disease: an expert consensus and review of key issues. Arch Neurol 2011; 68: 165.
3. Vance JM, Ali S, Bradley WG, et al. Gene-environment interactions in Parkinson's disease and other forms of parkinsonism. Neurotoxicology 2010; 31: 598–602.
4. Golbe LI. Alpha-synuclein and Parkinson's disease. Mov Disord 1999; 14: 6–9.
5. Funayama M, Hasegawa K, Kowa H, et al. A new locus for Parkinson's disease (PARK8) maps to chromosome 12p11.2-q13.1. Ann Neurol 2002; 51: 296–301.
6. Wszolek ZK, Uitti RJ, Markopoulou K. Familial Parkinson's disease and related conditions. Clinical genetics. Adv Neurol 2001; 86: 33–43.
7. Do CB, Tung JY, Dorfman E, et al. Web-based genome-wide association study identifies two novel loci and a substantial genetic component for Parkinson's disease. PLoS Genet 2011; 7: e1002141.
8. Gelb DJ, Oliver E, Gilman S. Diagnostic criteria for Parkinson disease. Arch Neurol 1999; 56: 33–9.
9. Dickson DW, Braak H, Duda JE, et al. Neuropathological assessment of Parkinson's disease: refining the diagnostic criteria. Lancet Neurol 2009; 8: 1150–7.
10. Uitti RJ, Calne DB, Dickson DW, et al. Is the neuropathological 'gold standard' diagnosis dead? Implications of clinicopathological findings in an autosomal dominant neurodegenerative disorder. Parkinsonism Relat Disord 2004; 10: 461–3.
11. Lazzarini AM, Myers RH, Zimmerman TR Jr, et al. A clinical genetic study of Parkinson's disease: evidence for dominant transmission. Neurology 1994; 44: 499–506.
12. Marder K, Tang MX, Mejia H, et al. Risk of Parkinson's disease among first-degree relatives: a community-based study. Neurology 1996; 47: 155–60.
13. Shino MY, McGuire V, Van Den Eeden SK, et al. Familial aggregation of Parkinson's disease in a multiethnic community-based case-control study. Mov Disord 2010; 25: 2587–94.
14. Rocca WA, McDonnell SK, Strain KJ, et al. Familial aggregation of Parkinson's disease: the Mayo clinic family study. Ann Neurol 2004; 56: 495–502.
15. De Michele G, Filla A, Volpe G, et al. Environmental and genetic risk factors in Parkinson's disease: a case-control study in southern Italy. Mov Disord 1996; 11: 17–23.
16. Uitti RJ, Shinotoh H, Hayward M, et al. "Familial Parkinson's disease": a case-control study of families. Can J Neurol Sci 1997; 24: 127–32.
17. Sveinbjornsdottir S, Hicks AA, Jonsson T, et al. Familial aggregation of Parkinson's disease in Iceland. N Engl J Med 2000; 343: 1765–70.
18. Maher NE, Golbe LI, Lazzarini AM, et al. Epidemiologic study of 203 sibling pairs with Parkinson's disease: the GenePD study. Neurology 2002; 58: 79–84.
19. Thacker EL, Ascherio A. Familial aggregation of Parkinson's disease: a meta-analysis. Mov Disord 2008; 23: 1174–83.
20. Simon DK, Lin MT, Pascual-Leone A. "Nature versus nurture" and incompletely penetrant mutations. J Neurol Neurosurg Psychiatry 2002; 72: 686–9.
21. Duvoisin RC, Eldridge R, Williams A, et al. Twin study of Parkinson disease. Neurology 1981; 31: 77–80.
22. Ward CD, Duvoisin RC, Ince SE, et al. Parkinson's disease in 65 pairs of twins and in a set of quadruplets. Neurology 1983; 33: 815–24.
23. Johnson WG, Hodge SE, Duvoisin R. Twin studies and the genetics of Parkinson's disease–a reappraisal. Mov Disord 1990; 5: 187–94.

24. Tanner CM, Ottman R, Goldman SM, et al. Parkinson disease in twins: an etiologic study. JAMA 1999; 281: 341–6.
25. Wirdefeldt K, Gatz M, Schalling M, et al. No evidence for heritability of Parkinson disease in Swedish twins. Neurology 2004; 63: 305–11.
26. Dickson D, Farrer M, Lincoln S, et al. Pathology of PD in monozygotic twins with a 20-year discordance interval. Neurology 2001; 56: 981–2.
27. Wirdefeldt K, Adami HO, Cole P, et al. Epidemiology and etiology of Parkinson's disease: a review of the evidence. Eur J Epidemiol 2011; 26: S1–58.
28. Laihinen A, Ruottinen H, Rinne JO, et al. Risk for Parkinson's disease: twin studies for the detection of asymptomatic subjects using [18F]6-fluorodopa PET. J Neurol 2000; 247: II110–13.
29. Piccini P, Burn DJ, Ceravolo R, et al. The role of inheritance in sporadic Parkinson's disease: evidence from a longitudinal study of dopaminergic function in twins. Ann Neurol 1999; 45: 577–82.
30. Gowers W. A Manual of Disease of the Nervous System. Philadelphia: P Blakiston, Son & Co, 1888.
31. Bell J, Clark A. A pedigree of paralysis agitans. Ann Eugenics 19251: 455–36.
32. Allen W. Inheritance of the shaking palsy. Arch Intern Med 1937; 60: 424–36.
33. Mjönes H. Paralysis agitans: a clinical and genetic study. Acta Psychiatry Neurol Scand 1949; 54(Suppl): 1–195.
34. Wszolek Z, Markopoulou K, Chase B. In: Watts R, Koller W, eds. Genetics of Parkinson's Disease and Parkinsonian Disorders, 2nd edn. New York: McGraw-Hill, 2004.
35. Golbe LI, Di Iorio G, Bonavita V, et al. A large kindred with autosomal dominant Parkinson's disease. Ann Neurol 1990; 27: 276–82.
36. Wszolek ZK, Cordes M, Calne DB, et al. Hereditary Parkinson disease: report of 3 families with dominant autosomal inheritance. Nervenarzt 1993; 64: 331–5.
37. Singleton AB. Exome sequencing: a transformative technology. Lancet Neurol 2011; 10: 942–6.
38. Polymeropoulos MH, Lavedan C, Leroy E, et al. Mutation in the alpha-synuclein gene identified in families with Parkinson's disease. Science 1997; 276: 2045–7.
39. Kitada T, Asakawa S, Hattori N, et al. Mutations in the parkin gene cause autosomal recessive juvenile parkinsonism. Nature 1998; 392: 605–8.
40. van Duijn CM, Dekker MC, Bonifati V, et al. Park7, a novel locus for autosomal recessive early-onset parkinsonism, on chromosome 1p36. Am J Hum Genet 2001; 69: 629–34.
41. Valente EM, Abou-Sleiman PM, Caputo V, et al. Hereditary early-onset Parkinson's disease caused by mutations in PINK1. Science 2004; 304: 1158–60.
42. Zimprich A, Biskup S, Leitner P, et al. Mutations in LRRK2 cause autosomal-dominant parkinsonism with pleomorphic pathology. Neuron 2004; 44: 601–7.
43. Ramirez A, Heimbach A, Grundemann J, et al. Hereditary parkinsonism with dementia is caused by mutations in ATP13A2, encoding a lysosomal type 5 P-type ATPase. Nat Genet 2006; 38: 1184–91.
44. Shojaee S, Sina F, Banihosseini SS, et al. Genome-wide linkage analysis of a Parkinsonian-pyramidal syndrome pedigree by 500 K SNP arrays. Am J Hum Genet 2008; 82: 1375–84.
45. Vilarino-Guell C, Wider C, Ross OA, et al. VPS35 mutations in Parkinson disease. Am J Hum Genet 2011; 89: 162–7.
46. Zimprich A, Benet-Pages A, Struhal W, et al. A mutation in VPS35, encoding a subunit of the retromer complex, causes late-onset Parkinson disease. Am J Hum Genet 2011; 89: 168–75.
47. Chartier-Harlin MC, Dachsel JC, Vilarino-Guell C, et al. Translation initiator EIF4G1 mutations in familial Parkinson disease. Am J Hum Genet 2011; 89: 398–406.
48. Polymeropoulos MH, Higgins JJ, Golbe LI, et al. Mapping of a gene for Parkinson's disease to chromosome 4q21-q23. Science 1996; 274: 1197–9.
49. Kruger R, Kuhn W, Muller T, et al. Ala30Pro mutation in the gene encoding alpha-synuclein in Parkinson's disease. Nat Genet 1998; 18: 106–8.
50. Zarranz JJ, Alegre J, Gomez-Esteban JC, et al. The new mutation, E46K, of alpha-synuclein causes Parkinson and Lewy body dementia. Ann Neurol 2004; 55: 164–73.

51. [Available from: http://www.molgen.ua.ac.be/PDmutDB/default.cfm?MT=0&ML= 0&Page=Home] [Cited 2011/11/16].

52. Ross OA, Braithwaite AT, Skipper LM, et al. Genomic investigation of alpha-synuclein multiplication and parkinsonism. Ann Neurol 2008; 63: 743–50.

53. Chartier-Harlin MC, Kachergus J, Roumier C, et al. Alpha-synuclein locus duplication as a cause of familial Parkinson's disease. Lancet 2004; 364: 1167–9.

54. Ibanez P, Lesage S, Janin S, et al. Alpha-synuclein gene rearrangements in dominantly inherited parkinsonism: frequency, phenotype, and mechanisms. Arch Neurol 2009; 66: 102–8.

55. Singleton AB, Farrer M, Johnson J, et al. Alpha-Synuclein locus triplication causes Parkinson's disease. Science 2003; 302: 841.

56. Irizarry MC, Kim TW, McNamara M, et al. Characterization of the precursor protein of the non-A beta component of senile plaques (NACP) in the human central nervous system. J Neuropathol Exp Neurol 1996; 55: 889–95.

57. Martin I, Dawson VL, Dawson TM. Recent advances in the genetics of Parkinson's disease. Annu Rev Genomics Hum Genet 2011; 12: 301–25.

58. Gasser T, Muller-Myhsok B, Wszolek ZK, et al. A susceptibility locus for Parkinson's disease maps to chromosome 2p13. Nat Genet 1998; 18: 262–5.

59. DeStefano AL, Lew MF, Golbe LI, et al. PARK3 influences age at onset in Parkinson disease: a genome scan in the GenePD study. Am J Hum Genet 2002; 70: 1089–95.

60. Pankratz N, Uniacke SK, Halter CA, et al. Genes influencing Parkinson disease onset: replication of PARK3 and identification of novel loci. Neurology 2004; 62: 1616–18.

61. Sharma M, Mueller JC, Zimprich A, et al. The sepiapterin reductase gene region reveals association in the PARK3 locus: analysis of familial and sporadic Parkinson's disease in European populations. J Med Genet 2006; 43: 557–62.

62. Sharma M, Maraganore DM, Ioannidis JP, et al. Role of sepiapterin reductase gene at the PARK3 locus in Parkinson's disease. Neurobiol Aging 2011; 32: 2108; e1–5.

63. Leroy E, Boyer R, Auburger G, et al. The ubiquitin pathway in Parkinson's disease. Nature 1998; 395: 451–2.

64. Lincoln S, Vaughan J, Wood N, et al. Low frequency of pathogenic mutations in the ubiquitin carboxy-terminal hydrolase gene in familial Parkinson's disease. Neuroreport 1999; 10: 427–9.

65. Healy DG, Abou-Sleiman PM, Casas JP, et al. UCHL-1 is not a Parkinson's disease susceptibility gene. Ann Neurol 2006; 59: 627–33.

66. Ragland M, Hutter C, Zabetian C, et al. Association between the ubiquitin carboxyl-terminal esterase L1 gene (UCHL1) S18Y variant and Parkinson's Disease: a HuGE review and meta-analysis. Am J Epidemiol 2009; 170: 1344–57.

67. Spillantini MG, Schmidt ML, Lee VM, et al. Alpha-synuclein in Lewy bodies. Nature 1997; 388: 839–40.

68. Liu Y, Fallon L, Lashuel HA, et al. The UCH-L1 gene encodes two opposing enzymatic activities that affect alpha-synuclein degradation and Parkinson's disease susceptibility. Cell 2002; 111: 209–18.

69. Paisan-Ruiz C, Jain S, Evans EW, et al. Cloning of the gene containing mutations that cause PARK8-linked Parkinson's disease. Neuron 2004; 44: 595–600.

70. Kachergus J, Mata IF, Hulihan M, et al. Identification of a novel LRRK2 mutation linked to autosomal dominant parkinsonism: evidence of a common founder across European populations. Am J Hum Genet 2005; 76: 672–80.

71. Di Fonzo A, Rohe CF, Ferreira J, et al. A frequent LRRK2 gene mutation associated with autosomal dominant Parkinson's disease. Lancet 2005; 365: 412–15.

72. Gilks WP, Abou-Sleiman PM, Gandhi S, et al. A common LRRK2 mutation in idiopathic Parkinson's disease. Lancet 2005; 365: 415–16.

73. Nichols WC, Pankratz N, Hernandez D, et al. Genetic screening for a single common LRRK2 mutation in familial Parkinson's disease. Lancet 2005; 365: 410–12.

74. Aasly JO, Vilarino-Guell C, Dachsel JC, et al. Novel pathogenic LRRK2 p.Asn1437His substitution in familial Parkinson's disease. Mov Disord 2010; 25: 2156–63.

75. Wider C, Dickson DW, Wszolek ZK. Leucine-rich repeat kinase 2 gene-associated disease: redefining genotype-phenotype correlation. Neurodegener Dis 2010; 7: 175–9.

76. Lesage S, Ibanez P, Lohmann E, et al. G2019S LRRK2 mutation in French and North African families with Parkinson's disease. Ann Neurol 2005; 58: 784–7.
77. Tomiyama H, Li Y, Funayama M, et al. Clinicogenetic study of mutations in LRRK2 exon 41 in Parkinson's disease patients from 18 countries. Mov Disord 2006; 21: 1102–8.
78. Mata IF, Hutter CM, Gonzalez-Fernandez MC, et al. Lrrk2 R1441G-related Parkinson's disease: evidence of a common founding event in the seventh century in Northern Spain. Neurogenetics 2009; 10: 347–53.
79. Nuytemans K, Rademakers R, Theuns J, et al. Founder mutation p.R1441C in the leucine-rich repeat kinase 2 gene in Belgian Parkinson's disease patients. Eur J Hum Genet 2008; 16: 471–9.
80. Johansen KK, White LR, Farrer MJ, et al. Subclinical signs in LRRK2 mutation carriers. Parkinsonism Relat Disord 2011; 17: 528–32.
81. Ross OA, Toft M, Whittle AJ, et al. Lrrk2 and Lewy body disease. Ann Neurol 2006; 59: 388–93.
82. Gasser T. Molecular genetic findings in LRRK2 American, Canadian and German families. J Neural Transm Suppl 2006: 231–4.
83. Wszolek ZK, Pfeiffer RF, Tsuboi Y, et al. Autosomal dominant parkinsonism associated with variable synuclein and tau pathology. Neurology 2004; 62: 1619–22.
84. Gaig C, Marti MJ, Ezquerra M, et al. G2019S LRRK2 mutation causing Parkinson's disease without Lewy bodies. J Neurol Neurosurg Psychiatry 2007; 78: 626–8.
85. Cookson MR. The role of leucine-rich repeat kinase 2 (LRRK2) in Parkinson's disease. Nat Rev Neurosci 2010; 11: 791–7.
86. Pankratz N, et al. Significant linkage of Parkinson disease to chromosome 2q36–37. Am J Hum Genet 2003; 72: 1053–7.
87. Lautier C, Goldwurm S, Durr A, et al. Mutations in the GIGYF2 (TNRC15) gene at the PARK11 locus in familial Parkinson disease. Am J Hum Genet 2008; 82: 822–33.
88. Bras J, Simon-Sanchez J, Federoff M, et al. Lack of replication of association between GIGYF2 variants and Parkinson disease. Hum Mol Genet 2009; 18: 341–6.
89. Giovannone B, Lee E, Laviola L, et al. Two novel proteins that are linked to insulin-like growth factor (IGF-I) receptors by the Grb10 adapter and modulate IGF-I signaling. J Biol Chem 2003; 278: 31564–73.
90. Craft S, Watson GS. Insulin and neurodegenerative disease: shared and specific mechanisms. Lancet Neurol 2004; 3: 169–78.
91. Nichols WC, Kissell DK, Pankratz N, et al. Variation in GIGYF2 is not associated with Parkinson disease. Neurology 2009; 72: 1886–92.
92. Strauss KM, Martins LM, Plun-Favreau H, et al. Loss of function mutations in the gene encoding Omi/HtrA2 in Parkinson's disease. Hum Mol Genet 2005; 14: 2099–111.
93. Kruger R, Sharma M, Riess O, et al. A large-scale genetic association study to evaluate the contribution of Omi/HtrA2 (PARK13) to Parkinson's disease. Neurobiol Aging 2011; 32: 548; e9-18.
94. Ross OA, Soto AI, Vilarino-Guell C, et al. Genetic variation of Omi/HtrA2 and Parkinson's disease. Parkinsonism Relat Disord 2008; 14: 539–43.
95. Simon-Sanchez J, Singleton AB. Sequencing analysis of OMI/HTRA2 shows previously reported pathogenic mutations in neurologically normal controls. Hum Mol Genet 2008; 17: 1988–93.
96. Hegde R, Srinivasula SM, Zhang Z, et al. Identification of Omi/HtrA2 as a mitochondrial apoptotic serine protease that disrupts inhibitor of apoptosis protein-caspase interaction. J Biol Chem 2002; 277: 432–8.
97. Jones JM, Datta P, Srinivasula SM, et al. Loss of Omi mitochondrial protease activity causes the neuromuscular disorder of mnd2 mutant mice. Nature 2003; 425: 721–7.
98. Wider C, Skipper L, Solida A, et al. Autosomal dominant dopa-responsive parkinsonism in a multigenerational Swiss family. Parkinsonism Relat Disord 2008; 14: 465–70.
99. Sheerin UM, Charlesworth G, Bras J, et al. Screening for VPS35 mutations in Parkinson's disease. Neurobiol Aging 2012; 33: 838; e1-5.

100. Matsumine H, Saito M, Shimoda-Matsubayashi S, et al. Localization of a gene for an autosomal recessive form of juvenile Parkinsonism to chromosome 6q25.2-27. Am J Hum Genet 1997; 60: 588–96.

101. Shimura H, Schlossmacher MG, Hattori N, et al. Ubiquitination of a new form of alpha-synuclein by parkin from human brain: implications for Parkinson's disease. Science 2001; 293: 263–9.

102. Valente EM, Bentivoglio AR, Dixon PH, et al. Localization of a novel locus for autosomal recessive early-onset parkinsonism, PARK6, on human chromosome 1p35-p36. Am J Hum Genet 2001; 68: 895–900.

103. Deas E, Wood NW, Plun-Favreau H. Mitophagy and Parkinson's disease: the PINK1-parkin link. Biochim Biophys Acta 2011; 1813: 623–33.

104. Geisler S, Holmstrom KM, Skujat D, et al. PINK1/Parkin-mediated mitophagy is dependent on VDAC1 and p62/SQSTM1. Nat Cell Biol 2010; 12: 119–31.

105. Bonifati V, Rizzu P, van Baren MJ, et al. Mutations in the DJ-1 gene associated with autosomal recessive early-onset parkinsonism. Science 2003; 299: 256–9.

106. Hedrich K, Djarmati A, Schafer N, et al. DJ-1 (PARK7) mutations are less frequent than Parkin (PARK2) mutations in early-onset Parkinson disease. Neurology 2004; 62: 389–94.

107. Cookson MR. Pathways to Parkinsonism. Neuron 2003; 37: 7–10.

108. Zhou W, Zhu M, Wilson MA, et al. The oxidation state of DJ-1 regulates its chaperone activity toward alpha-synuclein. J Mol Biol 2006; 356: 1036–48.

109. Hampshire DJ, Roberts E, Crow Y, et al. Kufor-Rakeb syndrome, pallido-pyramidal degeneration with supranuclear upgaze paresis and dementia, maps to 1p36. J Med Genet 2001; 38: 680–2.

110. Paisan-Ruiz C, Guevara R, Federoff M, et al. Early-onset L-dopa-responsive parkinsonism with pyramidal signs due to ATP13A2, PLA2G6, FBXO7 and spatacsin mutations. Mov Disord 2010; 25: 1791–800.

111. Lin CH, Tan EK, Chen ML, et al. Novel ATP13A2 variant associated with Parkinson disease in Taiwan and Singapore. Neurology 2008; 71: 1727–32.

112. Ning YP, Kanai K, Tomiyama H, et al. PARK9-linked parkinsonism in eastern Asia: mutation detection in ATP13A2 and clinical phenotype. Neurology 2008; 70: 1491–3.

113. Crosiers D, Ceulemans B, Meeus B, et al. Juvenile dystonia-parkinsonism and dementia caused by a novel ATP13A2 frameshift mutation. Parkinsonism Relat Disord 2011; 17: 135–8.

114. Gitler AD, Chesi A, Geddie ML, et al. Alpha-synuclein is part of a diverse and highly conserved interaction network that includes PARK9 and manganese toxicity. Nat Genet 2009; 41: 308–15.

115. Ugolino J, Fang S, Kubisch C, et al. Mutant Atp13a2 proteins involved in parkinsonism are degraded by ER-associated degradation and sensitize cells to ER-stress induced cell death. Hum Mol Genet 2011; 20: 3565–77.

116. Morgan NV, Westaway SK, Morton JE, et al. PLA2G6, encoding a phospholipase A2, is mutated in neurodegenerative disorders with high brain iron. Nat Genet 2006; 38: 752–4.

117. Paisan-Ruiz C, Bhatia KP, Li A, et al. Characterization of PLA2G6 as a locus for dystonia-parkinsonism. Ann Neurol 2009; 65: 19–23.

118. Sina F, Shojaee S, Elahi E, et al. R632W mutation in PLA2G6 segregates with dystonia-parkinsonism in a consanguineous Iranian family. Eur J Neurol 2009; 16: 101–4.

119. Paisan-Ruiz C, Li A, Schneider SA, et al. Widespread Lewy body and tau accumulation in childhood and adult onset dystonia-parkinsonism cases with PLA2G6 mutations. Neurobiol Aging 2012; 33: 814–23.

120. Tomiyama H, Yoshino H, Hattori N. Analysis of PLA2G6 in patients with frontotemporal type of dementia. Parkinsonism Relat Disord 2011; 17: 493–4.

121. Davison C. Pallido-pyramidal disease. J Neuropathol Exp Neurol 1954; 13: 50–9.

122. Di Fonzo A, Dekker MC, Montagna P, et al. FBXO7 mutations cause autosomal recessive, early-onset parkinsonian-pyramidal syndrome. Neurology 2009; 72: 240–5.

123. Zhao T, De Graaff E, Breedveld GJ, et al. Loss of nuclear activity of the FBXO7 protein in patients with parkinsonian-pyramidal syndrome. PARK15). PLoS One 2011; 6: e16983.

124. Hicks AA, Petursson H, Jonsson T, et al. A susceptibility gene for late-onset idiopathic Parkinson's disease. Ann Neurol 2002; 52: 549–55.
125. Scott WK, Nance MA, Watts RL, et al. Complete genomic screen in Parkinson disease: evidence for multiple genes. JAMA 2001; 286: 2239–44.
126. Oliveira SA, Li YJ, Noureddine MA, et al. Identification of risk and age-at-onset genes on chromosome 1p in Parkinson disease. Am J Hum Genet 2005; 77: 252–64.
127. Li YJ, Deng J, Mayhew GM, et al. Investigation of the PARK10 gene in Parkinson disease. Ann Hum Genet 2007; 71: 639–47.
128. Anderson LR, Betarbet R, Gearing M, et al. PARK10 candidate RNF11 is expressed by vulnerable neurons and localizes to Lewy bodies in Parkinson disease brain. J Neuropathol Exp Neurol 2007; 66: 955–64.
129. Haugarvoll K, Toft M, Ross OA, et al. ELAVL4, PARK10, and the Celts. Mov Disord 2007; 22: 585–7.
130. Haugarvoll K, Toft M, Skipper L, et al. Fine-mapping and candidate gene investigation within the PARK10 locus. Eur J Hum Genet 2009; 17: 336–43.
131. Satake W, Nakabayashi Y, Mizuta I, et al. Genome-wide association study identifies common variants at four loci as genetic risk factors for Parkinson's disease. Nat Genet 2009; 41: 1303–7.
132. Tan EK, Kwok HH, Tan LC, et al. Analysis of GWAS-linked loci in Parkinson disease reaffirms PARK16 as a susceptibility locus. Neurology 2010; 75: 508–12.
133. Ramirez A, Ziegler A, Winkler S, et al. Association of Parkinson disease to PARK16 in a Chilean sample. Parkinsonism Relat Disord 2011; 17: 70–1.
134. Tucci A, Nalls MA, Houlden H, et al. Genetic variability at the PARK16 locus. Eur J Hum Genet 2010; 18: 1356–9.
135. Mata IF, Yearout D, Alvarez V, et al. Replication of MAPT and SNCA, but not PARK16-18, as susceptibility genes for Parkinson's disease. Mov Disord 2011; 26: 819–23.
136. Valente EM, Brancati F, Ferraris A, et al. PARK6-linked parkinsonism occurs in several European families. Ann Neurol 2002; 51: 14–18.
137. Bardien S, Lesage S, Brice A, et al. Genetic characteristics of leucine-rich repeat kinase 2 (LRRK2) associated Parkinson's disease. Parkinsonism Relat Disord 2011; 17: 501–8.
138. Ross OA, Wu YR, Lee MC, et al. Analysis of Lrrk2 R1628P as a risk factor for Parkinson's disease. Ann Neurol 2008; 64: 88–92.
139. Farrer MJ, Stone JT, Lin CH, et al. Lrrk2 G2385R is an ancestral risk factor for Parkinson's disease in Asia. Parkinsonism Relat Disord 2007; 13: 89–92.
140. Di Fonzo A, Wu-Chou YH, Lu CS, et al. A common missense variant in the LRRK2 gene, Gly2385Arg, associated with Parkinson's disease risk in Taiwan. Neurogenetics 2006; 7: 133–8.
141. Tan EK, Tan LC, Lim HQ, et al. LRRK2 R1628P increases risk of Parkinson's disease: replication evidence. Hum Genet 2008; 124: 287–8.
142. Kim JM, Lee JY, Kim HJ, et al. The LRRK2 G2385R variant is a risk factor for sporadic Parkinson's disease in the Korean population. Parkinsonism Relat Disord 2010; 16: 85–8.
143. Ross OA, Soto-Ortolaza AI, Heckman MG, et al. Association of LRRK2 exonic variants with susceptibility to Parkinson's disease: a case-control study. Lancet Neurol 2011; 10: 898–908.
144. Mueller JC, Fuchs J, Hofer A, et al. Multiple regions of alpha-synuclein are associated with Parkinson's disease. Ann Neurol 2005; 57: 535–41.
145. Pals P, Lincoln S, Manning J, et al. alpha-Synuclein promoter confers susceptibility to Parkinson's disease. Ann Neurol 2004; 56: 591–5.
146. [Available from: www.pdgene.org] [Cited 2011/11/17].
147. Maraganore DM, de Andrade M, Elbaz A, et al. Collaborative analysis of alpha-synuclein gene promoter variability and Parkinson disease. JAMA 2006; 296: 661–70.
148. Hutton M, Lendon CL, Rizzu P, et al. Association of missense and 5′-splice-site mutations in tau with the inherited dementia FTDP-17. Nature 1998; 393: 702–5.
149. Pastor P, Ezquerra M, Munoz E, et al. Significant association between the tau gene A0/A0 genotype and Parkinson's disease. Ann Neurol 2000; 47: 242–5.

150. Ezquerra M, Pastor P, Gaig C, et al. Different MAPT haplotypes are associated with Parkinson's disease and progressive supranuclear palsy. Neurobiol Aging 2011; 32: 547; e11–6.
151. Tobin JE, Latourelle JC, Lew MF, et al. Haplotypes and gene expression implicate the MAPT region for Parkinson disease: the GenePD Study. Neurology 2008; 71: 28–34.
152. Wider C, Vilarino-Guell C, Jasinska-Myga B, et al. Association of the MAPT locus with Parkinson's disease. Eur J Neurol 2010; 17: 483–6.
153. Elbaz A, Ross OA, Ioannidis JP, et al. Independent and joint effects of the MAPT and SNCA genes in Parkinson disease. Ann Neurol 2011; 69: 778–92.
154. Grabowski GA. Gaucher disease. Enzymology, genetics, and treatment. Adv Hum Genet 1993; 21: 377–441.
155. Sidransky E, Nalls MA, Aasly JO, et al. Multicenter analysis of glucocerebrosidase mutations in Parkinson's disease. N Engl J Med 2009; 361: 1651–61.
156. Goker-Alpan O, Lopez G, Vithayathil J, et al. The spectrum of parkinsonian manifestations associated with glucocerebrosidase mutations. Arch Neurol 2008; 65: 1353–7.
157. Nishioka K, Ross OA, Vilarino-Guell C, et al. Glucocerebrosidase mutations in diffuse Lewy body disease. Parkinsonism Relat Disord 2011; 17: 55–7.
158. Goldwurm S, Di Fonzo A, Simons EJ, et al. The G6055A (G2019S) mutation in LRRK2 is frequent in both early and late onset Parkinson's disease and originates from a common ancestor. J Med Genet 2005; 42: e65.
159. Farrer M, Maraganore DM, Lockhart P, et al. alpha-Synuclein gene haplotypes are associated with Parkinson's disease. Hum Mol Genet 2001; 10: 1847–51.
160. Ahn TB, Kim SY, Kim JY, et al. Alpha-synuclein gene duplication is present in sporadic Parkinson disease. Neurology 2008; 70: 43–9.
161. Sinha R, Racette B, Perlmutter JS, et al. Prevalence of parkin gene mutations and variations in idiopathic Parkinson's disease. Parkinsonism Relat Disord 2005; 11: 341–7.
162. Maraganore DM, Farrer MJ, Hardy JA, et al. Case-control study of the ubiquitin carboxy-terminal hydrolase L1 gene in Parkinson's disease. Neurology 1999; 53: 1858–60.
163. Zhang J, Hattori N, Leroy E, et al. Association between a polymorphism of ubiquitin carboxy-terminal hydrolase L1 (UCH-L1) gene and sporadic Parkinson's disease. Parkinsonism Relat Disord 2000; 6: 195–7.
164. Valente EM, Salvi S, Ialongo T, et al. PINK1 mutations are associated with sporadic early-onset parkinsonism. Ann Neurol 2004; 56: 336–41.
165. Kumazawa R, Tomiyama H, Li Y, et al. Mutation analysis of the PINK1 gene in 391 patients with Parkinson disease. Arch Neurol 2008; 65: 802–8.
166. Abou-Sleiman PM, Healy DG, Quinn N, et al. The role of pathogenic DJ-1 mutations in Parkinson's disease. Ann Neurol 2003; 54: 283–6.
167. Gosal D, Ross OA, Wiley J, et al. Clinical traits of LRRK2-associated Parkinson's disease in Ireland: a link between familial and idiopathic PD. Parkinsonism Relat Disord 2005; 11: 349–52.
168. Maraganore DM, de Andrade M, Lesnick TG, et al. High-resolution whole-genome association study of Parkinson disease. Am J Hum Genet 2005; 77: 685–93.
169. Simon-Sanchez J, Schulte C, Bras JM, et al. Genome-wide association study reveals genetic risk underlying Parkinson's disease. Nat Genet 2009; 41: 1308–12.
170. Hamza TH, Zabetian CP, Tenesa A, et al. Common genetic variation in the HLA region is associated with late-onset sporadic Parkinson's disease. Nat Genet 2010; 42: 781–5.
171. Edwards TL, Scott WK, Almonte C, et al. Genome-wide association study confirms SNPs in SNCA and the MAPT region as common risk factors for Parkinson disease. Ann Hum Genet 2010; 74: 97–109.
172. Nalls MA, Plagnol V, Hernandez DG, et al. Imputation of sequence variants for identification of genetic risks for Parkinson's disease: a meta-analysis of genome-wide association studies. Lancet 2011; 377: 641–9.
173. Spencer CC, Plagnol V, Strange A, et al. Dissection of the genetics of Parkinson's disease identifies an additional association 5′ of SNCA and multiple associated haplotypes at 17q21. Hum Mol Genet 2011; 20: 345–53.

174. Plagnol V, Nalls MA, Bras JM, et al. (International Parkinson's Disease Genomics Consortium (IPDGC); Wellcome Trust Case Control Consortium 2 (WTCCC2)). A two-stage meta-analysis identifies several new loci for Parkinson's disease. PLoS Genet 2011; 7: e1002142.

175. Gandhi S, Wood NW. Genome-wide association studies: the key to unlocking neurodegeneration? Nat Neurosci 2010; 13: 789–94.

176. Hamza TH, Chen H, Hill-Burns EM, et al. Genome-wide gene-environment study identifies glutamate receptor gene GRIN2A as a Parkinson's disease modifier gene via interaction with coffee. PLoS Genet 2011; 7: e1002237.

177. Tang B, Xiong H, Sun P, et al. Association of PINK1 and DJ-1 confers digenic inheritance of early-onset Parkinson's disease. Hum Mol Genet 2006; 15: 1816–25.

178. Dächsel JC, Mata IF, Ross OA, et al. Digenic parkinsonism: investigation of the synergistic effects of PRKN and LRRK2. Neurosci Lett 2006; 410: 80–4.

179. Funayama M, Li Y, Tsoi TH, et al. Familial Parkinsonism with digenic parkin and PINK1 mutations. Mov Disord 2008; 23: 1461–5.

180. Charles P, Camuzat A, Benammar N, et al. Are interrupted SCA2 CAG repeat expansions responsible for parkinsonism? Neurology 2007; 69: 1970–5.

181. Klein C, Schlossmacher MG. Parkinson disease, 10 years after its genetic revolution: multiple clues to a complex disorder. Neurology 2007; 69: 2093–104.

182. Klein C, Chuang R, Marras C, et al. The curious case of phenocopies in families with genetic Parkinson's disease. Mov Disord 2011; 26: 1793–802.

183. Latourelle JC, Sun M, Lew MF, et al. The Gly2019Ser mutation in LRRK2 is not fully penetrant in familial Parkinson's disease: the GenePD study. BMC Med 2008; 6: 32.

184. [Available from: http://www.ncbi.nlm.nih.gov/sites/GeneTests/] [Cited 2011/11/28].

185. Beach TG, Adler CH, Lue L, et al. Unified staging system for Lewy body disorders: correlation with nigrostriatal degeneration, cognitive impairment and motor dysfunction. Acta Neuropathol 2009; 117: 613–34.

16

Environmental risk factors

Gill Nelson and Brad A. Racette

GENES VERSUS ENVIRONMENT

In 1949, Mjones conducted the first systematic study of the genetics of Parkinson's disease (PD) and concluded that the disease was autosomal dominant with 60% penetrance (1). Subsequent studies have found a substantially lower prevalence of familial PD, beginning an ongoing debate regarding the relative importance of genetic versus environmental factors in the pathogenesis of PD. There are several techniques that have been used to determine the genetic and environmental contributions to the etiology of PD, including family, twin, population kinship, and geographic information system (GIS) studies.

Family studies are designed to answer three basic questions: (*i*) Does the disease cluster in families? (*ii*) Is the clustering due to genetic, shared environmental, or cultural factors? (*iii*) How is genetic susceptibility inherited?

Genetic and Family Studies

Clinic-based studies have found that approximately 20% of patients with PD have a positive family history, suggesting that environmental factors play a primary role in the majority of cases (2). Family clusters of PD are rare, but were described for decades before molecular biology techniques enabling gene isolation were developed (3,4). However, the majority of patients with PD who have a family history are not members of large, multi-incident pedigrees. Reports of relative risks (RRs) for first-degree relatives of a PD patient vary from 2.3 to 14.6, depending on methodology (5,6). Studies involving direct examination of all cases and controls typically found a lower genetic risk (Table 16.1). One family study (7) compared the RR of first-degree relatives of early- and late-onset cases to controls, and found a RR for siblings of early-onset patients of 7.9 with no increased risk in parents. However, in late-onset families, siblings and parents had an increased risk of PD compared with controls (RR = 3.6 and 2.5, respectively). Therefore, the heritability of PD, the proportion of variation directly attributable to genetic differences among individuals relative to the total variation in the population, is relatively low in older patients. These findings, in addition to the predominance of young-onset disease in the known genetic parkinsonisms (8–10), suggest that younger-onset patients may have a different etiology.

Twin studies can provide evidence for genetic or environmental contributions by comparing the concordance of monozygotic (MZ) twins with that of dizygotic (DZ) twins. Since twins typically share the same early environment and MZ twins are genetically identical, significantly higher concordance in MZ versus DZ twins implies a genetic basis of the disease. On the other hand, similar concordance in disease rates between MZ and DZ twins implicates early-life, environmental exposures in the etiology of a disease. Appropriately designed twin studies can provide

TABLE 16.1 Relative Risk of Parkinson's Disease

Author	Examination of Relatives	Relative Risk	Odds Ratio
Payami et al. (6)	+	3.5	
Seidler et al. (54)	–		12.6
De Michele et al. (122)	+		14.6
Marder et al. (5)	+	2.3	

powerful evidence for the genetic or environmental contributions to the disease. However, large sample sizes may be difficult to obtain, and the twin environment is only controlled for approximately the first 20 years of life, confounding the interpretation of the environmental and gene–environmental contributions to the disease. Furthermore, most familial PD demonstrates age-dependent penetrance, making misclassification of phenotype possible without longitudinal follow-up of subjects. Early twin studies reporting higher concordance of PD in MZ twins compared with DZ twins (11,12) were not supported in larger non–population-based series (13,14). Subsequently, several population-based twin studies have found no difference in concordance between MZ and DZ twins in Finnish (15), Swedish (16), and American (17) populations. In one of these studies (17), the RR of PD in MZ twins was 6.0 for those with age at onset younger than 50 years. However, these findings were based on four concordant MZ, two concordant DZ, no discordant MZ, and 10 discordant DZ twins. Although these numbers are small, the findings are consistent with the family and linkage studies in which genetic contributions appear to be more common in younger-onset cases.

Another technique to determine the relative importance of genetic and environmental influences in the etiology of PD utilizes detailed knowledge of genealogies to calculate a kinship coefficient. The kinship coefficient is defined as the probability that two alleles at the same locus, drawn at random (one from each person), are identical by descent, providing a measure of the degree of relatedness between two individuals. A large study of an Icelandic genetic database found that subjects with PD were significantly more related to each other than controls from the same population (18), leading to the discovery of the PARK10 locus (19). However, the findings of this study are population specific and may not translate to other populations. For example, using the same methods, a study in an Amish community found that subjects with PD were less related to each other than subjects without evidence of PD (20). The authors concluded that adult environmental factors are the likely cause of PD in this community.

Geography and PD

Population-based prevalence and incidence studies can provide an indirect indication of potential environmental etiologies of PD, although it is impossible to compare between studies of different populations, given that genetic differences could account for the differing rates. Within a population, however, these studies can provide critical clues to environmental risk factors. A higher prevalence of PD in rural environments implicates regional farming practices, including use of pesticides and herbicides, and rural water sources. A higher prevalence of PD in urban environments potentially implicates byproducts of industrialization. Numerous studies demonstrate a higher risk of PD for individuals living in a rural environment in Alberta, Canada (21), Finland (22), the United States (23,24), and Italy (25). However, this relationship has not been found in all studies (26).

Although the findings are inconsistent, a higher prevalence of PD in urban areas argues for byproducts of industrialization as risk factors for PD. Several studies suggest that increasing industrialization may increase PD risk. Schoenberg et al. compared the prevalence of PD in Copiah County, Mississippi, U.S.A. (341/100,000 older than 39 years) to Igbo-Ora, Nigeria (67/100,000 older than 39 years) using similar methodology, in genetically similar populations. They concluded that environmental factors may be responsible for the observed higher prevalence in the industrialized U.S. population (27). In contrast, a study (28) of PD in Estonia found a similar prevalence of PD in urban and rural regions, although the definitions of "urban" and "rural" were unclear. A small study (26) conducted in a health district in Canada found a lower risk of PD in industrialized areas of the district. In a population-based mortality study, Rybicki et al. (29) demonstrated that counties in Michigan, U.S.A., with a higher concentration of industries, with potential for heavy metal exposures (iron, zinc, copper, mercury, magnesium, and manganese) had a higher PD death rate. Using levodopa prescription records as a surrogate for PD, Aquilonius and Hartvig found an increased risk of PD in areas with prominent employment in the wood pulp and steel alloy industries (30). Potential confounders to the surrogate diagnosis and study methodologies include inclusion of non-PD phenocopies and the inability to separate working in an environment from living in an environment. Similarly, a study (31) of annual state death rates of the U.S. World War II veterans found a higher PD death rate in a North–South gradient, with higher disease death rates in the more populated and industrialized Northern cities. Important methodologic limitations include inconsistent definitions of "rural living" and lack of information on timing of rural living, which may be critical determinants of PD risk. A study published in 2010 investigated rural–urban risk for PD using standard, population density–based definitions for rurality. Using population-based Medicare data to identify PD cases in the United States, a study of more than 500,000 prevalent PD cases older than 65 years found no dose-dependent relationship between rural living, as measured by the U.S. Department of Agricultural rural–urban continuum (32). However, these authors did find a significantly higher prevalence of PD in the most urban counties in the United States as compared with the most rural [prevalence in counties with population greater than 1 million: 1706.27; 95% confidence interval (CI) 1671.14–1741.26 vs prevalence in counties with population <2500: 1371.60; 95% CI 1303.23–1439.97].

If increasing world industrialization is a risk factor for PD, the incidence should be increasing throughout the last century. Only one study has addressed the incidence of PD over time. The yearly incidence of PD did not change significantly between 1967 and 1979 in Rochester, Minnesota, U.S.A. (33). However, it is unlikely that there was a substantial change in the industrialization of this relatively rural community over that period. The population prevalence of PD in the Midlands district of England increased between 1982 and 1992, potentially implicating greater regional industrialization or greater medical and public awareness of the disease (34). No preindustrial epidemiologic studies of PD exist, and many cases of PD likely went unrecognized in the beginning of industrialization in this country. It may be possible to reconcile these contradictory data with more attention to regional differences in industrial pollution and farming practices. A study in the

United States using Medicare for PD case identification found a strong geographic predominance in PD prevalence and incidence with regions of the Midwestern and Eastern United States demonstrating a 10-fold higher disease burden than the Western United States (32). Given the role of the Midwestern and Eastern United States in industrialization in the 20th century, this study provides compelling evidence for the importance of the environment in PD.

SPECIFIC ENVIRONMENTAL TOXINS

Although studies suggest that PD may be largely an environmentally mediated disease, the clinical characteristics are unusual for a toxic process—most notably the prominent asymmetry. Several toxins have been implicated in outbreaks of parkinsonism, including carbon disulfide (35), manganese (36), 1-methyl-4-phenyl-1,2,3,6-tetrahydropyridine (37), paraquat (38), and solvents (39). In general, these cases appear to be much more symmetric than sporadic and genetic PD, as would be expected from a toxic etiology (40). It is possible that the type of exposures, including chronicity, mode of entry, and genetic factors, influence neurodegeneration, but it remains unclear why environmentally mediated PD would be so strikingly asymmetric.

Manganese

Manganese was first recognized as a neurotoxin in the 19th century with the report of four manganese ore crushers developing a syndrome of a lower extremity predominant "muscular weakness," festination, postural instability, facial masking, hypophonia, and sialorrhea (41). The syndrome was more clearly delineated by Rodier (42) in 1955 when he described a group of Moroccan manganese miners with a neurologic illness, characterized by parkinsonism, gait disorder, dystonia, psychosis, and emotional lability. All of these individuals worked underground, and the majority mined manganese ore. The latency to symptom onset from work exposure was one month to more than 10 years. Rodier divided the syndrome into three phases: the prodromal period, the intermediate phase, and the established phase. The first phase was characterized by akinesia and apathy, followed by "manganese psychosis." During this phase, the gait was described as "staggering," and patients became aggressive. Early characteristics of the intermediate phase were hypophonia with vocal "freezing," facial masking, and emotional lability. In the final phase, the patients developed rigidity, bradykinesia, tremor, flexed posture, shuffling gait, and postural instability. Some patients developed a dystonic, wide-based gait described as a "cock gait." The disease progressed to total disability in most, despite discontinuing exposure. There are numerous other clinical reports of atypical parkinsonism in manganese-exposed workers (36,43).

Exposure to manganese at much lower levels may also be associated with parkinsonism. The Occupational Safety and Health Administration (OSHA) has a permissible exposure limit ceiling for manganese of $5\,mg/m^3$ (44). A cross-sectional epidemiologic study of workers in a manganese oxide and salt-producing plant found that workers exposed to low levels of manganese (approximately $1\,mg/m^3$) had slowed simple reaction times on a standardized reaction time test and increased hand tremor, as measured by a standardized hand steadiness assessment (45). Manganese-exposed foundry workers in Sweden (mean manganese exposure $0.18–0.41\,mg/m^3$)

demonstrated slower reaction time, reduced finger-tapping speed, reduced tapping endurance, and diadochokinesis (46–48). A larger, population-based study of workers in a manganese alloy facility found that exposed subjects had slower computerized finger-tapping scores and less hand steadiness (49). Lucchini et al. found an exposure-dependent increase in blood and urine manganese levels, and slowing of finger-tapping in workers in a ferroalloy plant exposed to low-level, chronic manganese (50). Even nonoccupational blood elevations in manganese are associated with an exposure-related slowing of motor tasks and difficulty with pointing tasks consistent with tremor (51).

Although high-level, acute exposures are clearly associated with parkinsonism and lower-level exposures are associated with parkinsonian motor abnormalities, evidence implicating manganese in the etiology of PD is contradictory. In a population-based case–control study using blinded industrial hygiene exposure assessment, Gorell et al. (52) found that occupational exposure to copper [odds ratio (OR) = 2.49] and manganese (OR = 10.61) for more than 20 years was associated with the diagnosis of PD. However, their study had only three cases and one control with long-duration manganese exposure (52,53). Zayed et al. (26) found an increased risk of PD in subjects exposed to a combination of manganese, iron, and aluminum for more than 30 years. They did not analyze the effects of individual metals, nor was there a dose–response relationship (the association was only significant with the longest duration of exposure). In addition, the study sample was small and occupational categories were broad. In a population-based German cohort, Seidler et al. (54) found no association between PD and occupational heavy metal exposure, categorized in a job-exposure matrix. Another population-based study, using self-reported occupational exposures, found no association between PD and manganese (55). Differences in study design, populations studied, and exposures, probably account for the discrepant findings in these studies.

There is a growing body of evidence for the association PD with environmental manganese exposure. Although a case–control study of 767 PD patients and 1989 controls in Scotland, Italy, Sweden, Romania, and Malta (56) did not demonstrate an association with manganese exposure, based on occupation, hobbies, and water supply, three subsequent large studies did report increased ORs. Finkelstein and Jerrett studied the association of PD with exposure to ambient manganese, using GIS coding and markers of exposure to vehicle exhausts and industrial emissions of manganese (57). They found no association with markers for traffic-generated air pollution, but they calculated an OR of 1.03 (95% CI 1.00–1.07) per 10 ng/m^3 increase in particulate manganese for those exposed to industrial emissions. In another GIS study, using Medicare for PD case identification and exposure lagging, Willis et al. found a higher neurologist-diagnosed incidence rate of PD in urban U.S. counties with high manganese release compared with those with no manganese release (RR = 1.78; 95% CI 1.54–2.07) (58). This was specific to manganese as there was no increased incidence in counties with high industrial lead or zinc emissions. These studies suggest that manganese may be a risk factor for PD, but another study suggested that manganese may modulate PD progression. A retrospective cohort study of 138,000 Medicare beneficiaries with incident PD demonstrated that patients living in urban areas with high industrial manganese emissions had a higher adjusted risk of death [hazard ratio (HR) = 1.19; 95% CI 1.10–1.29] than those living in areas with low emissions (59).

Lead

There is also evidence that long-term exposure to other heavy metals, such as lead, is a risk factor for PD. Lead in blood is a poor marker of exposure as it has a short half-life and is indicative only of recent exposure. The half-life of lead in bone, however, is measured in years and decades and, as such, is a good biomarker of cumulative exposure. Two epidemiologic studies have examined the association of lead stored in bone and the risk of PD. In a case–control study of 121 PD patients and 141 controls, Coon et al. (60) found an increased risk of PD for individuals exposed to the highest quartile, relative to the lowest, of estimated lifetime lead (OR = 2.27; 95% CI 1.13–4.55). Weisskopf et al. performed a similar study in 330 PD patients and 308 controls, and reported an elevated risk in the highest exposure quartile (OR = 3.21; 95% CI 1.17–8.83) (61). Willis and colleagues performed a GIS study to investigate the geographic clustering of PD in regions of the United States with industrial lead emissions (58). They found no relationship between industrial lead emissions and incident, neurologist diagnosed PD. This latter study should be viewed with caution given the multiple routes of environmental lead exposure.

Pesticides/Herbicides

Isolated reports of parkinsonism, developing after acute paraquat (38,62,63) and glyphosate (64) exposure, suggest a role of these pesticides as risk factors for PD. Ferraz et al. (65) performed a case–control study of parkinsonian features in a group of agricultural workers exposed to the manganese-containing fungicide, maneb. They found that the exposed workers (n = 50) were significantly more likely to have rigidity and a variety of constitutional symptoms than nonexposed workers (n = 19). There was no significant difference in other parkinsonian signs but the number of subjects was small.

Of studies reporting a relationship between pesticide exposure and PD, the ORs ranged from 1.77 to 10.0 with relatively wide CIs in many studies, reflecting small sample sizes (54,66). Only one peer-reviewed study reported a significant OR less than one for herbicides (67), and numerous studies found no relationship (23,26,68). If pesticide and herbicide exposures cause PD, those applying or working directly with the substances might be at a higher risk.

A few studies have investigated the relative frequency of PD in pesticide/herbicide workers compared with those living (but not working) in rural environments. Gorell et al. (69) performed a population-based case–control study of 144 PD subjects with occupational exposure to pesticides and herbicides in Michigan, U.S.A. They found that occupational exposure to insecticides (OR = 3.55) and herbicides (OR = 4.10) were significant risk factors for PD; fungicide use was not associated with PD. A case–control study, using California, U.S.A., mortality data from death certificates suggested that underlying PD mortality was significantly increased in counties using agricultural pesticides, with ORs ranging from 1.19 to 1.45 (70). Table 16.2 summarizes the positive case–control studies implicating pesticides as a risk factor for PD.

One of the major limitations of pesticide studies is that exposure is based on self-reported use. Two methods used to overcome this are GIS modeling and biomarkers. Costello et al. (71) and Ritz et al. (72) reported on a case–control study using GIS modeling to calculate residential exposure to maneb and paraquat in more than 300 incident PD patients and controls. Exposure to both pesticides increased PD risk significantly. Using the same methodology, they estimated potential well-water

TABLE 16.2 Positive Parkinson's Disease Case Control Studies for Pesticides[a]

Study	Exposure	Cases	Controls	Odds Ratio (95% CI)
Golbe et al. (123)	Pesticides	106	106	7.0 (1.61,63.46)
Semchuk et al. (97)	Herbicides	130	260	3.06 (1.34,7.00)
	Insecticides			2.05 (1.03,4.07)
Hubble et al. (24)	Pesticides	31	43	3.42 (1.27,7.32)
Liou et al. (95)	Pesticides	120	240	2.89 (2.28,3.66)
	Herbicides			3.22 (2.41,4.31)
Menegon et al. (77)	Pesticides	95	95	2.3 (1.2,4.4)
Duzcan et al. (124)	Pesticides			
	Insecticides/fungicides	36	108	2.96 (1.31,6.69)
				4.52 (1.83,11.2)
Seidler et al. (54)	Herbicides	380	755	1.97 (1.40,2.79)
	Insecticides			1.77 (1.28,2.43)
Gorell et al. (69)	Insecticides	144	464	3.55 (1.75,7.18)
	Herbicides			4.10 (1.37,12.24)
Frigerio et al. (125)	Pesticides	149	129	2.4 (1.1,5.4)
Dhillon et al. (66)	Pesticides	100	84	10.0 (2.9,34.3)
Ritz et al. (72)	Pesticides	324	334	2.32 (1.23,4.40)
Tanner et al. (126)	Pesticides	110	358	2.5 (1.4,4.7)

[a]Pesticides include all insecticides, herbicides, and fungicides.

pesticide contamination and found slightly raised ORs for the association of consumption of well-water contaminated with methomyl (OR = 1.67; 95% CI 1.00–2.78), chlorpyrifos (OR = 1.87; 95% CI 1.05–3.31), and propargite (OR = 1.92; 95% CI 1.15–3.20) and PD (73). Weisskopf et al. found little evidence for increased odds of PD with increasing prospective serum organochlorines in a nested case–control study, other than a possible association between PD and dieldrin (74). This was one of the few studies that provided objective evidence of historical exposures.

A few cohort studies have found associations between PD and pesticide use. Ascherio et al. reported an adjusted RR of 1.7 (95% CI 1.2–2.3) of PD in a large cohort of 7864 individuals exposed to pesticides, including farmers, ranchers, and fishermen (75). Another smaller cohort study found only weak associations between PD and pesticides (76). Several case–control studies suggest that gene variations may interact with occupational pesticide exposure to increased PD risk (72,77–79).

Carbon Disulfide

An outbreak of an atypical parkinsonism in grain workers implicated the fumigant, carbon disulfide, as the cause of a syndrome characterized by cerebellar signs, bradykinesia, rest tremor, and sensory neuropathy (35). Atypical features such as magnetic resonance imaging (MRI) abnormalities in some cases of paraquat exposure, and atypical clinical features in carbon disulfide exposure (cerebellar signs and neuropathy), argue for a primary causative effect (38).

Solvents

There are several case reports of parkinsonism in humans following solvent exposures. A patient who abused lacquer thinner developed acute onset of asymmetric parkinsonism with levodopa responsiveness, but normal positron emission tomography

(PET) with 6-[^{18}F] fluorodopa ([^{18}F]FDOPA PET) uptake (39). A patient exposed to occupational n-hexane also developed asymmetric parkinsonism with levodopa responsiveness and reduced [^{18}F]FDOPA PET uptake (80). A patient with mixed solvent exposures from petroleum waste developed transient parkinsonism associated with transient reduction in [^{18}F]FDOPA PET uptake, suggesting that there may be a critical duration of exposure beyond which the symptoms are irreversible (81). Although normal [^{18}F]FDOPA PET implies that the etiology of a patient's parkinsonism is not likely idiopathic PD, we do not know the sensitivity and specificity of [^{18}F]FDOPA PET for idiopathic PD. In case reports, it is difficult to elucidate causation from incidental, sporadic PD. Several case reports implicate the solvent trichloroethylene, commonly used as a degreasing agent, in patients with PD (82–84). The report by Gash et al. suggests that oral–buccal–lingual dyskinesia or impairment may be a distinguishing clinical feature.

A case–control study of 188 PD subjects drawn from a cohort study of occupational hydrocarbon exposures found that exposed subjects had a significantly earlier age of disease onset than PD controls, suggesting that hydrocarbons are an environmental accelerant (85). A population-based case–control study on 99 twin pairs discordant for PD showed an elevated odds of PD with exposure to trichloroethylene (OR = 6.1; 95% CI 1.2–33) (86). The sample size was small, however, and exposure assessments were based on job tasks that could have involved exposure to multiple agents. Follow-up studies with more detailed dose reconstruction and larger sample sizes are needed to confirm these findings, as solvents are common environmental toxins.

SPECIFIC OCCUPATIONS AND PARKINSONISM

Numerous epidemiologic studies have attempted to detect occupations at a high risk for developing PD. Fall et al. (87) performed an occupation case–control study and found an increased risk for PD in carpenters (OR = 3.9), cabinet-makers (OR = 11), and cleaners (OR = 6.7), compared with a population-based control group. Tanner et al. (88) performed a case–control study (non–population-based) of occupational exposures and PD in the People's Republic of China and found that occupations involving industrial chemical plants (OR = 2.39), printing plants (OR = 2.40), and quarries (OR = 4.50) were associated with a higher risk of PD. A population-based survey of PD in British Columbia found an association between PD and working in an orchard (adjusted OR = 2.30) or planer mill (adjusted OR = 4.97) (89). They hypothesized that industrial chemicals, including pesticides and herbicides, could be etiologic agents. Another non–population-based case–control study in the same region found that occupational categories, such as forestry, logging, mining, and oil/gas field work, had the highest ORs (90). Although referral bias of affected subjects may have influenced the results, the number of subjects studied (n = 414) was substantial. Another non–population-based case–control study in the Emilia-Romagna region of Italy found that occupational exposure to "industrial chemicals" was a risk factor for PD (OR = 2.13) (91). Among industrial chemicals, only organic solvents were identified as a risk factor (OR = 2.78). Limitations of this study include lack of specific information regarding occupations, small sample size, and subject selection bias.

Occupational exposure to magnetic fields may be a risk factor for PD (92). A death certificate (population-based) case–control study in Colorado, U.S.A., utilizing a tiered exposure matrix, found an adjusted OR of 1.76 for PD subjects exposed to magnetic fields. Occupations included in this study were electronic technicians and engineers, repairers of electronic equipment, telephone and telephone line installers and repairers, electric power installers and repairers, supervisors of electricians and power transmission installers, power plant operators, motion picture projectionists, broadcast equipment operators, and electricians (92). Another study of electrical workers in a similar group of occupations found a nonsignificant, elevated OR of 1.1 for PD compared with controls, but the study lacked power (93).

Several studies have investigated the association between residential exposures to industrial toxins and PD. Using standard industrial code classifications, Rybicki et al. (29) found that residential exposure to industrial chemicals, iron, and paper were significantly associated with the development of PD. The counties in Michigan, U.S.A., with the highest concentration of these industries had the greatest death rate from PD, suggesting that these individuals resided in an environmentally high-risk region. In a case–control study in China, subjects living near a rubber plant appeared to have a higher risk of PD; however, no specific data on those working in the plant were provided (94).

Most epidemiologic studies have focused on categories of exposure and not on specific occupations. A few occupations warrant specific attention, given the type of chemical exposures or the amount of data supporting these occupations in the etiology of PD.

Farming

Studies demonstrate both an association (69,95,96) and lack of an association (54,97,98) between PD and farming. Duration of plantation work was significantly associated with PD in the population-based Honolulu Heart study (99). In a non–population-based case–control study (89), orchard workers had a higher risk of PD. The association between rural residences is difficult to dissociate from farming as an occupation for the more traditional family farms. Not all studies corrected for established PD confounders, such as tobacco use, and less-established environmental confounders, such as pesticide/herbicide use, or well-water. Most of these studies used standard clinical criteria or expert diagnosis and had relatively small sample sizes. Furthermore, none of the studies reported detailed clinical information that might suggest clinical differences between exposed and nonexposed subjects.

Pesticide Applicators

One study investigated the risk of PD in nearly 80,000 pesticide applicators (76). The authors found a dose–response relationship between self-reported pesticide use and incident, but not prevalent, PD. However, there was no association between PD and use of specific pesticides, so uncertainty about the relationship between PD and pesticides persists.

Steel Industry

There is some evidence that acute exposures to fumes in the steel industry are associated with an atypical parkinsonian syndrome (100–102). The primary exposure in the steel industry is manganese. Wang et al. (102) described an outbreak of parkinsonism in a Taiwanese (Republic of China) ferromanganese smelter due to a defective ventilation control system. Of those subjects with brief, high-level exposure to inhaled manganese (>28.8 mg/m^3) six of eight subjects developed parkinsonism. Symptoms of affected individuals included bradykinesia, rigidity, gait abnormalities, and tremor. Only one subject developed a "cock gait," a dystonic gait disorder reportedly characteristic of manganese exposure (103). No details on disease asymmetry or characteristics of tremor were reported, but subjects were noted to experience 50% improvement in parkinsonism with levodopa (102). A follow-up assessment demonstrated disease progression at five years in four subjects.

Welding

Some materials safety data sheets (MSDS) for welding consumables list parkinsonism as a potential hazard of welding, although the data upon which this claim is based are unclear. There are several clinical reports (102,104–107) of parkinsonism in welders, although many patients had atypical features, including cognitive abnormalities, disturbances of sleep, peripheral nerve complaints, and mild motor slowing. In a study of magnetic field exposed workers, Noonan et al. found that welders were overrepresented in PD deaths (92). Blood manganese (105) and aluminum (106) levels may be elevated in welders, but no study convincingly demonstrates an association between motor signs and these metals. However, a small study (106) suggests that welders with exposure to manganese may be slower on peg-board and finger-tapping scores compared with welders without these exposures. In one study, 15 career welders were compared with consecutively ascertained and age-matched PD controls (107). Welders with PD were clinically identical to the control groups except for a significantly younger age of onset (46 years). A study in a large cohort of welders demonstrated that welders with parkinsonism had reductions in PD quality-of-life measures that were in the range of abnormalities found in newly diagnosed PD patients (108). Levodopa responsiveness of parkinsonism in welders has been questioned by other investigators. Koller et al. (109) performed a double-blind, placebo-controlled study of levodopa in 13 welders with parkinsonism and found no difference in motor function. The reason for the differences between these studies is unclear. A study of eight welders (110) described syndromes of parkinsonism, myoclonus, and cognitive abnormalities associated with MRI abnormalities typical of manganese neurotoxicity, suggesting a broader potential phenotype among workers exposed to welding fumes. A survey of three movement disorder clinics (111) found only three welders among 2249 consecutive patients with PD; however, it is possible that welders were underrepresented in these relatively white collar communities.

Studies of large welder cohorts and epidemiologic studies provide contradictory evidence regarding the relationship between welding and parkinsonism. A pilot epidemiologic study (112) suggested that occupational welding may be more common in PD patients compared with patients with other neurologic disorders; however, this study was not population-based and the number of subjects studied was small. Several studies (91,113–115) have been cited as evidence against a relationship between parkinsonism and welding. One population-based study (116) of veteran twins calculated an OR of 1.0 for welders, but this study was likely underpowered to detect a relationship, given that the investigators only identified eight welders. In a death certificate study (113) of neurodegenerative disease and PD, welding-related occupations were not listed among the highest ranked occupations in PD-related deaths. However, death certificates may substantially underestimate the true prevalence of parkinsonism or PD, given the long clinical course and rarity of death due to PD-related morbidity. A case–control study (114) of PD and occupational exposures found no relationship with occupational exposure to heavy metals. However, only 19 PD subjects with metal exposure were studied, and welding as an occupation was not specifically identified. Other studies (54,115) have used broad occupational categories or reported exposure only to metals and have not specifically investigated welding. A study of 1423 Alabama welders referred for medical-legal evaluation (117) found a substantially higher prevalence of parkinsonism in three standard occupational codes, using highly conservative assumptions. All patients were examined for parkinsonism with standardized videotaped assessments using the Unified Parkinson's Disease Rating Scale (UPDRS) motor scale. Patients provided information regarding exposure to welding fumes and job titles. Job titles were matched with Department of Labor Standard Occupational Codes (SOCs). Diagnoses for parkinsonism were assigned using quantitative criteria. The prevalence of parkinsonism in Alabama welders was calculated by using the number of active welders in this screening with parkinsonism as the numerator and the age-adjusted number of welders in each SOC as the denominator. This prevalence calculation was then compared with general population data from Copiah County, Mississippi, U.S.A. The estimated prevalence of parkinsonism among active male welders aged 40–69 years statewide was 977–1336 cases/100,000 population. The prevalence of parkinsonism was higher among welders when compared with age-standardized data for the general population (prevalence ratio 10.19, 95% CI 4.43–23.43). Lack of a contemporary control group and lack of blinding for welding trades as occupations were limitations. Most importantly, however, this study investigated parkinsonism, not PD, which may account for some of the discrepancies found in other studies.

A study of occupations in a national death certificate database (118) found an elevated mortality OR of PD below age 65 years in welders. However, there was no elevated mortality in the entire population of welders. A study of Danish metal-manufacturing employees' hospitalization rates (119) found no elevation in hospitalizations for PD. PD is not typically a primary cause of hospitalization or death, although parkinsonian symptoms may contribute to morbidity from other diseases. Therefore, mortality rates and hospitalizations may not be sensitive indicators of parkinsonism. Furthermore, the health and safety commitment in the Danish ship-yards may be substantially greater than in the United States. A Swedish study (120) found no relationship between welding and PD using nationwide, population-based registers. These methods may be more sensitive than hospitalization data, but the findings do not necessarily preclude a greater risk of parkinsonism using more sensitive methods or a greater risk in workplaces with less rigorous environmental controls.

Molecular imaging of manganese-exposed welders provides an opportunity to investigate the pathophysiology of manganese-associated neurotoxicity and to understand the relationship between manganese exposure and PD. [^{18}F]FDOPA PET imaging in two welders with PD demonstrated reduced [^{18}F]FDOPA uptake more prominent in the posterior putamen contralateral to the most affected side (107). The authors concluded that parkinsonism in welders is distinguished clinically from idiopathic PD only by age of onset, suggesting that it may accelerate the onset of the disease. A study of asymptomatic, active welders, published in 2011, found reductions in [^{18}F]FDOPA uptake preferentially involving the caudate with relative preservation of the posterior putamen (121). Workers imaged in this study had only mild abnormalities on UPDRS motor scores. Clearly, further work to investigate the spectrum of dopaminergic dysfunction in manganese-exposed workers is needed to understand the toxic effects of manganese on the substantia nigra.

CONCLUSIONS

There is compelling evidence that environmental risk factors are important mediators of PD risk. Twin studies and case clustering in the United States strongly argue for an environmental etiology. Numerous studies implicate pesticides as important risk factors for PD. In addition, several studies have added to the growing body of evidence that manganese may be an important substantia nigra neurotoxin. New study designs that include detailed residential and occupational histories, as well as state-of-the-art community level exposure modeling, are clearly the future of environmental health research. Finally, future studies need to include sample sizes that are an order of magnitude greater than previous studies.

ACKNOWLEDGMENTS

This study was supported by the National Institute for Environmental Health Sciences (R01 ES013743, K24 ES017765, P42ES04696), the Michael J. Fox Foundation, National Institute of Neurological Disorders and Stroke (NINDS) Grant Number 5T32NS007205-27, National Center for Research Resources (NCRR0) and National Institutes of Health (NIH) Roadmap for Medical Research Grant Number UL1 RR024992, the American Parkinson's Disease Association, and the St. Louis Chapter of the American Parkinson's Disease Association.

REFERENCES

1. Mjones H. Paralysis agitans. A clinical genetic study. Acta Psychiatr Neurol Scand 1949; 25: 1–195.
2. Bonifati V, Fabrizio E, Vanacore N, De Mari M, Meco G. Familial Parkinson's disease: a clinical genetic analysis. Can J Neurol Sci 1995; 22: 272–9.
3. Golbe LI, Di Lorio G, Sanges G, et al. Clinical genetic analysis of Parkinson's disease in the contursi kindred. Ann Neurol 1996; 40: 767–75.
4. Wszolek ZK, Pfeiffer B, Fulgham JR, et al. Western Nebraska family (Family D) with autosomal dominant Parkinsonism. Neurology 1995; 45: 502–5.
5. Marder K, Tang MX, Mejia H, et al. Risk of Parkinson's disease among first-degree relatives: a community-based study. Neurology 1996; 47: 155–60.
6. Payami H, Larsen K, Bernard S, Nutt J. Increased risk of parkinson's disease in parents and siblings of patients. Ann Neurol 1994; 36: 659–61.
7. Marder K, Levy G, Louis ED, et al. Familial aggregation of early- and late-onset Parkinson's Disease. Ann Neurol 2003; 54: 507–13.
8. Kitada T, Asakawa S, Hattori N, et al. Mutations in the parkin gene cause autosomal recessive juvenile Parkinsonism. Nature 1998; 392: 605–8.
9. Valente EM, Brancati F, Ferraris A, et al. PARK6-linked parkinsonism occurs in several european families. Ann Neurol 2002; 51: 14–18.
10. Bonifati V, Rizzu P, Van Baren MJ, et al. Mutations in the DJ-1 gene associated with autosomal recessive early-onset parkinsonism. Science 2003; 299: 256–9.
11. Koller W, O'Hara R, Nutt J, Young J, Rubino F. Monozygotic twins with Parkinson's disease. Ann Neurol 1986; 19: 402–5.
12. Pahwa R, Busenbark K, Gray C, Koller WC. Identical twins with similar onset of parkinson's disease: a case report. Neurology 1993; 43: 1159–61.

13. Ward CD, Duvoisin RC, Ince SE, et al. Parkinson's disease in 65 pairs of twins and in a set of quadruplets. Neurology 1983; 33: 815–24.
14. Vieregge P, Schiffke KA, Friedrich HJ, Muller B, Ludin HP. Parkinson's disease in twins. Neurology 1992; 42: 1453–61.
15. Marttila RJ, Kaprio J, Koskenvuo M, Rinne UK. Parkinson's disease in a nationwide twin cohort. Neurology 1988; 38: 1217–19.
16. Wirdefeldt K, Gatz M, Schalling M, Pedersen NL. No evidence for heritability of parkinson disease in Swedish twins. Neurology 2004; 63: 305–11.
17. Tanner CM, Ottman R, Goldman SM, et al. Parkinson's disease in twins: an etiologic study. J Am Med Assoc 1999; 281: 341–6.
18. Sveinbjornsdottir S, Hicks AA, Jonsson T, et al. Familial aggregation of parkinson's disease in Iceland. N Engl J Med 2000; 343: 1765–70.
19. Hicks AA, Petursson H, Jonsson T, et al. A susceptibility gene for late-onset idiopathic Parkinson's disease. Ann Neurol 2002; 52: 549–55.
20. Racette BA, Good LM, Kissel AM, Criswell SR, Perlmutter JS. A. Population-based study of parkinsonism in an Amish community. Neuroepidemiology 2009; 33: 225–30.
21. Svenson LW, Platt GH, Woodhead SE. Geographic variations in the prevalence rates of parkinson's disease in Alberta. Can J Neurol Sci 1993; 20: 307–11.
22. Marttila RJ, Rinne UK. Epidemiology of Parkinson's disease in Finland. Acta Neurol Scand 1976; 53: 81–102.
23. Koller W, Vetere-Overfield B, Gray C, et al. Environmental risk factors in Parkinson's disease. Neurology 1990; 40: 1218–21.
24. Hubble JP, Cao T, Hassanein RE, Neuberger JS, Koller WC. Risk factors for Parkinson's disease. Neurology 1993; 43: 1693–7.
25. Granieri E, Carreras M, Casetta I, et al. Parkinson's disease in Ferrara, Italy, 1967 through 1987. Arch Neurol 1991; 48: 854–7.
26. Zayed J, Ducic S, Campanella G, et al. Environmental factors in the etiology of Parkinson's disease. Can J Neurol Sci 1990; 17: 286–91.
27. Schoenberg BS, Osuntokun BO, Adeuja AO, et al. Comparison of the prevalence of Parkinson's disease in black populations in the rural United States and in rural Nigeria: door-to-door community studies. Neurology 1988; 38: 645–6.
28. Taba P, Asser T. Prevalence of Parkinson's disease in Estonia. Acta Neurol Scand 2002; 106: 276–81.
29. Rybicki BA, Johnson CC, Uman J, Gorell JM. Parkinson's disease mortality and the industrial use of heavy metals in Michigan. Mov Disord 1993; 8: 87–92.
30. Aquilonius SM, Hartvig PA. Swedish county with unexpectedly high utilization of anti-parkinsonian drugs. Acta Neurol Scand 1986; 74: 379–82.
31. Lux WE, Kurtzke JF. Is Parkinson's disease acquired? Evidence from a geographic comparison with multiple sclerosis. Neurology 1987; 37: 467–71.
32. Wright WA, Evanoff BA, Lian M, Criswell SR, Racette BA. Geographic and ethnic variation in parkinson disease: a population-based study of US medicare beneficiaries. Neuroepidemiology 2010; 34: 143–51.
33. Rajput AH, Offord KP, Beard CM, Kurland LT. Epidemiology of Parkinsonism: incidence, classification, and mortality. Ann Neurol 1984; 16: 278–82.
34. Sutcliffe RL, Meara JR. Parkinson's disease epidemiology in the Northampton district. England, 1992. Acta Neurol Scand 1995; 92: 443–50.
35. Peters HA, Levine RL, Matthews CG, Chapman LJ. Extrapyramidal and other neurologic manifestations associated with carbon disulfide fumigant exposure. Arch Neurol 1988; 45: 537–40.
36. Mena I, Marin O, Fuenzalida S, Cotzias GC. Chronic manganese poisoning: clinical pictures and manganese turnover. Neurology 1967; 17: 128–36.
37. Langston JW, Ballard P, Tetrud JW, Irwin I. Chronic parkinsonism in humans due to a product of meperidine-analog synthesis. Science 1983; 219: 979–80.
38. Sechi GP, Agnetti V, Piredda M, et al. Acute and persistent parkinsonism after use of Diquat. Neurology 1992; 42: 261–3.
39. Uitti RJ, Snow BJ, Shinotoh H, et al. Parkinsonism induced by solvent abuse. Ann Neurol 1994; 35: 616–19.

40. Lucking CB, Durr A, Bonifati V, et al. Association between early-onset Parkinson's disease and mutations in the parkin gene. French Parkinson's Disease Genetics Study Group. N Engl J Med 2000; 342: 1560–7.
41. Couper J. On the effects of black oxide of manganese when inhaled into the lungs. Br Ann Med Pharmacol 1837; 1: 41–2.
42. Rodier J. Manganese poisoning in Moroccan miners. Brit J Ind Med 1955; 12: 21–35.
43. Tanaka S, Lieben J. Manganese poisoning and exposure in Pennsylvania. Arch Environ Health 1969; 19: 674–84.
44. OSHA. Welding, cutting and brazing. OSHA archive. 2002. [Available from: Http:// www.Osha-Slc.Gov/Oshinfo/Priorities/Welding.Html]
45. Roels H, Lauwerys R, Buchet JP, et al. Epidemiological survey among workers exposed to manganese: effects on lung, central nervous system, and some biological indices. Am J Ind Med 1987; 11: 307–27.
46. Wennberg A, Iregren A, Struwe G, et al. Manganese exposure in steel smelters a health hazard to the nervous system. Scand J Work Environ Health 1991; 17: 255–62.
47. Wennberg A, Hagman M, Johansson L. Preclinical neurophysiological signs of parkinsonism in occupational manganese exposure. Neurotoxicology 1992; 13: 271–4.
48. Iregren A. Psychological test performance in foundry workers exposed to low levels of manganese. Neurotoxicol Teratol 1990; 12: 673–5.
49. Mergler D, Huel G, Bowler R, et al. Nervous system dysfunction among workers with long-term exposure to manganese. Environ Res 1994; 64: 151–80.
50. Lucchini R, Apostoli P, Perrone C, et al. Long-term exposure to "low levels" of manganese oxides and neurofunctional changes in ferroalloy workers. Neurotoxicology 1999; 20: 287–97.
51. Mergler D, Baldwin M, Belanger S, et al. Manganese neurotoxicity, a continuum of dysfunction: results from a community based study. Neurotoxicology 1999; 20: 327–42.
52. Gorell JM, Rybicki BA, Cole JC, Peterson EL. Occupational metal exposures and the risk of Parkinson's disease. Neuroepidemiology 1999; 18: 303–8.
53. Gorell JM, Johnson CC, Rybicki BA, et al. Occupational exposures to metals as risk factors for Parkinson's disease. Neurology 1997; 48: 650–8.
54. Seidler A, Hellenbrand W, Robra BP, et al. Possible environmental, occupational, and other etiologic factors for parkinson's disease: a case-control study in Germany. Neurology 1996; 46: 1275–84.
55. Semchuk KM, Love EJ, Lee RG. Parkinson's disease: a test of the multifactorial etiologic hypothesis. Neurology 1993; 43: 1173–80.
56. Dick FD, De PG, Ahmadi A, et al. Environmental risk factors for parkinson's disease and parkinsonism: the geoparkinson study. Occup Environ Med 2007; 64: 666–72.
57. Finkelstein MM, Jerrett M. A study of the relationships between Parkinson's disease and markers of traffic-derived and environmental manganese air pollution in two Canadian cities. Environ Res 2007; 104: 420–32.
58. Willis AW, Evanoff BA, Lian M, et al. Metal emissions and urban incident Parkinson disease: a community health study of medicare beneficiaries by using geographic information systems. Am J Epidemiol 2010; 172: 1357–63.
59. Willis AW, Schootman M, Kung N, et al. Predictors of survival in patients with Parkinson disease. Arch Neurol 2012.
60. Coon S, Stark A, Peterson E, et al. Whole-body lifetime occupational lead exposure and risk of Parkinson's disease. Environ Health Perspect 2006; 114: 1872–6.
61. Weisskopf MG, Weuve J, Nie H, et al. Association Of cumulative lead exposure with Parkinson's disease. Environ Health Perspect 2010; 118: 1609–13.
62. Bocchetta A, Corsini GU. Parkinson's Disease and pesticides. Lancet 1986; 2: 1163.
63. Sanchez-Ramos JR, Hefti F, Weiner WJ. Paraquat and Parkinson's Disease. Neurology 1987; 37: 728.
64. Barbosa ER, Leiros da Costa MD, Bacheschi LA, Scaff M, Leite CC. Parkinsonism after glycine-derivate exposure. Mov Disord 2001; 16: 565–8.
65. Ferraz HB, Bertolucci PH, Pereira JS, Lima JG, Andrade LA. Chronic exposure to the fungicide maneb may produce symptoms and signs of CNS manganese intoxication. Neurology 1988; 38: 550–3.

66. Dhillon AS, Tarbutton GL, Levin JL, et al. Pesticide/environmental exposures and parkinson's disease in east texas. J Agromedicine 2008; 13: 37–48.
67. Behari M, Srivastava AK, Das RR, Pandey RM. Risk factors of parkinson's disease in Indian patients. J Neurol Sci 2001; 190: 49–55.
68. Firestone JA, Smith-Weller T, Franklin G, et al. Pesticides and risk of parkinson disease: a population-based case-control study. Arch Neurol 2005; 62: 91–5.
69. Gorell JM, Johnson CC, Rybicki BA, Peterson EL, Richardson RJ. The risk of Parkinson's disease with exposure to pesticides, farming, well water, and rural living. Neurology 1998; 50: 1346–50.
70. Ritz B, Yu F. Parkinson's disease mortality and pesticide exposure in California 1984-1994. Int J Epidemiol 2000; 29: 323–9.
71. Costello S, Cockburn M, Bronstein J, Zhang X, Ritz B. Parkinson's disease and residential exposure to maneb and paraquat from agricultural applications in the central valley of california. Am J Epidemiol 2009; 169: 919–26.
72. Ritz BR, Manthripragada AD, Costello S, et al. Dopamine transporter genetic variants and pesticides in parkinson's disease. Environ Health Perspect 2009; 117: 964–9.
73. Gatto NM, Cockburn M, Bronstein J, Manthripragada AD, Ritz B. Well-water consumption and parkinson's disease in rural california. Environ Health Perspect 2009; 117: 1912–18.
74. Weisskopf MG, Knekt P, O'Reilly EJ, et al. Persistent organochlorine pesticides in serum and risk of parkinson disease. Neurology 2010; 74: 1055–61.
75. Ascherio A, Chen H, Weisskopf MG, et al. Pesticide exposure and risk for Parkinson's disease. Ann Neurol 2006; 60: 197–203.
76. Kamel F, Tanner C, Umbach D, et al. Pesticide exposure and self-reported Parkinson's disease in the agricultural health study. Am J Epidemiol 2007; 165: 364–74.
77. Menegon A, Board PG, Blackburn AC, Mellick GD, Le Couteur DG. Parkinson's disease, pesticides, and glutathione transferase polymorphisms. Lancet 1998; 352: 1344–6.
78. Elbaz A, Levecque C, Clavel J, et al. CYP2D6 polymorphism, pesticide exposure, and Parkinson's disease. Ann Neurol 2004; 55: 430–4.
79. Kelada SN, Checkoway H, Kardia SL, et al. 5' and 3' region variability in the dopamine transporter gene (slc6a3), pesticide exposure and Parkinson's disease risk: a hypothesis-generating study. Hum Mol Genet 2006; 15: 3055–62.
80. Pezzoli G, Antonini A, Barbieri S, et al. n-Hexane-induced parkinsonism: pathogenetic hypotheses. Mov Disord 1995; 10: 279–82.
81. Tetrud JW, Langston JW, Irwin I, Snow B. Parkinsonism caused by petroleum waste ingestion. Neurology 1994; 44: 1051–4.
82. Gash DM, Rutland K, Hudson NL, et al. Trichloroethylene: parkinsonism and complex 1 mitochondrial neurotoxicity. Ann Neurol 2008; 63: 184–92.
83. Guehl D, Bezard E, Dovero S, et al. Trichloroethylene and parkinsonism: a human and experimental observation. Eur J Neurol 1999; 6: 609–11.
84. Kochen W, Kohlmuller D, De BP, Ramsay R. The endogeneous formation of highly chlorinated tetrahydro-beta-carbolines as a possible causative mechanism in idiopathic Parkinson's disease. Adv Exp Med Biol 2003; 527: 253–63.
85. Pezzoli G, Canesi M, Antonini A, et al. Hydrocarbon exposure and Parkinson's disease. Neurology 2000; 55: 667–73.
86. Goldman SM, Quinlan PJ, Ross GW, et al. Solvent exposures and Parkinson disease risk in twins. Ann Neurol 2012; 776–84.
87. Fall PA, Fredrikson M, Axelson O, Granerus AK. Nutritional and occupational factors influencing the risk of parkinson's disease: a case-control study in Southeastern Sweden. Mov Disord 1999; 14: 28–37.
88. Tanner CM, Chen B, Wang W, et al. Environmental factors and parkinson's disease: a case-control study in China. Neurology 1989; 39: 660–4.
89. Hertzman C, Wiens M, Bowering D, Snow B, Calne D. Parkinson's disease: A case-control study of occupational and environmental risk factors. Am J Ind Med 1990; 17: 349–55.
90. Tsui JK, Calne DB, Wang Y, Schulzer M, Marion SA. Occupational risk factors in Parkinson's disease. Can J Public Health 1999; 90: 334–7.

91. Smargiassi A, Mutti A, De Rosa A, et al. A case-control study of occupational and environmental risk factors for Parkinson's disease in the Emilia-Romagna region of Italy. Neurotoxicology 1998; 19: 709–12.
92. Noonan CW, Reif JS, Yost M, Touchstone J. Occupational exposure to magnetic fields in case-referent studies of neurodegenerative diseases. Scand J Work Environ Health 2002; 28: 42–8.
93. Savitz DA, Loomis DP, Tse CK. Electrical occupations and neurodegenerative disease: analysis of U.S. mortality data. Arch Environ Health 1998; 53: 71–4.
94. Wang WZ, Fang XH, Cheng XM, Jiang DH, Lin ZJ. A case-control study on the environmental risk factors of Parkinson's disease in Tianjin, China. Neuroepidemiology 1993; 12: 209–18.
95. Liou HH, Tsai MC, Chen CJ, et al. Environmental risk factors and Parkinson's disease: a case-control study in Taiwan. Neurology 1997; 48: 1583–8.
96. Zorzon M, Capus L, Pellegrino A, Cazzato G, Zivadinov R. Familial and environmental risk factors in parkinson's disease: a case-control study in North-East Italy. Acta Neurol Scand 2002; 105: 77–82.
97. Semchuk KM, Love EJ, Lee RG. Parkinson's disease and exposure to agricultural work and pesticide chemicals. Neurology 1992; 42: 1328–35.
98. Rocca WA, Anderson DW, Meneghini F, et al. Occupation, education, and Parkinson's disease: a case-control study in an Italian population. Mov Disord 1996; 11: 201–6.
99. Petrovitch H, Ross GW, Abbott RD, et al. Plantation work and risk of Parkinson disease in a population-based longitudinal study. Arch Neurol 2002; 59: 1787–92.
100. Cook DG, Fahn S, Brait KA. Chronic manganese intoxication. Arch Neurol 1974; 30: 59–64.
101. Whitlock CM Jr, Amuso SJ, Bittenbender JB. Chronic neurological disease in two manganese steel workers. Am Ind Hyg Assoc J 1966; 27: 454–9.
102. Wang JD, Huang CC, Hwang YH, et al. Manganese induced parkinsonism: an outbreak due to an unrepaired ventilation control system in a ferromanganese smelter. Br J Ind Med 1989; 46: 856–9.
103. Huang CC, Lu CS, Chu NS, et al. Progression after chronic manganese exposure. Neurology 1993; 43: 1479–83.
104. Nelson K, Golnick J, Korn T, Angle C. Manganese encephalopathy: utility of early magnetic resonance imaging. Br J Ind Med 1993; 50: 510–13.
105. Chandra SV, Shukla GS, Srivastava RS, Singh H, Gupta VP. An exploratory study of manganese exposure to welders. Clin Toxicol 1981; 18: 407–16.
106. Sjogren B, Iregren A, Frech W, et al. Effects on the nervous system among welders exposed to aluminium and manganese. Occup Environ Med 1996; 53: 32–40.
107. Racette BA, Mcgee-Minnich L, Moerlein SM, et al. Welding-related parkinsonism: clinical features, treatment, and pathophysiology. Neurology 2001; 56: 8–13.
108. Harris RC, Lundin JI, Criswell SR, et al. Effects of parkinsonism on health status in welding exposed workers. Parkinsonism Relat Disord 2011; 672–6.
109. Koller WC, Lyons KE, Truly W. Effect of levodopa treatment for parkinsonism in welders: a double-blind study. Neurology 2004; 62: 730–3.
110. Josephs KA, Ahlskog JE, Klos KJ, et al. Neurologic manifestations in welders with pallidal MRI T1 hyperintensity. Neurology 2005; 64: 2033–9.
111. Goldman SM, Tanner CM, Olanow CW, et al. Occupation and parkinsonism in three movement disorders clinics. Neurology 2005; 65: 1430–5.
112. Wechsler LS, Checkoway H, Franklin GM, Costa LG. A pilot study of occupational and environmental risk factors for parkinson's disease. Neurotoxicology 1991; 12: 387–92.
113. Schulte PA, Burnett CA, Boeniger MF, Johnson J. Neurodegenerative diseases: occupational occurrence and potential risk factors, 1982 through 1991. Am J Public Health 1996; 86: 1281–8.
114. Hertzman C, Wiens M, Snow B, Kelly S, Calne D. A case-control study of parkinson's disease in a horticultural region of British Columbia. Mov Disord 1994; 9: 69–75.
115. Kirkey KL, Johnson CC, Rybicki BA, et al. Occupational categories at risk for Parkinson's disease. Am J Ind Med 2001; 39: 564–71.

116. Tanner C, Goldman SM, Quinlan P, et al. Occupation and risk of Parkinson's disease (pd) a preliminary investigation of standard occupational codes (SOC) in twins discordant for disease. Neurology 2003; 60: A415.
117. Racette BA, Tabbal SD, Jennings D, et al. Prevalence of parkinsonism and relationship to exposure in a large sample of Alabama welders. Neurology 2005; 64: 230–5.
118. Park RM, Schulte PA, Bowman JD, et al. Potential occupational risks for neurodegenerative diseases. Am J Ind Med 2005; 48: 63–77.
119. Fryzek JP, Hansen J, Cohen S, et al. A cohort study of parkinson's disease and other neurodegenerative disorders in danish welders. J Occup Environ Med 2005; 47: 466–72.
120. Fored CM, Fryzek JP, Brandt L, et al. Parkinson's disease and other basal ganglia or movement disorders in a large nationwide cohort of Swedish welders. Occup Environ Med 2006; 63: 135–40.
121. Criswell SR, Perlmutter JS, Videen TO, et al. Reduced uptake of [18F]FDOPA PET in asymptomatic welders with occupational manganese exposure. Neurology 2011; 76: 1296–301.
122. De Michele G, Filla A, Volpe G, et al. Environmental and genetic risk factors in parkinson's disease: a case-control study in Southern Italy. Mov Disord 1996; 11: 17–23.
123. Golbe LI, Farrell TM, Davis PH. Follow-up study of early-life protective and risk factors in Parkinson's disease. Mov Disord 1990; 5: 66–70.
124. Duzcan F, Zencir M, Ozdemir F, et al. Familial Influence on parkinsonism in a rural area of Turkey (Kizilcaboluk-Denizli): A community-based case-control study. Mov Disord 2003; 18: 799–804.
125. Frigerio R, Sanft KR, Grossardt BR, et al. Chemical exposures and parkinson's disease: a population-based case-control study. Mov Disord 2006; 21: 1688–92.
126. Tanner CM, Kamel F, Ross GW, et al. Rotenone, paraquat, and Parkinson's disease. Environ Health Perspect 2011; 119: 866–72.

17

Disease modification

Daniel E. Kremens

INTRODUCTION

Parkinson's disease (PD) is the second most common neurodegenerative condition after Alzheimer's disease, affecting at least one million people in the United States and four to six million people worldwide (1). The economic cost is estimated at $23 billion a year in the United States alone and, with the aging population, that cost is estimated to increase to $50 billion a year by 2040. Since its initial description by James Parkinson in 1817, the cardinal motor features of rest tremor, rigidity, brady-kinesia, and postural instability have characterized PD. This understanding was reinforced by the seminal work of Carlsson who suggested that dopamine deple-tion played a crucial role in the development of motor symptoms (2). By the 1960s Ehringer and Hornykiewicz (3) found that patients who had died of PD had marked depletion of dopamine in the substantia nigra and shortly thereafter Cotzias (4) demonstrated the profound beneficial effect of levodopa on motor symptoms. With time however, it became clear that dopamine replacement therapy was not a pana-cea. Patients developed motor complications and dyskinesia. More importantly, nonmotor symptoms, such as dementia, apathy, depression, and sleep disturbances emerged and did not respond to dopaminergic therapies (5,6). Indeed, as the dis-ease progresses, non-levodopa responsive nonmotor symptoms can be the most debilitating feature for both patients and caregivers (7).

Given the devastating effects of PD to the patients, caregivers, and society, therapies that can slow, stop, or reverse the underlying disease progress are argu-ably the greatest unmet need in PD (8). Although such therapies are often described as "neuroprotective," this term is a misnomer as it is currently impossible to measure dopaminergic cell survival in living humans (9,10). Moreover, so-called protected cells could survive but not function (9). Therefore, such therapies are more appropriately referred to as "disease modifying." That is, such therapies that "provide favorable changes in the clinical course of PD, in complement or even independently of their putative pathophysiological mechanism of action" (9).

Despite the promise of numerous compounds in the laboratory, the transla-tion into disease-modifying therapies in humans has remained an elusive goal. In 2009, Hart et al. published a systematic review of 23 clinical studies evaluating pos-sible disease-modifying agents (10). None of the agents examined were determined to be definitively disease modifying. Various factors, including the lack of validated biomarkers and study designs where symptomatic benefits potentially mimic or mask disease modifying effects have confounded the interpretation of disease-modifying studies. Thus while some agents cannot be determined definitively to be disease modifying, that possibility can also not be definitively excluded (11). This chapter examines the history of disease modification trials in PD, the limitations of study design, and the implications for the future of disease modification in PD.

THE FIRST TRIALS IN DISEASE MODIFICATION:
THE EMERGENCE OF SELEGILINE

The first disease modification trial was the result of a series of disparate coincidences involving monoamine oxidase (MAO) inhibition. Although MAOs were first described in the 1920s, it was not until the 1960s that Hornykiewicz suggested that MAO inhibition might be useful in the treatment of PD by delaying the degradation of dopamine (12). Initially, concerns of a reaction with dietary tyramine limited the use of MAOs. However, with the discovery that there were two isoforms of MAO, MAO-A and MAO-B, and that MAO-A was largely responsible for the tyramine reactions (13), clinicians began to investigate whether inhibition with the selective MAO-B inhibitor selegiline could result in clinical improvement in PD patients. In early studies, selegiline as monotherapy did not appear to have any clinical effect but as adjunctive therapy to levodopa, it appeared to lessen "wearing off" (14). By the early 1980s, Birkmayer published an uncontrolled retrospective study of patients treated with either levodopa alone or levodopa with adjunctive selegiline and suggested that selegiline had slowed the "evolution of the disease" (15,16).

Around the time of Birkmayer's studies in Europe, a group of intravenous drug users in California developed a parkinsonian syndrome after injecting what they believed to be a synthetic heroin (17,18). The actual substance injected was 1-methyl-4-phenyl-1,2,3,6-tetrahydropyridine (MPTP). Shortly thereafter it was discovered that MPTP itself was not toxic but its metabolite 1-methyl-4-phenylpyridium+ (MPP+), a mitochondrial complex I inhibitor, was toxic to cells in the substantia nigra and that the conversion of MPTP to MPP+ could be blocked by selegiline (19). In particular, it was thought that the blockade by selegiline would prevent the production of reactive oxidative species and their associated neurotoxic effects (19). Moreover, it was found that pretreating nonhuman primates with selegiline prevented the development of MPTP-induced parkinsonism in those animals (20).

There was emerging evidence that MAO-B inhibition with selegiline could protect against parkinsonism in an MPTP-induced animal model, and Birkmayer's early work suggested that as an adjunctive therapy, selegiline could result in prolonged longevity in PD patients. Tetrud and Langston embarked on the first clinical trial for disease modification in PD (21). In 1986, they enrolled 54 patients in a 36-month randomized study in which untreated early-stage patients received either selegiline 10 mg daily or placebo. The primary endpoint was the need for levodopa therapy. Forty-four patients completed the study and the time until levodopa was needed was 312 days in the placebo group and 549 days in the selegiline group. The authors concluded that selegiline may have neuroprotective effects but did not address whether there was a symptomatic benefit.

The results of the Tetrud and Langston study provided the foundation for the Deprenyl and Tocopherol Antioxidative Treatment of Parkinsonism (DATATOP) study (22). The DATATOP study was designed to evaluate selegiline 10 mg daily and/or tocopherol 2000 IU/day in 800 untreated early-stage PD patients. Patients were randomized to receive placebo, selegiline and tocopherol, active selegiline and tocopherol placebo, or selegiline placebo and active tocopherol. The primary endpoint was the onset of disability requiring the need for levodopa therapy. An interim analysis at 12 months demonstrated that 97 subjects receiving selegiline reached the endpoint compared with 176 patients receiving placebo. The risk of reaching the endpoint therefore was reduced by 57% at 12 months in the selegiline group. In addition, there was a significant benefit in the ability to continue full-time employment in the selegiline group.

The DATATOP results were then reported after up to 24 months of follow-up. Kaplan–Meier plots demonstrated that the probability of reaching the endpoint differed significantly between the selegiline-treated cohorts and the non–selegiline-treated cohorts (Fig. 17.1) (23). Selegiline appeared to delay the need for levodopa by 9 months compared with the non-selegiline cohorts, whereas no benefit was seen in the tocopherol-treated group.

Initially the authors concluded that selegiline either alone or in combination with tocopherol might "ameliorate the underlying process of Parkinson's disease" (22). On further analysis, however, it became apparent that selegiline had an unanticipated small but real symptomatic benefit. Patients randomized to the selegiline group had an improvement in motor scores of the Unified Parkinson's Disease Rating Scale (UPDRS) one month and three months after initiating therapy and that

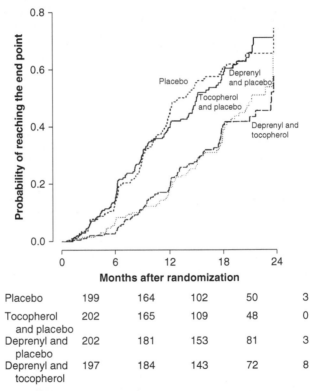

Placebo	199	164	102	50	3
Tocopherol and placebo	202	165	109	48	0
Deprenyl and placebo	202	181	153	81	3
Deprenyl and tocopherol	197	184	143	72	8

FIGURE 17.1 Kaplan–Meier estimate of the cumulative probability of reaching the endpoint, according to treatment group. The hazard ratio for the comparison of subjects taking deprenyl (with placebo or tocopherol) with subjects not taking deprenyl (placebo only or tocopherol with placebo) with respect to the risk of reaching the endpoint per unit of time is 0.50 ($P < 0.001$; 95% confidence interval, 0.41–0.62). The period of analysis was the time from baseline to the last evaluation during treatment. The number of subjects evaluated in each group is shown under each time point. *Source*: From Ref. 23.

when the drug was stopped, their scores worsened (23). This unanticipated symptomatic benefit confounded the suggestion that selegiline was disease modifying. In an attempt to answer this concern, the study was modified to include a one-month and later a two-month washout period at the end of the study. Although the selegiline group did not deteriorate as would be expected if the benefits were solely symptomatic, it is likely that selegiline has a prolonged biological effect and that even a two-month washout period may be too short. This argument was supported by a later analysis of cerebrospinal fluid of these patients that demonstrated elevated homovanillic acid levels two to four months after stopping selegiline (24).

Olanow et al. attempted to answer the question of the confounding symptomatic benefits of selegiline versus disease modification by employing a washout design in the SINDEPAR (Sinemet vs Deprenyl in PD) study (25). In SINDEPAR, 101 early PD patients were randomized to either selegiline or placebo and to symptomatic treatment with either bromocriptine or carbidopa/levodopa and followed for 14 months. The primary endpoint was change in UPDRS from baseline to the final visit following a two-month washout period for selegiline or placebo and a seven-day washout of bromocriptine or carbidopa/levodopa. At the end of the washout, the UPDRS score of the group that received placebo worsened by 5.8 points, whereas the group treated with selegiline worsened by only 0.4 points ($P < 0.001$). These results suggested that treatment with selegiline resulted in a reduction in the rate of worsening in the UPDRS. Although such a result is consistent with disease modification, it may also be the result of a prolonged symptomatic effect in the setting of an inadequate washout period.

While the DATATOP study was confounded by the symptomatic benefits of selegiline, a long-term extension to DATATOP found that of 368 patients who required levodopa and underwent a second randomization to selegiline or placebo, the selegiline-treated group had less freezing of gait and less worsening of their UPDRS scores than the placebo group (26). Similarly, in a long-term study done in Sweden, Palhagen et al. found that patients treated with selegiline required lower doses of levodopa, had better scores on the UPDRS, and had a lower rate of motor fluctuations than the patients receiving placebo (27). Although these results are consistent with possible disease modification, they are not conclusive and may reflect either symptomatic benefit or a survivor effect.

One study suggested that rather than being disease modifying, selegiline, in combination with levodopa, lead to increased mortality (28). Lees followed 520 early PD patients and found that mortality was 28% for those treated with levodopa and selegiline versus 18% for those treated with levodopa alone. However, in a follow-up study where the patient population was increased to 624, although increased mortality was again seen, the hazard ratio was no longer statistically significant (29). Moreover, a meta-analysis demonstrated no difference in mortality between patients treated with selegiline and those treated with levodopa (30).

NEUROIMAGING AS A SURROGATE BIOMARKER

DATATOP and the other selegiline studies highlighted the difficulty of demonstrating disease modification using clinical endpoints in drugs with symptomatic benefits. Rather than use clinical milestones another study paradigm using biomarkers as a surrogate endpoint was proposed. A biomarker is "a characteristic that is objectively measured as an indicator of normal biologic processes, pathogenic processes or pharmacological response to treatment" (9). Similarly a surrogate endpoint is "a biomarker that is meant to substitute for a clinical endpoint and that is expected to predict clinical benefit (or harm or lack of benefit/harm)" (9). The most commonly proposed biomarker to date in PD is functional neuroimaging. Neuroimaging can be used as a marker for the nigrostriatal system by measuring striatal uptake of either 18(F)-dopa with positron emission tomography (PET) or 2 beta-carboxyme-thoxy-3 beta-(4-idodophenyl) tropane (beta-CIT) uptake with single photon emission computerized tomography (SPECT). 18(F)-dopa PET measures the ability of dopaminergic neurons to store dopamine, whereas beta-CIT SPECT quantifies density of dopamine transporters (DAT) on presynaptic dopamine terminals. Functional neuroimaging is theoretically superior to clinical endpoints in that it is objective, not confounded by a drug's symptomatic benefits and possibly more sensitive in early disease (9).

The first two studies to use neuroimaging as a biomarker involve dopamine agonists. Since the introduction of bromocriptine, dopamine agonists have been used for the treatment of PD. They provide a significant symptomatic benefit while reducing the risk of dyskinesia compared with treatment with levodopa. Dopamine agonists have also been shown both in vivo and in vitro laboratory studies to protect dopaminergic neurons (8). Possible disease-modifying mechanisms of dopamine agonists include that they are antioxidants, that they reduce the formation of reactive oxidative species through the decreased turnover of levodopa, that they may decrease excitotoxicity due to increased activity in the subthalamic nucleus in PD and that they have demonstrated antiapoptotic activity in a number of cell models (8,31).

In the Comparison of the Agonist Pramipexole versus Levodopa on Motor Complications of Parkinson's Disease (CALM-PD-CIT) trial, 82 patients with early PD were randomized to receive either pramipexole or carbidopa/levodopa for 48 months and received beta-CIT scans at baseline and then at 22, 34, and 46 months (32). The primary endpoint was the percent change in beta-CIT uptake and the secondary endpoint was change in the UPDRS. Supplemental open-label levodopa was allowed for either group. At 46 months, patients randomized to the pramipexole arm had a 36% reduction in the rate of decline of beta-CIT striatal uptake compared with patients randomized to levodopa. Similarly, in the Ropinirole as Early Therapy versus L-dopa-PET (REAL-PET) study, 162 de novo patients were randomized to either ropinirole or carbidopa/levodopa for two years (33). Patients received 18(F)-dopa PET scans at initiation and at 24 months. The primary outcome was the mean reduction in 18(F)-Dopa PET uptake at two years and the secondary outcome was change in UPDRS. Patients randomized to ropinirole had a 35% reduction in the rate of decline of striatal uptake on PET scan compared with the levodopa arm. While both the CALM-PD-CIT and REAL-PET studies demonstrated significant decrease in the rate of decline of the surrogate neuroimaging biomarker of striatal function in the patients receiving dopamine agonists, no similar benefit was seen in clinical outcomes as measured by the UPDRS. Indeed in both the studies, patients randomized to levodopa were more clinically improved compared with the patients receiving dopamine agonists.

The interpretation of these studies is controversial. First, there was no placebo arm in either study. While the decline in the rate of loss of a surrogate biomarker is consistent with disease modification, the lack of a corresponding clinical benefit is confounding. It has been suggested that the time course of the trials may be too short to "permit such an effect in the context of viable compensatory mechanisms and powerful symptomatic agents" (31). Nevertheless, no clear clinical benefit of the dopamine agonists has appeared in long-term follow-up of these studies.

Another possible explanation is that the effects of levodopa and dopamine agonists seen in the REAL-PET and CALM-PD-CIT studies are not related to neurodegeneration but instead reflect a pharmacological effect that levodopa or dopamine agonists may have on SPECT or 18(F)-dopa metabolism (34). Studies looking at the effect of levodopa and dopamine agonists on DAT in SPECT scans have been inconsistent and have shown no clear pattern on whether striatal DAT levels are upregulated or downregulated by dopaminergic drugs (31). Data looking at the effect of dopamine agonists and levodopa on 18(F)-dopa metabolism are similarly limited. 18(F)-dopa PET imaging "reflects ligand uptake into dopamine nerve terminals, dopa decarboxylase activity and dopamine storage, suggesting that drug effects at any of these steps might alter the signal" (5). Therefore, levodopa may "induce greater internalization or down regulation of the biomarker than the dopamine agonist, thereby accounting for reduced uptake and creating a false impression that there is a greater loss of dopaminergic neurons in levodopa treated patients" (1). In an attempt to clarify the effects of dopaminergic agents on imaging, Jennings et al conducted the Investigating the Effects of Short Term Treatment with Pramipexole or Levodopa on [123-I]Beta-CIT and SPECT Imaging in Early PD (INSPECT) trial (35). Patients were randomized to receive levodopa, pramipexole, or placebo with a primary endpoint of change in DAT binding between baseline and 12 weeks. This study found no evidence of a pharmacological effect to explain the difference in the imaging between levodopa and dopamine agonists seen in the CALM-PD or REAL-PET studies. Nevertheless, this study was only 12 weeks, involved a relatively small number of patients and thus does not exclude the possibility of a pharmacological effect emerging later. Therefore while the imaging studies involving the dopamine agonists are intriguing, they are confounded by the limitations of imaging and neither prove or disprove a disease-modifying effect.

LEVODOPA: TOXIC OR DISEASE MODIFYING

Another possible interpretation of the REAL-PET and CALM-PD studies to explain the greater decrease in DAT binding in the levodopa-treated group is not that the dopamine agonists are disease modifying but rather that levodopa is toxic to dopaminergic neurons. This concern led to the Early versus Later Levodopa Therapy in PD (ELLDOPA) trial (36). The ELLDOPA study used a washout design in which early, drug-naïve PD patients were randomized to receive placebo or carbidopa/levodopa 150, 300, or 600 mg daily for 40 weeks followed by a two-week washout period. The primary endpoint was change in the total UPDRS scores. At the conclusion of the study, the mean difference in UPDRS scores from baseline to week 42 worsened by 7.8 points for placebo, 1.9 for the 150 mg group, and 1.9 for the 300 mg group and improved by 1.4 for the 600 mg group (Fig. 17.2). Thus levodopa, in a dose–response pattern, significantly reduced worsening of PD compared with placebo as measured by the UPDRS. The observation that levodopa continued to have a benefit after the washout is arguably consistent with disease modification. This conclusion, however, must be tempered by the fact that subsequent studies have demonstrated that the benefits of levodopa may persist for weeks to even months after washout (1). Moreover, these results might also be explained by the development of

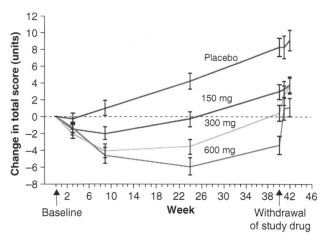

FIGURE 17.2 Changes in total scores on the Unified Parkinson's Disease Rating Scale from baseline through week 42. *Source*: From Ref. 36.

compensatory mechanisms as a result of early treatment with a symptomatic drug rather than a true disease-modifying effect.

The interpretation of the ELLDOPA trial was further complicated by the imaging results of a subset of patients. Beta-CIT scanning was completed in 116 patients to assess striatal DAT density at baseline and at 40 weeks (36). Initial analysis demonstrated no significant difference in loss of uptake for any dose of levodopa versus placebo. However, on re-examination, 19 patients had no evidence of dopaminergic deficit at baseline or at nine months. When these patients were excluded from the analysis, the percent decline of Beta-CIT uptake at 40 weeks was significantly greater in the levodopa groups than the placebo group (–7.2%, –4%, –6%, and –1.4% for the 600, 300, 150 mg/day and placebo groups, respectively). Nevertheless, the same limitations with neuroimaging observed in the dopamine agonist studies are present in ELLDOPA. Whether the decline in uptake is a result of actual cell loss or instead a pharmacological effect on nuclear ligands is unknown and therefore no firm conclusions regarding disease modification can be drawn.

As in the studies involving dopamine agonists, the clinical data in ELLDOPA is at odds with the imaging data. Clinically, levodopa appears to slow the progression of PD or have a prolonged symptomatic effect while neuroimaging suggests levodopa accelerates loss of nigrostriatal dopamine nerve terminals. This confound highlights the difficulties of using clinical endpoints and biomarkers in disease modification studies involving drugs with symptomatic benefit.

THE DELAYED START DESIGN AND RASAGILINE

With no reliable biomarkers available and with the limitations of the washout design in disease modification trials, it became apparent that a new trial design was necessary. In 1997, Dr. Paul Leber, head of the neuropharmacology division of the Food and Drug Administration (FDA), proposed an alternative approach in a paper addressing study design in Alzheimer's disease (37). Dr. Leber examined the difficulties of the washout design, including determining the amount of time necessary to account for a prolonged symptomatic effect and the problems of withdrawal of potentially effective treatments and how this would affect patients. Leber instead proposed that studies employ a "wash-in" or "delayed start" design that would eliminate the need for any washout period. In the delayed start design, there are two phases. In the first phase, subjects are randomized to either placebo (the delayed start group) or active treatment (the early start group) for a predetermined period. This period must be long enough to allow for a symptomatic effect but short enough so that there is not an unacceptable amount of drop out especially from the placebo arm. At the end of the first phase, if the drug has a symptomatic benefit, the early start group will have less disability than the delayed start group. In the second phase, the early start group continues on active treatment and the delayed start group is switched to active treatment and followed for another predetermined period. If the delayed start group improves to the same level as the early start group, this would suggest that the drug has only symptomatic benefits. If the delayed start group improves but not to the same level as the early start group, this suggests that the drug has a disease modifying effect.

This delayed-start design was used in the Rasagiline Mesylate (TVP-1012) in Early Monotherapy for Parkinson's Disease Outpatients (TEMPO) study to evaluate whether rasagiline, an MAO-B inhibitor, was disease modifying (38). Similar to selegiline, rasagiline has a propargylamine side chain and has been demonstrated to have antiapoptotic effects in vitro and in vivo (39). Unlike selegiline, however, rasagiline does not generate amphetamine metabolites that are thought to be potentially neurotoxic (8). The TEMPO trial was originally conceived to test the efficacy and safety of rasagiline in early PD patients but ultimately incorporated a delayed start design. The primary outcome would be change in UPDRS scores between baseline and six months. In the first phase, 404 early, untreated PD patients were randomized to receive placebo (the delayed start group) or rasagiline 1 or 2 mg daily (the early start groups) and followed for six months. At the end of the six-month period, the patients in the early start groups showed similar clinical benefit, whereas the delayed start group worsened by 16% on UPDRS scores (38). The second phase of the study included 371 patients. In this phase, the early start groups continued on rasagiline and the delayed start group was switched from placebo to rasagiline 2 mg daily and was followed for another six months. At the end of the second phase, the UPDRS scores of both early start groups and the delayed start group had worsened but a significant advantage was demonstrated between the 1 mg early start group versus the delayed treatment group (mean total UPDRS difference −1.82; 95% CI −3.64, 0.01; $P = 0.05$) and the 2 mg early start group versus the delayed treatment group (mean total UPDRS difference −2.29; 95% CI −4.11, −0.48; $P = 0.01$). These results suggested that the effects of rasagiline could not be explained fully by its symptomatic effect and were potentially consistent with a disease-modifying effect (5).

Given that PD is a chronic slowly progressive condition, it is not clear whether a 12-month study is long enough to demonstrate a disease-modifying effect and that if followed for a longer period, the delayed start group would in fact "catch up" to the early start group. To address this question, the TEMPO cohorts were followed for 6.5 years in an open-label extension study (40). There were 117 remaining in the study at 6.5 years. At all times throughout the study, the early start group performed better on the UPDRS compared with the delayed start group with a 16% difference at 6.5 years. These data however must be interpreted with caution. Only 117 out of the original 404 subjects completed the extension study, other medications were allowed during the extension study and TEMPO was not powered initially to test for disease modification (5). Despite these limitations, the data from TEMPO and its long-term extension were sufficiently robust to support performing a larger trial designed to determine specifically whether rasagiline was disease modifying.

The Attenuation of Disease Progression with Azilect (rasagiline) Given Once-daily (ADAGIO) study was a prospective, randomized, delayed start, double-blind, placebo-controlled study that followed 1176 patients with early, untreated PD for 18 months (41). Patients were randomized to one of four arms. Two arms received placebo (the delayed start groups), one arm received rasagiline 1 mg daily and one arm received 2 mg daily (the early start groups). At the end of 36 weeks, the placebo arms were switched to either rasagiline 1 or 2 mg daily and the early start groups continued on rasagiline 1 or 2 mg daily for another 36 weeks. In order to demonstrate disease modification, the FDA, independent statisticians, and the steering committee determined that there would be three primary endpoints that would have to be met in a hierarchical manner involving complex slope analysis of the UPDRS at various points in the trial (41). The three hierarchical endpoints were (*i*) superiority of slope from weeks 12 to 36 (i.e., were the curves diverging so that the placebo arm was deteriorating faster); (*ii*) superiority in change from baseline to week 72 (i.e., was there a gap between the early start and the delayed start groups at week 72 suggesting greater worsening in the delayed group); and (*iii*) noninferiority of slopes during weeks 48–72 (i.e., both groups were on the medication and the curves were not converging demonstrating an enduring effect consistent with disease modification).

The 1 mg dose groups met all three endpoints in a hierarchical fashion consistent with disease modification (Fig. 17.3) (42). The 2 mg dose groups met the first endpoint with a more rapid worsening in the placebo arm between weeks 12 and 36. The 2 mg dose groups, however, failed to meet the second endpoint as there was no statistically significant sustained superiority between the early start and the delayed start groups (Fig. 17.4).

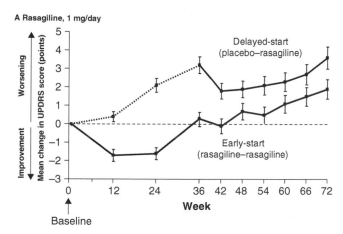

FIGURE 17.3 Changes in scores on the Unified Parkinson's Disease Rating Scale in the 1 mg/day rasagiline-delayed (placebo) and early-start groups in the ADAGIO study. *Source*: From Ref. 42.

Why did the 2 mg dose fail to meet the second endpoint in ADAGIO when the 1 mg dose succeeded in ADAGIO and TEMPO and the 2 mg dose succeeded in TEMPO? One possible explanation is that the success of the 1 mg dose is a false positive or conversely that the 2 mg result is a false negative. Given the hierarchical design of the study and the multiple endpoints, the likelihood of either false-positive or false-negative results, while possible, is unlikely. The authors of the ADAGIO study suggested that a marked symptomatic effect of the 2 mg dose might have masked a modest disease-modifying effect in a population with only mild disease and low UPDRS scores (42). A post hoc analysis was performed to look at the 289 patients taking the 2 mg/day dose in the upper quartile of UPDRS scores (>25.5) at baseline to see if the primary endpoints would be met in a population with more advanced disease. In this more advanced population, all three primary endpoints were met, suggesting a possible "floor effect" limited the ability to detect the disease-modifying effect in a population with milder disease (Fig. 17.5).

The ADAGIO and TEMPO studies have been criticized for a number of reasons, including that the UPDRS is insensitive and that the differences in UPDRS scores between the early start and delayed start groups is small and clinically irrelevant (43). For example, in the ADAGIO study the difference between the delayed start and early start 1 mg groups was 1.7 points at 72 weeks. It should be remembered that the 1.7-point difference is between two groups receiving active treatment, and not active treatment versus placebo. Nevertheless, this difference represents a 38% reduction in the rate of decline in the early treatment arm (5). Moreover, delayed start studies are not designed to assess the clinical magnitude of a treatment but are instead designed to determine if a study drug can provide benefits that cannot be accounted for by symptomatic treatment alone and is therefore consistent with disease modification (11).

An additional criticism of delayed start trials is that starting any treatment early will provide a positive result by either maintaining a compensatory mechanism in the basal ganglia or preventing maladaptive compensatory responses (9). This criticism, however, was recently challenged by the results of the Pramipexole On Underlying Disease (PROUD) study. The PROUD study was a randomized delayed

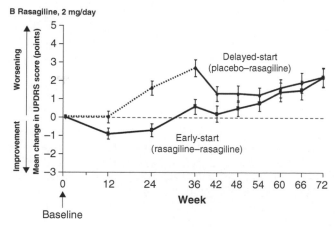

FIGURE 17.4 Changes in scores on the Unified Parkinson's Disease Rating Scale in the 2 mg/day rasagiline-delayed (placebo) and early-start groups in the ADAGIO study. *Source*: From Ref. 42.

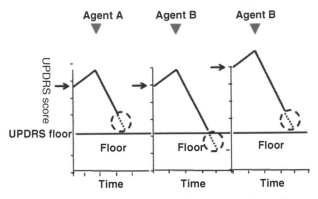

FIGURE 17.5 Schematic illustration of how a floor effect in UPDRS could theoretically interfere with detection of a disease-modifying effect in a delayed-start study. The left panel illustrates agent A with symptomatic and disease-modifying effects that can be detected because the combined effect does not extend beyond the floor of the UPDRS. The center panel illustrates agent B with symptomatic effects that extend to the UPDRS floor and thereby mask detection of any additional benefit due to a disease-modifying effect. The right panel illustrates that the disease-modifying effect of agent B can be detected if subjects with higher baseline UPDRS scores are used in the trial. (Arrow = baseline UPDRS score. Arrowhead = introduction of agent. Circle with dotted line = disease modifying effects due to early start. Red line = UPDRS floor: maximum benefit that can be recorded with the UPDRS scale). *Abbreviation*: UPDRS, Unified Parkinson's Disease Rating Scale. *Source*: From Ref. 11.

start placebo-controlled study evaluating whether pramipexole was disease modifying in early PD patients (44). In the first phase, 535 untreated PD patients were randomized to receive pramipexole 0.5 mg three times daily or placebo for six to nine months. In the second phase, the placebo group was then switched to pramipexole and the active treatment group was continued on pramipexole. The primary endpoint was change in UPDRS at 15 months. Moreover, a subgroup of 150 patients underwent DAT SPECT scanning at baseline and 15 months. At 15 months, there was no difference in UPDRS or SPECT scanning between the early start and the delayed start groups thus confirming that simply starting any therapy in a delayed-start design will not result in positive results (45).

A ROAD MAP TO THE FUTURE

Without valid biomarkers and given the confounding limitations of using clinical endpoints in drugs with symptomatic benefits, trial design to demonstrate disease modification in PD remains an enormous challenge. Olanow and Kiebertz have recently proposed a "road map" for developing putative disease-modifying therapies (Table 17.1) (11). In this road map, drugs initially are identified in the laboratory for possible disease-modifying effects. Phase I studies are then conducted to ensure that promising drugs are safe and tolerable and therefore would not be from approval by regulatory agencies. "Futility" or "Nonsuperiority" trials would then be conducted on those drugs found to be safe and tolerable.

TABLE 17.1 Road map for Defining a Disease-Modifying Agent in PD

- Identify candidate agent based on laboratory studies
- Phase I studies to determine safety and tolerability
- Futility study
- Delayed-start study
- Long-term simple study

Source: From Ref. 11.

In a futility trial, drugs are screened for nonsuperiority in comparison to placebo or a natural history comparator with the null hypothesis being that the drug is superior to the placebo or comparator. If the study is negative, the null hypothesis is rejected and the drug is deemed futile. If the study is positive, the null hypothesis is not rejected and the drug should be considered for further investigation (11). Futility trials allow for the rapid and relatively inexpensive screening of multiple promising therapies thereby avoiding more expensive long-term trials in drugs with no reasonable chance of success.

The National Institutes of Health's consortium, Neuroprotection Exploratory Trials in PD (NET-PD) investigators recently employed the futility design to evaluate a number of potential disease-modifying agents in PD. The first of these studies evaluated creatine and minocycline with the futility threshold being a 30% reduction in UPDRS progression based on the placebo/tocopherol arm of the DATATOP study (46). Neither creatine nor minocycline were rejected as futile. A second futility study looked a Coenzyme Q10 and GPI-1485, a neuroimmunophilin, and both agents were found to be nonfutile when compared with the DATATOP cohort (45,47). However, when a separate analysis was done using a current control cohort (rather than the DATATOP cohort), only creatine was found to be nonfutile.

Indeed, the finding of futility with respect to Coenzyme Q10 was recently confirmed in the Effects of CoQ10 in Parkinson's disease study (QE3). Coenzyme Q10 was thought to have potential disease-modifying benefits in PD because it acts as an electron acceptor for complexes I and II and is an antioxidant and PD patients have been shown to have reduced mitochondrial complex I activity (48,49). QE3 was a large double-blind placebo-controlled study in which 600 patients were randomized to placebo or Coenzyme Q10 at 1200 or 2400 mg daily. The primary endpoint was change in UPDRS at 16 months. The study was terminated early when an interim release of data demonstrated that it would be unlikely to show any difference between the placebo and Coenzyme Q10 (45).

The next step in the road map is to perform a delayed start design study. This step would determine if the drug has benefits that cannot be explained by symptomatic effects alone. The final step in the road map would be to perform a long-term simple study (LTSS). In an LTSS, patients are randomized to receive the study drug or placebo for an extended period (i.e., years) during which time they may receive any other PD therapies that their physician deems appropriate (11). The endpoint can be a composite of multiple measures of cumulative disability, including change in UPDRS and non-dopaminergic features and quality of life. An LTSS is not designed to explain the mechanism of any observed benefit but instead to elicit the effect of a study drug on long-term disability. The NET-PD investigators used the LTSS design to evaluate creatine in the LS-1 study (45). In this ongoing study, 1720 PD patients have been randomized to placebo or creatine 5 g daily and are now being followed for five years. The primary endpoints include quality of life, activities of daily living, motor function, gait, falling, and cognition. Although an LTSS is relatively cheap and easy to perform, they require large numbers of patients and a long duration to see any disease-modifying effect.

CONCLUSION

In 1817, James Parkinson recognized the importance of disease modification and was hopeful that such a therapy could be found. In his "Essay on the Shaking Palsy" he wrote, "...although at present, uninformed as to the precise nature of the disease, still it ought not to be considered as one against which there exists no countervailing remedy. On the contrary, there appears to be sufficient reason for hoping that some remedial process may be discovered, by which, at least, the progress of the disease may be stopped" (50). Nearly 200 years later, Parkinson's words still ring true.

Disease modification remains the greatest unmet need in PD. Beginning with the early selegiline trials through the neuroimaging trials and most recently with the delayed start design trials, there are signals of possible disease modification. Although the results of the DATATOP, ELLDOPA, TEMPO, and ADAGIO trials are arguably consistent with disease modification, they are not conclusive and each of the study designs is subject to criticism. Without a reliable, valid biomarker, absolute proof of disease modification appears stymied. Perhaps the best hope to demonstrate disease modification at the current time is to use the cumulative results of the "road map" approach, rather than relying on any single study design.

REFERENCES

1. Olanow CW, Stern MB, Sethi K. The scientific and clinical basis for the treatment of Parkinson disease. Neurology 2009; 72: S1–136.
2. Carlsson A. The occurrence, distribution and physiological role of catecholamines in the nervous system. Pharmacol Rev 1959; 11: 490–3.
3. Ehringer H, Hornykiewicz O. Distribution of noradrenaline and dopamine (3-hydroxytyramine) in the human brain and their behavior in diseases of the extrapyramidal system. Klin Wochenschr 1960; 38: 1236–9.
4. Cotzias GC, Van Woert MH, Schiffer LM. Aromatic amino acids and modification of parkinsonism. N Engl J Med 1967; 276: 374–9.
5. Henchcliffe C, Severt WL. Disease modification in Parkinson's disease. Drugs Aging 2011; 28: 605–15.
6. Langston JW. The Parkinson's complex: parkinsonism is just the tip of the iceberg. Ann Neurol 2006; 59: 591–6.
7. Chaudhuri KR, Healy DG, Schapira AH. Non-motor symptoms of Parkinson's disease: diagnosis and management. Lancet Neurol 2006; 5: 235–45.
8. Olanow CW. Can we achieve neuroprotection with currently available anti-parkinsonian interventions? Neurology 2009; 72: S59–64.
9. Rascol O. "Disease-modification" trials in Parkinson disease: target populations, endpoints and study design. Neurology 2009; 72: S51–8.
10. Hart RG, Pearce LA, Ravina BM, et al. Neuroprotection trials in Parkinson's disease: systematic review. Mov Disord 2009; 24: 647–54.
11. Olanow CW, Kieburtz K. Defining disease-modifying therapies for PD–a road map for moving forward. Mov Disord 2010; 25: 1774–9.
12. Hornykiewicz O. Dopamine (3-hydroxytyramine) in the central nervous system and its relation to the Parkinson syndrome in man. Dtsch Med Wochenschr 1962; 87: 1807–10.

13. Johnson AG. Monoamine oxidase inhibitors. Br Med J 1968; 2: 433.
14. Birkmayer W, Riederer P, Youdim MB, et al. The potentiation of the anti akinetic effect after L-dopa treatment by an inhibitor of MAO-B, Deprenil. J Neural Transm 1975; 36: 303–26.
15. Birkmayer W. Deprenyl (selegiline) in the treatment of Parkinson's disease. Acta Neurol Scand Suppl 1983; 95: 103–5.
16. Birkmayer W, Knoll J, Riederer P, et al. (-)-Deprenyl leads to prolongation of L-dopa efficacy in Parkinson's disease. Mod Probl Pharmacopsychiatry 1983; 19: 170–6.
17. Langston JW, Ballard P, Tetrud JW, et al. Chronic Parkinsonism in humans due to a product of meperidine-analog synthesis. Science 1983; 219: 979–80.
18. Ballard PA, Tetrud JW, Langston JW. Permanent human parkinsonism due to 1-methyl-4-phenyl-1,2,3,6-tetrahydropyridine (MPTP): seven cases. Neurology 1985; 35: 949–56.
19. Schapira AH. Monoamine oxidase B inhibitors for the treatment of Parkinson's disease: a review of symptomatic and potential disease-modifying effects. CNS Drugs 2011; 25: 1061–71.
20. Cohen G, Pasik P, Cohen B, et al. Pargyline and deprenyl prevent the neurotoxicity of 1-methyl-4-phenyl-1,2,3,6-tetrahydropyridine (MPTP) in monkeys. Eur J Pharmacol 1984; 106: 209–10.
21. Tetrud JW, Langston JW. The effect of deprenyl (selegiline) on the natural history of Parkinson's disease. Science 1989; 245: 519–22.
22. Parkinson Study Group. Effect of deprenyl on the progression of disability in early Parkinson's disease. N Engl J Med 1989; 321: 1364–71.
23. Parkinson Study Group. Effect of tocopherol and deprenyl on the progression of disability in early Parkinson's disease. N Engl J Med 1993; 328: 176–83.
24. Parkinson Study Group. Cerebrospinal fluid homovanillic acid in the DATATOP study on Parkinson's disease. Arch Neurol 1995; 52: 237–45.
25. Olanow CW, Hauser RA, Gauger L, et al. The effect of deprenyl and levodopa on the progression of Parkinson's disease. Ann Neurol 1995; 38: 771–7.
26. Shoulson I, Oakes D, Fahn S, et al. Impact of sustained deprenyl (selegiline) in levodopa-treated Parkinson's disease: a randomized placebo-controlled extension of the deprenyl and tocopherol antioxidative therapy of parkinsonism trial. Ann Neurol 2002; 51: 604–12.
27. Palhagen S, Heinonen E, Hagglund J, et al. Selegiline slows the progression of the symptoms of Parkinson disease. Neurology 2006; 66: 1200–6.
28. Lees AJ; Parkinson's Disease Research Group of the United Kingdom. Comparison of therapeutic effects and mortality data of levodopa and levodopa combined with selegiline in patients with early, mild Parkinson's disease. BMJ 1995; 311: 1602–7.
29. Ben-Shlomo Y, Churchyard A, Head J, et al. Investigation by Parkinson's Disease Research Group of United Kingdom into excess mortality seen with combined levodopa and selegiline treatment in patients with early, mild Parkinson's disease: further results of randomised trial and confidential inquiry. BMJ 1998; 316: 1191–6.
30. Olanow CW, Myllyla VV, Sotaniemi KA, et al. Effect of selegiline on mortality in patients with Parkinson's disease: a meta-analysis. Neurology 1998; 51: 825–30.
31. Schapira AH, Olanow CW. Neuroprotection in Parkinson disease: mysteries, myths, and misconceptions. JAMA 2004; 291: 358–64.
32. Parkinson Study Group. Dopamine transporter brain imaging to assess the effects of pramipexole vs levodopa on Parkinson disease progression. JAMA 2002; 287: 1653–61.
33. Whone AL, Watts RL, Stoessl AJ, et al. Slower progression of Parkinson's disease with ropinirole versus levodopa: The REAL-PET study. Ann Neurol 2003; 54: 93–101.
34. Pavese N, Kiferle L, Piccini P. Neuroprotection and imaging studies in Parkinson's disease. Parkinsonism Relat Disord 2009; 15:S33–7.
35. Jennings DL, Tabamo R, Seibyl JP. InSPECT: investigating the effect of short-term treatment with pramipexole or levodopa on [123-I] Beta-CIT and SPECT imaging. Mov Disord 2007; 22: S143.
36. Parkinson Study Group. Levodopa and the progression of Parkinson's disease. N Engl J Med 2004; 351: 2498–508.

37. Leber P. Slowing the progression of Alzheimer disease: methodologic issues. Alzheimer Dis Assoc Disord 1997; 11: S10–21.
38. Parkinson Study Group. A controlled trial of rasagiline in early Parkinson disease: the TEMPO Study. Arch Neurol 2002; 59: 1937–43.
39. Olanow CW. Rationale for considering that propargylamines might be neuroprotective in Parkinson's disease. Neurology 2006; 66: S69–79.
40. Hauser RA, Lew MF, Hurtig HI, et al. Long-term outcome of early versus delayed rasagiline treatment in early Parkinson's disease. Mov Disord 2009; 24: 562–71.
41. Olanow CW, Hauser RA, Jankovic J, et al. A randomized, double-blind, placebo-controlled, delayed start study to assess rasagiline as a disease modifying therapy in Parkinson's disease (the ADAGIO study): rationale, design, and baseline characteristics. Mov Disord 2008; 23: 2194–201.
42. Olanow CW, Rascol O, Hauser R, et al. A double-blind, delayed-start trial of rasagiline in Parkinson's disease. N Engl J Med 2009; 361: 1268–78.
43. Ahlskog JE, Uitti RJ. Rasagiline, Parkinson neuroprotection, and delayed-start trials: still no satisfaction? Neurology 2010; 74: 1143–8.
44. Schapira AH, Albrecht S, Barone P, et al. Rationale for delayed-start study of pramipexole in Parkinson's disease: the PROUD study. Mov Disord 2010; 25: 1627–32.
45. Lew MF. The evidence for disease modification in Parkinson's disease. Int J Neurosci 2011; 121: 18–26.
46. NINDS NET-PD Investigators. A randomized, double-blind, futility clinical trial of creatine and minocycline in early Parkinson's disease. Neurology 2006; 66: 664–71.
47. NINDS NET-PD Investigators. A randomized clinical trial of coenzyme Q10 and GPI-1485 in early Parkinson's disease. Neurology 2007; 68: 20–8.
48. Parker WD Jr, Boyson SJ, Parks JK. Abnormalities of the electron transport chain in idiopathic Parkinson's disease. Ann Neurol 1989; 26: 719–23.
49. Shults CW, Haas RH, Passov D, et al. Coenzyme Q10 levels correlate with the activities of complexes I and II/III in mitochondria from parkinsonian and nonparkinsonian subjects. Ann Neurol 1997; 42: 261–4.
50. Parkinson J. Essay on the Shaking Palsy. London: Whittingham and Rowland for Sherwood, Neeley and Jones, 1817.

18 Amantadine and anticholinergics

Khashayar Dashtipour, Joseph S. Chung,
Allan D. Wu, and Mark F. Lew

INTRODUCTION

Amantadine and anticholinergics have been used for several decades as therapy for Parkinson's disease (PD). In spite of reduced interest in these compounds with the advent of more specific dopaminergic therapies, there remain clinical situations where amantadine and anticholinergics retain clinical usefulness and a role in the contemporary treatment of PD. In fact, in the last few years, amantadine is being prescribed more frequently to treat patients experiencing dyskinesia.

AMANTADINE
History

Amantadine (Symmetrel®) was approved by the Food and Drug Administration of the United States in 1966 and was marketed as an antiviral agent. Its use as an antiparkinsonian agent was first described in 1969 when a woman with advanced PD serendipitously noted transient relief of tremor, rigidity, and bradykinesia, during a six-week course of flu prophylaxis with amantadine (1). Since that time, further studies confirmed a mild antiparkinsonian effect with amantadine (2). The use of amantadine has been limited, likely due to the development of dopamine agonists and other antiparkinsonian medications, better tolerance of levodopa with the advent of carbidopa, and the misconception of transient benefit, known as tachyphylaxis. Investigators have sought to examine the potential clinical uses for amantadine in the management of PD. Modulating effects of amantadine on motor complications in later-stage PD have been documented in several studies (3–5).

Many different mechanisms of action have been proposed for the antiparkinsonian effects of amantadine, but clear attribution has remained obscure. Traditional mechanisms for amantadine were usually ascribed to dopaminergic or anticholinergic mechanisms such as the proposed promotion of endogenous dopamine release (6). However, further studies have demonstrated a variety of biologic effects beyond these systems. For instance, studies have suggested that amantadine possesses glutamate-blocking activity (7).

Pharmacokinetics and Dosing

Amantadine is an aliphatic primary amine formulated as a hydrochloride salt for clinical use, as an oral preparation. It is a relatively inexpensive drug available as a 100-mg tablet or capsule and a 50-mg/mL liquid. Other than some anticholinergics and apomorphine, it is also one of the few PD medications available in a parenteral formulation (amantadine-sulfate). This intravenous preparation, however, is not available for use in the United States (8). Intravenous amantadine has been shown to be safe and effective in PD patients who undergo surgery and medications cannot be administered orally (9).

The bioavailability of amantadine is 86% in the elderly and more than 90% in young adults in oral form (10). It is excreted virtually unmetabolized via the kidneys and has a large volume of distribution. In fasting, healthy patients, peak plasma concentration was found 1–4 hours after a single oral dose of 2.5–5 mg/kg. Plasma half-life in healthy elderly men has been reported between 18 and 45 hours, suggesting that steady state may take up to nine days (11). It crosses the blood–brain barrier and the placenta, and is excreted into the breast milk. Serum amantadine levels are not routinely drawn and are probably of limited clinical utility. Pharmacological studies have reported serum levels between 0.2 and 0.9 μg/mL at dosages of 200 mg/day (12). Fahn et al. (13) reported a patient with psychosis following acute intoxication with amantadine who had a level of 2.37 μg/mL.

A few drug interactions have been reported with amantadine. Ethanol in combination with amantadine can increase central nervous system (CNS) side effects, such as dizziness, confusion, and orthostatic hypotension (14). Antimuscarinics and medication with significant anticholinergic activity may increase the anticholinergic side effects of amantadine (14). A potential interaction of amantadine with bupropion has been reported (14,15). Affected patients develop restlessness, agitation, gait disturbance, and dizziness, and may require hospitalization depending on the severity. There is also a case report, suggesting amantadine toxicity from an interaction with hydrochlorothiazide–triamterene (16).

Routine dosing starts at 100 mg twice daily. Doses up to 500 mg have been reported for controlling motor complications in PD patients (17). The maximum tolerable doses are suggested at 400–500 mg each day, in patients with normal renal function (18); however, doses over 400 mg have no added benefit and have an increased incidence of side effects.

Clinical Uses

Early Parkinson's Disease

Amantadine is generally considered a mild antiparkinsonian agent, with effects on tremor, rigidity, and bradykinesia, and a well-tolerated side-effect profile. It is used in early PD when considering levodopa sparing strategies or when symptoms are mild enough not to warrant more aggressive therapy. Amantadine has been studied in early PD as monotherapy, and in combination with anticholinergics in limited series and small controlled studies, with relatively short follow-up (19–21). However, a review of randomized, controlled trials of amantadine does not reveal sufficient evidence to support its efficacy in the treatment of early PD (22,23). The 2002 American Academy of Neurology (AAN) guidelines for the initiation of PD treatment did not discuss the use of amantadine (24).

Part of the rationale for considering amantadine monotherapy are suggestions that it may have neuroprotective properties to slow the progression of PD. Uitti et al. found that amantadine use was an independent predictor of improved survival in a retrospective analysis of all parkinsonism patients (92% PD) treated with amantadine compared with those not using this medication. The results are suggestive of either an ongoing symptomatic improvement or the presence of inherent neuroprotection (25). Because of a nonrandomized design and nonindependent outcome assessment, this study was graded Class IV in the most recent practice guideline about neuroprotective strategies for PD (26). The quality standards subcommittee of the AAN concluded lack of sufficient evidence to support or refute the use of amantadine for neuroprotection (26).

Advanced Parkinson's Disease

The use of amantadine in managing PD motor complications was first described in 1987 by Shannon et al. (4) in a small open-label study. They reported improved motor fluctuations using a qualitative scale, examining on and off function in 20 PD patients. This notion has gained further support from Metman et al. who reported the results of double-blind, placebo-controlled, cross-over studies of amantadine in a small cohort of 14 PD patients. There was a 60% reduction in both peak dose dyskinesia and severity of off periods, along with a decreased duration of off time (27). One year later, these patients had maintained significant benefit (6). The Cochrane database systematically reviewed randomized, controlled studies (28) that evaluated amantadine versus placebo in the treatment of levodopa-induced dyskinesia, and reported a lack of evidence to support the efficacy of amantadine. Thomas et al. (29) conducted a double-blind, placebo-controlled study in 40 PD patients and concluded that 300 mg of amantadine was effective to control levodopa-induced dyskinesia by approximately 45%; however, the effect was maintained for less than eight months in all patients. Another randomized, double-blind, controlled study (30) of 18 PD patients found that the duration of levodopa-induced dyskinesia was reduced by using amantadine. A more recent randomized control trial evaluated the long-term antidyskinetic effect of amantadine in 32 PD subjects with dyskinesia (31). This study confirmed the result of prior studies that amantadine is efficacious for the treatment of dyskinesia. In a separate double-blind, randomized, placebo-controlled, cross-over trial the efficacy of amantadine in PD patients suffering from dyskinesia were assessed (32). This study showed the efficacy of amantadine against dyskinesia in 60–70% of patients. Multivariate logistic analysis demonstrated that higher age-of-onset and use of dopamine agonists were positively associated with the response to amantadine (32). The recognition of different dyskinesia phenomenology may be important in the response to amantadine. For instance, dystonic dyskinesia has shown varied interindividual effects in a few studies (3,4). Also, specific efficacy for sudden on–offs or biphasic dyskinesia has not been formally investigated. Based on AAN practice parameter recommendations, amantadine may be considered to reduce dyskinesia (Level C) (33) but the National Guideline Clearinghouse (NGC) according to the European Federation of Neurological Societies (FENS) criteria recommended to add amantadine for peak-dose dyskinesia (Level A) (34). Because there is insufficient scientific evidence, a consensus statement (good practice point) was made regarding wearing-off symptoms and the NGC recommended amantadine, may improve wearing-off symptoms in some cases (34).

Recent evidence suggests that amantadine produces its antidyskinetic effects via a glutamate N-methyl-D-aspartate (NMDA) antagonism (35). This independence from dopaminergic mechanisms was proposed as an explanation for the ability of amantadine to ameliorate levodopa-induced dyskinesia without worsening parkinsonism (27). Clinical trials are underway evaluating the use of an extended release formulation of amantadine to treat patients with PD and severe dyskinesia.

Freezing of gait is one of the disabling motor complications of PD during the advanced stages of disease. In an open and uncontrolled study IV amantadine was used in six patients with PD and induced improvement in freezing of gait resistant to dopaminergic medications (36).

Miscellaneous Considerations

One frequent assumption about amantadine is that it offers only transient efficacy that typically lasts less than a year. However, this apparent loss of efficacy for amelio-rating parkinsonian symptoms was reviewed and attributed largely to the progres-sion of the disease itself. It has also been reported that early-stage PD patients may be treated effectively for years with amantadine, and still find that their symptoms noticeably worsen following drug withdrawal (17).

Side Effects

Amantadine is generally well tolerated. The most common side effects include livedo reticularis and pedal edema. Livedo reticularis is a mottled bluish-red reticu-lar skin discoloration, which blanches to pressure. It is observed in more than 5% of patients receiving amantadine. It is more common in women (37) and is usually predominant in the lower extremities. The appearance is nonspecific, and skin biop-sies of the area are normal (38). Livedo reticularis usually appears after weeks of treatment and it can occur up to one year from initiation of therapy. The etiology of livedo reticularis is unclear, but it is believed to be caused by abnormal widespread dilatation of dermal blood vessels due to depletion of catecholamines at the periph-eral nerve terminals (39). The cosmetic appearance is usually far more apparent than any physical adverse effects. Pedal edema can also appear, and is independent of either renal or cardiac failure. Its presence has generally been attributed to a redistribution of fluid and does not appear to represent excess fluid. Quinn et al. (40) reported a few cases of congestive heart failure occurring in association with the use of amantadine, but this appears to be an exception to routine clinical use.

The presence of either livedo reticularis or pedal edema does not always necessitate discontinuation of amantadine. There is no specific treatment for the cosmetic discoloration associated with livedo reticularis. Symptoms are generally expected to resolve with discontinuation of the drug, but may take up to several weeks. Rarely, these conditions may be severe and associated with leg ulceration and peripheral neuropathy (41). A prudent combination of discontinuing the drug and providing appropriate referrals to exclude important secondary causes, such as a superimposed renal failure, cardiac failure, autoimmune or vasculitic livedo, and deep vein thrombosis, must be an important part of continued clinical follow-up for patients on amantadine.

Rimantadine is an alpha-methyl derivative of amantadine. An open-label trial showed the effectiveness of rimantadine in controlling motor symptoms in PD (42). A retrospective study of seven patients with moderate-to-severe PD revealed that rimantadine was an effective alternative to amantadine, in patients experiencing amantadine-induced peripheral side effects such as livedo reticularis and lower limb edema (43). Side effects did not develop on rimantadine and patients showed good clinical efficacy.

Amantadine-induced peripheral neuropathy has been rarely reported (44). It was hypothesized that amantadine transfers the blood supply to the peripheral nerves because of its effect on catecholamine storage (44). Nonspecific symptoms, such as lightheadedness, insomnia, jitteriness, depression, and concentration diffi-culties, are potential side effects of amantadine (11). Amantadine also possesses mild anticholinergic properties, which contribute to side effects such as dry mouth, orthostatic hypotension, constipation, dyspepsia, and urinary retention. Therefore, reasonable care should be taken when administering amantadine in conjunction with anticholinergics (45). One report (8) noted cardiac arrhythmias with amantadine. Amantadine is not recommended during pregnancy, as it has more teratogenic potential than the other PD medications (46).

There are reports of ocular side effects, such as corneal lesions and edema, associated with the use of amantadine (47–49). Corneal side effects can occur within a few weeks to a few years after initiation of therapy and are generally reversible within a week of stopping the medication.

Impulse control disorders were reported in a 50-year-old woman with a 15-year history of PD after initiation of amantadine (50). On the other hand the efficacy of amantadine in the control of pathologic gambling was assessed in a double-blind crossover study with amantadine 200 mg/day versus placebo. This study showed that pathologic gambling could be abolished in 2 to 3 days by amantadine (51). Later a secondary analysis of a large cross-sectional study of impulse control disorders including pathologic gambling in patients with PD treated with amantadine was performed. The results of this study showed that amantadine was positively associated with the occurrence of impulse control disorders (52).

Acute toxicity presenting as delirium (19), seizure (53), and psychosis (13) has been reported. Abrupt withdrawal has been described to produce delirium (54), as well as neuroleptic malignant syndrome (55). In many of these cases, patients either had baseline cognitive deficits, psychiatric background, or excess amantadine use beyond clinical recommendations. In general, the cognitive side effects such as confusion and concentration difficulties are more common in those with underlying, pre-existing cognitive dysfunction. In advanced PD, amantadine may even carry comparable propensity for cognitive side effects to levodopa (56). As such, conservative use in the elderly and avoidance of use even in the mildly cognitively impaired patient is necessary.

Because of the renal predominant excretion of amantadine, patients with impaired kidney function carry a higher risk of toxicity. Dosing schedules have been developed for patients with poor renal function according to creatinine clearance (57). It is best to avoid the use of amantadine in patients with poor renal clearance. In the event of suspected toxicity, dialysis is not helpful in decreasing toxic levels, probably due to extensive tissue binding (58).

Mechanisms of Action
Many studies have suggested putative mechanisms of action for amantadine that may explain antiparkinsonian effects, but the clinical significance of any given individual mechanism remains uncertain. It seems likely that amantadine has a combination of multiple effects on both dopaminergic and nondopaminergic systems.

Dopaminergic mechanisms described for amantadine include findings of increased dopamine release (59), increased dopamine synthesis (60), inhibition of dopamine reuptake (61), and modulation of dopamine D2 receptors, producing a high-affinity state (62). This latter effect may speculatively play a role in modulating levodopa-induced dyskinesia. The relevance of these dopaminergic mechanisms is uncertain, given that studies have demonstrated that the antiparkinsonian effects can occur without changes in brain concentrations of dopamine or its metabolites (63) and without evidence for dopamine synthesis or release (64).

Other neurotransmitter effects reported with amantadine include serotonergic, noradrenergic (65), anticholinergic, and antiglutaminergic properties (66). The anticholinergic properties suggest a well-described antiparkinsonian interaction (67,68).

In the past decade, renewed interest has arisen in the antiglutamate properties of amantadine (69). This can be attributed to two important clinical implications. First, it may provide a putative neuroprotective mechanism. Second, converging lines of evidence provide support to the idea that the antiglutamate properties of amantadine may be important for modulating motor complications in late-stage PD, particularly dyskinesia.

Amantadine possesses mild anti-NMDA properties that have led to the suggestion that the drug may contribute to a possible neuroprotective effect in PD (70). Glutamate excitotoxicity, mediated via persistent or sustained activation of NMDA receptors, produces an excess calcium influx, activating a cascade of molecular events leading to the common final pathway of neuronal death. Blockade of NMDA glutamate receptors has been shown to experimentally diminish the excitotoxic effects of this cascade of reactions (71,72). In cell cultures, pre-exposure of substantia nigra dopaminergic neurons to glutamate antagonists provided protection when subsequently exposed to 1-methyl-4-phenyl-pyridium ion, the active metabolite of 1-methyl-4-phenyl-1,2,3,6-tetrahydropyridine (MPP+), a common specific nigral toxin used to produce animal models of PD (73). Extension of these preclinical findings to clinical applicability in PD patients remains speculative, but probably best serves a role to stimulate future studies.

The anti-NMDA properties of amantadine have also been implicated in its role-modulating motor complications, such as dyskinesia (74–76). Evidence has accumulated that glutamate NMDA receptors may play a significant role in the pathogenesis of motor complications. Loss of striatal dopamine and nonphysiologic stimulation by extrinsic levodopa, both cause sensitization of NMDA receptors on striatal medium spiny neurons in animal models (31). This sensitization may play a key role in altering normal basal ganglia responses to cortical glutaminergic input and produce the disordered motor output, which leads to motor complications. Recent studies have reported that striatal injection or systemic administration of glutamate antagonists in primate and rodent models of PD can decrease levodopa motor complications with-out decreasing benefits of dopaminergic treatment (7,77–80).

Using cultured microglial cells, a recent study showed the microglia-inhibiting activity of amantadine. Amantadine reduced the production of proinflammatory mediators in bacterial lipopolysaccharide-stimulated microglia cells (81). This effect was also demonstrated in animal models of PD. These findings suggest that amantadine may act on microglia in the central nervous system and attenuate neuroinflammation (81).

Summary

With improved management options for PD, patients are living longer and, as a result, more are suffering from long-term complications of disease and therapy. Although the influx of new medications has changed the landscape of pharmacologic options for PD patients, a re-examination of the older medications such as amantadine can offer benefit.

Amantadine retains its primary utility as a mild antiparkinsonian agent to be used mostly as adjunctive therapy, and occasionally in early monotherapy when PD symptoms are mild. Most recently, it is frequently being utilized as the only available antiparkinsonian agent to diminish dyskinesia and offer improvement of PD symptoms simultaneously (82).

ANTICHOLINERGICS
History
Anticholinergics are the earliest class of pharmaceuticals used for the management of PD. Naturally occurring anticholinergics, such as the belladonna alkaloids, have been used for centuries to treat a variety of ailments. Since the mid-1900s and until the modern development of dopaminergic agents, anticholinergics were a major component of therapy for PD (83). In the 1940s, synthetic anticholinergics were introduced with trihexyphenidyl (Artane®) and similar agents, replacing impure herbal preparations of belladonna alkaloids in the treatment of PD. Eventually, a wide variety of anticholinergics, each with varying receptor specificities, blood–brain barrier penetration, and side effect profiles, became available. Historically and by physician's preference, certain medications have gained popularity or notoriety for particular use in treating PD (84). This has varied throughout the decades. For instance, benzhexol was used as an antiparkinsonian medication in 1972 (84), but is not in common use today.

With recent developments in PD therapy, anticholinergics have been relegated to a distinctly less prominent role. In particular, levodopa, dopamine agonists, and MAO-B inhibitors have largely replaced anticholinergics. Contemporary reviews and investigations continue to support anticholinergic use in certain clinical situations, such as PD-associated tremor or dystonia. Side effects have always been a prominent concern with anticholinergics, particularly in susceptible individuals such as the elderly. As such, careful risk–benefit assessment in anticholinergic use remains a prudent routine practice in PD patients.

Pharmacokinetics and Dosing
Anticholinergics are a diverse group of medications. The majority of the anticholinergic medications have good oral absorption, but precise figures on many are not known. In general, most have half-lives requiring at least twice and usually three times a day dosing. The antiparkinsonian effect of anticholinergics is largely attributed to centrally acting acetylcholine receptors (85). Most synthetic (tertiary) anticholinergics used in PD are predominantly in this class: biperiden (Akineton®), trihexyphenidyl (Artane®), benztropine (Cogentin®), and procyclidine (Kemadrin®). Benztropine was formulated as a combination of the anticholinergic, atropine, and an antihistamine, diphenhydramine (Benadryl®). Benztropine has useful central effects that can be used for PD management and is more potent than trihexyphenidyl, but has less sedating effects than antihistamines (86). Recommended doses and choice of a particular anticholinergic vary by practitioner, but one rule is to start with a low dose and increase slowly and conservatively (Table 18.1).

Clinical Uses
Since the advent of levodopa therapy for PD in the 1960s, the usefulness and popularity of anticholinergics waned dramatically. However, an evidence-based review by the Cochrane Collaboration concluded that anticholinergics are effective in improving motor function in parkinsonian patients as monotherapy and adjunct therapy. The current data are not sufficient to allow comparison in efficacy or tolerability between individual anticholinergic medications (87).

Tremor-Predominant Parkinson's Disease
The most recognized use of anticholinergics is to treat tremor in early- or young-onset PD representing a levodopa-sparing strategy. In general, it appears that

TABLE 18.1 Common Anticholinergics Used in Parkinson's Disease

Name	Mechanisms	Preparations	Initial Dose	Escalation Schedule	Maximum Dose/Day	Comments
Primary anticholinergics						
Trihexyphenidyl (Artane®)	Central antimuscarinic	2, 5 mg tablets; 2 mg/5 mL elixir	1 mg qd–bid	Increase to tid; every 3–4 days increase by 0.5–1 mg each dose	2–3 mg tid	First synthetic anticholinergic
Benztropine (Cogentin®)	Central antimuscarinic	0.5, 1, 2 mg tablets; injection 1 mg/mL	0.5 mg bid	Increase to tid; every 3–4 days increase by 0.5–1 mg each dose	2 mg tid	Also available parenterally
Biperiden (Akineton®)	Central antimuscarinic	2 mg tablets; 5 mg/mL ampules	1 mg bid	Increase to tid; every 3–4 days increase by 0.5–1 mg each dose	3 mg tid	Also available parenterally
Ethopropazine (Parsidol®, Parsitan®)	Central antimuscarinic	50 mg tablets	12.5 mg tid/qid	Increase to tid; every 3–4 days increase by 12.5 mg each dose	50 mg tid–qid	Not available in the United States
Secondary anticholinergic effects						
Diphenhydramine (Benadryl®)	Antihistamine	12.5, 25 mg tablets; 12.5 mg liquid	25 mg qhs	Increase by 25 mg every 3–4 days	25 mg tid or 25–100 mg qhs	H1 blocker
Amitryptiline (Elavil®)	Tricyclic antidepressant	10, 25, 50, 75, 100, 150 tablets; injection 10 mg/mL	12.5 mg qhs	Increase by 12.5 mg every 2–3 nights	150 mg	Also available parenterally
Clozapine (Clozaril®)	Atypical antipsychotic	25 mg tablets	6.25–12.5 mg	Increase by 6.25–12.5 mg every 2–3 nights	100 mg	May cause increased salivation

anticholinergics help tremor, but do not significantly affect bradykinesia or rigidity of PD. Anticholinergic agents may be used as initial therapy of tremor-predominant PD (83). Schrag et al. (88) found equivalent reductions in tremor with a single dose of either a dopamine agonist (apomorphine) or an anticholinergic (biperiden), but only apomorphine reduced rigidity and akinesia. Although anticholinergics do not appear to have significant effects on akinesia and rigidity, deterioration of all parkinsonian symptoms has been described following abrupt withdrawal (89).

Anticholinergics are useful in the early treatment of tremor-predominant PD in young or mild patients if the primary indication for symptomatic therapy is tremor, and there are relatively minimal associated signs of rigidity or bradykinesia. Anticholinergics should be avoided in patients with baseline cognitive deficits, significant orthostatic hypotension, or urinary retention, as they are at higher risk for exacerbation of these symptoms.

Parkinson's Disease-Associated Dystonia
Dystonia can occur in several clinical circumstances in association with PD. Anticholinergics can play an adjunctive role in managing such dystonia. Most PD-associated dystonia occurs in the context of motor complications, but can occur even in levodopa-naïve patients. Most commonly, an off-period dystonia characteristically causes painful foot- and toe-posturing when dopaminergic medication wears off in the morning. Levodopa-induced on-period dystonia can follow either biphasic or peak-dose patterns. Poewe et al. suggested that anticholinergics can play a role in helping relieve the severity of episodic dystonia in PD. However, limb dystonia as an early symptom in levodopa-naïve patients tended not to respond as well compared with dystonia associated with motor fluctuations (90).

In practice, dopamine agonists seem more useful in treating most forms of PD-associated dystonia. Anticholinergics can be used as adjunctive therapy if dystonia persists despite dopaminergic therapy. Theoretically, on-period dystonia may be more amenable to anticholinergics, as dopaminergic agents risk prolonging peak-dose effects.

Miscellaneous Considerations
Often anticholinergic agents can be used to treat miscellaneous indications. In this setting, agents are often chosen on the basis of secondary anticholinergic side effects. For example, if antidepressants are needed, a tricyclic antidepressant such as amitriptyline might be chosen for its anticholinergic properties to assist with insomnia or PD-related tremor. Diphenhydramine is an antihistamine commonly prescribed for allergies or insomnia, and possesses mild anticholinergic side effects that can be used for PD-associated sialorrhea and may help reduce tremor. Regarding sialorrhea, atropine drops in 1% solution administered sublingually twice daily has been reported as beneficial with no significant mental state changes (91).

Another class of medications commonly used in PD is the atypical antipsychotics. Quetiapine (Seroquel®), olanzapine (Zyprexa®), and clozapine (Clozaril®) all have anticholinergic properties that may contribute to side effects and may be of only modest benefit. Clozapine, in particular, has significant anticholinergic-attributed sedation, but also can reduce tremor (92) and produce increased salivation and drooling. Amantadine also has modest anticholinergic properties, although its antiparkinsonian use is commonly chosen on its own merits (93). A partial list of commonly used medications with either primary or secondary anticholinergic properties and their use is shown in Table 18.1.

Side Effects

Side effects of anticholinergic agents are a significant clinical concern, which can limit their usefulness in the treatment of PD symptoms. Most antiparkinsonian effects are assumed to be mediated via central muscarinic acetylcholine receptors. Side effects may occur as either unintended central muscarinic effects or as incidental autonomic effects, attributed to peripheral binding to muscarinic and nicotinic acetylcholine receptors. In general, most effects are dose-dependent and respond to dose reductions.

Central Side Effects

Sedation, confusion, memory difficulties, and psychosis are well-described adverse events attributed to central nervous system anticholinergic toxicity. Scopolamine (Transderm-Scop®), an anticholinergic, was found to have effects on cognitive activities requiring rapid information processing in normal controls (94). Bedard et al. (95) found a transient induction of executive dysfunction in nondemented PD subjects with an acute subclinical dose of scopolamine. These findings underscore the necessity of being aware that, even in early PD patients with no clinical intellectual dysfunction, anticholinergics may have adverse effects on cognition. These drug-induced cognitive deficits are reversible, and persistent cognitive deficits off medications tend to be due to the progression of underlying disease rather than a direct adverse anticholinergic effect. In patients taking anticholinergics who develop psychosis, increased memory difficulties, and confusion, anticholinergic agents should be withdrawn promptly. Furthermore, in elderly parkinsonian patients, long-term use of anticholinergic medications has been associated with an increase in amyloid plaque densities and neurofibrillary tangles (96).

Peripheral Side Effects

Peripheral anticholinergic effects can produce a variety of autonomic dysfunction, including dry mouth, orthostatic hypotension, and urinary retention. Rare but potentially serious side effects such as narrow-angle glaucoma have also been described.

Similar to central effects, peripheral effects are often exacerbated in PD patients due to an underlying baseline autonomic dysfunction or an increased susceptibility due to advanced age. Concomitant dopaminergic medications may further exacerbate anticholinergic symptoms, such as orthostatic hypotension, constipation, or sedation. Orthostatic hypotension is a common problem in PD and can be exacerbated by the addition of anticholinergic agents. Conservative therapies begin by considering a dose reduction of either the anticholinergic or other hypotensive medications (including dopaminergic agents).

Dry mouth due to parasympathetic depression of salivary glands is a common and potentially uncomfortable side effect. In some patients with drooling, this effect may be advantageous. For excessive dry mouth, symptomatic oral moisturizing gel and other over-the-counter preparations such as specially formulated gum, mouthwash, and toothpaste may be used. Sipping ice water and sugarless sucking candies may also be helpful. The severity of dry mouth also improves with a decrease in anticholinergic dose and may improve with prolonged exposure. The addition of pyridostigmine (Mestinon®), which does not cross the blood–brain barrier has been reported as helpful (97). Anticholinergics are often used to treat urinary frequency, a symptom of PD-associated autonomic dysfunction. These include medications such as oxybutynin (Ditropan® 5 mg bid or tid), tolterodine (Detrol® 1–2 mg bid), hyoscyamine (Anaspaz® 0.125–0.25 mg q4h), darifenacin (Enablex® 7.5–15 mg daily), trospium (Sanctura® 20 mg bid), flavoxate (Urispas® 100–200 mg tid/qid), and Solife-nacine (VESIcare® 5–10 mg daily). Anticholinergics can also result in urinary retention due to excess parasympathetic inhibition, so caution must be exercised. Risks are particularly great in elderly men due to bladder outlet obstruction from benign prostate hypertrophy. If there is any history of urinary hesitancy or urgency, a urology evaluation is reasonable prior to initiation of anticholinergic therapy.

Blurred vision is another common side effect with anticholinergics. This symptom is often attributed to relatively reduced accommodation due to parasympathetic blockade, and excessive dryness of the cornea may also contribute. For persistent symptoms, consultation with an ophthalmologist may be appropriate. The use of pyridostigmine can be helpful. Rarely, anticholinergic therapy can precipitate narrow-angle glaucoma (closed-angle glaucoma), an ophthalmic emergency. The acute increase in intraocular pressure presents with pain and redness in the affected eye. In practice, this condition is extremely rare. Risk of narrow-angle glaucoma is minimal if there are normal pupillary responses and intact vision. Ophthalmology consultation should be sought during anticholinergic treatment if vision diminishes or pupillary responses become abnormal. In contrast, the more common open-angle glaucoma presents minimal risk for treatment with anticholinergics (84).

Careful consideration of risk–benefit analysis is needed when prescribing anticholinergic medications. Patients should be counseled about the potential for side effects and instructed to call with any problems. In younger patients without comorbidity besides mild PD, anticholinergics are generally very well tolerated and represent a viable option for tremor-predominant symptoms. In more susceptible patients with clinically relevant autonomic dysfunction, cognitive dysfunction, or advanced age, anticholinergics should be used very sparingly.

Mechanisms of Action

Antiparkinsonian benefit is generally attributed to inhibition of central muscarinic acetylcholine receptors. For instance, Duvoisin and Katz reported an antiparkinsonian benefit to benztropine and scopolamine, both centrally acting anticholinergics, with an exacerbation of parkinsonism after a trial of physostigmine, a centrally acting anticholinesterase inhibitor. In contrast, peripheral anticholinergics (methyl scopolamine and propantheline) and a peripheral anticholinesterase (edrophonium) did not affect parkinsonian symptoms (85). Details of how centrally acting anticholinergics can modify PD symptoms usually attributed to dopaminergic deficiency remain unclear.

Abnormalities in the central acetylcholine neurotransmitter system have been described in PD patients (98,99). An oversimplified, but clinically useful, conceptualization is that the anticholinergic use corrects an imbalance between dopamine and acetylcholine (100). The depleted nigrostriatal dopaminergic system in PD causes a relative increase in striatal acetylcholine–dopamine ratio, which can be normalized by the use of anticholinergics. The clinical consequences of disrupted neurotransmitter ratios are not precisely known. Other proposed mechanisms include inhibition of dopamine reuptake (101) and mild NMDA glutamate antagonism (102). The clinical significance of these findings remains to be determined.

Summary
Anticholinergics have relatively few clinical uses in PD other than the treatment of tremor in young-onset patients. Anticholinergics can be used in younger patients with PD-associated dystonia unresponsive to or intolerant of dopaminergic medications. Secondary anticholinergic effects may occasionally be helpful for sialorrhea or increased urinary frequency. Appropriate caution remains in judging risks of side effects versus benefits in anticholinergic use, particularly in patients who may be more susceptible to either the central or peripheral anticholinergic effects.

CONCLUSION
With the advent of specific dopaminergic agents, amantadine and anticholinergics have taken a back seat. Traditional uses still dominate with amantadine used as a mild antiparkinsonian agent, with a well-tolerated side-effect profile and anticholinergics used to treat tremor-predominant PD. In addition, there is evidence that amantadine has efficacy in the modulation of later-stage PD motor complications. Careful judgment of use of both of these agents related to their respective side effect profiles remains a concern, particularly with anticholinergics in susceptible elderly patients. In summary, amantadine and anticholinergics are helpful agents in the practicing clinician's arsenal when dealing with particular clinical PD scenarios.

REFERENCES
1. Schwab RS, England AC Jr, Poskanzer DC, Young RR. Amantadine in the treatment of Parkinson's disease. JAMA 1969; 208: 1168–70.
2. Danielczyk W. Twenty-five years of amantadine therapy in Parkinson's disease. J Neural Transm 1995; 46: 399–405.
3. Shannon KM, Goetz CG, Carroll VS, Tanner CM, Klawans HL. Amantadine and motor fluctuations in chronic Parkinson's disease. Clin Neuropharmacol 1987; 10: 522–6.
4. Adler CH, Stern MB, Vernon G, Hurtig HI. Amantadine in advanced Parkinson's disease: good use of an old drug. J Neurol 1997; 244: 336–7.
5. Metman LV, Del Dotto P, LePoole K, et al. Amantadine for levodopa-induced dyskinesias: a 1-year follow-up study. Arch Neurol 1999; 56: 1383–6.
6. Farnebo LO, Fuxe K, Goldstein M, Hamberger B, Ungerstedt U. Dopamine and noradrenaline releasing action of amantadine in the central and peripheral nervous system: a possible mode of action in Parkinson's disease. Eur J Pharmacol 1971; 16: 27–38.
7. Greenamyre JT, O'Brien CF. N-methyl-D-aspartate antagonists in the treatment of Parkinson's disease. Arch Neurol 1991; 48: 977–81.
8. Ruzicka E, Streitova H, Jech R, et al. Amantadine infusion in treatment of motor fluctuations and dyskinesias in Parkinson's disease. J Neural Transm 2000; 107: 1297–306.
9. Kim YE, Kim HJ, Yun JY, et al. Intravenous amantadine is safe and effective for the perioperative management of patients with Parkinson's disease. J Neurol 2011; 258: 2274–5.
10. Deeter RG, Khanderia U. Recent advances in antiviral therapy. Clin Pharm 1986; 5: 961–76.
11. Aoki FY, Sitar DS. Clinical pharmacokinetics of amantadine hydrochloride. Clin Pharmacokinet 1988; 14: 35–51.

12. Pacifici GM, Nardini M, Ferrari P, et al. Effect of amantadine on drug-induced parkinsonism: relationship between plasma levels and effect. Br J Clin Pharmacol 1976; 3: 883–9.

13. Fahn S, Craddock G, Kumin G. Acute toxic psychosis from suicidal overdosage of amantadine. Arch Neurol 1971; 25: 45–8.

14. Symmetrel® (amantadine) package insert. Chadds Ford, PA: Endo Pharmaceuticals, 2003.

15. Trappler B, Miyashiro AM. Bupropion-amantadine associated neurotoxicity. J Clin Psychiatry 2000; 61: 61–2.

16. Wilson TW, Rajput AH. Amantadine-dyazide interaction. Can Med Assoc J 1983; 129: 974–5.

17. Factor SA, Molho ES. Transient benefit of amantadine in Parkinson's disease: the facts about the myth. Mov Disord 1999; 14: 515–17.

18. Greulich W, Fenger E. Amantadine in Parkinson's disease: pro and contra. J Neural Transm 1995; 46: 415–21.

19. Butzer JF, Silver DE, Sahs AL. Amantadine in Parkinson's disease. A double-blind, placebo-controlled, crossover study with long-term follow-up. Neurology 1975; 25: 603–6.

20. Dallos V, Heathfield K, Stone P, Allen FA. Use of amantadine in Parkinson's disease. Results of a double-blind trial. Br Med J 1970; 4: 24–6.

21. Mann DC, Pearce LA, Waterbury LD. Amantadine for Parkinson's disease. Neurology 1971; 21: 958–62.

22. Crosby N, Deane KH, Clarke CE. Amantadine in Parkinson's disease. Cochrane Database Syst Rev 2003: CD003468.

23. Goetz CG, Poewe W, Rascol O, et al. Evidence-based medical review update: pharmacological and surgical treatments of Parkinson's disease: 2001 to 2004. Mov Disord 2005; 20: 523–39.

24. Miyasaki JM, Martin W, Suchowersky O, Weiner WJ, Lang AE. Practice parameter: Initiation of treatment for Parkinson's disease: An evidence-based review: Report of the Quality Standards Subcommittee of the American Academy of Neurology. Neurology 2002; 58: 11–17.

25. Uitti RJ, Rajput AH, Ahlskog JE, et al. Amantadine treatment is an independent predictor of improved survival in Parkinson's disease. Neurology 1996; 46: 1551–6.

26. Suchowersky O, Gronseth G, Perlmutter J, et al. Practice Parameter: neuroprotective strategies and alternative therapies for Parkinson disease (an evidence-based review): report of the Quality Standards Subcommittee of the American Academy of Neurology. Neurology 2006; 66: 976–82.

27. Verhagen Metman L, Del Dotto P, van den Munckhof P, et al. Amantadine as treatment for dyskinesias and motor fluctuations in Parkinson's disease. Neurology 1998; 50: 1323–6.

28. Crosby NJ, Deane KH, Clarke CE. Amantadine for dyskinesia in Parkinson's disease. Cochrane Database Syst Rev 2003: CD003467.

29. Thomas A, Iacono D, Luciano AL, et al. Duration of amantadine benefit on dyskinesia of severe Parkinson's disease. J Neurol Neurosurg Psychiatry 2004; 75: 141–3.

30. da Silva-Junior FP, Braga-Neto P, Sueli Monte F, et al. Amantadine reduces the duration of levodopa-induced dyskinesia: a randomized, double-blind, placebo-controlled study. Parkinsonism Relat Disord 2005; 11: 449–52.

31. Wolf E, Seppi K, Katzenschlager R, et al. Long-term antidyskinetic efficacy of amantadine in Parkinson's disease. Mov Disord 2010; 25: 1357–63.

32. Sawada H, Oeda T, Kuno S, et al. Amantadine for dyskinesias in Parkinson'sdisease: a randomized controlled trial. PLoS One 2010; 5: e15298.

33. Pahwa R, Factor SA, Lyons KE, et al. Practice Parameter: treatment of Parkinson disease with motor fluctuations and dyskinesia (an evidence-based review): report of the Quality Standards Subcommittee of the American Academy of Neurology. Neurology 2006; 66: 983–95.

34. Horstink M, Tolosa E, Bonuccelli U, et al. Review of the therapeutic management of Parkinson's disease. Report of a joint task force of the EFNS and the MDS-ES. Part II: late (complicated) Parkinson's disease. Eur J Neurol 2006; 13: 1186–202.

35. Chase TN, Oh JD. Striatal mechanisms and pathogenesis of parkinsonian signs and motor complications. Ann Neurol 2000; 47: S122–9; discussion S129–S130.
36. Kim YE, Yun JY, Jeon BS. Effect of intravenous amantadine on dopaminergic-drug-resistant freezing of gait. Parkinsonism Relat Disord 2011; 17: 491–2.
37. Timberlake WH, Vance MA. Four-year treatment of patients with parkinsonism using amantadine alone or with levodopa. Ann Neurol 1978; 3: 119–28.
38. Vollum DI, Parkes JD, Doyle D. Livedo reticularis during amantadine treatment. Br Med J 1971; 2: 627–8.
39. Sladden MJ, Nicolaou N, Johnston GA, et al. Livedo reticularis induced by amantadine. Br J Dermatol 2003; 149: 656–8.
40. Quinn NP. Anti-parkinsonian drugs today. Drugs 1984; 28: 236–62.
41. Shulman LM, Minagar A, Sharma K, Weiner WJ. Amantadine-induced peripheral neuropathy. Neurology 1999; 53: 1862–5.
42. Evidente VG, Adler CH, Caviness JN, et al. A pilot study on the motor effects of rimantadine in Parkinson's disease. Clin Neuropharmacol 1999; 22: 30–2.
43. Singer C, Papapetropoulos S, Gonzalez MA, et al. Rimantadine in Parkinson's disease patients experiencing peripheral adverse effects from amantadine: report of a case series. Mov Disord 2005; 20: 873–7.
44. Shulman LM, Minagar A, Sharma K, et al. Amantadine-induced peripheral neuropathy. Neurology 1999; 53: 1862–5.
45. Schwab RS, Poskanzer DC, England AC Jr, Young RR. Amantadine in Parkinson's disease. Review of more than two years' experience. JAMA 1972; 222: 792–5.
46. Hagell P, Odin P, Vinge E. Pregnancy in Parkinson's disease: a review of the literature and a case report. Mov Disord 1998; 13: 34–8.
47. Hughes B, Feiz V, Flynn SB, et al. Reversible amantadine-induced corneal edema in an adolescent. Cornea 2004; 23: 823–4.
48. Fraunfelder FT, Fraunfelder FW. Drug-Induced Side Effects and Drug Interactions, 5th edn. Boston: Butterworth and Heinemann, 2001: 421–2.
49. Blanchard DL. Amantadine caused corneal edema. Cornea 1990; 9: 181.
50. Walsh RA, Lang AE. Multiple impulse control disorders developing in Parkinson's disease after initiation of amantadine. Mov Disord 2012; 27: 326.
51. Thomas A, Bonanni L, Gambi F, et al. Pathological gambling in Parkinson disease is reduced by amantadine. Ann Neurol 2010; 68: 400–4.
52. Weintraub D, Sohr M, Potenza MN, et al. Amantadine use associated with impulse control disorders in Parkinson disease in cross-sectional study. Ann Neurol 2010; 68: 963–8.
53. Ohta K, Matsushima E, Matsuura M, et al. Amantadine-induced multiple spike waves on an electroencephalogram of a schizophrenic patient. World J Biol Psychiatry 2000; 1: 59–64.
54. Factor SA, Molho ES, Brown DL. Acute delirium after withdrawal of amantadine in Parkinson's disease. Neurology 1998; 50: 1456–8.
55. Simpson DM, Davis GC. Case report of neuroleptic malignant syndrome associated with withdrawal from amantadine. Am J Psychiatry 1984; 141: 796–7.
56. Cummings JL. Behavioral complications of drug treatment of Parkinson's disease. J Am Geriatr Soc 1991; 39: 708–16.
57. Wu MJ, Ing TS, Soung LS, et al. Amantadine hydrochloride pharmacokinetics in patients with impaired renal function. Clin Nephrol 1982; 17: 19–23.
58. Blye E, Lorch J, Cortell S. Extracorporeal therapy in the treatment of intoxication. Am J Kidney Dis 1984; 3: 321–38.
59. Stromberg U, Svensson TH. Further studies on the mode of action of amantadine. Acta Pharmacol Toxicol (Copenh) 1971; 30: 161–71.
60. Scatton B, Cheramy A, Besson MJ, Glowinski J. Increased synthesis and release of dopamine in the striatum of the rat after amantadine treatment. Eur J Pharmacol 1970; 13: 131–3.
61. Von Voigtlander PF, Moore KE. Dopamine: release from the brain in vivo by amantadine. Science 1971; 174: 408–10.

62. Allen RM. Role of amantadine in the management of neuroleptic-induced extrapyramidal syndromes: overview and pharmacology. Clin Neuropharmacol 1983; 6: S64–73.

63. Quack G, Hesselink M, Danysz W, Spanagel R. Microdialysis studies with amantadine and memantine on pharmacokinetics and effects on dopamine turnover. J Neural Transm 1995; 46: 97–105.

64. Grelak RP, Clark R, Stump JM, et al. Amantadine-dopamine interaction: possible mode of action in Parkinsonism. Science 1970; 169: 203–4.

65. Maj J, Sowinska H, Baran L. The effect of amantadine on motor activity and catalepsy in rats. Psychopharmacologia 1972; 24: 296–307.

66. Huber TJ, Dietrich DE, Emrich HM. Possible use of amantadine in depression. Pharmacopsychiatry 1999; 32: 47–55.

67. Stoof JC, Booij J, Drukarch B, Wolters EC. The anti-parkinsonian drug amantadine inhibits the N-methyl-D-aspartic acid-evoked release of acetylcholine from rat neostriatum in a non-competitive way. Eur J Pharmacol 1992; 213: 439–43.

68. Lupp A, Lucking CH, Koch R, Jackisch R, Feuerstein TJ. Inhibitory effects of the antiparkinsonian drugs memantine and amantadine on N-methyl-D-aspartate-evoked acetylcholine release in the rabbit caudate nucleus in vitro. J Pharmacol Exp Ther 1992; 263: 717–24.

69. Danysz W, Parsons CG, Kornhuber J, Schmidt WJ, Quack G. Aminoadamantanes as NMDA receptor antagonists and antiparkinsonian agents—preclinical studies. Neurosci Biobehav Rev 1997; 21: 455–68.

70. Kornhuber J, Bormann J, Hubers M, Rusche K, Riederer P. Effects of the 1-amino-adamantanes at the MK-801-binding site of the NMDA-receptor-gated ion channel: a human postmortem brain study. Eur J Pharmacol 1991; 206: 297–300.

71. Albin RL, Greenamyre JT. Alternative excitotoxic hypotheses. Neurology 1992; 42: 733–8.

72. Blandini F, Porter RH, Greenamyre JT. Glutamate and Parkinson's disease. Mol Neurobiol 1996; 12: 73–94.

73. Turski L, Bressler K, Rettig KJ, Loschmann PA, Wachtel H. Protection of substantia nigra from MPP neurotoxicity by N-methyl-D-aspartate antagonists. Nature 1991; 349: 414–18.

74. Rajput A, Wallukait M, Rajput AH. 18 month prospective study of amantadine (Amd) for dopa (LD) induced dyskinesias (DK) in idiopathic Parkinson's disease. Can J Neurol Sci 1997; 24: S23.

75. Snow BJ, Macdonald L, Mcauley D, Wallis W. The effect of amantadine on levodopa-induced dyskinesias in Parkinson's disease: a double-blind, placebo-controlled study. Clin Neuropharmacol 2000; 23: 82–5.

76. Luginger E, Wenning GK, Bosch S, et al. Beneficial effects of amantadine on L-dopa-induced dyskinesias in Parkinson's disease. Mov Disord 2000; 15: 873–8.

77. Shoulson I, Penney J, McDermott M, et al. A randomized, controlled trial of remacemide for motor fluctuations in Parkinson's disease. Neurology 2001; 56: 455–62.

78. Marin C, Papa S, Engber TM, et al. MK-801 prevents levodopa-induced motor response alterations in parkinsonian rats. Brain Res 1996; 736: 202–5.

79. Papa SM, Boldry RC, Engber TM, Kask AM, Chase TN. Reversal of levodopa-induced motor fluctuations in experimental parkinsonism by NMDA receptor blockade. Brain Res 1995; 701: 13–18.

80. Blanchet PJ, Konitsiotis S, Chase TN. Amantadine reduces levodopa-induced dyskinesias in parkinsonian monkeys. Mov Disord 1998; 13: 798–802.

81. Kim JH, Lee HW, Hwang J, et al. Microglia-inhibiting activity of Parkinson's disease drug amantadine. Neurobiol Aging 2012; 33: 2145–59.

82. Ferreira JJ, Rascol O. Prevention and therapeutic strategies for levodopa-induced dyskinesias in Parkinson's disease. Curr Opin Neurol 2000; 13: 431–6.

83. Olanow CW, Watts RL, Koller WC. An algorithm (decision tree) for the management of Parkinson's disease (2001): treatment guidelines. Neurology 2001; 56: S1–S88.

84. Friedman Z, Neumann E. Benzhexol-induced blindness in Parkinson's disease. Br Med J 1972; 1: 605.

85. Duvoisin RC, Katz R. Reversal of central anticholinergic syndrome in man by physo-stigmine. JAMA 1968; 206: 1963–5.
86. de Leon J, Canuso C, White AO, Simpson GM. A pilot effort to determine benztropine equivalents of anticholinergic medications. Hosp Community Psychiatry 1994; 45: 606–7.
87. Katzenschlager R, Sampaio C, Costa J, et al. Anticholinergics for symptomatic management of Parkinson's disease. Cochrane Database Syst Rev 2003: CD003735.
88. Schrag A, Schelosky L, Scholz U, Poewe W. Reduction of Parkinsonian signs in patients with Parkinson's disease by dopaminergic versus anticholinergic single-dose challenges. Mov Disord 1999; 14: 252–5.
89. Weiner WJ, Lang AE. Parkinson's disease. In: Movement Disorders, a Complete Survey. New York: Futura Publishing Co, 1989: 95.
90. Poewe WH, Lees AJ, Stern GM. Dystonia in Parkinson's disease: clinical and pharmacological features. Ann Neurol 1988; 23: 73–8.
91. Hyson HC, Jog MS, Johnson A. Sublingual atropine for sialorrhea secondary to parkinsonism. Parkinsonism Relat Disord 2001; 7(Suppl): 194.
92. Marjama-Lyons J, Koller W. Tremor-predominant Parkinson's disease. Approaches to treatment. Drugs Aging 2000; 16: 273–8.
93. Nastuk WL, Su P, Doubilet P. Anticholinergic and membrane activities of amantadine in neuromuscular transmission. Nature 1976; 264: 76–9.
94. Wesnes K, Warburton DM. Effects of scopolamine and nicotine on human rapid information processing performance. Psychopharmacology (Berl) 1984; 82: 147–50.
95. Bedard MA, Lemay S, Gagnon JF, Masson H, Paquet F. Induction of a transient dysexecutive syndrome in Parkinson's disease using a subclinical dose of scopolamine. Behav Neurol 1998; 11: 187–95.
96. Perry EK, Kilford L, Lees AJ, et al. Increased Alzheimer pathology in Parkinson's disease related to antimuscarinic drugs. Ann Neurol 2003; 54: 235–8.
97. Burke RE, Fahn S. Pharmacokinetics of trihexyphenidyl after short-term and long-term administration to dystonic patients. Ann Neurol 1985; 18: 35–40.
98. Whitehouse PJ, Hedreen JC, White CL 3rd, Price DL. Basal forebrain neurons in the dementia of Parkinson disease. Ann Neurol 1983; 13: 243–8.
99. Ruberg M, Ploska A, Javoy-Agid F, Agid Y. Muscarinic binding and choline acetyl-transferase activity in Parkinsonian subjects with reference to dementia. Brain Res 1982; 232: 129–39.
100. Barbeau A. The pathogenesis of Parkinson's disease: a new hypothesis. Can Med Assoc J 1962; 87: 802–7.
101. Coyle JT, Snyder SH. Antiparkinsonian drugs: inhibition of dopamine uptake in the corpus striatum as a possible mechanism of action. Science 1969; 166: 899–901.
102. Olney JW, Price MT, Labruyere J, et al. Anti-parkinsonian agents are phencyclidine agonists and N-methyl- aspartate antagonists. Eur J Pharmacol 1987; 142: 319–20.

19 Levodopa

David Salat and Eduardo Tolosa

INTRODUCTION

The precursor of dopamine, levodopa, is an aromatic amino acid, which occurs naturally in a number of leguminous plants. The highest concentration is found in the bean plant mucuna pruriens, which has been used in Ayurvedic medicine since 1500 BC for conditions resembling parkinsonism (1,2). Synthetic levodopa was introduced into Western medicine in the early 1960s, and has since remained the gold standard among antiparkinsonian drugs due to the degree of symptom relief it is capable of providing. Levodopa continues to be the most powerful orally active antiparkinsonian drug with only subcutaneous apomorphine matching its effects on motor function.

HISTORICAL OVERVIEW

In 1967, George Cotzias presented for the first time the results of administering levodopa in patients with Parkinson's disease (PD). He had tried to remelanize the substantia nigra in PD by administering melanocyte stimulating hormone and several precursors of melanin to PD patients. When these failed, he tried oral levodopa, given initially at small doses and then gradually increased to larger doses. The same year he published the remarkable results of these investigations in the seminal paper "Aromatic aminoacids and modification of parkinsonism" (3). Cotzias and his colleagues were the first to describe how levodopa induced a sustained improvement in parkinsonism and that the price for this improvement was the frequent development of abnormal involuntary movements, motor fluctuations, and occasional mental aberrations. He later introduced the peripheral dopa decarboxylase inhibitors (DDI) into standard therapy, a step that proved to have great practical and theoretical consequences (4).

The introduction by Cotzias and colleagues of levodopa followed the remarkable discoveries in the 1950s by Arvid Carlsson (5) that levodopa rescued animals with parkinsonian symptoms, work that led Carlsson to a Nobel Prize. In the 1960s Hornykiewicz and colleagues demonstrated that dopamine in the striatum-mediated movements and that its concentrations were markedly decreased in the striatum of PD patients. In 1961 Birkmayer administered levodopa intravenously to PD patients and observed a spectacular antibradykinetic effect (6,7). By 1966 most neurologists had concluded that the changes observed after intravenous or oral levodopa were barely more than a placebo effect (8) and it was not until the work of Cotzias and colleagues demonstrating the remarkable effect of oral levodopa that the neurological community recognized that "there seems no longer any question that the addition of levodopa to the Parkinson armamentarium is the single most effective advance in the almost two centuries since James Parkinson described the disease" (9). Soon after Cotzias' publications, in 1969, Yahr published the first double-blind levodopa study, establishing objectively the amino acid's superior effectiveness as an antiparkinson agent (9). Cotzias' work opened a new field of incredible consequences for patients and changing the way we understand treatment of neurodegenerative disorders.

PHARMACOLOGY OF LEVODOPA

In humans, the aromatic amino acid L-3,4-dihydroxy phenylalanine (Fig. 19.1), is only found as an intermediary metabolite in the synthetic pathway of dopamine. Salient aspects of the pharmacology of levodopa (10) are briefly outlined in the following sections.

Pharmacokinetics

Levodopa is actively absorbed in the duodenum and proximal jejunum. The rate at which this takes place is largely influenced by factors such as gastric pH and emptying, the amino acid content of recently ingested meals, and intestinal bacterial overgrowth. Absorbed levodopa may be metabolized to dopamine by the aromatic amino acid decarboxylase (AAD) of intestinal epithelial cells or to 3-O-methyldopa by the catechol-O-methyl transferase (COMT) in the liver, muscles, kidneys, and red blood cells. If these enzyme activities are not inhibited, only a small fraction of levodopa, estimated to be in the range of 1–5%, will reach the central nervous system, while their inhibition allows for about 25% of the ingested drug to do so. With currently

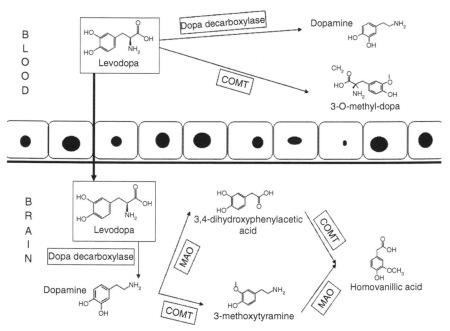

FIGURE 19.1 Peripheral and central metabolic pathways for levodopa. *Abbreviations*: COMT, cathecol-O-methyl transferase; MAO, monoamine oxidase.

available LD/AAD inhibitor preparations (benserazide and carbidopa), peak plasma levels are achieved within 30–60 minutes, and plasma half-life is in the range of 90 minutes (these may be further increased by the concomitant administration of a COMT inhibitor). The clinical effects of orally disintegrating tablets of carbidopa/ levodopa are similar to the immediate release carbidopa/levodopa. The variability of the pharmacokinetics of levodopa was exemplified by the results of a study (11) in which plasma concentrations of the drug were determined serially in 20-minute intervals during the waking hours in 10 parkinsonian patients. Both mean plasma concentrations (0.45–7.07 µg/mL) and peak plasma concentrations (0.95–13.75 µg/mL) were found to have substantial intra- and interindividual differences. Levodopa crosses the blood–brain barrier through the same active transport system used for intestinal absorption. In the central nervous system it is taken up mainly by dopaminergic *substantia nigra* pars compacta cells and very efficiently converted to dopamine by aromatic AAD. In advanced stages of the disease, dopaminergic neurons are depleted and serotoninergic neurons (which also contain aromatic AAD) may progressively overtake their role in the conversion of levodopa to dopamine (12). Levodopa itself is biologically inactive, and in order to exert its desired clinical effects it must be converted to dopamine, which will be stored in vesicles in the axon terminals of the nigrostriatal projections and released in proximity of striatal dopaminergic receptors in response to adequate stimuli.

Preparations

Levodopa has been marketed as an oral suspension, tablets, and capsules. Different doses of levodopa (ranging from 100 to 250 mg) with either benserazide (in a ratio of 4:1) or carbidopa (in a ratio of 10:1 or 4:1), and regular and extended release formulations are commercially available (Table 19.1). Different mechanisms are used to achieve delayed absorption and extended release with each of the AAD inhibitors: Carbidopa/levodopa is embedded in a slowly dissolving matrix (13,14), whereas levodopa/benserazide floats on the surface of gastric content (15). Not all of these presentations, however, can be found in every country, and regional prescription practices must conform to this limitation. Madopar™ (Roche) and Sinemet™ (MSD) are the most widely used brand names for levodopa, the first one with benserazide and the latter with carbidopa, but in certain countries levodopoa/ benserazide is also marketed under the name of Prolopa™, and carbidopa/levodopa may be found as Atamet™, Carbidopum™, or Parcopa™ (this latter one is the only available orally disintegrating preparation).

A COMT inhibitor (most typically entacapone) may be added to the combination of levodopa and an AAD inhibitor. This strategy has been found to slowdown the peripheral degradation of levodopa and thus prolong its plasma levels without significantly increasing or delaying its peak plasma concentration, and may be useful for advanced patients with motor fluctuations. These agents and their clinical use are discussed in chapter 22.

THE THERAPEUTIC RESPONSE OF LEVODOPA
Efficacy and Side Effects

Levodopa is used for the management of those motor aspects, which are related to the dopaminergic deficit in PD, in particular the cardinal motor signs, tremor, bradykinesia, and rigidity. Severe motor impairment may occur, particularly in the later stages of the disease, independently of dopaminergic function; for instance, freezing and loss of balance. For these problems levodopa and other dopaminergic drugs typically have a very limited role.

The efficacy of levodopa is firmly established from over 30 years of use (16–18). In many patients levodopa leads to substantial or nearly complete reversal of symptoms, including tremor, and is generally well tolerated. In some patients tremor may not respond to levodopa. This may be a dose-dependent phenomenon and increasing the drug to high doses may result in marked tremor suppression. Rarely truly levodopa-resistant tremor occurs. A double-blind, placebo-controlled trial [the Early vs Later Levodopa (ELLDOPA) trial] in treatment-naïve PD patients showed a dose-dependent improvement in motor scores with levodopa, compared with patients receiving placebo, after nine months of treatment. In studies of up to five years follow-up comparing the effect of other antiparkinsonian agents, such as the dopamine agonists with levodopa, the results in levodopa only treated patients consistently showed improvements of motor function of up to 30%. These results were better than those in patients receiving dopamine agonists (19). Supplementation of levodopa to other antiparkinsonian medications in stable PD is common clinical practice to improve symptomatic control.

Levodopa increases the duration of time the patients remain independent and employable, and there is evidence to suggest a beneficial effect on life expectancy, although this has not been confirmed in all studies. A number of symptomatic treatment options are available, but virtually all patients will at some stage require levodopa.

TABLE 19.1   Commercially Available Formulations of Levodopa

Carbidopa/levodopa	10/100 mg 25/100 mg 25/250 mg	Sinemet
	25/100 mg extended release 50/200 mg extended release	Sinemet CR
	10/100 mg orally disintigrating tablets 25/100 mg orally disintigrating tablets 25/250 mg orally disintigrating tablets	Parcopa
Levodopa/benserazide	50/12.5 mg 100/125 mg 200/50 mg 250/50 mg	Madopar
	100/25 mg	Madopar HBS
	50/12.5 mg dispersible tablets 100/125 mg dispersible tablets	Madopar LT
Levodopa/carbidopa/entacapone	50/12.5/200 mg 75/18.75/200 mg 100/25/200 mg 125/31.25/200 mg 150/37.5/200 mg 200/50/200 mg	Stalevo
Levodopa/carbidopa enteral gel	2/0.5 g/100 mL	Duodopa

The clinical response of the core motor features of parkinsonism to levodopa treatment is considered to persist throughout the course of the disease, although with the passage of time progressive predominance of non–levodopa-responsive symptoms occurs (20). Bonnet et al (21) prospectively studied a group of 19 patients who started levodopa therapy within three years of symptom onset. These patients were periodically evaluated during 12 years, and compared with two historical cohorts that had been started on levodopa between four and six years and between seven and nine years, respectively. Disability scores at treatment initiation were found to be significantly different in the three groups. These differences persisted throughout the study period, but disappeared if patients were matched for disease duration. The authors concluded that worsening of symptoms is a function of disease progression and not related to levodopa treatment. This concept has been corroborated by the results of the Sidney Multicentre Study of Parkinson's Disease. This study prospectively evaluated 136 newly diagnosed PD patients and published reports at 10, 15, and 20 years of follow-up (22–24). End-of-dose failure and dyskinesia were experienced by up to 95% of patients and were considered surrogate markers of persistent response to levodopa in this population.

Long-term use of levodopa is associated with the emergence of treatment-related complications, including dyskinesia. In contrast, with respect to short-term tolerability it offers a favorable side effect profile compared with the other classes of antiparkinsonian agents. As with any dopaminergic drug, it can induce typical dopaminergic adverse effects, such as orthostatic hypotension, nausea, vomiting, and anorexia. The addition of decarboxylase inhibitors has greatly limited some of these side effects such as nausea but has not had any effect on orthostatic hypotension. Unplanned episodes of sleep during daytime, including while driving a vehicle, were originally described in nonergot dopamine agonists but have now been shown to also be associated with other agonists and they may rarely occur with levodopa monotherapy (Table 19.2) (25).

Rare side effects include hemolytic anemia due to an uncommon positive Coombs test, pupillary dilation, and dark discoloration of the urine, sweat, and

TABLE 19.2   Side Effects of Levodopa

Orthostatic hypotension
Nausea, vomiting
Anorexia[a]
Bitter, unpleasant, taste[a]
Drenching sweats
Insomnia, excessive daytime somnolence, occasionally sleep attacks
Hemolytic anemia (+Coombs test)[b]
Pupillary dilatation[b]
Dark discoloration of the urine, sweat, and saliva[b]
Peripheral neuropathy[a]
Anxiety, depression, hypomania
Vivid dreams, delusions, hallucinations, psychosis
Impulse control disorders
Dopamine dysregulation syndrome, punding
Motor and nonmotor response fluctuations

[a]Uncommon.
[b]Rare.

saliva. Also, a reduction in serum folate levels and a modest elevation of homocysteine have been reported. It is unknown whether the increase in plasma homocysteine increases the risk for other medical problems (26). Epidemiological studies have shown that PD patients have an increased prevalence of malignant melanoma (27) but no association between levodopa therapy and the incidence of melanoma has been found (28).

Some reports have linked chronic levodopa treatment to a peripheral neuropathy. Rajabally et al. (29) detected a neuropathy in 14 of 37 of their PD patients (37.8%) and found a correlation between cumulative levodopa exposure and neuropathy severity. Neuropathy in patients on chronic levodopa treatment has been linked to elevated plasma levels of homocysteine and methylmalonic acid (30) and with reduced vitamin B12 levels (29). Additional studies are needed to evaluate a causative link between levodopa exposure in PD and neuropathy.

RESPONSE FLUCTUATIONS AND DYSKINESIA
Phenomenology of Motor and Nonmotor Fluctuations
The re-emergence of parkinsonian signs before the next levodopa dose is termed "end of dose deterioration" or "wearing-off," and it is associated with troughs in plasma levodopa levels. An early sign of this phenomenon that may be recognized in some patients is termed "early morning akinesia," and consists in the presence of signs and symptoms of parkinsonism preceding the first daily dose of levodopa, and significant improvement thereof with the drug. With disease progression, periods when the motor symptoms are reversed by administered therapies (on-periods) become shorter and less predictable. Transition to an off phase does not require the re-emergence of the full-blown parkinsonian syndrome. Not infrequently, patients become markedly akinetic, with little or no rigidity or tremor. Furthermore, tremor is often related to environmental factors, such as anxiety or fatigue, and may be present irrespective of whether the patient is in an "on" or an "off" phase. Besides these phenomena of loss of therapeutic effect of the administered drug, in later stages of PD certain doses may take longer than expected to become clinically effective (delayed on) or may never do so (dose failure, no-on). Some patients may experience a transient worsening of their tremor (beginning of dose deterioration), which is also recognized as a type of motor fluctuation. Finally, some patients in the advanced stages experience a complex sequence of initial symptomatic improvement preceded or followed by clinical worsening that reaches the greatest degree of functional impairment before returning to the patient's baseline (super off) (Table 19.3) (31). Motor fluctuations, and most notably the unpredictable transition between the on and off phases, have been recognized as important determinants of quality of life among PD patients (32,33).

Although levodopa therapy will generally improve gait abnormalities in PD patients, its use may result in freezing episodes during on-periods (34). These are uncommon, short-lived motor blocks that generally occur upon gait initiation when other features of the parkinsonian syndrome are responding to the administered treatment.

Nonmotor symptoms are being increasingly recognized as important features of the off period that significantly contribute to patients' distress (35,36). In one study (35), all patients who had motor fluctuations experienced at least one nonmotor problem during off phases. The most frequently reported of these symptoms

TABLE 19.3   Fluctuations in Motor Disability in PD

Levodopa Related
Wearing-off: Re-emergence of parkinsonian symptoms (either motor or nonmotor) before the following scheduled treatment dose
Delayed ON: Significantly prolonged time to experience improvement of parkinsonian symptoms after a given treatment dose
Dose failure (no ON): Lack of improvement of parkinsonian symptoms after a given treatment dose, despite its correct administration
Unpredictable ON/OFF: Rapid and erratic transitions between periods with and periods without improvement in parkinsonian symptoms
Beginning of dose deterioration: transient worsening of tremor as the first manifestation of a given dose of levodopa
Early morning akinesia: parkinsonism occurring when awakening in the morning that usually improves after the first levodopa dose
Unrelated to treatment
Sleep benefit
Freezing of gait
Stress related tremor
Nocturnal immobility
Akathisia

were anxiety, drenching sweats, slowness of thought, fatigue, akathisia, irritability, and hallucinations, whereas nocturia, fatigue, and sialorrhea were the most frequently reported nonmotor symptoms related to the off phase in another study (37). These symptoms generally respond to treatment changes directed to achieve a more continuous drug delivery to the brain.

Phenomenology of Dyskinesia

Levodopa-induced dyskinesia are generally choreic or dystonic movements, while ballism, tic-like movements and myoclonus are seen much less often. They may be classified according to their temporal relation to drug ingestion and clinical state as peak-dose, beginning- and end-of-dose (diphasic) or off-period dyskinesia (Table 19.4).

At the time of initial presentation, dyskinesia tends to involve the musculature of the buccolingual area or the distal limbs and present in an apparently random fashion. Unless levodopa dose can be reduced, with the passage of time they frequently spread to other body regions, become more intense and tend to occur at fairly predictable times of the day. Most patients will exhibit a specific pattern of dyskinesia (including both phenomenology and location) that persists for as long as levodopa therapy is maintained. Levodopa-induced dyskinesia typically worsen with stress, and frequently during volitional movements.

Peak dose dyskinesia are choreoathetotic involuntary movements that appear at the time of maximal symptomatic effect of a given levodopa dose (38,39). In some patients dyskinesia may progress to occur through the entire period of antiparkinsonian effect of a given dose (square wave dyskinesia). On period dyskinesia are the most common types of involuntary movements observed in PD patients on chronic levodopa therapy. They cause variable degrees of disability, depending both on their intensity and the muscle groups involved, and may interfere with speech,

TABLE 19.4   Levodopa-Induced Dyskinesia in PD

On period dyskinesia
  Occur during peak effect of a levodopa dose (peak dose); at times during
    the entire on (square dose)
  Limb and trunk; mostly choreic movements
  Craneocervical: mostly dystonic movements
Biphasic dyskinesia
  Occur at onset or wearing off (or both) of clinical benefit from a dose of levodopa
  Stereotyped, ballistic, or dystonic movements
  May be accompanied by worsening of tremor
Off period dystonia
  Mostly distal in one leg
  Frequently painful
  May occur only in early morning (early morning dystonia)
  Worsen with walking

---

stance, gait, and with various activities of daily living (such as writing, feeding, or dressing). They are also frequently distressing, because they can be socially embarrassing. Several studies have documented the negative impact that dyskinesia have on the patient's quality of life (40–42) and their cost (43,44).

Some patients experience dyskinesia shortly after the ingestion of levodopa, when its antiparkinsonian effect begins, and/or hours later, when the effect of the drug is beginning to wane. These phenomena were first described in 1975 (38), and are frequently called diphasic. They are transient, usually lasting for only 10–15 minutes, and they are followed by either an on (in the case of beginning-of-dose episodes) or an off (in the case of end-of-dose episodes) phase (45). In most patients, they occur predictably either at the beginning or the end of the doses. Although they are often mild and tolerable (38), patients may present with severe ballistic painful spasms, at times accompanied by profuse sweating, tachycardia, and incapacitating feelings of anxiety and prostration. Beginning-of-dose dyskinesia may coexist with a worsening of the patient's rest tremor.

Off-period dystonia is a late complication of levodopa therapy that tends to appear after at least four or five years of continuous administration (46,47). A study evaluated the prevalence of dyskinesia in a community-based population of patients with PD, and documented off-period dystonia in 10% of patients in their sample. Off-period dystonia was reported by 2% of patients treated with levodopa for five years or less, by 12% of those treated between six and nine years and by 56% of those treated for 10 or more years. Patients with both off-period and diphasic dyskinesia, had a younger age at onset of PD. Early morning dystonia can be precipitated by anxiety or attempts to walk. Many patients with early morning dystonia also display wearing off phenomena, peak dose or diphasic dyskinesia, and, in some cases, dystonic spasms of the legs recurring during daytime off periods (48).

Off dystonia can occur as an early side effect of levodopa treatment in some cases of genetic PD, such as in those associated with mutations in the parkin gene (PARK2) (49) or in PINK-1 (PARK6) (50,51). Withdrawal of levodopa and continuous intravenous or duodenal infusion levodopa formulations effectively relieve off-period dystonia.

Prevalence and Pathopysiology of Motor Complications and Dyskinesia

A meta-analysis of published prospective studies quantified the risk of motor fluctuations and dyskinesia after four to six years of levodopa treatment to be around 40% (52). In individual studies, the percentage of patients with fluctuations and dyskinesia ranges between 10% and 60% at five years, and may rise up to 80% or 90% in later years (17,53). Although generally regarded as occurring in advanced disease response fluctuations may be an early phenomenon when subtle and nonmotor signs are also considered (36). Younger age at disease onset, longer disease duration, and levodopa therapy have been identified as risk factors for their development (17,53–60). Levodopa dose appears to be a driving factor for the development of motor complications. In the ELLDOPA trial, wearing-off and dyskinesia occurred in 30% and 16% of patients, respectively, in de novo patients receiving 600 mg/day of levodopa. In contrast, the incidence of wearing-off and dyskinesia in those receiving smaller doses of levodopa (150 or 300 mg/day) was similar to that of the placebo arm (61).

In the early stages of disease, adequate symptom control occurs with levodopa throughout the day, even if the drug is given only three times a day. With time, however, both the onset and termination of the clinical response to a levodopa dose are altered, reflecting the fluctuation of levodopa plasma levels that occurs in advanced disease (38,39). This variability is generally regarded as the consequence of erratic drug absorption and competition of levodopa with other amino acids for the neutral amino acid transport system (involved in the absorption of the drug from the proximal gastrointestinal tract and in crossing the blood–brain barrier).

Their pathophysiology is complex and incompletely understood. Peripheral pharmacokinetic factors are unlikely to be responsible alone for the emergence of fluctuations since they are present from the beginning of treatment and do not change, and the peripheral pharmacokinetic profile of plasma levodopa is not different in those with early disease and a stable response from those with fluctuations either of the "wearing-off" or "on–off" type (62–64). Progressive cell loss in the substantia nigra hinders levodopa uptake as well as its metabolism to dopamine and storage in presynaptic terminals (65,66). In this situation, striatal dopamine levels are increasingly dependent on the amount of levodopa that reaches the brain. Given the fact that levodopa is administered in repeated doses and that it has a short plasma half-life, stimulation of dopamine receptors becomes intermittent (67). In animal experiments, pulsatile stimulation of spiny neurons in the caudate nucleus results in the upregulation of intracellular messengers involved in the function of γ-aminobutyric acid efferents and, finally, alteration in the pattern of firing and synchronization of different structures in the basal ganglia (67,68). As shown in different animal models, some of these changes occur only if levodopa administration is pulsatile, and they may even be reversed by continuous dopaminergic stimulation (69). Consequently, the hypothesis has been put forward that dyskinesia may be caused by this pulsatile stimulation of striatal dopamine receptors.

COGNITIVE EFFECTS AND NEUROPSYCHIATRIC COMPLICATIONS OF LEVODOPA

The potential impact of replacement therapy with levodopa on cognitive function has been extensively evaluated, but evidence to support their association is scarce. Research focused on the various cognitive domains suggests that levodopa treatment may improve working memory and spatial span (70), while attention, verbal fluency, immediate recall and recognition memory (71) and visuospatial perception (70), are unaffected by levodopa therapy. Reports on the effect of replacement therapy on executive functions are conflicting, and studies suggesting a beneficial effect (70), a variable effect (72), and no significant effect (71) have been published.

The list of potential neuropsychiatric complications of dopaminergic replacement therapy is extensive. The most frequent of these symptoms are hallucinations (usually visual, fairly stereotyped, and consisting of fully formed human figures or animals). Although they initially occur during the night hours and are rarely perceived as threatening, the frequency of episodes progressively increases and they become worrisome to both the patient and caregivers (73). Patients may also present with auditory, tactile, or gustatory hallucinations (alone or associated to the visual misperception), although this seldom occurs. The conviction experienced by some patients that there is someone in their proximity (without a clear-cut perceptual experience to support it) is referred to, as "sense of presence hallucination" and is probably not infrequent, but rarely self-reported by patients. Not infrequently, sensory perceptual abnormalities are followed by delusions, which very often have a nonbizarre persecutory content.

Depression is common in PD, and it may either precede or follow the onset of its motor symptoms. Although levodopa is not considered to have an antidepressive effect, its initiation may result in improvement of mood (sometimes thought to be due to its effect on the motor symptoms of the disease and the functional impairment they cause). On rare occasions, however, depressive symptoms or hypomania may emerge shortly after levodopa initiation and remit with drug withdrawal (74). Moreover, affective symptoms, including depression and anxiety, may be prominent constituents of the nonmotor off state; hypomania during the on phase has also been reported.

Complex behavioral disorders are increasingly being recognized as side effects of long-term treatment with dopamine replacing agents. All of them fall into the category of impulsive-compulsive behaviors, but they may be classified as either impulse control disorders or the dopamine dysregulation syndrome.

Impulse control disorders (of which pathological gambling, compulsive sexual behavior, compulsive buying, or binge eating are prominent examples), are more often seen in patients on dopamine agonists (75,76). A six-month prevalence of impulse control disorders of 13.6% was found in the DOMINION study (76). This study disclosed a strong association between therapy with dopamine agonists (irrespective of their dose) and the development of these behavioral disturbances. Moreover, levodopa was found to have a weak association with their occurrence only when taken in the higher dose range. Reports of impulse control disorders with levodopa monotherapy are scarce and focus almost exclusively on hypersexuality (77).

The dopamine dysregulation syndrome, on the other hand, is most often associated with the use of shorter-acting dopaminergic compounds, such as levodopa and apomorphine. This condition is characterized by compulsive dopaminergic drug use (patients begin to take increasing quantities of medication, well beyond those required to control their motor symptoms, and continue to request dose escalation). This occurs despite the emergence of drug-induced motor complications, in particular dyskinesia, and has potentially harmful behavioral consequences (78,79). Patients with young age at disease onset, high dopaminergic drug intake, past drug use, depression, novelty seeking personality traits, and alcohol intake seem to be especially prone to develop this symptom complex (80).

"Punding," first described in amphetamine addicts, is a complex stereotyped behavior characterized by an intense fascination with repetitive manipulations of technical equipment, the continual handling, examining, and sorting of objects, grooming, hoarding, pointless driving, walkabouts or using a computer, often associated with dopamine dysregulation syndrome (80–82). Initially patients may engage themselves in these activities mainly at night. They are carried out during on phases, and are often associated with dyskinesia. Punding is acknowledged as disruptive and unproductive by the patients, but attempts to interrupt the behavior typically lead to irritability and dysphoria. Patients rarely report punding behavior spontaneously. Punding, which needs to be distinguished from obsessive-compulsive and manic disorders, is believed to result from the dysfunction of ventral striatal and frontal lobe structures (closely linked to reward responses), and subsequent inability to control automatic response mechanisms, induced by dopaminergic replacement therapy.

LIMITATIONS OF LEVODOPA THERAPY AND THE ISSUE OF LEVODOPA TOXICITY

Levodopa maintains its symptomatic effect on the cardinal motor signs of PD for many years after its initiation (22–24). Its long-term use, however, requires a progressive dose escalation and has been classically linked to the development of various types of motor fluctuations and dyskinesia. Moreover, levodopa therapy has little effect on certain nonmotor features of the disease (such as dementia or autonomic dysfunction), and may even contribute to the emergence of additional clinical problems (on-period gait disturbance and freezing) (Table 19.5).

The observation of treatment-related complications following the introduction of levodopa, led to speculations about a potential negative "toxic" effect of the drug at a cellular level. Clinical studies (21,61) suggest that worsening of symptoms in PD can be comprehensively explained by disease progression, and argue against any meaningful deleterious effect of levodopa. Importantly, their findings are largely in accordance with nonclinical research. Basic science has provided conflicting results, since either noxious or protective effects on dopaminergic neurons have been demonstrated, depending on the experimental conditions

TABLE 19.5 Limitations of Levodopa Therapy

Correction of classic motor symptoms is at times partial
Development of motor and nonmotor fluctuations
Development of dyskinesia
Limited or no response of some motor symptoms: e.g., freezing of gait, dysarthria
Limited response of nonmotor symptoms: e.g., dysautonomia, cognitive deterioration, sleep disturbances REM sleep behavior disorder (RBD), apathy
Occurrence of non-motor adverse events: nausea, orthostatic hypotension, sleepiness, dysautonomic and neuropsychiatric problems
Rare development of on period gait disturbances
Is not neuroprotective

---

such as levodopa concentration and the presence or absence of glia cells and ascorbic acid (83–85).

On the other hand, exposure to levodopa in various animal models has not resulted in dopaminergic cell death in healthy animals (86) nor additional cell death in lesioned animals (87,88), and even a trophic effect of levodopa on this cellular population has been reported (89). Similarly, neuropathological studies in humans without PD who had been on chronic high-dose levodopa regimes, found no evidence of nigral degeneration (90).

This debate, however, was recently fueled by the results of functional neuro-imaging studies using positron emission tomography (PET) and single photon emission computed tomography (SPECT) in early PD patients, in whom a slower decline in tracer uptake (considered to be a surrogate marker of nigrostriatal function) was found among patients on dopamine agonists compared with those on levodopa (91,92). The lack of a placebo-control arm in these studies, however, hampers the possibility of drawing causal conclusions, as these findings could result not from a direct "toxic" effect of levodopa, but from a drug-related pharmacologic response or a neuroprotective effect of dopamine agonists. Moreover, some authors (93,94) have questioned whether PET and SPECT scans reliably estimate the degree of neurodegeneration.

Current consensus is that the short half-life of levodopa and the manner of its administration are much more likely to be related to the development of motor complications than any intrinsic property of the molecule itself (68,89,95,96).

PRACTICAL ASPECTS OF LEVODOPA TREATMENT
Initiating Treatment
In early PD, administration of a monoamine oxidase type B (MAO-B) inhibitor is frequently considered when disability is minimal, but when a significant symptomatic effect needs to be achieved, a dopamine agonist or levodopa are the drugs of choice when starting treatment. Dopamine agonists are used widely as initial therapy because of their symptomatic effect and because they have been shown to reduce the risk of motor complications when compared with levodopa. However, clinical trials have shown that two years after the initiation of monotherapy with a dopamine agonist, about 50% of patients have received additional levodopa (97). Dopamine agonists, on the other hand, can cause sleepiness, behavioral side effects, and symptomatic postural hypotension more frequently than levodopa, even in early stages of treatment, and more commonly in elderly patients and those with cognitive impairment. Starting treatment with a dopamine agonist is considered justified though, and is frequently implemented in patients with early onset of motor symptoms because these subjects have a higher risk for the development of motor complications (55,90,98).

Often treating physicians delay levodopa and start with a dopamine agonist or another antiparkinsonian agent in patients younger than 60 years. Levodopa is generally employed instead of dopamine agonists when starting treatment in elderly patients. It is important, though, to keep in mind that the trials comparing early levodopa and agonist treatment consistently showed significantly better and longer lasting motor improvement in the levodopa arms. The consequences of undertreatment in younger patients may ultimately hamper employability and may lead to social withdrawal or, at later stages, to complications associated with bradykinesia such as falls.

No special benefit has been shown to occur from starting levodopa therapy with controlled-release formulations (99) or with a levodopa decarboxylase inhibitor plus entacapone (100). For each patient, the best initial dose of levodopa should be determined individually. In recently diagnosed patients or when first adding levodopa, daily doses are usually 300 mg/day. As the disease progresses, adaptations should be made as required and as tolerated. The patient´s current needs in terms of symptom control, including employment status, should be weighed against factors such as age that have an impact on the individual risk of motor complications. It may take several weeks before patients have a significant motor benefit. Patients should therefore not expect a dramatic, quick response to levodopa initiation, particularly at lower doses. If a patient has started on an MAO-B inhibitor, amantadine, anticholinergic, a dopamine agonist, or a combination of these drugs, a stage will come when, because of worsening motor symptoms, levodopa is generally required. Nearly all patients started on an MAO-B inhibitor or a dopamine agonist will need levodopa within the following two to three years for adequate control of motor symptoms.

In most instances, initiation of treatment with levodopa is followed by a period of good response, which may last from months to years. In these initial months of treatment the patient does not experience clinically significant motor fluctuations and consequently, the patient is said to be in the stable phase. Even during this stable phase, though, repeated adjustments of treatment according to tolerability and symptoms are necessary as the disease progresses. In stable patients requiring additional symptomatic treatment, adding a COMT inhibitor is another consideration since studies have shown that in these subjects COMT inhibitors can improve secondary outcome measures including activities of daily living and quality-of-life data. UPDRS motor scores were not significantly improved in all studies but this may be related to a reduction in the levodopa dose.

Levodopa used for the treatment of motor symptoms can influence some non-motor manifestations of PD. While its effects upon such symptoms as cognition or autonomic symptoms, are generally minimal it can improve sleep quality (101), REM behavior disorder (102,103), and central pain (104).

OPTIMIZATION OF LEVODOPA TREATMENT IN MODERATE AND ADVANCED-STAGE PARKINSON'S DISEASE

Motor complications are generally considered the main feature that indicates transition into a moderate-to-advanced phase of the disease (105). It is unclear how many patients initiated on dopaminergic therapy remain clinically stable, that is, without clinically significant response fluctuations of the wearing off type. While studies on clinic or drug trial-based populations suggest that the majority develop clinically relevant fluctuations, other studies (such as long-term trial studies (99,106) and community-based studies) (107) show that the majority of patients remain free of clinically significant fluctuations for prolonged periods of time. In the study by Larsen et al. (107) only 22% of patients had fluctuations, perhaps reflecting the higher age of the unselected group of patients. Despite having a stable drug response on motor function, these patients had more distress, neuropsychiatric manifestations, fatigue, and problems with their daily life activities than healthy elderly people.

In patients with motor fluctuations, linked mostly to an intermittent and irregular arrival of levodopa to the brain, achieving stable levodopa plasma levels within a therapeutic window (clinically defined by an on-state without disabling dyskinesia) becomes a major objective, which becomes in some patients increasingly challenging (108). The following paragraphs outline management options that may be considered if any motor complications ensue.

Wearing Off

When the patients develop motor fluctuations of the wearing off type, fragmentation of the total daily levodopa intake into smaller and more frequent quanta may be attempted. This approach, however, is often unsuccessful, because the lower doses fail to provide adequate symptom control. For this reason, if dyskinesia are not worrisome, increasing the levodopa dose whenever wearing off is occurring is frequently required. With progressing disease, levodopa may even need to be administered in 2-hour intervals, and the cumulative daily dose could be up to 2000 mg per day. After adjustment of levodopa doses, the addition of COMT inhibitors, dopamine agonists, or MAO-B inhibitors should be considered. Several trials have shown that dopamine agonists such as pergolide (109–111), pramipexole (112–115), or ropinirole (116,117) effectively reduce off time in patients with levodopa-related motor fluctuations. Less convincing evidence exists for bromocriptine (112,118,119) and cabergoline (120). Reported evidence (bromocriptine vs cabergoline, lisuride vs pergolide) suggests that efficacy is similar among the various agonists. The same was true when comparing bromocriptine (121) and pergolide (122) to the COMT inhibitor tolcapone. No other comparisons have been published.

Adding a COMT or MAO-B inhibitor results on average in a reduction in off time of about 1–1.5 hours. However, tolcapone is potentially hepatotoxic and is only recommended in patients in whom all other available medications have failed. Both types of drugs increase and prolong the presence of dopamine in the striatum and therefore carry a risk of increasing dyskinesia. This is best handled by attempting to reduce levodopa first. A combined add-on treatment of COMT and MAO-B inhibitors is possible and useful as there is no evidence of a ceiling effect reached when one enzymatic pathway is blocked.

The standard oral formulation of selegiline has been shown to improve PD symptoms in patients with motor fluctuations, but a consistent effect in reducing off time in patients with wearing off has not been shown (16). A study with orally disintegrating tablets of selegiline (123) showed that this formulation of selegiline significantly reduces off time when used as adjunctive therapy with levodopa in patients with motor fluctuations. Two double-blind, placebo-controlled, randomized clinical trials have assessed the efficacy of rasagiline in patients with PD experiencing levodopa-related motor fluctuations, the Parkinson's Rasagiline: Efficacy and Safety in the Treatment of "Off" (PRESTO) and the Lasting effect in Adjunct therapy with Rasagiline Given Once-daily (LARGO) trials (124,125). A significant reduction in daily off time of about 20% occurred in both trials in patients receiving rasagiline relative to placebo. Although the LARGO study was not designed to directly compare rasagiline and entacapone, the results clearly demonstrate that the clinical effects on "off" time were similar with these two compounds.

Delayed on and Dose Failure

With disease progression a prolonged latency or complete lack of clinical improvement after a dose of levodopa is ingested is not uncommon. These problems are attributed to the known erratic absorption of levodopa and the fact that the drug competes with other amino acids to cross both the gastrointestinal mucosa and the blood–brain barrier. Modifications in the way the medication is ingested are usually the first measures to be tried. Among the usual recommendations are chewing the tablets instead of swallowing them, taking the medication on an empty stomach or taking it with carbonated beverages. Dietary protein restriction is often recommended, but patients should be closely monitored to ensure that it does not contribute to worsening malnutrition. If these measures fail, short-acting agents (such as soluble levodopa or apomorphine) may provide an alternative to achieve adequate symptom control.

Unpredictable Motor Fluctuations

From a conceptual point of view, these may be considered as the coexistence of wearing off and dose failure in a single patient. Its management, therefore, requires a combination of the previously suggested strategies. The clinical state of a patient in this situation is often unpredictable. As a consequence, the patient's clinical state may not be significantly improved, even after expertise and sound clinical judgement are merged to make adjustments in the medication schemes. If the patient remains functionally impaired, advanced therapies [continuous duodenal infusion of levodopa gel, subcutaneous apomorphine pump, or deep brain stimulation (DBS)] need be considered.

Management of Dyskinesia

Treatment of involuntary movements should be considered if they significantly impact daily functioning or are a source of social embarrassment. Overall, except for young-onset patients, dyskinesia are troublesome in about 40% of patients and only about 10% cannot be managed by medication adjustments (126).

Peak-dose dyskinesia usually improve by reducing the individual doses of levodopa. This may result in aggravation of parkinsonism and the patients may need to take more frequent levodopa doses. In this scenario, the addition of alternative dopamine stimulating agents such as dopamine agonists may allow for a reduction in the dose of levodopa and improved control in dyskinesia. Still, in some patients with dyskinesia who are taking multiple dopaminergic drugs, reducing adjuvant treatments, such as dopamine agonists, MAO-B, or COMT inhibitors, results in less dyskinesia.

If adjustment of dopaminergic treatment does not result in sufficient control of dyskinesia, specific treatment with amantadine can be tried. Clozapine may also be used (127,128) but potential hematologic toxicity limits its use. Several clinical trials have shown that amantadine can improve dyskinesia in patients taking levodopa (129–132). The antidyskinetic effect is dose dependent and patients often require 300–400 mg/day. In one study (133), improvement in dyskinesia was reported to last only from three to eight months. Several subjects treated with amantadine experienced a rebound in dyskinesia severity after drug discontinuation.

If these pharmacological treatments are unsuccessful, patients may be considered for more complex therapies, such as DBS (134), the enteral infusion of levodopa gel (135), or the subcutaneous administration of apomorphine (136).

The management of biphasic dyskinesia is challenging and the previously proposed treatments may worsen them. Higher doses of levodopa have been proposed (137), but it only works for very short time periods and worsens peak dose dyskinesia. Decreasing the individual doses of levodopa reduces the intensity of the involuntary movements but almost invariably worsens parkinsonism. Patients with intense beginning and end-of-dose dyskinesia may skip one or more doses of levodopa remaining in an off state for several hours, to avoid the paroxysms.

Dystonic spasms usually occur when plasma levodopa is low such as early in the morning before the first dose of levodopa. Off period dystonia can occur anytime when the patient is off. All strategies used for the management of wearing off can be helpful in alleviating early morning and off period dystonia. Supplementing levodopa with a dopamine agonist can be useful and possibly also using controlled release levodopa or levodopa plus entacapone at bedtime. In some patients, taking a dose of levodopa one hour or two before getting out of bed in the morning can prevent early morning "off" and accompanying dystonia. In selected cases, the injection of botulinum toxin can result in improvement in off period dystonia, such as blepharospasm or painful toe extension spasms.

MANAGEMENT OF PSYCHIATRIC SIDE EFFECTS
Psychotic symptoms such as hallucinations and delusions, or impulse control disorders such as hypersexuality are not uncommon in patients on chronic levodopa therapy and are frequently difficult to manage. Unless they appear with changes in levodopa dose it is difficult to know what role this drug may be playing in their causation since all of the medications used in PD have been linked to the development of these complications. Levodopa, though, has been less so than other antiparkinsonian agents (89,138). The management of these problems should start with the exclusion of any precipitating factor (metabolic derangements, infection, stroke, drugs other than antiparkinsonian therapies). Once the medications given for PD are considered as potentially responsible for the episode reduction and eventual discontinuation of the drugs (in clinical practice the sequence anticholinergics, amantadine, dopamine agonists, COMT inhibitors, MAO-B inhibitors, and levodopa) is often recommended. For psychosis which does not respond to the above measures, no treatment may be required if psychotic features are not troublesome to the patient. In more severe psychosis, and also if patients do not tolerate drug withdrawal because of worsening parkinsonism, antipsychotic medication should be considered. Typical antipsychotics exacerbate PD and should not be used. Two atypical neuroleptics, quetiapine and clozapine, are frequently needed in the management of psychosis in PD. Quetiapine is an atypical antipsychotic, which has a similar structure to clozapine, but has the advantage of not requiring blood monitoring. It combines a strong antagonism of 5HT2 receptors with a weak antagonism of D2 receptors. The only placebo controlled study that has documented the effectiveness of quetiapine in PD psychosis (139, in contrast to the results of 140–143) excluded patients with delusions. In spite of that many physicians believe that quetiapine is effective and the American Academy of Neurology's task force on PD treatment recommended quetiapine as a treatment option after clozapine has been considered (144).

In patients with dopamine dysregulation syndrome levodopa is the initial agent to wean with a subsequent increase in dopamine agonist treatment if motor symptoms worsen. Patients with this syndrome often are not compliant, and therefore external control of doses by the families/caregivers is important. As far as additional pharmacological options, antidepressants for obsessive thoughts, and antipsychotic treatment for manic or aberrant behavioral, may be considered (78).

The pathophysiological mechanisms underlying punding have not been understood, in consequence the therapeutic strategies are not clear. A reduction in the dose of levodopa or dopamine agonist is the first step. Atypical antipsychotics or selective serotonin reuptake inhibitors (SSRIs) have been suggested (145,146).

DBS to the subthalamic nucleus may allow dopaminergic drug reduction and therefore improvement in these symptoms. Patients with refractory symptoms may therefore be considered for this procedure. Rarely though dopamine dysregulation syndrome and impulse control disorders may worsen or develop for the first time after DBS surgery (147,148).

RECENT DEVELOPMENTS IN TREATMENT WITH LEVODOPA
Intraduodenal Levodopa Therapy
Erratic gastric emptying has been recognized as a significant determinant of levodopa plasma level variability (149), and continuous intraduodenal levodopa delivery was developed as an attempt to overcome this problem. Ever since the first reports of its clinical use (150,151), multiple studies (152–155) have shown that compared with orally administered levodopa, the enteral infusion of the drug achieves more stable plasma levels of levodopa (variability falling from 34% to 14% in one study), reduces daily off-time and increases daily on-time without dyskinesia (off time reduction from 50% to 11% and disabling dyskinesia from 13% to 3%). A beneficial effect on nonmotor symptoms (including cognitive impairment, fatigue, autonomic dysfunction, sleep disturbance, and pain) and quality of life (156,157) has also been reported.

Enteral levodopa therapy may be considered in advanced PD patients with severe motor fluctuations and/or disabling dyskinesia that have not been controlled with optimization of standard pharmacological therapies. Candidates must have a good response to levodopa therapy, and lack certain exclusion criteria (most notably severe comorbidities that adversely impact functional status or life expectancy, ongoing neuropsychiatric symptoms, and contraindications for abdominal surgery). Although a formal direct comparison between enteral levodopa infusion and DBS has not been carried out, there is some clinical evidence that both procedures have similar indications and outcomes. It should be noted, however, that advanced age might be a less stringent exclusion criteria for enteral levodopa infusion, and mild cognitive impairment does not contraindicate this procedure.

Levodopa/carbidopa in a 20 mg/5 mg per milliliter water-soluble suspension in methylcellulose (Duodopa™) is commercially available in Europe in 100 mL containers. This treatment modality requires a gastrostomy for the insertion of a cannula with the tip placed in the duodenum and an external pump, which delivers the levodopa gel according to certain operator-defined parameters. A standard therapeutic scheme includes a morning dose (typically 100–200 mg of levodopa administered in 10–30 minutes), a maintenance dose (40–120 mg of levodopa hourly for a period of about 16 hours) and rescue doses (10–40 mg of levodopa, to be administered in case of unexpected off-periods). Dosages and schedules, however, should be tailored to individual patient's needs (e.g., continuing drug administration throughout the night in patients with disabling nocturnal symptoms).

Reports on emergent complications in the course of enteral levodopa infusion are relatively scarce. At least 60% of patients on this therapy have been reported to continue on this therapy after extensive periods of time. A recently published follow-up study of 135 patients (158) found that 81 continued on enteral levodopa after a variable time span, which extended up to 16 years (this same group (159) had reported that at least 75% of patients continue on this modality after two years, and about 50% after six years). Reported complications may be related to the gastrostomy (decubitus ulcer of the gastrointestinal mucosa, granuloma, or infection of the ostomy), to the mechanical device (kinking, displacement, or rupture of the cannula), or to levodopa therapy (dyskinesia, neuropsychiatric disturbances, mixed axonal neuropathy). Device-related adverse events are the most frequent events and their incidence has been calculated to reach two episodes per patient-year (159). The first two classes of complications usually require repeat radiologic or endoscopic procedures, and the replacement of parts or the whole infusion system. Regarding the complications related to levodopa itself, those that are attributable to excessive dopaminergic stimulation require dose adjustments, while neuropathy is thought to originate from cobalamine deficiency and is usually managed with vitamin B12 supplementation. Although results from clinical trials have shown that this approach is clinically effective, it should be noted that its clinical use is hindered by elevated costs, invasiveness and, most of all, technical complexity (160).

Newer Levodopa Formulations
Levodopa remains the mainstay of treatment for PD patients 40 years after its introduction in clinical practice. Nevertheless, its use has certain drawbacks, among which are a relatively short duration of clinical effect, and the eventual development of motor complications (fluctuations and dyskinesia). Refinements in treatment strategies have largely focused on achieving a state of "continuous drug delivery." Adjustments in the dose or schedule of levodopa are generally effective only in the early stages of the disease, and in more advanced stages add-on medications (including dopamine agonists, COMT inhibitors, or MAO-B inhibitors) are generally required. The use of extended-release levodopa formulations has met with conflicting results. If these strategies fail, advanced therapies (which include DBS, the duodenal infusion of levodopa gel, and the apomorphine pump) may be considered.

There is ongoing research with different levodopa prodrugs and derivatives (IPX066 and XP21279) and a transdermal levodopa patch (97) to attain more sustained plasma levels, and melevodopa (161) has been shown to have a shorter latency to clinical effect as compared to regular carbidopa/levodopa. In general, however, the significance of these results remains to be determined.

REFERENCES
1. Manyam BV. Paralysis agitans and levodopa in "Ayurveda": ancient Indian medical treatise. Mov Disord 1990; 5: 47–8.
2. Katzenschlager R, Evans A, Manson A, et al. Mucuna pruriens in Parkinson's disease: a double blind clinical and pharmacological study. J Neurol Neurosurg Psychiatry 2004; 75: 1672–7.
3. Cotzias GC, Van Woert MH, Schiffer LM. Aromatic amino acids and modification of parkinsonism. N Engl J Med 1967; 276: 374–9.
4. Cotzias GC, Papavasiliou PS, Gellene R. Modification of Parkinsonism–chronic treatment with L-dopa. N Engl J Med 1969; 280: 337–45.
5. Carlsson A, Lindqvist M, Magnusson T. 3,4-Dihydroxyphenylalanine and 5-hydroxytryptophan as reserpine antagonists. Nature 1957; 180: 1200.

6. Birkmayer W, Hornykiewicz O. The L-3,4-dioxyphenylalanine (DOPA)-effect in Parkinson-akinesia. Wien Klin Wochenschr 1961; 73: 787–8.

7. Hornykiewicz O. L-DOPA: from a biologically inactive amino acid to a successful therapeutic agent. Amino Acids 2002; 23: 65–70.

8. Barbeau A. L-dopa therapy in Parkinson's disease: a critical review of nine years' experience. Can Med Assoc J 1969; 101: 59–68.

9. Yahr MD, Duvoisin RC, Schear MJ, Barrett RE, Hoehn MM. Treatment of parkinsonism with levodopa. Arch Neurol 1969; 21: 343–54.

10. Juncos JL. Levodopa: pharmacology, pharmacokinetics, and pharmacodynamics. Neurol Clin 1992; 10: 487–509.

11. Nyholm D, Lennernas H, Gomes-Trolin C, Aquilonius SM. Levodopa pharmacokinetics and motor performance during activities of daily living in patients with Parkinson's disease on individual drug combinations. Clin Neuropharmacol 2002; 25: 89–96.

12. Tanaka H, Kannari K, Maeda T, et al. Role of serotonergic neurons in L-DOPA-derived extracellular dopamine in the striatum of 6-OHDA-lesioned rats. Neuroreport 1999; 10: 631–4.

13. LeWitt PA, Nelson MV, Berchou RC, et al. Controlled-release carbidopa/levodopa (Sinemet 50/200 CR4): clinical and pharmacokinetic studies. Neurology 1989; 39: 45–53; discussion 9.

14. Yeh KC, August TF, Bush DF, et al. Pharmacokinetics and bioavailability of Sinemet CR: a summary of human studies. Neurology 1989; 39: 25–38.

15. Erni W, Held K. The hydrodynamically balanced system: a novel principle of controlled drug release. Eur Neurol 1987; 27: 21–7.

16. Goetz CG, Koller WC, Poewe W, et al. Management of Parkinson's disease: an evidence-based review. Mov Disord 2002; 17:S1–166.

17. Levine CB, Fahrbach KR, Siderowf AD, et al. Diagnosis and treatment of Parkinson's disease: a systematic review of the literature. Evid Rep Technol Assess (Summ) 2003; 1–4.

18. Tolosa E, Katzenschlager R. Pharmacological Management of Parkinson's disease. In: Jankovic J, Tolosa E, eds. Parkinson's Disease & Movement Disorders, 5th edn. Philadelphia: Lippincott Williams & Wilkins, 2007: 110–45.

19. Horstink M, Tolosa E, Bonuccelli U, et al. Review of the therapeutic management of Parkinson's disease. Report of a joint task force of the European federation of neurological societies and the movement disorder society-European section. Part I: early (uncomplicated) Parkinson's disease. Eur J Neurol 2006; 13: 1170–85.

20. Klawans HL. Individual manifestations of Parkinson's disease after ten or more years of levodopa. Mov Disord 1986; 1: 187–92.

21. Bonnet AM, Loria Y, Saint-Hilaire MH, Lhermitte F, Agid Y. Does long-term aggravation of Parkinson's disease result from nondopaminergic lesions? Neurology 1987; 37: 1539–42.

22. Hely MA, Morris JG, Traficante R, et al. The Sydney multicentre study of Parkinson's disease: progression and mortality at 10 years. J Neurol Neurosurg Psychiatry 1999; 67: 300–7.

23. Hely MA, Morris JG, Reid WG, Trafficante R. Sydney multicenter study of Parkinson's disease: non-L-dopa-responsive problems dominate at 15 years. Mov Disord 2005; 20: 190–9.

24. Hely MA, Reid WG, Adena MA, Halliday GM, Morris JG. The Sydney multicenter study of Parkinson's disease: the inevitability of dementia at 20 years. Mov Disord 2008; 23: 837–44.

25. Ferreira JJ, Thalamas C, Montastruc JL, Castro-Caldas A, Rascol O. Levodopa monotherapy can induce "sleep attacks" in Parkinson's disease patients. J Neurol 2001; 248: 426–7.

26. Postuma RB, Lang AE. Homocysteine and levodopa: should Parkinson disease patients receive preventative therapy? Neurology 2004; 63: 886–91.

27. Olsen JH, Friis S, Frederiksen K. Malignant melanoma and other types of cancer preceding Parkinson disease. Epidemiology 2006; 17: 582–7.

28. Constantinescu R, Romer M, Kieburtz K. Malignant melanoma in early Parkinson's disease: the DATATOP trial. Mov Disord 2007; 22: 720–2.

29. Rajabally YA, Martey J. Neuropathy in Parkinson disease: prevalence and determinants. Neurology 2011; 77: 1947–50.
30. Toth C, Breithaupt K, Ge S, et al. Levodopa, methylmalonic acid, and neuropathy in idiopathic Parkinson disease. Ann Neurol 2010; 68: 28–36.
31. Nutt JG, Gancher ST, Woodward WR. Does an inhibitory action of levodopa contribute to motor fluctuations? Neurology 1988; 38: 1553–7.
32. Souza RG, Borges V, Silva SM, Ferraz HB. Quality of life scale in Parkinson's disease PDQ-39 - (Brazilian Portuguese version) to assess patients with and without levodopa motor fluctuation. Arq Neuropsiquiatr 2007; 65: 787–91.
33. Rahman S, Griffin HJ, Quinn NP, Jahanshahi M. Quality of life in Parkinson's disease: the relative importance of the symptoms. Mov Disord 2008; 23: 1428–34.
34. Espay AJ, Fasano A, van Nuenen BF, et al. "On" state freezing of gait in Parkinson disease: a paradoxical levodopa-induced complication. Neurology 2012; 78: 454–7.
35. Witjas T, Kaphan E, Azulay JP, et al. Nonmotor fluctuations in Parkinson's disease: frequent and disabling. Neurology 2002; 59: 408–13.
36. Stacy M, Bowron A, Guttman M, et al. Identification of motor and nonmotor wearing-off in Parkinson's disease: comparison of a patient questionnaire versus a clinician assessment. Mov Disord 2005; 20: 726–33.
37. Martinez-Martin P, Rodriguez-Blazquez C, Kurtis MM, Chaudhuri KR. The impact of non-motor symptoms on health-related quality of life of patients with Parkinson's disease. Mov Disord 2011; 26: 399–406.
38. Tolosa ES, Martin WE, Cohen HP, Jacobson RL. Patterns of clinical response and plasma dopa levels in Parkinson's disease. Neurology 1975; 25: 177–83.
39. Muenter MD, Sharpless NS, Tyce GM, Darley FL. Patterns of dystonia ("I-D-I" and "D-I-D-") in response to l-dopa therapy for Parkinson's disease. Mayo Clin Proc 1977; 52: 163–74.
40. Damiano AM, McGrath MM, Willian MK, et al. Evaluation of a measurement strategy for Parkinson's disease: assessing patient health-related quality of life. Qual Life Res 2000; 9: 87–100.
41. Chapuis S, Ouchchane L, Metz O, Gerbaud L, Durif F. Impact of the motor complications of Parkinson's disease on the quality of life. Mov Disord 2005; 20: 224–30.
42. Pechevis M, Clarke CE, Vieregge P, et al. Effects of dyskinesias in Parkinson's disease on quality of life and health-related costs: a prospective European study. Eur J Neurol 2005; 12: 956–63.
43. LePen C, Wait S, Moutard-Martin F, Dujardin M, Ziegler M. Cost of illness and disease severity in a cohort of French patients with Parkinson's disease. Pharmacoeconomics 1999; 16: 59–69.
44. Dodel RC, Berger K, Oertel WH. Health-related quality of life and healthcare utilisation in patients with Parkinson's disease: impact of motor fluctuations and dyskinesias. Pharmacoeconomics 2001; 19: 1013–38.
45. Lhermitte F, Agid Y, Signoret JL. Onset and end-of-dose levodopa-induced dyskinesias. Possible treatment by increasing the daily doses of levodopa. Arch Neurol 1978; 35: 261–3.
46. Melamed E. Early-morning dystonia. A late side effect of long-term levodopa therapy in Parkinson's disease. Arch Neurol 1979; 36: 308–10.
47. Schrag A, Quinn N. Dyskinesias and motor fluctuations in Parkinson's disease. A community-based study. Brain 2000; 123: 2297–305.
48. Poewe WH, Lees AJ, Stern GM. Dystonia in Parkinson's disease: clinical and pharmacological features. Ann Neurol 1988; 23: 73–8.
49. Khan NL, Graham E, Critchley P, et al. Parkin disease: a phenotypic study of a large case series. Brain 2003; 126: 1279–92.
50. Valente EM, Abou-Sleiman PM, Caputo V, et al. Hereditary early-onset Parkinson's disease caused by mutations in PINK1. Science 2004; 304: 1158–60.
51. Albanese A, Valente EM, Romito LM, et al. The PINK1 phenotype can be indistinguishable from idiopathic Parkinson disease. Neurology 2005; 64: 1958–60.
52. Ahlskog JE, Muenter MD. Frequency of levodopa-related dyskinesias and motor fluctuations as estimated from the cumulative literature. Mov Disord 2001; 16: 448–58.

53. Olanow CW, Watts RL, Koller WC. An algorithm (decision tree) for the management of Parkinson's disease (2001): treatment guidelines. Neurology 2001; 56: S1–S88.

54. Poewe WH, Lees AJ, Stern GM. Treatment of motor fluctuations in Parkinson's disease with an oral sustained-release preparation of L-dopa: clinical and pharmacokinetic observations. Clin Neuropharmacol 1986; 9: 430–9.

55. Kostic V, Przedborski S, Flaster E, Sternic N. Early development of levodopa-induced dyskinesias and response fluctuations in young-onset Parkinson's disease. Neurology 1991; 41: 202–5.

56. Blanchet PJ, Allard P, Gregoire L, Tardif F, Bedard PJ. Risk factors for peak dose dyskinesia in 100 levodopa-treated parkinsonian patients. Can J Neurol Sci 1996; 23: 189–93.

57. Denny AP, Behari M. Motor fluctuations in Parkinson's disease. J Neurol Sci 1999; 165: 18–23.

58. Grandas F, Galiano ML, Tabernero C. Risk factors for levodopa-induced dyskinesias in Parkinson's disease. J Neurol 1999; 246: 1127–33.

59. Kumar N, Van Gerpen JA, Bower JH, Ahlskog JE. Levodopa-dyskinesia incidence by age of Parkinson's disease onset. Mov Disord 2005; 20: 342–4.

60. Jankovic J. Motor fluctuations and dyskinesias in Parkinson's disease: clinical manifestations. Mov Disord 2005; 20: S11–16.

61. Fahn S, Oakes D, Shoulson I, et al. Levodopa and the progression of Parkinson's disease. N Engl J Med 2004; 351: 2498–508.

62. Fabbrini G, Juncos J, Mouradian MM, Serrati C, Chase TN. Levodopa pharmacokinetic mechanisms and motor fluctuations in Parkinson's disease. Ann Neurol 1987; 21: 370–6.

63. Nutt JG. On-off phenomenon: relation to levodopa pharmacokinetics and pharmacodynamics. Ann Neurol 1987; 22: 535–40.

64. Nutt JG, Woodward WR, Anderson JL. The effect of carbidopa on the pharmacokinetics of intravenously administered levodopa: the mechanism of action in the treatment of parkinsonism. Ann Neurol 1985; 18: 537–43.

65. de la Fuente-Fernandez R, Lu JQ, Sossi V, et al. Biochemical variations in the synaptic level of dopamine precede motor fluctuations in Parkinson's disease: PET evidence of increased dopamine turnover. Ann Neurol 2001; 49: 298–303.

66. de la Fuente-Fernandez R, Sossi V, Huang Z, et al. Levodopa-induced changes in synaptic dopamine levels increase with progression of Parkinson's disease: implications for dyskinesias. Brain 2004; 127: 2747–54.

67. Chase TN. Levodopa therapy: consequences of the nonphysiologic replacement of dopamine. Neurology 1998; 50: S17–25.

68. Obeso JA, Rodriguez-Oroz MC, Rodriguez M, DeLong MR, Olanow CW. Pathophysiology of levodopa-induced dyskinesias in Parkinson's disease: problems with the current model. Ann Neurol 2000; 47: S22–32; discussion S-4.

69. Stocchi F. The concept of continuous dopaminergic stimulation: what we should consider when starting Parkinson's disease treatment. Neurodegener Dis 2010; 7: 213–15.

70. Lange KW, Robbins TW, Marsden CD, et al. L-dopa withdrawal in Parkinson's disease selectively impairs cognitive performance in tests sensitive to frontal lobe dysfunction. Psychopharmacology (Berl) 1992; 107: 394–404.

71. Gotham AM, Brown RG, Marsden CD. 'Frontal' cognitive function in patients with Parkinson's disease 'on' and 'off' levodopa. Brain 1988; 111: 299–321.

72. Pascual-Sedano B, Kulisevsky J, Barbanoj M, et al. Levodopa and executive performance in Parkinson's disease: a randomized study. J Int Neuropsychol Soc 2008; 14: 832–41.

73. Wolters E. PD-related psychosis: pathophysiology with therapeutical strategies. J Neural Transm Suppl 2006: 31–7.

74. Eskow Jaunarajs KL, Angoa-Perez M, Kuhn DM, Bishop C. Potential mechanisms underlying anxiety and depression in Parkinson's disease: consequences of L-dopa treatment. Neurosci Biobehav Rev 2011; 35: 556–64.

75. Stamey W, Jankovic J. Impulse control disorders and pathological gambling in patients with Parkinson disease. Neurologist 2008; 14: 89–99.

76. Weintraub D, Koester J, Potenza MN, et al. Impulse control disorders in Parkinson disease: a cross-sectional study of 3090 patients. Arch Neurol 2010; 67: 589–95.

77. van Deelen RA, Rommers MK, Eerenberg JG, Egberts AC. Hypersexuality during use of levodopa. Ned Tijdschr Geneeskd 2002; 146: 2095–8.
78. Giovannoni G, O'Sullivan JD, Turner K, Manson AJ, Lees AJ. Hedonistic homeostatic dysregulation in patients with Parkinson's disease on dopamine replacement therapies. J Neurol Neurosurg Psychiatry 2000; 68: 423–8.
79. Lawrence AD, Evans AH, Lees AJ. Compulsive use of dopamine replacement therapy in Parkinson's disease: reward systems gone awry? Lancet Neurol 2003; 2: 595–604.
80. Evans AH, Lawrence AD, Potts J, Appel S, Lees AJ. Factors influencing susceptibility to compulsive dopaminergic drug use in Parkinson disease. Neurology 2005; 65: 1570–4.
81. Friedman JH. Punding on levodopa. Biol Psychiatry 1994; 36: 350–1.
82. Evans AH, Katzenschlager R, Paviour D, et al. Punding in Parkinson's disease: its relation to the dopamine dysregulation syndrome. Mov Disord 2004; 19: 397–405.
83. Michel PP, Hefti F. Toxicity of 6-hydroxydopamine and dopamine for dopaminergic neurons in culture. J Neurosci Res 1990; 26: 428–35.
84. Mytilineou C, Han SK, Cohen G. Toxic and protective effects of L-dopa on mesencephalic cell cultures. J Neurochem 1993; 61: 1470–8.
85. Mena MA, Casarejos MJ, Garcia de Yebenes J. The effect of glia-conditioned medium on dopamine neurons in culture. Modulation of apoptosis, tyrosine hydroxylase expression and 1-methyl-4-phenylpyridinium toxicity. J Neural Transm 1999; 106: 1105–23.
86. Pearce RK, Heikkila M, Linden IB, Jenner P. L-dopa induces dyskinesia in normal monkeys: behavioural and pharmacokinetic observations. Psychopharmacology (Berl) 2001; 156: 402–9.
87. Murer MG, Dziewczapolski G, Menalled LB, et al. Chronic levodopa is not toxic for remaining dopamine neurons, but instead promotes their recovery, in rats with moderate nigrostriatal lesions. Ann Neurol 1998; 43: 561–75.
88. Datla KP, Blunt SB, Dexter DT. Chronic L-DOPA administration is not toxic to the remaining dopaminergic nigrostriatal neurons, but instead may promote their functional recovery, in rats with partial 6-OHDA or FeCl(3) nigrostriatal lesions. Mov Disord 2001; 16: 424–34.
89. Olanow CW, Agid Y, Mizuno Y, et al. Levodopa in the treatment of Parkinson's disease: current controversies. Mov Disord 2004; 19: 997–1005.
90. Quinn N, Parkes D, Janota I, Marsden CD. Preservation of the substantia nigra and locus coeruleus in a patient receiving levodopa (2 kg) plus decarboxylase inhibitor over a four-year period. Mov Disord 1986; 1: 65–8.
91. Marek K, Jennings D, Seibyl J. Do dopamine agonists or levodopa modify Parkinson's disease progression? Eur J Neurol 2002; 9: 15–22.
92. Whone AL, Watts RL, Stoessl AJ, et al. Slower progression of Parkinson's disease with ropinirole versus levodopa: The REAL-PET study. Ann Neurol 2003; 54: 93–101.
93. Morrish PK. How valid is dopamine transporter imaging as a surrogate marker in research trials in Parkinson's disease? Mov Disord 2003; 18: S63–70.
94. Ravina B, Eidelberg D, Ahlskog JE, et al. The role of radiotracer imaging in Parkinson disease. Neurology 2005; 64: 208–15.
95. Chase TN, Oh JD. Striatal mechanisms and pathogenesis of parkinsonian signs and motor complications. Ann Neurol 2000; 47: S122–9; discussion S9–30.
96. Nutt JG. Clinical pharmacology of levodopa-induced dyskinesia. Ann Neurol 2000; 47: S160–4; discussion S4–6.
97. Hauser RA, Ellenbogen AL, Metman LV, et al. Crossover comparison of IPX066 and a standard levodopa formulation in advanced Parkinson's disease. Mov Disord 2011; 26: 2246–52.
98. Quinn N, Critchley P, Marsden CD. Young onset Parkinson's disease. Mov Disord 1987; 2: 73–91.
99. Block G, Liss C, Reines S, Irr J, Nibbelink D; The CR First Study Group. Comparison of immediate-release and controlled release carbidopa/levodopa in Parkinson's disease. A multicenter 5-year study. Eur Neurol 1997; 37: 23–7.
100. Stocchi F, Rascol O, Kieburtz K, et al. Initiating levodopa/carbidopa therapy with and without entacapone in early Parkinson disease: the STRIDE-PD study. Ann Neurol 2010; 68: 18–27.

101. Stocchi F, Barbato L, Nordera G, Berardelli A, Ruggieri S. Sleep disorders in Parkinson's disease. J Neurol 1998; 245: S15–18.
102. Tan A, Salgado M, Fahn S. Rapid eye movement sleep behavior disorder preceding Parkinson's disease with therapeutic response to levodopa. Mov Disord 1996; 11: 214–16.
103. Iranzo A, Molinuevo JL, Santamaria J, et al. Rapid-eye-movement sleep behaviour disorder as an early marker for a neurodegenerative disorder: a descriptive study. Lancet Neurol 2006; 5: 572–7.
104. Schestatsky P, Kumru H, Valls-Sole J, et al. Neurophysiologic study of central pain in patients with Parkinson disease. Neurology 2007; 69: 2162–9.
105. Gershanik OS. Clinical problems in late-stage Parkinson's disease. J Neurol 2010; 257: S288–91.
106. Larsen JP, Boas J, Erdal JE. The Norwegian-Danish Study Group. Does selegiline modify the progression of early Parkinson's disease? Results from a five-year study. Eur J Neurol 1999; 6: 539–47.
107. Larsen JP, Karlsen K, Tandberg E. Clinical problems in non-fluctuating patients with Parkinson's disease: a community-based study. Mov Disord 2000; 15: 826–9.
108. Harder S, Baas H. Concentration-response relationship of levodopa in patients at different stages of Parkinson's disease. Clin Pharmacol Ther 1998; 64: 183–91.
109. Sage JI, Duvoisin RC. Long-term efficacy of pergolide in patients with Parkinson's disease. Clin Neuropharmacol 1986; 9: 160–4.
110. Jankovic J, Orman J. Parallel double-blind study of pergolide in Parkinson's disease. Adv Neurol 1987; 45: 551–4.
111. Olanow CW, Fahn S, Muenter M, et al. A multicenter double-blind placebo-controlled trial of pergolide as an adjunct to Sinemet in Parkinson's disease. Mov Disord 1994; 9: 40–7.
112. Guttman M; International Pramipexole-Bromocriptine Study Group. Double-blind comparison of pramipexole and bromocriptine treatment with placebo in advanced Parkinson's disease. Neurology 1997; 49: 1060–5.
113. Lieberman A, Ranhosky A, Korts D. Clinical evaluation of pramipexole in advanced Parkinson's disease: results of a double-blind, placebo-controlled, parallel-group study. Neurology 1997; 49: 162–8.
114. Pinter MM, Pogarell O, Oertel WH. Efficacy, safety, and tolerance of the non-ergoline dopamine agonist pramipexole in the treatment of advanced Parkinson's disease: a double blind, placebo controlled, randomised, multicentre study. J Neurol Neurosurg Psychiatry 1999; 66: 436–41.
115. Mizuno Y, Yanagisawa N, Kuno S, et al. Randomized, double-blind study of pramipexole with placebo and bromocriptine in advanced Parkinson's disease. Mov Disord 2003; 18: 1149–56.
116. Rascol O, Lees AJ, Senard JM, et al. Ropinirole in the treatment of levodopa-induced motor fluctuations in patients with Parkinson's disease. Clin Neuropharmacol 1996; 19: 234–45.
117. Lieberman A, Olanow CW, Sethi K, et al. Ropinirole Study Group. A multicenter trial of ropinirole as adjunct treatment for Parkinson's disease. Neurology 1998; 51: 1057–62.
118. Hoehn MM, Elton RL. Low dosages of bromocriptine added to levodopa in Parkinson's disease. Neurology 1985; 35: 199–206.
119. Toyokura Y, Mizuno Y, Kase M, et al. Effects of bromocriptine on parkinsonism. A nation-wide collaborative double-blind study. Acta Neurol Scand 1985; 72: 157–70.
120. Hutton JT, Koller WC, Ahlskog JE, et al. Multicenter, placebo-controlled trial of cabergoline taken once daily in the treatment of Parkinson's disease. Neurology 1996; 46: 1062–5.
121. Tolcapone Study Group. Efficacy and tolerability of tolcapone compared with bromocriptine in levodopa-treated parkinsonian patients. Mov Disord 1999; 14: 38–44.
122. Koller W, Lees A, Doder M, Hely M. Randomized trial of tolcapone versus pergolide as add-on to levodopa therapy in Parkinson's disease patients with motor fluctuations. Mov Disord 2001; 16: 858–66.

123. Waters CH, Sethi KD, Hauser RA, Molho E, Bertoni JM. Zydis selegiline reduces off time in Parkinson's disease patients with motor fluctuations: a 3-month, randomized, placebo-controlled study. Mov Disord 2004; 19: 426–32.

124. The Parkinson Study Group. Effect of deprenyl on the progression of disability in early Parkinson's disease. N Engl J Med 1989; 321: 1364–71.

125. Rascol O, Brooks DJ, Melamed E, et al. Rasagiline as an adjunct to levodopa in patients with Parkinson's disease and motor fluctuations (LARGO, Lasting effect in Adjunct therapy with Rasagiline Given Once daily, study): a randomised, double-blind, parallel-group trial. Lancet 2005; 365: 947–54.

126. Van Gerpen JA, Kumar N, Bower JH, Weigand S, Ahlskog JE. Levodopa-associated dyskinesia risk among Parkinson disease patients in Olmsted County, Minnesota, 1976–1990. Arch Neurol 2006; 63: 205–9.

127. Bennett JP Jr, Landow ER, Schuh LA. Suppression of dyskinesias in advanced Parkinson's disease. II. Increasing daily clozapine doses suppress dyskinesias and improve parkinsonism symptoms. Neurology 1993; 43: 1551–5.

128. Durif F, Debilly B, Galitzky M, et al. Clozapine improves dyskinesias in Parkinson disease: a double-blind, placebo-controlled study. Neurology 2004; 62: 381–8.

129. Verhagen Metman L, Del Dotto P, van den Munckhof P, et al. Amantadine as treatment for dyskinesias and motor fluctuations in Parkinson's disease. Neurology 1998; 50: 1323–6.

130. Metman LV, Del Dotto P, LePoole K, et al. Amantadine for levodopa-induced dyskinesias: a 1-year follow-up study. Arch Neurol 1999; 56: 1383–6.

131. Snow BJ, Macdonald L, McAuley D, Wallis W. The effect of amantadine on levodopa-induced dyskinesias in Parkinson's disease: a double-blind, placebo-controlled study. Clin Neuropharmacol 2000; 23: 82–5.

132. Luginger E, Wenning GK, Bosch S, Poewe W. Beneficial effects of amantadine on L-dopa-induced dyskinesias in Parkinson's disease. Mov Disord 2000; 15: 873–8.

133. Thomas A, Iacono D, Luciano AL, et al. Duration of amantadine benefit on dyskinesia of severe Parkinson's disease. J Neurol Neurosurg Psychiatry 2004; 75: 141–3.

134. Guridi J, Obeso JA, Rodriguez-Oroz MC, Lozano AA, Manrique M. L-dopa-induced dyskinesia and stereotactic surgery for Parkinson's disease. Neurosurgery 2008; 62: 311–23; discussion 23–5.

135. Nyholm D. Enteral levodopa/carbidopa gel infusion for the treatment of motor fluctuations and dyskinesias in advanced Parkinson's disease. Expert Rev Neurother 2006; 6: 1403–11.

136. Katzenschlager R, Hughes A, Evans A, et al. Continuous subcutaneous apomorphine therapy improves dyskinesias in Parkinson's disease: a prospective study using single-dose challenges. Mov Disord 2005; 20: 151–7.

137. Lhermitte F, Agid Y, Feuerstein C, et al. Abnormal movements caused by L-DOPA in patients with Parkinson's disease: correlation with the plasma concentrations of DOPA and O-methyl-DOPA. Rev Neurol (Paris) 1977; 133: 445–54.

138. Hubble JP. Long-term studies of dopamine agonists. Neurology 2002; 58:S42–50.

139. Fernandez HH, Okun MS, Rodriguez RL, et al. Quetiapine improves visual hallucinations in Parkinson disease but not through normalization of sleep architecture: results from a double-blind clinical-polysomnography study. Int J Neurosci 2009; 119: 2196–205.

140. Ondo WG, Tintner R, Voung KD, Lai D, Ringholz G. Double-blind, placebo-controlled, unforced titration parallel trial of quetiapine for dopaminergic-induced hallucinations in Parkinson's disease. Mov Disord 2005; 20: 958–63.

141. Rabey JM, Prokhorov T, Miniovitz A, Dobronevsky E, Klein C. Effect of quetiapine in psychotic Parkinson's disease patients: a double-blind labeled study of 3 months' duration. Mov Disord 2007; 22: 313–18.

142. Shotbolt P, Samuel M, Fox C, David AS. A randomized controlled trial of quetiapine for psychosis in Parkinson's disease. Neuropsychiatr Dis Treat 2009; 5: 327–32.

143. Kurlan R, Cummings J, Raman R, Thal L. Quetiapine for agitation or psychosis in patients with dementia and parkinsonism. Neurology 2007; 68: 1356–63.

144. Miyasaki JM, Shannon K, Voon V, et al. Practice parameter: evaluation and treatment of depression, psychosis, and dementia in Parkinson disease (an evidence-based review): report of the quality standards subcommittee of the American academy of neurology. Neurology 2006; 66: 996–1002.
145. Bandini F, Primavera A, Pizzorno M, Cocito L. Using STN DBS and medication reduction as a strategy to treat pathological gambling in Parkinson's disease. Parkinsonism Relat Disord 2007; 13: 369–71.
146. Miwa H, Morita S, Nakanishi I, Kondo T. Stereotyped behaviors or punding after quetiapine administration in Parkinson's disease. Parkinsonism Relat Disord 2004; 10: 177–80.
147. Lim SY, O'Sullivan SS, Kotschet K, et al. Dopamine dysregulation syndrome, impulse control disorders and punding after deep brain stimulation surgery for Parkinson's disease. J Clin Neurosci 2009; 16: 1148–52.
148. Broen M, Duits A, Visser-Vandewalle V, Temel Y, Winogrodzka A. Impulse control and related disorders in Parkinson's disease patients treated with bilateral subthalamic nucleus stimulation: a review. Parkinsonism Relat Disord 2011; 17: 413–17.
149. Fernandez N, Garcia JJ, Diez MJ, et al. Effects of slowed gastrointestinal motility on levodopa pharmacokinetics. Auton Neurosci 2010; 156: 67–72.
150. Kurlan R, Rubin AJ, Miller C, et al. Duodenal delivery of levodopa for on-off fluctuations in parkinsonism: preliminary observations. Ann Neurol 1986; 20: 262–5.
151. Sage JI, Schuh L, Heikkila RE, Duvoisin RC. Continuous duodenal infusions of levodopa: plasma concentrations and motor fluctuations in Parkinson's disease. Clin Neuropharmacol 1988; 11: 36–44.
152. Nilsson D, Nyholm D, Aquilonius SM. Duodenal levodopa infusion in Parkinson's disease–long-term experience. Acta Neurol Scand 2001; 104: 343–8.
153. Odelowo OO, Naab T, Dewitty RL. Metastatic choriocarcinoma presenting as a bleeding duodenal ulcer. J Assoc Acad Minor Phys 2001; 12: 144–8.
154. Nyholm D, Askmark H, Gomes-Trolin C, et al. Optimizing levodopa pharmacokinetics: intestinal infusion versus oral sustained-release tablets. Clin Neuropharmacol 2003; 26: 156–63.
155. Nyholm D, Jansson R, Willows T, Remahl IN. Long-term 24-hour duodenal infusion of levodopa: outcome and dose requirements. Neurology 2005; 65: 1506–7.
156. Antonini A, Mancini F, Canesi M, et al. Duodenal levodopa infusion improves quality of life in advanced Parkinson's disease. Neurodegener Dis 2008; 5: 244–6.
157. Honig H, Antonini A, Martinez-Martin P, et al. Intrajejunal levodopa infusion in Parkinson's disease: a pilot multicenter study of effects on nonmotor symptoms and quality of life. Mov Disord 2009; 24: 1468–74.
158. Nyholm D, Klangemo K, Johansson A. Levodopa/carbidopa intestinal gel infusion long-term therapy in advanced Parkinson's disease. Eur J Neurol 2012.
159. Nyholm D, Lewander T, Johansson A, et al. Enteral levodopa/carbidopa infusion in advanced Parkinson disease: long-term exposure. Clin Neuropharmacol 2008; 31: 63–73.
160. Syed N, Murphy J, Zimmerman T Jr, Mark MH, Sage JI. Ten years' experience with enteral levodopa infusions for motor fluctuations in Parkinson's disease. Mov Disord 1998; 13: 336–8.
161. Stocchi F, Zappia M, Dall'Armi V, et al. Melevodopa/carbidopa effervescent formulation in the treatment of motor fluctuations in advanced Parkinson's disease. Mov Disord 2010; 25: 1881–7.

20 Dopamine agonists

Valerie Suski and Mark Stacy

INTRODUCTION

Dopamine agonists have been used to treat Parkinson's disease (PD) since the late 1970s (1). These agents were initially introduced as adjunctive therapy to levodopa. In the last 30 years, dopamine agonists have demonstrated therapeutic benefit in all stages of PD, both in combination with levodopa and as monotherapy. Clinical, neuroimaging, animal, and cellular data suggest not only a levodopa-sparing effect and a delay in the incidence of motor fluctuations, but also a potential neuroprotective effect (2–5). A number of hypotheses have been proposed including a reduction of free radical formation by limiting levodopa exposure or an increase in the activity of radical-scavenging systems, perhaps by changing mitochondrial membrane potential. In addition, some investigators suggest that dopamine agonists may provide neurotrophic activity. However, there is currently no definitive evidence of disease modification beyond the delay of levodopa-induced motor complications.

This chapter reviews the history of dopamine agonists in the treatment of PD and provides a summary of data concerning efficacy, treatment approaches, and comparisons between commonly prescribed dopamine agonists. Similarly designed clinical trials are discussed, including direct comparative trials, in an effort to better define the relative efficacies of these agents.

DOPAMINE AGONISTS AND DOPAMINE RECEPTORS

The dopamine agonists used in the treatment of PD include ergoline-derived (bromocriptine, carbergoline, lisuride, and pergolide) and nonergoline-derived (apomorphine, pramipexole, ropinirole, and rotigotine). All of these agents activate D_2 receptors, whereas pergolide has been shown to be a mild D_1 agonist, and pramipexole may have higher affinity for D_3 receptors (Table 20.1). Five subtypes of dopamine agonist receptors have been identified and may be classified into striatal (D_1 and D_2) receptors or cortical (D_3, D_4, and D_5) receptors. The D_{3-5} receptors are present in the mesolimbic and mesocortical dopaminergic pathways. The D_1-receptor ($D_{1,5}$) family is associated with activation of adenylate cyclase and dopamine, and dopamine agonists activate the D_2-receptor family (D_{2-4}) (6). Postmortem examination of brains of patients with PD revealed upregulation of striatal D_2 and downregulation of the D_1 receptors. It is postulated that these changes lead to alteration of the indirect D_2-mediated pathway and disinhibition of the subthalamic nucleus (STN). Studies comparing apomorphine, a rapid-acting dopamine agonist, to deep brain stimulation (DBS) found comparable changes in Unified Parkinson's Disease Rating Scale (UPDRS) scores and intracortical inhibition with STN stimulation, globus pallidus stimulation, and apomorphine infusion, suggesting a connection between the nigral dopaminergic pathway and the thalamocortical motor pathway (7).

TABLE 20.1 Dopamine Agonists in Parkinson's Disease

Dopamine Agonist	D_1	D_2	D_3	D_4	D_5	5-HT	NE	ACh
Dopamine	+	++	+++	++	+++	0	0	0
Bromocriptine	−	++	+	+	+	−	+	0
Pergolide	+	+++	+++	+++	+	0	+	0
Pramipexole	0	+++	+++	++	0	+	+	+
Ropinirole	0	+++	+++	0	0	0	0	0
Apomorphine	−	++	++	+++	++	−	+	0

Abbreviations: 5-HT, 5-hydroxytryptamine; Ach, acetylcholine; D, dopamine; NE, norepinephrine.
Source: From Ref. 6.

Apomorphine

The United States Food and Drug Administration (FDA)–approved apomorphine, a nonergoline dopamine agonist, as a subcutaneously injected treatment for severe off episodes in 2004. It was first used in the 1930s as an emetic and was found to have benefit for PD over 50 years ago. Although the mechanism of action is unclear, it is thought that apomorphine ameliorates symptoms of PD by stimulating D_2 receptors within the caudate nucleus and putamen. It has a high affinity for D_4 receptors; moderate affinity for D_2, D_3, and D_5; moderate affinity for adrenergic receptors; and low affinity for D_1 and 5-hydroxytryptamine (5-HT) receptors (Table 20.1). In addition to the FDA-approved formulation administered subcutaneously, it has also been administered as an intravenous infusion, intranasal spray, sublingual tablet, and as a rectal suppository (8). Although intravenous administration of apomorphine results in consistent motor control, allowing for a reduction in oral medications, unanticipated intravascular thrombotic complications secondary to apomorphine crystal accumulation have led to termination of this route of administration (9). Subcutaneously administered apomorphine has a rapid onset of 7.3–14 minutes after administration and a short half-life of 45–90 minutes. The rate of uptake after apomorphine injection is influenced by factors such as location, temperature, depth of injection, and body fat. Plasma protein binding of apomorphine is approximately 30%, and its metabolism is unclear (Table 20.2) (10).

Apomorphine may be given subcutaneously every two hours. A test dose of 2 mg is administered to determine the initial dosing, and may be titrated to an effective dosage by 1 mg increments up to a maximum single exposure of 6 mg (11). There are limited data for dosing over five times per day, and at this dosing frequency, continuous subcutaneous infusion should be considered. Common side effects of apomorphine include nausea, vomiting, QT-interval prolongation on electrocardiogram, angina, somnolence, and hypotension. With the subcutaneous formulation of apomorphine, the injection site can experience tenderness, ecchymosis, hardening of the skin, necrosis, ulceration, and pruritis, which can be reduced by changing the injection site. Because of the powerful emetic action of apomorphine, treatment is initiated three days after beginning antiemetic agents—domperidone or trimethobenzamide (12). Apomorphine should not be administered with antiemetic serotonin type 3 receptor (5HT3) antagonists, such as ondansetron, granisetron, dolasetron, and palonosetron, because of the risks of severe hypotension and syncope. QT-interval prolongation has been found to be insignificant with doses less than 6 mg.

TABLE 20.2 Dopamine Agonists in Parkinson's Disease

Dopamine Agonist	$t^{1/2}$	Metabolism	N	S	H	OH	RPF
Bromocriptine	3–8 hr	Hepatic	37	8	12	44	2–5%
Pergolide	27 hr	Hepatic	24	6	14	2	2–5%
Pramipexole	8–12 hr	Renal	18	13	19	16	0
Ropinirole	4–6 hr	Hepatic	20	12	15	17	0
Apomorphine	40 min	Unclear	30	35	10	20	0

Abbreviations: H, hallucinations; N, nausea; OH, orthostatic hypotension; RPF, retroperitoneal or pulmonary fibrosis; S, somnolence.
Source: From Ref. 1. Additional data are collected from published package inserts.

Dewey et al. (13) demonstrated a 62% improvement in off-state UPDRS scores in subjects with advanced PD, 20 minutes after administering apomorphine in a 2:1 randomized, placebo-controlled trial. Subcutaneously administered apomorphine was also shown to be effective in 30 patients for up to five years of therapy (14).

Bromocriptine

Bromocriptine was approved in the United States in 1978. This ergot alkaloid is a partial D_2 agonist and a mild adrenergic agonist. It also has mild D_1 and 5-HT-antagonist properties (Table 20.1). When taken orally, bromocriptine is rapidly absorbed and 90% degraded through first-pass hepatic metabolism. Peak drug levels are achieved in 70–100 minutes, and it has a half-life of 3–8 hours. Less than 5% of the drug is excreted into the urine, and it is highly protein bound (Table 20.2). Bromocriptine is formulated into 2.5 mg-scored tablets and 5 mg capsules (1). Bromocriptine is initiated at 1.25 mg/day and is generally increased to 20 mg/day in three divided doses over the course of seven weeks; however, some patients may require dosages higher than 60 mg/day (15).

Although the side effects of all dopamine agonists are similar, only the ergot-derived compounds have been associated with retroperitoneal fibrosis—a rare but serious condition associated with severe pulmonary and renal complications (16). Erythromelalgia, a painful reddish discoloration usually involving the lower extremities, may also be more prevalent in patients taking ergoline dopamine agonists. The side effects of nausea, vomiting, sleepiness, orthostatic hypotension, and hallucinations are common to all dopamine agonists and in pivotal trials these side effects were 8–12% more common with bromocriptine than with placebo (Table 20.2) (17).

Bromocriptine has been investigated in de novo and levodopa-treated PD patients (18–22). A systematic review of all randomized, controlled trials of bromocriptine monotherapy compared with levodopa monotherapy in PD found that methodological factors or lack of control populations have led to a lack of evidence to guide clinical decisions (19–21). From 1974 to 1999, six studies randomizing more than 850 PD patients to bromocriptine or levodopa were reported, but only two trials used a double-blind design (19–21). These studies indicated a reduced frequency of dyskinesia and a trend toward less wearing off with bromocriptine. However, the larger number of dropouts in the bromocriptine group leaves these data subject to varied interpretations. In the treatment of early PD, bromocriptine may be beneficial in delaying motor complications and dyskinesia with comparable effects on impairment and disability in patients who tolerate the drug.

Numerous studies have demonstrated the benefits of bromocriptine in advanced PD. A double-blind, placebo-controlled, multicenter trial of bromocriptine in patients with motor fluctuations reported a 14% improvement in UPDRS activities of daily living (ADL), a 23.8% improvement in UPDRS motor scores, and a 29.7% reduction in off time after nine months, with a mean daily dosage of 22.8 mg of bromocriptine (22).

Pergolide

Pergolide, an ergoline-derived dopamine agonist, was approved in the United States in 1989. Like bromocriptine, pergolide has high affinity for the D_2 receptor and mild α_2-adrenergic activity, but it does not have 5-HT activity. In addition, pergolide has significant D_3 activity and mild D_1-agonist activity (Table 20.1) (1). Pergolide is available in three tablet sizes, 0.05, 0.25, and 1.0 mg, and is usually titrated to an effective dosage or an initial maximum dosage of 3 mg/day in three divided doses over the course of six to eight weeks (15). If clinical benefit is seen at 3 mg/day, this dosage may be increased if needed to a maximum of 6 to 8 mg/day. This agent is rapidly absorbed from the gut and reaches a peak plasma concentration in 1–3 hours. Although the duration of action is typically 4–8 hours, the half-life ranges from 15 to 42 hours with a mean of 27 hours. Pergolide is highly protein bound, and greater than 50% of the drug is excreted through the kidney (1). Side effects of pergolide are similar to bromocriptine, and include retroperitoneal fibrosis, erythromelalgia, somnolence, orthostatic hypotension, and hallucinations. These side effects are 2–12% higher with pergolide than with placebo (Table 20.2) (15,23).

Pergolide has been demonstrated to be effective in both early and advanced PD (24,25). A de novo PD study, Pergolide versus L-Dopa Monotherapy and Positron Emission Tomography trial (PELMOPET), with randomization to levodopa or pergolide and concurrent positron emission tomography (PET) scanning was completed. In this double-blind study, 294 subjects were randomized to pergolide or levodopa and treated without levodopa rescue for 36 months (4). Seventy-seven subjects (52%) receiving pergolide compared with 90 subjects (61.6%) treated with levodopa completed the study. The mean dosage of pergolide was 3.23 mg/day, whereas subjects receiving levodopa averaged 504 mg/day. Although differences were noted in change from baseline UPDRS motor score (13.4 ± 8.8 pergolide vs 18.1 ± 10.1 levodopa), dyskinesia was three times more frequent in the levodopa group. In addition, 88 subjects were followed by ^{18}F-Dopa PET scans. There was a decrease in uptake in the putamen of 7.9% in the pergolide group and 14.5% in the levodopa group, but these were not significant differences ($P = 0.288$).

Olanow et al. reported a 24-week, double-blind trial of 377 PD subjects with motor fluctuations randomized to pergolide or placebo. Significant improvements were seen in UPDRS motor scores and off time, and levodopa dosages were reduced by approximately 25% in the pergolide group (26).

A database review, comparing efficacy in adjunct therapy trials of pergolide and bromocriptine, found that pergolide was superior to bromocriptine with regard to motor function and ADLs. In addition, more subjects recorded a marked or moderate improvement with pergolide than with bromocriptine. However, no significant differences in motor fluctuations, dyskinesia, levodopa dose reduction, dropouts, or adverse events were found (19).

Cardiopulmonary fibrosis has been reported in patients on long-term pergolide therapy. One patient with no previous underlying pulmonary disease was reported to develop pulmonary symptoms 16 years after the start of bromocriptine and 11 years after starting pergolide. Chest radiograph and computed tomography defined a mass in the right upper lobe, and a biopsy revealed pleural and parenchymal fibrosis. The patient improved after a change from pergolide to pramipexole (27). A subsequent chart review compared 55 patients taking pergolide to 63 control patients (28). Echocardiograms revealed aortic regurgitation in 45% of the pergolide group compared with 21% in the control group ($P = 0.006$). In the pergolide group, other diseases affected the tricuspid (11%) and mitral (13%) valves, and the aortic valve involvement was judged to be moderate to severe in 13% of subjects. There was also some suggestion of a dosage effect with higher daily doses of pergolide, possibly associated with moderate to severe aortic regurgitation ($P = 0.05$). Moderate to severe valvular changes have been reported in 23–28% of PD patients exposed to pergolide versus 10% in ropinirole, pramipexole, or control groups (29). Because of this potential risk, pergolide was voluntarily withdrawn the United States and Canadian markets, but remains available in other countries.

Pramipexole

Pramipexole was approved in the United States in 1997 and is a synthetic, nonergot dopamine agonist. Like the ergot-derived dopamine agonists, this agent is active at the D_2, D_3, and D_4 receptors. Pramipexole also has affinity for α- and β-adrenoreceptors, acetylcholine receptors, and 5-HT receptors (Table 20.1). The drug is available as immediate release (IR) or extended release (ER). The IR preparation is available in 0.125, 0.25, 0.5, 0.75, 1.0, and 1.5 mg tablets, and the usual dosage is 3.0 mg/day in three divided doses titrated over five weeks (15). This drug reaches peak plasma levels within 1–3 hours and has an elimination half-life of 8–12 hours. The agent is excreted mostly unchanged in the urine and less than 20% is protein bound. Therefore, pramipexole levels may be increased by renally excreted basic drugs (e.g., cimetidine, verapamil, and quinidine) (30). Pivotal trials with pramipexole report that nausea, vomiting, somnolence, and orthostatic hypotension were 0–13% higher than in subjects randomized to placebo (Table 20.2) (2,29–32). Since pramipexole has come to market, unexpected sleep episodes and increased impulsivity, such as pathological gambling, have been reported, and although seen with other dopamine agents, are most often associated with this agent (33–38).

Pramipexole has been studied in de novo and advanced PD populations. A large dose-ranging trial of 264 subjects found that most patients tolerated dosages of 6 mg/day or less of pramipexole IR. In this 10-week study, 98% (placebo), 81% (1.5 mg/day), 92% (3.0 mg/day), 78% (4.5 mg/day), and 67% (6.0 mg/day) of subjects tolerated the drug. A 20% benefit in UPDRS motor scores was seen in all active treatment groups, and it was determined that the optimum dosage range was 1.5–4.5 mg/day (31). Supporting these results, in another six-month study, 335 subjects were randomized to pramipexole or placebo. Investigators reported a greater than 20% improvement in the UPDRS ADL and motor scores in the active treatment group (32). Moller et al. (2005) compared pramipexole (IR) to placebo in 363 advanced PD patients with motor fluctuations as add-on therapy during a 24-week period. UPDRS ADL scores showed a significant improvement with pramipexole versus placebo (4.3 vs 1.8, respectively, P < 0.0001) and UPDRS motor scores improved with pramipexole versus placebo (10.3 from a baseline mean score of 27.5 vs 4.43 from a baseline mean score of 29.8, respectively, P < 0.0001) (39).

The CALM-PD trial compared pramipexole IR to levodopa in early PD (2,31,32). In this trial, 301 subjects were randomized to pramipexole IR or levodopa and were followed for four years. At the conclusion of the trial, 52% of pramipexole and 74% of levodopa subjects reached the primary endpoint of motor complications. Furthermore, dyskinesia occurred in 25% on pramipexole and 54% on levodopa, and wearing off occurred in 47% of the pramipexole group and 67% of the levodopa group. However, UPDRS assessments demonstrated significant improvements (~4 points) in subjects receiving levodopa (31). Eighty-two subjects in the CALM-PD cohort also underwent single photon emission computed tomography (SPECT) imaging with β-CIT to assess striatal uptake of this dopamine transporter (2). Comparisons between the pramipexole IR group and the levodopa group found significant differences ranging from 6.4% to 9.5% in transporter uptake at 22, 34, and 46 months, suggesting less functional decline with pramipexole. Supplemental levodopa was allowed in the CALM-PD study. The dosages of pramipexole averaged 2.78 mg/day with 48% of subjects receiving a mean levodopa supplement of 264 mg/day, whereas 36% of the levodopa-treated subjects required levodopa supplementation with a mean dosage of 509 mg/day.

In a 12-week study by Kieburtz et al. (2010), 311 patients with early PD were randomized to monotherapy of fixed dosages of pramipexole IR (0.5 or 0.75 mg twice daily or at 0.5 mg three times a day) versus placebo. The monoamine oxidase B (MAO-B) inhibitors, amantadine, and anticholinergics were allowed if kept stable. There was a 4.7-point improvement with 0.75 mg twice a day, 4.4 points with 0.5 mg twice a day, and 4.4 points with 0.5 mg three times a day from baseline in UPDRS total scores (all pramipexole groups compared with placebo $P < 0.0001$). Epworth Sleepiness Scale was greater in the 0.75 mg group than the 0.5 mg groups as well as placebo. Quality of life on the Parkinson's Disease Questionnaire was improved with 0.75 mg twice a day and 0.5 mg three times a day but not with placebo or 0.5 mg twice a day (33).

Two randomized trials of pramipexole IR in levodopa-treated patients demonstrated significant benefit in off time (31% and 15%), ADLs (22% and 27%), motor function (25% and 35%), and levodopa dosage reduction (27%) (32,37). The mean dosage of pramipexole was 3.36 mg/day, and side effects included dyskinesia, orthostatic hypotension, dizziness, insomnia, hallucinations, nausea, confusion, and headache (32,37) (Table 20.2). Moller et al. (2005) showed pramipexole improved motor fluctuations, reducing "off" time by 2.5 hours compared with placebo with 10 minutes of "off" time reduction (39).

Pramipexole ER is a once daily, oral preparation available in the United States since October 2009. It is available as 0.375, 0.75, 1.5, 2.25, 3, 3.75, and 4.5 mg tablets. Starting initial monotherapy, it is recommended to start with 0.375 mg daily, followed by titration of 0.375 mg per week based on efficacy and tolerability to a maximum dosage of 4.5 mg/day (34). Converting a patient over from IR to ER may be done because of the convenience and compliance of taking a once daily medication versus dosing several times a day as well as trying to reduce the side effects that may be observed with the peak plasma levels with an IR preparation. The switch usually occurs successfully overnight in a 1:1 conversation (e.g., 0.25 mg IR tid = 0.75 mg ER qd) in 83–85% of patients (38,40).

In a study by Hauser et al, 259 subjects with early PD were randomized to pramipexole ER once daily, pramipexole IR three times daily, or placebo in a ratio of 2:2:1. Levodopa rescue was required more by the placebo group (14%) than in the pramipexole ER (2.9%) and pramipexole IR (1%) groups. Adjusted mean change in UPDRS ADL + motor scores from baseline to week 18, including postlevodopa rescue evaluations, was −5.1 (SD = 1.3) in the placebo group, −8.1 (1.1) in the pramipexole ER group ($P = 0.0282$), and −8.4 (1.1) in the pramipexole IR group ($P = 0.0153$). Adjusted mean (SE) change in UPDRS ADL + motor scores, censoring postlevodopa rescue data, was −2.7 (1.3) in the placebo group, −7.4 (1.1) in the pramipexole ER group ($P = 0.0010$), and −7.5 (1.1) in the pramipexole IR group ($P = 0.0006$). Adverse events were more common with pramipexole ER than placebo but no different than pramipexole IR, including somnolence, nausea, constipation, and fatigue (41).

Pramipexole ER may also reduce "off" time. Among 507 patients after 18 weeks, UPDRS ADL + motor scores decreased (from baseline means of 40.0–41.7) by an adjusted mean of −11.0 for pramipexole ER and −12.8 for pramipexole IR versus −6.1 for placebo ($P = 0.0001$ and $P < 0.0001$) and off-time decreased (from baseline means of 5.8–6.0 hours/day) by an adjusted mean of −2.1 (pramipexole ER) and −2.5 (pramipexole IR) versus −1.4 (placebo) hours/day ($P = 0.0199$ and $P < 0.0001$) (42).

Ropinirole

Ropinirole was approved in the United States in 1998. This dopamine agonist is a nonergot compound with affinity for the D_2 family of receptors, but not the D_1 or D_5 receptors. In addition, unlike pergolide or pramipexole, ropinirole lacks affinity for adrenergic, cholinergic, or serotonergic receptors (Table 20.1). This drug is also rapidly absorbed from the gut with peak plasma concentrations occurring in 1–2 hours and 40% remaining protein bound (1). The elimination half-life is 6 hours. The P450 CYP1A2 hepatic enzyme pathway metabolizes the drug. Ropinirole is available in 0.25, 0.5, 1.0, 2.0, 3.0, 4.0, and 5.0 mg tablets, and is initially titrated to 9 mg/day in three divided doses over an eight-week period. Clinical improvement is usually not seen until patients are taking at least 6 mg/day. Due to the longer dosing range, up to 24 mg/day, this agent is often prescribed at subtherapeutic doses (Table 20.2) (15). The common side effects are similar to those seen with the other dopamine agonists, including nausea, somnolence, hallucinations, and orthostatic hypotension (Table 20.2) (43). Ropinirole drug interaction can be seen with CYP1A2 inhibitors (e.g., ciprofloxacin) (44,45).

Ropinirole has been evaluated in early and advanced PD. Adler et al. (46) randomized 241 de novo subjects to ropinirole ($n = 116$) or placebo ($n = 125$) in a 24-week trial. Responders were defined as subjects achieving at least a 30% improvement in UPDRS total and motor scores. In addition, subjects were assessed for time to levodopa initiation by a clinical global improvement scale. With an average dosage of 15.7 mg/day, 47% of ropinirole subjects were identified as responders, whereas only 20% of subjects responded in the placebo arm. The mean changes in UPDRS scores were significant with a 24% improvement in the ropinirole group and 3% with placebo. Time to levodopa initiation significantly differed with 11% of ropinirole subjects and 29% of placebo subjects, requiring additional therapy. Requirement for levodopa therapy for the ropinirole subjects was 16%, 27%, and 40% at one, two, and three years, respectively (46).

A five-year clinical trial randomized 268 subjects to ropinirole or levodopa in a 2:1 fashion, allowing add-on levodopa. In this study, 85 subjects in the ropinirole group (47%) and 45 subjects in the levodopa group (51%) completed the study. In the ropinirole group, 29 subjects (34%) had not received levodopa supplementation at five years. The analysis of the time to dyskinesia showed a significant difference in favor of ropinirole and, at five years, the cumulative incidence of dyskinesia, regardless of levodopa supplementation, was 20% in the ropinirole group and 45% in the levodopa group. The mean daily dose of ropinirole at the end of the study was 16.5 mg/day. The average dosage for levodopa supplementation was 427 mg/day. The subjects randomized to levodopa received an average of 753 mg/day (47).

The results of a PET analysis comparing ropinirole to levodopa have been reported (REAL-PET) (3). This two-year randomized trial found a significant difference in striatal uptake, comparing ropinirole to levodopa in 186 subjects. Of these subjects, 162 had abnormal baseline ^{18}F-dopa PET scans (ropinirole $n = 87$; levodopa $n = 75$). There was a 75% completion rate for each group. The mean dosage in the ropinirole group was 12.2 mg/day and in the levodopa group 559 mg/day. Fifteen out of the 87 subjects taking ropinirole needed levodopa supplementation some time during the two-year trial. Subjects in the ropinirole group had a slower decline in putamenal F-dopa uptake Ki compared to the levodopa group [−14.1% ($n = 68$) vs −22.9% ($n = 59$); $P < 0.001$]. Subjects in the ropinirole group worsened by 0.70 points on the UPDRS motor scale from baseline, compared with an improvement of 5.64 points in the levodopa group. The ropinirole group also had dyskinesia at a significantly decreased rate when compared with the levodopa group after two years (3.4% vs 26.7%; $P < 0.001$).

Lang et al. reviewed ropinirole data to assess the risk of the development of dyskinesia in subjects exposed to early dopamine agonist monotherapy. They found that once levodopa was initiated, the time to the development of dyskinesia was similar, regardless of whether levodopa was preceded by a dopamine agonist (48).

A six-month, placebo-controlled trial of 149 PD subjects with motor fluctuations randomized to ropinirole ($n = 95$) or placebo ($n = 54$) examined the reduction in levodopa and off time. In this study, levodopa dosage was reduced on an average of 31% in ropinirole subjects compared with 6% in placebo subjects. "Off" time was reduced by 12% in the ropinirole group and 5% in the placebo group, which was a decrease in "off" time of slightly more than 1 hr/day (43).

A 24-hour prolonged release formulation of ropinirole has been developed to allow for once per day dosing—an easier and more rapid titration schedule than immediate release ropinirole. The prolonged release preparation is available in the United States in 2, 4, 6, 8, and 12 mg tablets. Ropinirole prolonged release is initiated at 2 mg once daily for one to two weeks, followed by increases of 2 mg/day at one-week intervals as appropriate for efficacy and tolerability for a maximum dose of 24 mg/day. Converting to the prolonged release preparation of ropinirole should closely match the total daily dose of the immediate-release formulation and should then be adjusted based on therapeutic response and tolerability.

A six-month study involving 393 PD subjects not optimally controlled with levodopa reported a significant decrease in daily "off" time of 2.1 hours with ropinirole 24-hour prolonged release (mean daily dose, 18.8 mg/day), compared with a decrease of 0.3 hours in the placebo group. There were also significant improvements with ropinirole prolonged release in daily "on" time, "on" time without troublesome dyskinesia, and UPDRS ADL and motor scores, compared with placebo. Adverse events were as expected for a dopamine agonist, including dyskinesia, nausea, dizziness, somnolence, hallucinations, and orthostatic hypotension. UPDRS motor scores were improved by 6.5 + 1.81 with ropinirole prolonged release compared with 1.7 + 1.83 with placebo ($P < 0.0001$) (49).

Cabergoline

Cabergoline is a once daily ergot-derived dopamine agonist, commonly used in Europe, but available in the United States for the treatment of hyperprolactinemia.

Cabergoline has been evaluated in de novo and advanced PD populations. In a double-blind, 2:1 placebo-controlled trial of 188 PD subjects taking levodopa, the addition of cabergoline allowed for an 18% reduction in levodopa and a 16% improvement in motor scores (50). In a larger placebo-controlled comparison of 419 treatment-naive subjects randomized to receive either cabergoline or levodopa, similar benefit was found. Motor complications were significantly delayed ($P = 0.0175$) and occurred less frequently with cabergoline than with levodopa (22.3% vs 33.7%). Similar to other studies, the levodopa-treated subjects demonstrated significantly ($P < 0.001$) greater improvement in motor disability. Cabergoline-treated patients experienced a significantly higher frequency of peripheral edema (16.1% vs 3.4%, respectively; $P < 0.0001$) (51).

Clarke and Deane (52) compared cabergoline to bromocriptine in a meta-analysis of five randomized, double-blind, parallel-group studies in 1071 subjects. Cabergoline produced benefits similar to bromocriptine in off-time reduction, motor impairment, disability ratings, and levodopa dose reduction over the first three months of therapy. Dyskinesia and confusion were increased with cabergoline, but otherwise the frequency of adverse events and withdrawals from treatment were similar with the two agonists. Side effects of cabergoline are similar to other dopamine agonists, but also include severe restrictive mitral regurgitation and male sexual dysfunction (53).

Rotigotine

Rotigotine is a novel, nonergoline dopamine agonist, which is unique in that it is delivered through a silicone-based, transdermal system. It affects all of the dopamine receptors, with a 20-fold prevalence for D_3 over D_2 and 100-fold prevalence of D_2 over D_1 receptors. Rotigotine also exhibits antagonistic activity on alpha-2 receptors and agonistic activity on 5-HT1A receptors comparable to that of D_2 and D_1 receptors (54). Administration of this drug through a transdermal application can deliver a stable drug release and a steady-state plasma concentration over a 24-hour period, reduce peak dose or wearing-off adverse effects, and circumvent gastrointestinal metabolism (55). Side effects for rotigotine are similar to other dopamine agonists, but also include skin reactions (erythema, pruritis, and dermatitis) as well as green nail dyschromia (56). Changing the application sites for the transdermal system can reduce the skin reactions.

Rotigotine has been used as monotherapy in early PD. In a multicenter, dose-ranging trial of rotigotine versus placebo, 242 subjects with early, untreated, idiopathic PD (average duration of PD 1.3 years) were assessed. For 11 weeks, subjects were randomly assigned to treatment with patches containing 4.5, 9.0, 13.5, or 18.0 mg of active or placebo monotherapy. The primary outcome was the change in the sum of the UPDRS ADL and motor scales between baseline and the 11-week visit. ADL scores were significantly improved relative to placebo in the 18.0 mg group only, whereas the motor score was improved in both the 13.5 and 18.0 mg groups. There was a dose–response relationship from 4.5 to 13.5 mg, with a plateau between 13.5 and 18.0 mg. The sum scores of UPDRS ADL and motor subscales showed significant improvement by week 4 in the 9.0, 13.5, and 18.0 mg groups and persisted throughout the maintenance phase (57).

Rotigotine has been shown to be efficacious as monotherapy for symptomatic motor control of PD. Watts et al. performed a six-month study of 277 early-onset PD (less than five years since onset of symptoms) in which they found rotigotine at 5.7 mg/day improved the baseline UPDRS ADL + motor scores by 3.98 + 0.71 points compared with a worsening of the placebo group by 1.31 + 0.96 ($P < 0.001$) (58). In a study by Giladi et al., rotigotine was compared with ropinirole in 561 patients with early PD. Patients were randomized to 2:2:1 to rotigotine 8 mg/day, ropinirole 24 mg/day, or placebo. The primary outcome was a >20% decrease in UPDRS ADL+motor scores from baseline. The rotigotine group had a higher rate of improvement compared with placebo (52% vs 30%, respectively, $P < 0.0001$). In an analysis of noninferiority, rotigotine was found to be inferior to ropinirole. However, the absolute improvement in UPDRS ADL + motor scores between baseline and end of treatment was significant between rotigotine and placebo (−2.2 + 10.2 placebo vs −7.2 + 2.2 rotigotine; $P < 0.0001$) (59).

Studies evaluating the efficacy of rotigotine in patients with advanced PD as an adjunctive therapy to levodopa have also demonstrated efficacy. One multicenter study of 351 subjects with advanced PD inadequately controlled with levodopa randomized subjects to rotigotine (18 or 27 mg/day) or placebo in a 29-week study. Those who received rotigotine at 27 mg had a decrease in off time of 2.1 hours, the 18 mg group had a decrease of 2.7 hours, and the placebo group had a decrease of 0.9 hours. There was no increase in troublesome dyskinesia (60). The results were supported by the another study that showed there was a significant decrease in the mean "off" time with rotigotine in two doses compared with placebo in advanced PD. The rotigotine dose of 8 mg/24 hours group had 1.8 hours/day decrease in "off" time and 1.2 hours/day for the 12 mg/24 hours group (61).

In a multinational trial, 287 PD patients with unsatisfactory early-morning motor symptoms were randomized to receive rotigotine (2–16 mg/24 hours) or placebo. Patients were examined in the early morning prior to medications, using the UPDRS motor subscale and the modified Parkinson's Disease Sleep Scale (PDSS-2) after eight weeks of medication titration and four weeks of dose maintenance. Nineteen percent of the rotigotine group were not taking levodopa compared with 18% of the control group. Rotigotine showed a 7-point improvement in UPDRS motor scores from baseline compared with 3.9 points with placebo ($P = 0.0002$) and a 5.9-point improvement in PDSS-2 scores compared with a 1.9-point improvement with placebo ($P \leq 0.0001$). Therefore rotigotine showed a benefit with both motor function and nocturnal sleep disturbances (62).

In 2008, the rotigotine transdermal patch was recalled in the United States and in some places in Europe because of problems with the delivery system. The medication had a tendency to crystalize on the patch, especially if not refrigerated (63). Rotigotine was reintroduced to the European market using a cold chain storage process. Subsequently, the crystalization problem was resolved so that cold chain storage was not necessary, and in 2012, rotigotine was approved by the United States FDA for the treatment of both early and advanced PD.

Piribedil

Piribedil is a piperazine derived, nonergoline-selective D_2/D_3 agonist with alpha-1 antagonist activity. Oral doses of this medication range between 80 and 250 mg/day. Once blood levels are stabilized with a piribedil dose of at least 150 mg/day, it has a mean half-life of approximately 21 hours.

Several studies demonstrated the efficacy of piribedil as monotherapy and as an adjunct to levodopa. Rascol et al. compared piribedil monotherapy to placebo. Over a seven-month period, 401 early, untreated PD patients were randomized to piribedil (mean average dose of 244 mg/day) or placebo. UPDRS motor scores improved on piribedil by 4.9 points compared with a worsening with placebo of 2.6 points ($P < 0.0001$). The proportion of patients requiring supplemental levodopa after the seven-month period versus those remaining on monotherapy was smaller in the piribedil group (17%) versus the placebo group (40%) ($P < 0.001$) (64). Castro-Caldas et al. performed a 12-month, randomized, double-blind study evaluating the benefit of piribedil (150 mg/day) on motor function compared with bromocriptine (25 mg/day) as adjunct therapy with levodopa in 425 PD subjects. There were no significant differences between piribedil (58.4% response) and bromocriptine (55.3%) in UPDRS motor scores, response rate, or cognitive performance. Subjects randomized to piribedil required less levodopa increase than those on bromocriptine (7.6 ± 121.9 mg vs 16.7 ± 91.3 mg), although this was not clinically significant (65).

COMPARISONS BETWEEN DOPAMINE AGONISTS

Tan and Jankovic (6) summarized 15 comparative trials between dopamine agonists, and reported conversion factors of 10:1 for bromocriptine to pergolide, 1:1 for pergolide to pramipexole, 1:6 for pergolide to ropinirole, and 10:6 for bromocriptine to ropinirole. Hanna et al. (66) followed 21 stable subjects on pergolide and switched them to pramipexole in a 1:1 ratio. Although not significant, levodopa dosages were reduced by 16.5%, and 13 of the 21 (62%) subjects reported improvement with the change in regimen. Hauser et al. reported the conversion of stable subjects on levodopa and pramipexole to levodopa and ropinirole in a 1:3 mg ratio. A gradual transition was better tolerated than a rapid change (67). However, in retrospect, the difficulties reported by subjects may have been improved with a higher conversion factor for ropinirole.

Although there are obvious difficulties when making direct comparisons in studies to determine dosage equivalence, a reasonable equation of relative dopamine agonist potency would suggest bromocriptine × 10 = pergolide = pramipexole = ropinirole × 6 on a mg:mg basis. Perhaps a better measure of treatment response is to review similar trials of dopamine agonist therapy. In the early PD population, UPDRS data are similar. Placebo-controlled studies of pramipexole and ropinirole found remarkably similar benefit. Another potential comparison is to evaluate trials comparing two active interventions, such as a dopamine agonist and levodopa. In the imaging trials of pergolide, pramipexole, and ropinirole, subjects treated with an agonist demonstrated similar benefit, which was less than that with levodopa.

The PELMOPET, CALM-PD, ropinirole 056, and REAL-PET trials may represent the most rigorous and careful information gathered about these compounds, and it is therefore useful to compare them (2–4). Subjects treated with pergolide at an average dosage of 3.23 mg/day demonstrated a UPDRS motor scale worsening of 3 points over 36 months, whereas subjects randomized to levodopa demonstrated an improvement of 2.5 points in the same time interval. Although the dopamine agonist/levodopa trials using pramipexole and ropinirole allowed for levodopa supplementation and had different durations, like the 5.5-point difference seen between pergolide and levodopa in the PELMOPET trial, the differences between pramipexole (−3.4) and levodopa (−7.3) at 23.5 months (difference = 3.9 points) and ropinirole (−0.8) and levodopa (−4.8) at 60 months (difference = 4 points) are similar. The neuroimaging data from these investigations are also similar for dosages of pergolide 3.23 mg/day, pramipexole 2.78 mg/day, and ropinirole 16.5 mg/day. Modifications of these data to reflect a ratio of dopamine agonist to levodopa striatal decline produce percentages ranging from 52.6% to 65%. F-dopa PET demonstrates ropinirole striatal decline 65% of levodopa at 24 months and pergolide striatal decline 54.5% of levodopa at 36 months. SPECT imaging with β-CIT demonstrates 52.6%, 55.6%, and 62.7% pramipexole to levodopa decline at 22, 34, and 46 months of treatment, respectively. The imaging impact of added levodopa in the pramipexole and ropinirole groups is unknown.

A study by Thomas et al. was performed comparing wearing-off episodes during dopamine agonist monotherapy. Sixty de novo patients with PD were randomized to either ropinirole IR 15 mg per day versus pramipexole IR 2.1 mg per day. The dopamine agonist doses could be increased for the following two years; however, levodopa could not be added until the study ended. Eighteen patients (30%) experienced wearing off 15–21 months after beginning monotherapy. No differences were observed between dopamine agonists. Wearing off was observed 3.4 ± 0.3 hours after intake of the morning or afternoon dose and consisted of UPDRS score worsening by 11.1 ± 2.1 points. There were no differences in UPDRS scores in the "on" phase of their treatment between dopamine agonists (68).

In summary, similar designs between pergolide, pramipexole, and ropinirole demonstrate similar benefits in terms of levodopa dosage reduction, levodopa percent reduction, treatment responders, and decrease in off time in adjunctive therapy trials. In these studies, subject selection, methodological design, and data collected differed to the point that trends are less reliable than in the early patient studies, but, in general, similar improvements in all variables are seen.

INITIATION OF DOPAMINE AGONIST THERAPY

Dopamine agonists provide substantial improvement in PD symptoms while delaying the development of motor fluctuations and dyskinesia (36,47,69). Similar trials comparing dopamine agonists (pergolide, pramipexole, ropinirole) to levodopa in a randomized fashion suggest possible long-term benefit according to functional imaging measures (2,3). The reduction in striatal and nigral decline in F-dopa and β-CIT uptake suggest these agents have some benefit over levodopa for up to 46 months of treatment. In a clinical setting of a 30-year-old patient, it is compelling to delay levodopa therapy in favor of a dopamine agonist because of the potentially long clinical horizon (70). Conversely, in an 80-year-old patient with other health concerns, treatment with levodopa may be better tolerated. The decisions regarding initial therapy in the 50 years between these two examples is dependent on the health of the patient, the side-effect profiles, and cost of the drugs (Table 20.2).

Dopaminergic medications have similar side effect profiles: nausea, sleepiness, confusion, orthostatic hypotension, and hallucinations among others (Table 20.2). Besides these problems, lower extremity edema, hair loss, and weight gain have also been seen with dopamine agonist use. The ergoline-derivatives, bromocriptine, cabergoline, and pergolide, also have a slight risk of erythromelalgia and pulmonary and retroperitoneal fibrosis, which have been reported in 2%–5% of patients exposed to these agents (1). This class of dopamine agonists should not be used in patients with serious inflammation, fibrosis, or cardiac valvulopathy. If these ergot dopamine agonists are started, periodic monitoring for valvulopathy is recommended. With all dopaminergic agents, it is possible that excessive daytime sleepiness, unexpected sleep episodes, and reduced impulse control leading to behaviors such as pathological gambling could occur in a small percentage of patients (71–76). The incidence of impulse control disorders has been reported (77) as between 5.6% and 13.8% and is higher (13.5%) with dopamine agonists compared with levodopa alone (0.7%) (78,79). Therefore, patients should be educated to be vigilant about any of these potential side effects and notify their physician if they occur. The side effects of these agents may be quite similar, but vary from patient to patient, so it is important for a patient to understand that if he or she does not tolerate the first dopamine agonist; there is no reason to expect that none of the medications in this class will provide benefit.

Initiation of dopamine agonist therapy is somewhat dependent on the needs and emotional state of the patient. Each of the dopamine agonists requires a titration period from four to eight weeks. In the healthy patient seeking to improve quickly, initiation of a rapidly titrated agent may be preferred, whereas the more slowly titrated schedules may suit the needs of a patient reluctant to take any drugs. Each patient should be reminded that the differences in titration time usually are less than three weeks, a brief period of time in the context of a 20-year treatment horizon.

CONCLUSIONS

The development of dopamine agonists, particularly, pramipexole and ropinirole, has gradually shifted treatment paradigms in PD. In the last 20 years, many PD specialists have moved from using dopamine agonists only as adjunctive therapy to levodopa to initiating antiparkinson therapy with one of these agents (69). Imaging data with SPECT and PET scanning has produced debate regarding the possible "neuroprotective" advantages of dopamine agonists when compared with levodopa (2–4). In this regard, some have questioned whether these agents should be initiated sooner in the disease course, perhaps before obvious disability develops. Regardless of when dopamine agonist therapy is initiated, patients benefit from the choice of several agents for treating PD symptoms.

REFERENCES

1. Factor SA. Dopamine agonists. Med Clin North Am 1999; 83: 415–43.
2. Parkinson Study Group. Dopamine transporter brain imaging to assess the effects of pramipexole vs. levodopa on Parkinson disease progression. JAMA 2002; 287: 1653–61.
3. Whone AL, Watts RL, Stoessl AJ, et al. Slower progression of Parkinson's disease with ropinirole versus levodopa: The REAL-PET study. Ann Neurol 2003; 54: 93–101.
4. Oertel WH, Wolters E, Sampaio C, et al. Pergolide versus levodopa monotherapy in early Parkinson's disease patients: The PELMOPET study. Mov Disord 2006; 21: 343–53.
5. Le WD, Jankovic J. Are dopamine receptor agonists neuroprotective in Parkinson's disease? Drugs Aging 2001; 18: 389–96.
6. Tan EK, Jankovic J. Choosing dopamine agonists in Parkinson's disease. Clin Neuropharmacol 2001; 24: 247–53.
7. Pierantozzi M, Palmieri MG, Mazzone P, et al. Deep brain stimulation of both subthalamic nucleus and internal globus pallidus restores intracortical inhibition in Parkinson's disease paralleling apomorphine effects: a paired magnetic stimulation study. Clin Neurophysiol 2002; 113: 108–13.

8. Koller W, Stacy M. Other formulations and future considerations for apomorphine for subcutaneous injection therapy. Neurology 2004; 62: S22–6.
9. Manson AJ, Hanagasi H, Turner K, et al. Intravenous apomorphine therapy in Parkinson's disease: clinical and pharmacokinetic observations. Brain 2001; 124: 331–40.
10. Lewitt PA. Subcutaneously administered apomorphine: pharmacokinetics and metabolism. Neurology 2004; 62: S8–S11.
11. Bowron A. Practical considerations in the use of apomorphine injectable. Neurology 2004; 62: S32–6.
12. Poewe W, Wenning GK. Apomorphine: an underutilized therapy for Parkinson's disease. Mov Disord 2000; 15: 789–94.
13. Dewey RB Jr, Hutton JT, LeWitt PA, et al. A randomized, double-blind, placebo-controlled trial of subcutaneously injected apomorphine for parkinsonian off-state events. Arch Neurol 2001; 58: 1385–92.
14. Stocchi F, Vacca L, De Pandis MF, et al. Subcutaneous continuous apomorphine infusion in fluctuating patients with Parkinson's disease: long-term results. Neurol Sci 2001; 22: 93–4.
15. Pahwa R, Lyons KE. Solving the puzzle of Parkinson's therapy. Pract Neurol 2002; 1: 17–18; 22–24.
16. Goetz CG, Tanner CM, Glantz RH, et al. Chronic agonist therapy for Parkinson's disease: a 5-year study of bromocriptine and pergolide. Neurology 1985; 35: 749–51.
17. Physician's Desk Reference, 60th edn. Montvale, NJ: Thomson PDR, 2006.
18. Factor SA, Weiner WJ. Viewpoint: early combination therapy with bromocriptine and levodopa in Parkinson's disease. Mov Disord 1993; 8: 257–62.
19. Clarke CE, Speller JM. Pergolide versus bromocriptine for levodopa-induced motor complications in Parkinson's disease. Cochrane Database Syst Rev 2000: CD000236.
20. Ramaker C, van Hilten JJ. Bromocriptine versus levodopa in early Parkinson's disease. Cochrane Database Syst Rev 2000: CD002258.
21. van Hilten JJ, Ramaker C, Van de Beek WJ, et al. Bromocriptine for levodopa-induced motor complications in Parkinson's disease. Cochrane Database Syst Rev 2000: CD001203.
22. Guttman M. International Pramipexole-Bromocriptine Study Group. Double-blind comparison of pramipexole and bromocriptine treatment with placebo in advanced Parkinson's disease. Neurology 1997; 49: 1060–5.
23. Jankovic J. Long-term study of pergolide in Parkinson's disease. Neurology 1985; 35: 296–9.
24. Bonuccelli U, Colzi A, Del Dotto P. Pergolide in the treatment of patients with early and advanced Parkinson's disease. Clin Neuropharmacol 2002; 25: 1–10.
25. Mizuno Y, Kondo T, Narabayashi H. Pergolide in the treatment of Parkinson's disease. Neurology 1995; 45(Suppl): S13–21.
26. Olanow CW, Fahn S, Muenter M, et al. A Multicenter double-blind placebo controlled trial of pergolide as adjunct to Sinemet in the treatment of Parkinson's disease. Mov Disord 1994; 9: 40–7.
27. Tintner R, Manian P, Gauthier P, et al. Pleuropulmonary fibrosis after long-term treatment with the dopamine agonist pergolide for Parkinson Disease. Arch Neurol 2005; 62: 1290–5.
28. Waller EA, Kaplan J, Heckman MG. Valvular heart disease in patients taking pergolide. Mayo Clin Proc 2005; 80: 1016–20.
29. Simonis G, Fuhrmann JT, Strasser RH. Meta-analysis of heart valve abnormalities in Parkinson's disease patients treated with dopamine agonists. Mov Disord 2007; 22: 1936–42.
30. Mirapex [Package Insert]. Ridgefield, CT: Boehringer Ingelheim, 2009.
31. Hubble JP, Koller WC, Cutler NR, et al. Pramipexole in patients with early Parkinson's disease. Clin Neuropharmacol 1995; 18: 338–47.
32. Lieberman AN, Ranhosky A, Korts D. Clinical evaluation of pramipexole in advanced Parkinson's disease: Results of a randomized, placebo-controlled, parallel group study. Neurology 1997; 49: 162–8.
33. Kieburtz K. Twice-daily, low-dose pramipexole in early Parkinson's disease: a randomized, placebo-controlled trial. Mov Disord 2011; 26: 37–44.
34. Mirapex ER [Package Insert]. Ridgefield, CT: Boehringer Ingelheim, 2010.

35. Parkinson Study Group. Pramipexole vs. levodopa as and initial treatment for Parkinson disease. JAMA 2000; 284: 1931–8.
36. Holloway RG, Shoulson I, Fahn S, et al. Pramipexole vs. levodopa as initial treatment for Parkinson disease: a 4-year randomized controlled trial. Arch Neurol 2004; 61: 1044–53.
37. Pinter MM, Pogarell O, Oertel WH. Efficacy, safety, and tolerance of the non-ergoline dopamine agonist pramipexole in the treatment of advanced Parkinson's disease: a double blind, placebo controlled, randomised, multicentre study. J Neurol Neurosurg Psychiatry 1999; 66: 436–41.
38. Rascol O, Barone P, Debieuvre CD, et al. Overnight switching from immediate- to extended-release pramipexole in early Parkinson's disease. Neurology 2009; 72: A320.
39. Moller JC, Oertel WH, Koster J, et al. Longterm efficacy and safety of pramipexole in advanced Parkinson's disease: results from a European multicenter trial. Mov Disord 2005; 20: 602–10.
40. Mizuno Y, Yamamoto M, Kuno S, et al. Efficacy of pramipexole extended release (ER) and switching from pramipexole immediate release (IR) to ER in Japanese advanced Parkinson's disease (PD) patients. Proceeding of the 18th WFN World Congress on Parkinson's Disease and Related Disorders, Miami Beach, Fla, USA, 2009; poster 2.192.
41. Hauser RA, Schapira AH, Rascol O, et al. Randomized, double-blind, multicenter evaluations of pramipexole extended release once daily in early Parkinson's disease. Mov Disord 2010; 25: 2542–9.
42. Schapira AH, Barone P, Hauser RA, et al. Extended-release pramipexole in advanced Parkinson disease. Neurology 2011; 77: 767–74.
43. Lieberman A, Olanow CW, Sethi K, et al. A multicenter trial of ropinirole as adjunct treatment for Parkinson's disease. Neurology 1998; 51: 1057–61.
44. Requip [Package Insert]. Research Triangle Park, NC: GlaxoSmithKline, 2009.
45. Requip XL [Package Insert]. Research Triangle Park, NC: GlaxoSmithKline, 2009.
46. Adler CH, Sethi KD, Hauser RA, et al. Ropinirole for the treatment of early Parkinson's disease. Neurology 1997; 49: 393–9.
47. Rascol O, Brooks DJ, Korczyn AD, et al; 056 Study Group. A five-year study of the incidence of dyskinesia in patients with early Parkinson's disease who were treated with ropinirole or levodopa. N Engl J Med 2000; 342: 1484–91.
48. Lang AE, Rascol O, Brooks DJ, et al. The development of dyskinesias in Parkinson's disease patients receiving ropinirole and given supplemental l-dopa. Neurology 2002; 58: A82.
49. Pahwa R, Stacy MA, Factor SA, et al. Ropinirole 24-hour prolonged release: randominzed, controlled study in advanced Parkinson disease. Neurology 2007; 68: 1108–15.
50. Hutton JT, Koller WC, Ahlskog JE, et al. Multicenter, placebo-controlled trial of cabergoline taken once daily in Parkinson's disease. Neurology 1996; 46: 1062–5.
51. Bracco F, Battaglia A, Chouza C, et al. The long-acting dopamine receptor agonist cabergoline in early Parkinson's disease: final results of a 5-year, double-blind, levodopa-controlled study. CNS Drugs 2004; 18: 733–46.
52. Clarke CE, Deane KD. Cabergoline versus bromocriptine for levodopa-induced complications in Parkinson's disease. Cochrane Database Syst Rev 2001: CD001519.
53. Pinero A, Marcos-Alberca P, Fortes J. Cabergoline-related severe restrictive mitral regurgitation. N Engl J Med 2005; 353: 1976–7.
54. Jenner P. A novel dopamine agonist for the transdermal treatment of Parkinson's disease. Neurology 2005; 65: S3–5.
55. Pfeiffer RF. A promising new technology for Parkinson's disease. Neurology 2005; 65: S6–S10.
56. Teive HA, Munhoz RP. Rotigotine-induced nail dyschromia in a patient with Parkinson Disease. Neurology 2011; 76: 1605.
57. Parkinson Study Group. A controlled trial of rotigotine monotherapy in early Parkinson's disease. Arch Neurol 2003; 60: 1721–8.
58. Watts RL, Jankovic J, Waters C, et al. Randomized, blind, controlled trial of transdermal rotigotine in early Parkinson disease. Neurology 2007; 68: 272–6.
59. Giladi N, Boroojerdi B, Korczyn AD, et al. Rotigotine transdermal patch in early Parkinson's disease: a randomized, double-blind, controlled study versus placebo and ropinirole. Mov Disord 2007; 22: 2398–404.

60. LeWitt P, Nausieda P, Chang F-L, et al. Rotigotine transdermal system in a multicenter trial of patients with advanced-stage Parkinson's disease as adjunctive therapy to levodopa. Neurology 2006; 66: A184–5.
61. LeWitt PA, Lyons KE, Pahwa R. Advanced Parkinson disease treated with rotigotine transdermal system: PREFER Study. Neurology 2007; 68: 1262–7.
62. Trenkwalder C, Kies B, Rudzinska M, et al. Rotigotine effects on early morning motor function and sleep in Parkinson's disease: a double-blind, randomized, placebo-controlled study (RECOVER). Mov Disord 2011; 26: 90–9.
63. U.S. Food and Drug Administration. Neupro (rotigotine transdermal system). [Available from: www.fda.gov/Safety/MedWatch/SafetyInformation/SafetyAlertsforHumanMedicalProducts/ucm094861.htm]
64. Rascol O, Dubois B, Caldas AC, et al. Early piribedil monotherapy of Parkinson's disease: a planned seven-month report of the REGAIN study. Mov Disord 2006; 21: 2110–15.
65. Castro-Caldas A, Delwaide P, Jost W, et al. The Parkinson-Control study: A 1-year randomized, double-blind trial comparing piribedil (150mg/d) with bromocriptine (25mg/d) in early combination with levodopa in Parkinson's disease. Mov Disord 2006; 21: 500–9.
66. Hanna PA, Ratkos L, Ondo WG, et al. A comparison of the therapeutic efficacy of pergolide and pramipexole in Parkinson's disease. J Neural Transm 2001; 108: 63–70.
67. Hauser R, Reider C, Stacy M, et al. Acute vs. gradual pramipexole to ropinirole switch. Mov Disord 1998; 15(Suppl): 133.
68. Thomas A, Bonanni L, DiIorio A, et al. End-of-dose deterioration in non ergolinic dopamine agonist monotherapy of Parkinson's disease. J Neurol 2006; 253: 1633–9.
69. Olanow CW, Koller WC. An algorithm for the management of Parkinson's disease. Neurology 1998; 50(Suppl): S10–14.
70. Poewe W. Should treatment of Parkinson's disease be started with a dopamine agonist? Neurology 1998; 51(Suppl): S21–4.
71. Frucht S, Rogers JD, Greene PE, et al. Falling asleep at the wheel; motor vehicle mishaps in persons taking pramipexole and ropinirole. Neurology 1999; 52: 1908–10.
72. Stacy M. Sleep disorders in Parkinson's disease: Epidemiology and management. Drugs Aging 2002; 19: 733–9.
73. Rissling I, Geller F, Bandmann O, et al. Dopamine receptor gene polymorphisms in Parkinson's disease patients reporting "sleep attacks". Mov Disord 2004; 19: 1279–84.
74. Samanta JES, Stacy M. Pathologic Gambling in Parkinson's disease. Mov Disord 1998; 15: 111.
75. Gschwandtner U, Astar J, Renard S, Fuhr P. Pathologic gambling in patients with Parkinson's disease. Clin Neuropharmacol 2001; 24: 170–2.
76. Dodd ML, Kloss KJ, Bower KH, et al. Pathological gambling caused by drugs used to treat Parkinson's disease. Arch Neurol 2005; 62: 1–5.
77. Weintraub D, Koester J, Potenza MN, et al. Impulse control disorders in Parkinson disease: a cross-sectional study of 3090 patients. Arch Neurol 2010; 67: 589–95.
78. Voon V, Hassan K, Zurowski M, et al. Prospective prevalence of pathologic gambling and medication association in Parkinson diseasee. Neurology 2006; 66: 1750–2.
79. Weintraub D, Siderowf AD, Potenza MN, et al. Association of dopamine agonist use with impulse control disorders in Parkinson disease. Arch Neurol 2006; 63: 969–73.

Monoamine oxidase inhibitors

Alex Rajput, Theresa Zesiewicz, and Robert A. Hauser

INTRODUCTION

The monoamines include the catecholamine neurotransmitters dopamine, norepinephrine, and 5-hydroxytryptamine. Monoamine oxidases (MAOs) are intracellular enzymes found in the outer mitochondrial membrane that catabolize these amines (1). The first MAO identified was tyramine oxidase in 1928 (2). Monoamine oxidase inhibitors (MAOIs) inhibit the action of MAOs.

In the 1950s and 1960s, patients were reported to "dance in the hall" following treatment with antituberculosis drugs (3). One of these medications, iproniazid, was noted to have potent MAO inhibitory properties (4). An open-label trial of iproniazid found significant mood improvement in institutionalized depressed patients (5) and it was later introduced as the first antidepressant medication (6).

In 1965, Knoll and Ecseri synthesized phenylisopropyl-N-methylpropinylamine or E-250 (7,8). E-250 was a strong, irreversible MAOI that metabolized tyramine (9), phenylethylamine (9), and benzylamine (8). The compound was separated into two isomers, and the L-form was named deprenyl. In 1968, Johnston synthesized a compound structurally similar to deprenyl, 2,3-dichlorophenoxy-propyl-N-methylpropinylamine, or clorgyline (10). He arbitrarily called the MAO with greater affinity for clorgyline MAO-A and for deprenyl MAO-B.

MECHANISMS OF ACTION

MAOs are intracellular enzymes found throughout the body, with most bound tightly to the outer mitochondrial membrane (11,12). The MAOs oxidatively deaminate monoamines in the presence of oxygen (13). MAO-A is the primary form in intestine, pancreas, and spleen, and is the sole form in human placenta (14–16). MAO-B predominates in skin and skeletal muscle, and is the sole form in platelets. While the human liver contains both forms, MAO is absent in plasma and red blood cells (17). Human brain MAO is 70–80% type B (18).

While both MAO subtypes can be detected throughout the brain (19), MAO-A localizes to cell groups containing catecholamines—the locus coeruleus, the nucleus subcoeruleus in the lateral pontine tegmentum, and the substantia nigra (20). MAO-B preferentially localizes to midline serotoninergic brain regions (19,20)—the raphe nucleus and the nucleus centralis superior (20). The lateral and posterior hypothalamic regions stain for both MAO-A and MAO-B (20). MAO-B is also found in high concentrations in astrocytes (but not oligodendrocytes) (19,21).

Striatal ratios of MAO-A to MAO-B vary widely depending on species: high in rat (due to large amounts of MAO-A), low in humans (large amounts of MAO-B), and intermediate in the pig and cat (21). With increasing age, MAO-B activity in the human brain increases, whereas MAO-A activity remains unchanged (21). This also varies according to brain region, with the largest increase (20–30% per decade) noted in the caudate, putamen, nucleus accumbens, and substantia nigra (21). In neurodegenerative diseases there is also an increase in MAO-B activity, including a roughly 25% increase in the substantia nigra of those with Parkinson's disease (PD) (22). This increased MAO-B activity is almost entirely due to an increase in the extraneuronal component of the enzyme, most likely due to glial (astrocytic) contributions (21).

Both MAO-A and MAO-B catabolize dopamine, epinephrine, norepinephrine, tyramine, tryptamine, 3-methoxytyramine, and kynuramine (23). While MAO-A primarily catabolizes serotonin and octopamine, MAO-B metabolizes benzylamine, phenylethylamine, milacemide, and N-methylhistamine. MAO-B also converts the pro-toxin 1-methyl-4-phenyl-1,2,3,6-tetrahydropyridine (MPTP) to MPP+ (23). MAO-A and MAO-B are structurally similar, and the flavin sites on each are identical (24). True selectivity of most MAO inhibitors is present only at low concentrations (25).

HYPERTENSIVE CRISIS

Tyramine is a sympathomimetic amine normally metabolized by gut MAO-A. When tyramine-rich foods such as red wines, pickled herring, or aged cheeses are ingested by someone taking an irreversible MAO-A inhibitor (clorgyline) or nonselective MAO inhibitor (e.g., phenelzine, tranylcypromine), the tyramine is absorbed rather than metabolized; this results in norepinephrine release from postganglionic sympathetic nerve fibers and may lead to a hypertensive crisis (26). This is known as the "cheese effect." Levodopa is contraindicated with MAO-A or nonselective MAO inhibitors as it may cause a similar hypertensive crisis.

The MAO-B selective inhibitor selegiline (deprenyl) at oral doses of 10 mg/ day is safe to be taken with levodopa and requires no dietary restrictions. Transient blood pressure changes have been reported with selegiline doses of 20 mg/day; doses above 10 mg/day are usually not recommended as selectivity may be lost. The second-generation MAO-B selective inhibitor rasagiline was approved by the European Union in 2005 and by the Food and Drug Administration (FDA) in the United States in 2006. The risk of a tyramine reaction with rasagiline also appears to be very low at recommended dosages. In clinical trials there were no tyramine reactions observed even when there were no dietary restrictions. A dose finding study of 179 healthy volunteers showed no evidence of increased tyramine sensitivity for either selegiline 10 mg/day or rasagiline 1 mg/day (27). In December 2009, the FDA relaxed dietary recommendations with rasagiline, but continues to recommend avoidance of foods with very high amounts (>150 mg) of tyramine, such as aged cheese because of the potential for a hypertensive reaction even with the maximum recommended daily dose of rasagiline 1 mg. In the postmarketing period, rare cases of hypertensive crises have been reported in individuals taking unknown quantities of tyramine-rich food on the recommended dosages of rasagiline.

NEUROPROTECTIVE EFFECTS OF MAO INHIBITORS

Neuroprotective effects of the MAO-B inhibitors selegiline and rasagiline are dependent on their propargyl moiety and independent of their MAO inhibitory properties. The selegiline metabolite, desmethylselegiline, is responsible for the majority of the neuroprotective effects of selegiline. The S-isomer of rasagiline, TVP 1022, is one thousand times less potent at inhibiting MAO-B yet demonstrates similar neuroprotective effects to rasagiline (28). Both selegiline and rasagiline have demonstrated neuroprotection in multiple in vitro and animal models (28–43). Selegiline and rasagiline inhibit apoptosis, or programmed cell death, in cell lines (29,31,35,36,44). While the selegiline metabolite L-methamphetamine inhibits the antiapoptotic activities of selegiline and rasagiline, the rasagiline metabolite aminoindan does not (45).

The mitochondrial permeability transition pore (MPTp) appears only in the setting of apoptosis (28). The antiapoptotic proteins stabilize the MPTp, whereas the proapoptotic proteins allow pore opening, with loss of mitochondrial membrane potential (28,42). This causes an apoptotic cascade including release of cytochrome c and activation of caspases, particularly caspase-3. MAOIs increase the antiapoptotic proteins Bcl-2, Bcl-XL, and Bcl-w, and downregulate the proapoptotic proteins Bad, Bax, and Fas (28,44). The "death receptor" Fas and its ligand FasL (which interact with proapoptotic proteins on the outer mitochondrial membrane) are downregulated by MAOIs (28,46).

Oxygen free radical (OFR) scavenging proteins, superoxide dismutase 1 (SOD1), superoxide dismutase 2 (SOD2), catalase, and glutathione are all increased with MAOIs (33,47). The MAOIs themselves may possess OFR scavenging ability (48). Trophic factors including glial-derived neurotrophic factor (GDNF), brain-derived neurotrophic factor (BDNF), nerve growth factor (NGF), and basic fibroblast growth factor (FGF2) are also increased by MAOIs (38,49).

Other mechanisms of neuroprotection mediated by MAOIs include protein kinase C (PKC) α and ε activation, which inhibit formation of the activated cleaved form of caspase-3; the cleavage of PARP-1, a caspase substrate; and Fas, the conversion of amyloid precursor protein (APP) into soluble (nonamyloidogenic) APPα, which itself has neurotrophic and neuroprotective properties; and the inhibition of nuclear translocation of glyceraldehyde-3-phosphate dehydrogenase (28,46). Rasagiline has also been reported to reduce the synaptic expression of glutamate receptors in the striatum and hippocampus (50).

Models in which neuroprotection by either rasagiline or selegiline has been demonstrated include glutamate toxicity in hippocampal neurons (51), focal brain ischemia in rats (40,41), memory and learning tasks following anoxic brain injury (52) and motor and spatial memory in a rodent closed head injury model (53), optic nerve crush injury (54), rescue of dorsal root ganglia sensory neurons (55) and of axotomized motoneurons (56), and protection against cell death in rat pheochromocytoma PC-12 cells deprived of oxygen and glucose (57). Selegiline given after intrathecal injection of rat pups with cerebrospinal fluid from human amyotrophic lateral sclerosis (ALS) subjects protects against anterior horn cell loss (58). Pretreatment with rasagiline is neuroprotective in primate MPTP (59) and rodent 6-OHDA models of PD (39). Primates treated with selegiline and MPTP simultaneously do not develop parkinsonism (60).

SELEGILINE

Selegiline is a lipophilic, relatively selective MAO-B inhibitor, which is readily absorbed from the gastrointestinal (GI) tract. Maximal concentrations occur 30–120 minutes after ingestion (61), and over 90% is bound to plasma proteins (62). Platelet

MAO-B activity is inhibited by more than 85% within 4 hours after selegiline 5 mg, and by almost 98% within 24 hours after selegiline 10 mg (63). Selegiline passes through the blood–brain barrier and accumulates in MAO-B-rich brain areas, including the striatum, thalamus, cortex, and brain stem (64). Selegiline is considered a "suicide inhibitor" as it forms an irreversible covalent bond with MAO-B. Enzyme activity returns only when new MAO-B is produced.

Selegiline is primarily metabolized by the liver P-450 system with some extrahepatic metabolism (65). Three metabolites are identified in serum and urine: l-(–)-methamphetamine, l-(–)-amphetamine, and (–)-desmethylselegiline (66). Desmethylselegiline has neuroprotective activity (35) and also irreversibly inhibits MAO-B (although less so than selegiline) (67–69).

Symptomatic benefit from selegiline in PD is mediated through MAO-B inhibition, thereby inhibiting catabolism of dopamine, both endogenous and exogenous (from levodopa). Selegiline may also inhibit dopamine reuptake (69) and block presynaptic dopamine receptors (70). Amphetamine metabolites of selegiline may also promote dopamine release.

Oral selegiline is generally very well tolerated. The usual dose is 5 mg twice daily (breakfast and lunch). Potential adverse effects include nausea, dizziness, confusion, anxiety, dry mouth, and hallucinations. Selegiline is not recommended after early afternoon because of potential insomnia from its amphetamine metabolites. With concomitant levodopa use, orthostatic hypotension may be significant. Selegiline added to levodopa may worsen dyskinesia. Dopaminergic side effects, including dyskinesia, can usually be managed by lowering the dose of levodopa. Serotonin syndrome may occur when selegiline is combined with selective serotonin reuptake inhibitors (SSRIs); however, this interaction is rare (71). Selegiline may produce altered mental state, rigidity, and fever in some patients receiving meperidine (72). Concomitant use of selegiline with meperidine is contraindicated, and this contraindication is often extended to other opioids.

CLINICAL TRIALS OF SELEGILINE
DATATOP

The Deprenyl and Tocopherol Antioxidative Therapy of Parkinsonism (DATATOP) study (73) evaluated 800 PD subjects randomized to receive selegiline 10 mg/day or placebo. Total Unified Parkinson's Disease Rating Scale (UPDRS) scores were improved in the selegiline-treated group compared with placebo at one month (2.1 vs 0.1; $P < 0.001$) and at three months (1.6 vs –1.3; $P < 0.001$) (73). Motor UPDRS scores also improved significantly in the selegiline compared with the placebo group at one month (1.40 vs 0.01; $P < 0.001$) and at three months (0.9 vs –0.8; $P < 0.001$) (73). In the DATATOP trial, selegiline delayed the need for levodopa by approximately nine months compared with placebo. Following selegiline withdrawal, there was no loss of benefit at one month but at two months, total UPDRS had worsened 3.2 points in selegiline-treated patients compared with 0.5 in placebo-treated patients ($P < 0.001$). Selegiline monotherapy slowed decline in parkinsonian disability in the DATATOP (73) trial and other clinical trials (74,75) as measured by motor or total UPDRS scores or other standardized rating scales (76).

One DATATOP open-label extension study (77) evaluated subjects who had reached endpoint (need for levodopa) in the original DATATOP trial (73). Three hundred fifty-two of 371 subjects completed the 18-month follow-up (77); all were treated with selegiline 10 mg/day and levodopa as needed. Patients originally treated with selegiline (73) had taken levodopa for a significantly shorter period of time ($P < 0.0001$) and received significantly lower total cumulative levodopa dosages ($P < 0.02$) over that 18-month period (77) than those initially randomized to placebo in the DATATOP trial (73). However, the total daily levodopa dosage at final evaluation was similar between groups (77) and wearing off, dyskinesia, and freezing occurred in the same proportion of patients originally treated with selegiline compared with placebo.

Subjects who completed the original DATATOP trial but did not reach endpoint (i.e., did not require levodopa) were initially withdrawn from selegiline or placebo for two months, and then were placed on open-label selegiline 10 mg/day (78) in another extension study. The original treatment blind was maintained. Although subjects treated with selegiline had better total UPDRS scores than placebo subjects prior to selegiline withdrawal, after the two-month wash-out period, total UPDRS scores were not different between the groups. These two open-label DATATOP extension studies (77,78) suggest a symptomatic rather than neuroprotective benefit of selegiline.

Original DATATOP subjects ($n = 368$) who had required levodopa therapy and were on open-label selegiline underwent an independent second randomization (79). A half were assigned to continue selegiline 10 mg/day and the other half received placebo. Subjects were followed over two years. There was no significant overall difference between the two groups in the primary outcome measure of occurrence of motor fluctuations. There was a nonsignificant difference in wearing off (52% placebo vs 41% selegiline), however dyskinesia occurred significantly more often in subjects assigned to selegiline compared with placebo (34% vs 19%; $P = 0.006$). Secondary outcome measures included time until motor fluctuations, freezing of gait, confusion, and dementia. Gait freezing was reported in 29% of the placebo group versus 16% of selegiline-treated subjects ($P = 0.0003$). In addition, there was significantly less decline in total UPDRS ($P = 0.0002$), motor ($P = 0.0006$), and ADL ($P = 0.0045$) subscales in the selegiline-treated group. These results again appear to suggest a symptomatic benefit of selegiline with better UPDRS scores and less likelihood of freezing, but a higher rate of dyskinesia when compared with placebo (79).

Other Trials in Early PD

Palhagen et al. reported a study of selegiline in 157 de novo PD subjects (75). Selegiline 10 mg/day delayed the need for levodopa by four months compared with placebo ($P = 0.028$). There was a "wash-in" effect at six weeks and three months, with total and motor UPDRS scores significantly better in the selegiline group ($P < 0.01$ and $P < 0.05$, respectively). At six months, rate of disease progression was significantly slower for both total UPDRS (-1.9 vs 3.5; $P < 0.001$) and motor UPDRS (-1.5 vs 2.5; $P < 0.001$) (negative numbers refer to improvement and positive numbers refer to worsening). Between baseline and the end of an eight-week wash-out period there was significantly slower progression of total UPDRS scores in the selegiline group (11.3) compared with the placebo group (14.2) when length of time to reach the endpoint was used as a covariate ($P = 0.033$) (75).

A seven-year extension (80) of the original (75) Palhagen study reported 140 of the original 157 PD subjects who participated in the initial study; all were treated with levodopa and randomized to receive selegiline 10 mg/day or placebo. Selegiline slowed disease progression as measured by UPDRS total scores ($P = 0.003$), motor scores ($P = 0.002$) and ADL scores ($P = 0.0002$) compared with placebo. After five years, subjects on placebo had a mean worsening UPDRS total scores of 10 points ($P = 0.07$) and were receiving 19% more levodopa ($P = 0.0002$) than those treated with selegiline. Wearing off fluctuations were experienced by 27% of subjects, with a trend for fluctuations to be less common (20% vs 34%; $P = 0.053$) and appear later ($P = 0.076$) in the selegiline group over the entire seven years. Dyskinesia developed in 37% of subjects, with no significant difference in frequency (selegiline 35%, placebo 40%) or time to appearance between groups. Nausea, but not hallucinations or diarrhea, was more common in the selegiline group (24% vs 10%, $P = 0.033$). This study provides evidence of long-term benefit and suggests that selegiline may reduce progression of disability in PD (80). The remarkable difference between patients treated with placebo versus selegiline over 5–7 years suggests either an increasing symptomatic benefit over time or possible slowing of disease progression.

The French Selegiline Multicenter Trial (FSMT) (81) randomized 93 de novo PD subjects to selegiline 10 mg/day or placebo. Significant improvements in total and motor UPDRS scores were noted at one and three months. In a small double-blind randomized trial (74) of 54 early PD patients, selegiline 10 mg/day delayed the need for levodopa by eight months (log rank test, $P < 0.002$), and delayed disease progression as assessed by five different scales (including UPDRS motor score) by 40–83% per year compared with placebo. The Finnish Study of selegiline monotherapy (76) found that selegiline delayed the need for levodopa by nearly six months ($P = 0.03$), and disability at 12 months was reduced with selegiline compared with placebo. At the end of two years on levodopa, the selegiline group was receiving significantly lower daily levodopa dosages compared with placebo (358 vs 543 mg; $P < 0.001$). The selegiline group could also be managed with fewer mean daily doses of levodopa compared with placebo (3.5 vs 4.5, $P = 0.01$) (76).

In the Sinemet–Deprenyl–Parlodel (SINDEPAR) study (82), 101 untreated PD patients were randomized to selegiline or placebo, in addition to being randomized to symptomatic treatment with bromocriptine or levodopa [i.e., four treatment arms – (selegiline or placebo) + (levodopa or bromocriptine)]. After a two-month wash-out of selegiline and a one-week wash-out of bromocriptine and levodopa, endpoint evaluation at 14 months revealed significantly less worsening of total UPDRS scores with selegiline compared to placebo regardless of the symptomatic treatment used (0.4 vs 5.8; $P < 0.001$) (82).

Advanced PD

Selegiline has mild-to-moderate benefit as adjunct therapy to levodopa in advanced PD patients and is approved by the FDA in the United States for this indication. In a small double-blind placebo-controlled trial (83) of selegiline 10 mg/day in PD subjects ($n = 38$) on stable levodopa doses, selegiline reduced daily levodopa dosage requirements ($P < 0.05$) and significantly improved tremor ($P = 0.02$) over eight weeks. Thirty subjects (selegiline $n = 18$, placebo $n = 12$) completed a 16-month follow-up (83). Both mean levodopa dosage (-133 mg/day; $P < 0.001$) and dosing frequency (-1.1 times/day; $P < 0.001$) were significantly reduced in the selegiline-treated group.

Significantly less end of dose akinesia was reported in double-blind crossover trials with selegiline (84,85). Golbe et al. (86) randomized 96 PD patients with motor fluctuations that could not be improved with levodopa adjustments to selegiline

10 mg/day or placebo. Mean hourly symptom control in subjects randomized to selegiline was significantly improved compared with placebo (58% vs 26%; $P < 0.01$). On average, patients had one hour more on time with selegiline 10 mg/day (86). Adjunct use of selegiline reduces daily levodopa requirements by 10–25% (83–86). Selegiline may worsen levodopa-induced dyskinesia, but once levodopa dosage adjustments are made, dyskinesia are typically no worse than baseline. Nearly 60% of subjects receiving selegiline and 30% treated with placebo reported worsened dyskinesia within three days after starting treatment (86), with most subjects reporting improvement after reduction of the levodopa dose.

SELEGILINE AND MORTALITY

The Parkinson's Disease Research Group of the United Kingdom (87) reported increased mortality rate in PD patients randomized to levodopa and selegiline compared with levodopa alone. Forty-four (17.7%) deaths were observed in the levodopa group, compared with 76 (28%) deaths in the levodopa plus selegiline group after a mean duration of 5.6 years ($P = 0.015$). Methodologic questions were raised (88), and both groups had higher than expected mortality rates. After a 14-year follow-up of those assigned to levodopa with selegiline compared with levodopa alone, there was no significant difference in mortality between groups (89). Other studies have not reported higher mortality with selegiline. Analysis of the DATATOP trial and subsequent open-label extensions revealed an overall death rate of 17.1% (137 of 800), or 2.1% per year through a mean of 8.2 years of observation (90), and mortality rate was not affected by any of the treatments. Cumulative exposure to selegiline was not associated with increased mortality in the 13-year follow-up of the DATATOP cohort (91). Overall, there is no definitive evidence linking selegiline use to increased mortality.

ZYDIS SELEGILINE

Orally disintegrating Zydis selegiline (Zelapar®) was approved by the U.S. FDA in 2006 as an adjunct for PD patients treated with carbidopa/levodopa who exhibited deterioration in response to therapy (e.g., wearing off). The recommended dose is 1.25 mg once daily, which can be increased to 2.5 mg once daily after six weeks if necessary. It dissolves within seconds after being placed on the tongue (92) and is rapidly absorbed through the buccal mucosa. It is recommended that Zydis selegiline be taken before breakfast and without liquid. Nearly one-third of a Zydis selegiline 10 mg dose is absorbed pre-gastrically within one minute in healthy volunteers (93). Zydis selegiline produces nearly five times higher plasma selegiline concentrations and significantly lower (>90%) plasma concentrations of selegiline metabolites compared with oral selegiline (93), as the mucosal absorption allows Zydis selegiline to avoid first pass metabolism in the liver.

Clarke and colleagues (94) reported three studies of Zydis selegiline. In the first study, both 1.25 mg/day and 10 mg/day Zydis formulations were compared with oral selegiline 10 mg/day. In those who switched from oral selegiline 10 mg/day to Zydis selegiline 1.25 mg/day, the mean adjusted total UPDRS score was improved slightly at 12 weeks (−2.50, $P = 0.01$); however, there was no difference in subjects who switched from oral selegiline 10 mg/day to Zydis selegiline 10 mg/day. In the second study, more PD patients preferred the Zydis formulation to standard oral selegiline irrespective of swallowing and salivation problems (94). Tyramine pressor effect was measured in healthy volunteers in the third study (94). After 14 days of Zydis selegiline 1.25 mg/day there was no change in pressor response to 400 mg tyramine. In contrast, after 14 days oral selegiline 10 mg/day the threshold for pressor response was reduced to 200 mg tyramine (90).

In a three-month study, Zydis selegiline significantly reduced off time (95). PD patients ($n = 140$) with a minimum of 3 hours daily off time were randomized 2:1 to Zydis selegiline or placebo (95). Initial dosage of Zydis selegiline was 1.25 mg/day, and this was increased to 2.5 mg/day after six weeks. Overall, the drug was well tolerated and over 90% of each group completed the trial. Drug-related adverse events occurred in 32% of Zydis selegiline and 21% of placebo subjects. The most frequent adverse events in the Zydis selegiline group were dizziness, dyskinesia, hallucinations, headache, and dyspepsia. At weeks four to six, off time was reduced 1.4 hours with Zydis selegiline 1.25 mg/day compared with 0.5 hours for placebo ($P = 0.003$); at weeks 10–12, off time was reduced by 2.2 hours with Zydis selegiline 2.5 mg/day compared with 0.6 hours for placebo ($P < 0.001$). Dyskinesia-free on time was also significantly increased at weeks 6 and 12. There was no significant difference in daily on time with dyskinesia in the Zydis and placebo groups at weeks 6 and 12 (95). In an identically designed study, 150 PD patients with at least three hours daily off time were randomized in a 2:1 ratio to Zydis selegiline or placebo (96). The primary outcome of percentage in off time reduction for weeks 10–12 was not met in this study, with only a 0.3-hour improvement in off time favoring Zydis selegiline. Completion rate, frequency, and type of adverse effects were similar between the two trials (95,96). The failure of benefit for this trial (96) was felt to possibly be due to a larger than expected placebo response rate. However, a pooled analysis of these two studies showed a reduction of daily off time of 12.4% in the Zydis selegiline group compared with 6.9% for the placebo group ($P = 0.003$), which correlates to an hour less off time per day with Zydis selegiline (97). Open-label follow-up of PD patients using Zydis selegiline 2.5 mg/day up to two years confirmed its safety, efficacy, and tolerability (98).

RASAGILINE

Rasagiline [R(+)-N-propargyl-1-aminoindan] mesylate (Azilect®) was approved by the U.S. FDA in 2006 as monotherapy in early disease and as an adjunct to levodopa in more advanced disease. The recommended daily dose is 1 mg for monotherapy; for adjunct therapy it is recommended to start at 0.5 mg and increase to 1 mg as needed.

Rasagiline produces selective irreversible MAO-B inhibition (99). Platelet MAO-B inhibition is dose dependent; 1 hour after ingestion, platelet MAO-B inhibition is 35% with 1 mg rasagiline and 99% with 10 mg rasagiline. By day 6, rasagiline 2 mg/day inhibits over 99% of platelet MAO-B (99). It takes approximately two weeks for MAO-B activity to return to baseline values (99). The area under the curve and maximum concentration (C_{max}) increase linearly with rasagiline dosage. The plasma half-lives of rasagiline and its active metabolite 1(R)-aminoindan are 3.5 and 11 hours, respectively. As rasagiline irreversibly inhibits MAO-B, the serum (pharmacokinetic) half-life does not correlate with its functional (pharmacodynamic) half-life.

Rasagiline up to 20 mg/day was well tolerated in healthy male volunteers (99). Dry mouth, headache, nausea, thirst, and abdominal discomfort were the most common adverse effects but tended to be mild. There were no significant effects on vital signs, laboratory test values, physical examination, or electrocardiogram.

CLINICAL TRIALS OF RASAGILINE
TEMPO

Subjects with early PD (n = 404) were evaluated in a phase III study called TEMPO [Rasagiline Mesylate (TVP-1012) in Early Monotherapy for Parkinson's Disease Outpatients] (100). Subjects were randomized to receive rasagiline 1 mg/day (n = 134), rasagiline 2 mg/day (n = 132) or placebo (n = 138), with the change in total UPDRS scores between baseline and 26 weeks as the primary outcome measure. Significant improvements in total UPDRS scores were observed for both rasagiline 1 mg/day and rasagiline 2 mg/day (–4.2 units and –3.6 units, respectively) compared with placebo, P < 0.001 for each comparison) (100). Two-thirds of both rasagiline groups compared with approximately half of the placebo group were responders (defined as less than 3 points worsening in total UPDRS scores from baseline to week 26; P < 0.01 for each rasagiline group compared with placebo). Secondary endpoints including UPDRS motor and ADL subscales, and the Parkinson's Disease Quality of Life scale (PDQUALIF), all significantly favored both dosages of rasagiline compared with placebo. The need for levodopa did not differ among the groups (16.7% for placebo, 11.2% for rasagiline 1 mg, and 16.7% for rasagiline 2 mg). Rasagiline was very well tolerated.

The TEMPO study included an open treatment phase in which all subjects who completed 26 weeks of the double-blind placebo-controlled phase were placed on rasagiline. Those treated with rasagiline 1 or 2 mg/day from the start remained on that dosage for the full 12 months, while subjects initially treated with placebo for the first six months were then treated with rasagiline 2 mg/day (delayed start) (101). There were 380 subjects enrolled, and the intention-to-treat cohort consisted of 371 subjects. The primary outcome measure was the change in total UPDRS from baseline to 12 months. Subjects treated with rasagiline 2 mg/day for one year were 2.29 points better on the total UPDRS than subjects initially treated with placebo for six months followed by rasagiline 2 mg/day for six months (P = 0.01). Subjects who received rasagiline 1 mg/day for one year also experienced less worsening of total UPDRS scores than those treated with placebo for six months followed by rasagiline 2 mg/day for 6 months (1.82 units better total UPDRS in the 1 mg/day group; P = 0.05). The better outcome of patients who took rasagiline for the full year suggested that rasagiline may slow the progression of disability in PD. An open-label extension of TEMPO was offered, and 306 subjects agreed to participate; 177 received rasagiline for more than five years. Sustained benefit was seen over the entire 6.5-year follow-up period, with subjects who had received early–start rasagiline scoring better on the total UPDRS than those who had received delayed-start rasagiline, irrespective of subsequent treatment (2.5 points better; P = 0.006) (102).

ADAGIO

The Attenuation of Disease Progression with Azilect Given Once daily (ADAGIO) study sought to verify the promising results of the delayed start TEMPO study and determine whether rasagiline has a disease-modifying effect in early PD (103). A total of 1176 subjects were randomized to one of four groups: early or delayed treatment with rasagiline 1 mg/day; or early or delayed treatment with rasagiline 2 mg/day. All subjects were on no other antiparkinsonian medication. The groups with delayed treatment received rasagiline at week 36 and subjects were followed over 72 weeks. To determine whether rasagiline had a disease-modifying and not simply a symptomatic effect, the early treatment groups had to meet three primary endpoints (as they relate to the total UPDRS score): (i) superiority to placebo in rate of change of UPDRS score between weeks 12 and 36; (ii) superiority to the delayed-start group in change of UPDRS score between baseline and week 72; and (iii) noninferiority to the delayed-start group in rate of change of UPDRS score between weeks 48 and 72. The group receiving 1 mg rasagiline as initial therapy outperformed the delayed 1 mg rasagiline group in all three categories—rate of change between weeks 12 and 36 [0.09 ± 0.02 points/week vs 0.14 ± 0.01 points/week, $P = 0.01$ (smaller values means less worsening)], less increase (worsening) in UPDRS score at week 72 (2.82 ± 0.53 vs 4.52 ± 0.56 points, $P = 0.02$), and noninferiority in rate of change in UPDRS score between weeks 48 and 72 (0.085 ± 0.02 vs 0.085 ± 0.02 per week for each, $P < 0.001$). The group receiving 2 mg rasagiline as initial therapy failed to meet all three endpoints. While the rate of change between weeks 12 and 36 was better (0.07 ± 0.02 vs 0.14 ± 0.01 (less worsening with early 2 mg rasagiline) $P < 0.001$) and there was noninferiority in the rate of change between weeks 48 and 72 (0.094 ± 0.01 points/wk in early start vs 0.065 ± 0.02 points/week in delayed start; $P < 0.001$), there was no difference in change in UPDRS from baseline to week 72 (early start 3.47 ± 0.50 vs delayed start 3.11 ± 0.50; $P = 0.60$).

The authors conducted a post hoc subgroup analysis comparing those with the highest quartile UPDRS scores (>25.5 points at baseline) with those in the other three quartiles. Both rasagiline 1 and 2 mg doses met all three endpoints in this analysis, while neither dose met all three endpoints in the lower three quartiles (103). The likelihood of needing additional antiparkinsonian therapy was reduced by approximately 60% in both the rasagiline 1 mg ($P = 0.0002$) and 2 mg ($P = 0.0001$) groups compared with placebo (delayed start group) (104). At 36 weeks, both rasagiline groups had significantly improved UPDRS motor subscores compared with placebo (−1.88 for rasagiline 1 mg, −2.18 for rasagiline 2 mg; $P < 0.0001$ for each comparison), and the ADL subscore (−0.86 for rasagiline 1 mg, −0.88 for rasagiline 2 mg; $P < 0.0001$). In addition, the Parkinson Fatigue Scale at 36 weeks was improved in both the rasagiline 1 mg (−0.14; $P = 0.0032$) and 2 mg (−0.19; $P < 0.0001$) groups. However, the only significant difference between early- and late-start groups at week 72 was for the ADL subscore with rasagiline 1 mg (−0.62; $P = 0.035$) (104).

The results and methodology of this study have generated considerable debate about whether rasagiline does indeed have disease-modifying properties aside from its symptomatic benefits. In October 2011, a 17-member committee of the United States FDA ruled unanimously that rasagiline not be indicated as a "disease-modifying" therapy for PD based on the available data. In part this decision was likely based on the lack of a clear explanation for why the 1 mg dose result in the ADAGIO study was consistent with a disease-modifying effect, whereas the 2 mg dose was not.

PRESTO

The Parkinson's Rasagiline: Efficacy and Safety in the Treatment of Off (PRESTO) study evaluated rasagiline as an adjunct in PD patients with motor fluctuations on levodopa (105). In this study, 472 PD patients with at least 2.5 hours of daily off time were randomized to rasagiline 0.5 mg/day, 1 mg/day, or placebo. The primary outcome was the change in off time as measured by patients' home diaries from baseline to 26 weeks. Mean adjusted off time (in hours) improved with each treatment: rasagiline 1 mg/day (1.85 hours), rasagiline 0.5 mg/day (1.41 hours), and placebo (0.91 hours). Compared with placebo, the differences were significant for both rasagiline 1 mg/day ($P < 0.001$) and rasagiline 0.5 mg/day ($P = 0.02$). There was a small but significant increase in on time with troublesome dyskinesia in the rasagiline 1 mg group ($P = 0.03$). The secondary endpoints of UPDRS ADL "off," motor UPDRS "on," and clinical global impression were all significantly improved with both dosages of rasagiline (105), and 1 mg/day rasagiline was also associated with significant improvement on the Schwab and England scale during off time (105).

LARGO

The Lasting Effect in Adjunct therapy with Rasagiline Given Once daily (LARGO) study evaluated once daily rasagiline and entacapone administered with each levodopa dose, compared with placebo in patients with motor fluctuations. In this 18-week, double-blind, parallel-group trial, 687 subjects were randomized to receive rasagiline 1 mg daily, entacapone 200 mg with each levodopa dose, or placebo (106). Off hours were significantly reduced in both the rasagiline (−1.18 hours; $P = 0.0001$) and entacapone (−1.2 hours; $P < 0.0001$) groups compared with placebo (−0.4 hours). In addition, both active treatment groups did better on the secondary outcomes of clinical global impression, UPDRS ADL scores in the off state, and UPDRS motor scores in the on state, compared with placebo. Neither rasagiline nor entacapone caused any worsening of dyskinesia. Rasagiline, but not entacapone, improved three exploratory UPDRS subscores: postural instability/gait disorder, freezing, and motor score in the practically defined off state. While the placebo group had a slight increase (+5 mg) in mean daily levodopa dosage at the end of 18 weeks, both rasagiline (−24 mg, $P = 0.0003$ vs placebo) and entacapone (−19 mg, $P = 0.0024$ vs placebo) were associated with small but significant reductions in daily levodopa requirement. Benefits of rasagiline were independent of age and concomitant dopamine agonist therapy, and post hoc analysis revealed no increase in dopaminergic adverse effects in those over age 70 years (106).

Gait freezing was examined in an auxiliary study of LARGO (107). Advanced PD subjects ($n = 454$) who had been randomized to rasagiline (1 mg/day; $n = 150$), entacapone (200 mg with each dose of levodopa; $n = 150$), or placebo ($n = 154$) were evaluated with a Freezing of Gait Questionnaire (FOG-Q) (98). Compared with baseline, the rasagiline and entacapone groups demonstrated a mean FOG-Q improvement of 1.2 points ($P = 0.045$) and 1.1 points ($P = 0.066$), respectively, at 10 weeks compared with 0.5-point improvement in the placebo group.

In a small substudy of LARGO (rasagiline $n = 32$, entacapone $n = 36$, placebo $n = 37$), the UPDRS motor "off" score was significantly better with rasagiline (5.63; $P = 0.0013$) than placebo; the improvement with entacapone was not significant (3.22; $P = 0.14$) (108).

An open-label study of 272 PD patients compared time to onset of benefit with those using rasagiline 1 mg/day monotherapy ($n = 123$) and rasagiline 0.5 mg/day adjunct therapy ($n = 149$). Benefit was seen within one week, with maximal benefit at two weeks; this benefit was sustained at four and 12 weeks. Both groups had similar time to onset of benefit and similar magnitude of benefit (109).

RASAGILINE ADVERSE EVENTS

Adverse events were no more common with rasagiline than placebo in the TEMPO (100) study of early patients; the two most common adverse events were infection and headache. In the active treatment phase, there were no significant differences in the most common adverse events occurring in the second six months of the study (infection, headache, unintentional injury, and dizziness). There were eight newly diagnosed malignancies detected over the 12 months of the TEMPO study including six skin cancers (three squamous cell, two melanoma, one basal cell carcinoma). Although this may be higher than would be expected in the general population, it appears that the risk of skin cancers is higher in PD patients and does not appear to be specifically related to rasagiline. Given the potential interaction between tyramine and MAO inhibition, a subset of patients on rasagiline also underwent uneventful tyramine challenge tests and blood pressures were generally unchanged after 75 mg of tyramine (110).

In the ADAGIO study, the three most common adverse events with rasagiline in the placebo-controlled phase were headache, back pain, and fatigue. Those related to dopaminergic therapy in the placebo-controlled phase were nausea or vomiting, hypertension, and somnolence. In the active phase the most common adverse events were falls, back pain, nasopharyngitis, arthralgia, and headache. Both dosages of rasagiline were well tolerated and there was no difference in the rate of adverse events among the study groups. No tyramine or serotonin reactions were reported. There was a single case of melanoma detected at week 72 in a subject on rasagiline 1 mg/day (103).

In the PRESTO study of advanced patients (105), balance difficulty was more common with rasagiline 0.5 mg/day than placebo, and weight loss, anorexia, and vomiting were each more common with rasagiline 1 mg/day than placebo ($P < 0.05$ for each). The safety of rasagiline in elderly (70 years and older) PD patients was reported (111). The authors analyzed the data (including both 1 and 2 mg/day dosages of rasagiline) from the PRESTO (105) and TEMPO (101) studies. They found that older subjects were more prone to develop serious adverse effects than younger subjects, but this was irrespective of treatment with rasagiline or placebo (111). In the PRESTO study, the total number of adverse effects was higher with rasagiline compared with placebo ($P = 0.03$) and more subjects experienced dyskinesia with rasagiline ($P = 0.02$), but this was seen in both older and younger subjects. Elderly subjects in both TEMPO ($P = 0.06$) and PRESTO ($P = 0.01$) were more prone to develop hallucinations regardless of treatment. Although the authors acknowledge that this was a secondary analysis and not specifically powered to detect age–rasagiline interactions directly, no significant interaction between age and rasagiline use was identified as a risk factor for adverse effects (111).

While no cases of serotonin syndrome were reported in the clinical trials, a 76-year-old woman with PD who accidentally took rasagiline 4 mg/day for four days before developing serotonin syndrome has been reported (112). A rare movement disorder, Pisa syndrome (sustained lateral trunk flexion), has been reported in four PD patients on rasagiline, which resolved after discontinuing treatment (113).

CONCLUSION

MAO inhibitors provide symptomatic benefit in PD. Selegiline monotherapy delays the need for levodopa by approximately nine months, and permits lower levodopa dosages once levodopa is required. As an adjunct to levodopa, selegiline reduces off time and improves symptom control in more advanced disease. Dopaminergic side effects and dyskinesia may worsen with selegiline and require reduction of levodopa dosage. Zydis selegiline is rapidly absorbed in the buccal mucosa and was approved as an adjunct to levodopa. Rasagiline is about 10 times more potent than selegiline. It was approved by the FDA for monotherapy in early PD and as an adjunct to levodopa in moderate-to-advanced PD. Rasagiline is very well tolerated in early disease and generally well tolerated in advanced disease and in the elderly (70 years and older). Some delayed start studies suggest that rasagiline provides more than a simple symptomatic effect, and long-term selegiline trials suggest increasing benefit with increasing duration of treatment. These observations are potentially consistent with a disease-modifying effect or an increasing symptomatic benefit over time. Long-term studies that evaluate nondopaminergic features of PD and include imaging and other biomarkers may be able to shed more light on these issues.

REFERENCES

1. Nicoll RA. Introduction to the pharmacology of CNS drugs, chapter 21. In: Katzung BG, ed. Basic and Clinical Pharmacology, 8th edn. New York: Lange Medical Books/McGraw-Hill, 2000: 351–63.
2. Hare MLC. Tyramine oxidase. A new enzyme system in liver. Biochem J 1928; 22: 968–79.
3. Pletscher A. The discovery of antidepressants: a winding path. Experientia 1991; 47: 4–8.
4. Zeller EA, Barsky J. In vivo inhibition of liver and brain monoamine oxidase by 1-isonicotinyl-2-isopropyl hydrazine. Proc Soc Exp Biol Med 1952; 81: 459–61.
5. Loomer HP, Saunders JC, Kline NS. A clinical and pharamcodynamic evaluation of iproniazid as a psychic energizer. Psychiatr Res Rep Am Psychiatr Assoc 1957; 8: 129–41.
6. Loomer HP, Saunders JC, Kline NS. Iproniazid, an amine oxidase inhibitor, as an example of a psychic energizer. Congres Rec 1957; 1382–90.
7. Knoll J, Magyar K. Some puzzling pharmacological effects of monoamine oxidase inhibitors. Adv Biochem Psychopharmacol 1972; 5: 393–408.
8. Knoll H, Ecseri Z, Kelemen K, et al. Phenylisopropyl methylpropinylamine (E-250), a new spectrum psychic energizer. Arch Int Pharmacodyn Ther 1965; 155: 154–64.
9. Yang HYT, Neff NH. The monoamine oxidases of brain: selective inhibition with drugs and the consequences for the metabolism of the biogenic amines. J Pharmacol Exp Ther 1974; 189: 733–40.
10. Johnston JP. Some observations upon a new inhibitor of monoamine oxidase in brain tissue. Biochem Pharmacol 1968; 17: 1285–97.
11. Pugh CEM, Quastel JH. Oxidation of amines by animal tissues. Biochem J 1937; 31: 2306–21.
12. Quastel JH. Amine oxidases. In: Lajta A, ed. Handbook of Neurochemistry. New York: Plenum, 1970: 285–312.
13. Davison AN. Physiological role of monoamine oxidase. Physiol Rev 1958; 38: 729–47.
14. Lewinsohn R, Glover V, Sandler M. Development of benzylamine oxidase and monoamine oxidase A and B in man. Biochem Pharmacol 1980; 29: 1221–30.
15. Riederer P, Reynolds GP, Youdim MBH. Selectivity of MAO inhibitors in human brain and their clinical consequences. In: Youdim MBH, Paykel ES, eds. Monoamine Oxidase Inhibitors: The State of the Art. Chichester: Wiley & Sons, 1981: 63–76.
16. White HL, Tansik RL. Characterization of multiple substrate binding sites of MAO. In: Singer TP, von Korff RW, Murphy DL, eds. Monoamine Oxidase: Structure, Function, Altered Functions. New York: Academic Press, 1979: 129–44.
17. Blaschko H. Amine oxidase and amine metabolism. Pharmacol Rev 1952; 4: 415–58.

18. Reynolds GP, Riederer P, Rausch WD. Dopamine metabolism in human brain: effects of monoamine oxidase inhibition in vitro by (–)deprenyl and (+) and (–) tranylcypromine. J Neural Transm Suppl 1980; 16: 173–8.

19. Levitt P, Pintar JE, Breakefield XO. Immunocytochemical demonstration of monoamine oxidase B in brain astrocytes and serotonergic neurons. Proc Natl Acad Sci USA 1982; 79: 6385–9.

20. Westlund KN, Kenney RM, Kochersperger LM, et al. Distinct monoamine oxidase A and B populations in primate brain. Science 1985; 230: 181–3.

21. Oreland L. Monoamine oxidase, dopamine and Parkinson's disease. Acta Neurol Scand 1991; 84: 60–5.

22. Riederer P, Konradi C, Hebenstreit G, et al. Neurochemical perspectives to the function of monoamine oxidase. Acta Neurol Scand 1989; 126: 41–5.

23. May T, Strauss S, Rommelspacher H. [3H] Harman labels selectively and with high affinity the active site of monoamine oxidase (EC1.4.3.4) subtype A (MAO-A) in rat, marmoset, and pig. J Neural Transm Suppl 1990; 32: 93–102.

24. Nagy J, Salach JI. Identity of the active site flavin-peptide fragments from the human "A"-form and the bovine "B"-form of monoamine oxidase. Arch Biochem Biophys 1981; 208: 388–94.

25. Dahlstrom A, Fuxe K. Evidence for the existence of monoamine-containing neurons in the central nervous system. I. Demonstration of monoamines in the cell bodies of brain-stem neurons. Acta Physiol Scand 1965; 62: 1–55.

26. Blackwell B, Marley E, Price J, et al. Hypertensive interactions between monoamine oxidase inhibitors and foodstuffs. Br J Psychiatry 1967; 113: 349–65.

27. Goren T, Adar L, Sasson N, et al. Clinical pharmacology tyramine challenge study to determine the selectivity of the monoamine oxidase type B (MAO-B) inhibitor rasagiline. J Clin Pharmacol 2010; 50: 1420–8.

28. Youdim MBH, Bar Am O, Yogev-Falach M, et al. Rasagiline: neurodegenerative, neuro-protection, and mitochondrial permeability transition. J Neurosci Res 2005; 79: 172–9.

29. Finberg JP, Takeshima T, Johnston JM, et al. Increased survival of dopaminergic neurons by rasagiline, a monoamine oxidase B inhibitor. Neuroreport 1998; 9: 703–7.

30. Maruyama W, Akao Y, Youdim MBH, et al. Transfection-enforced Bcl-2 overexpression and an anti-Parkinson drug, rasagiline, prevent nuclear accumulation of glyceraldehyde-3-phosphate dehydrogenase induced by an endogenous dopaminergic neurotoxin, N-methyl(R)salsolinol. J Neurochem 2001; 78: 727–35.

31. Maruyama W, Akao Y, Carrillo MC, et al. Neuroprotection by propargylamines in Parkinson's disease: suppression of apoptosis and induction of prosurvival genes. Neurotoxicol Teratol 2002; 24: 675–82.

32. Sanz E, Romera M, Bellik L, et al. Indolalkylamines derivatives as antioxidant and neuroprotective agents in an experimental model of Parkinson's disease. Med Sci Monit 2004; 10: 477–84.

33. Takahata K, Shimazu S, Katsuki H, et al. Effects of selegiline on antioxidant systems in the nigrostriatum in rat. J Neural Transm 2006; 113: 151–8.

34. Szende B, Bokonyi Gy, Bocsi J, et al. Anti-apoptotic and apoptotic action of (–)-deprenyl and its metabolites. J Neural Transm 2001; 108: 25–33.

35. Szende B, Magyar K, Szegedi Z. Apoptotic and antiapoptotic effect of (–)deprenyl and (–)-desmethyl-deprenyl on human cell lines. Neurobiology (Bp) 2000; 8: 249–55.

36. Sharma SK, Carlson EC, Ebadi M. Neuroprotective actions of Selegiline in inhibiting 1-methyl, 4-phenyl, pyridinium ion (MPP+)-induced apoptosis in SK-N-SH neurons. J Neurocytol 2003; 32: 329–43.

37. Muralikrishnan D, Samantaray S, Mohanakumar KP. D-deprenyl protects nigrostriatal neurons against 1-methyl-4-phenyl-1,2,3,6-tetrahydropyridine-induced dopaminergic neurotoxicity. Synapse 2003; 50: 7–13.

38. Mizuta I, Ohta M, Ohta K, et al. Selegiline and desmethylselegiline stimulate NGF, BDNF, and GDNF synthesis in cultured mouse astrocytes. Biochem Biophys Res Commun 2000; 279: 751–5.

39. Blandini F, Armentero MT, Fancellu R, et al. Neuroprotective effect of rasagiline in a rodent model of Parkinson's disease. Exp Neurol 2004; 187: 455–9.

40. Simon L, Szilagyi G, Bori Z, et al. (–)-D-Deprenyl attenuates apoptosis in experimental brain ischaemia. Eur J Pharmacol 2001; 430: 235–41.
41. Speiser Z, Mayk A, Eliash S, et al. Studies with rasagiline, a MAO-B inhibitor, in experimental focal ischemia in the rat. J Neural Transm 1999; 106: 593–606.
42. Blandini F. Neuroprotection by rasagiline: a new therapeutic approach to Parkinson's disease? CNS Drug Rev 2005; 11: 183–94.
43. Xiao H, Lv F Xu W, et al. Deprenyl prevents MPP(+)-induced oxidative damage in PC12 cells by the upregulation of Nrf2-mediated NQO1 expression through the activation of PI3K/Akt and Erk. Toxicology 2011; 290: 286–94.
44. Abu-Raya S, Tabakman R, Blaugrund E, Trembovler V, Lazarovici P. Neuroprotective and neurotoxic effects of monoamine oxidase-B inhibitors and derived metabolites under ischemia in PC12 cells. Eur J Pharmacol 2002; 434: 109–16.
45. Bar Am O, Amit T, Youdim MBH. Contrasting neuroprotective and neurotoxic actions of respective metabolites of anti-Parkinson drugs rasagiline and selegiline. Neurosci Lett 2004; 355: 169–72.
46. Mandel S, Weinreb O, Amit T, et al. Mechanism of neuroprotective action of the anti-Parkinson drug rasagiline and its derivatives. Brain Res Brain Res Rev 2005; 48: 379–87.
47. Carrillo MC, Minami C, Kitani K, et al. Enhancing effect of rasagiline on superoxide dismutase and catalase activities in the dopaminergic system in the rat. Life Sci 2000; 67: 577–85.
48. Wu RM, Chiueh CC, Pert A, et al. Apparent antioxidant effect of L-deprenyl on hydroxyl radical formation and nigral injury elicited by MPP+ in vivo. Eur J Pharmacol 1993; 243: 241–7.
49. Riva MA, Molteni R, Racagni G. L-deprenyl potentiates cAMP-induced elevation of FGF-2 mRNA levels in rat cortical astrocytes. Neuroreport 1997; 8: 2165–8.
50. Gardoni F, Zianni E, Eramo A, et al. Effect of rasagiline on the molecular composition of the excitatory postsynaptic density. Eur J Pharmacol 2011; 670: 458–63.
51. Finberg JP, Lamensdorf I, Weinstock M, et al. Pharmacology of rasagiline (N-propargyl-1R-aminoindan). Adv Neurol 1999; 80: 495–9.
52. Speiser Z, Katzir O, Rehavi M, et al. Sparing by rasagiline (TVP-1012) of cholinergic functions and behavior in the postnatal anoxia rat. Pharmacol Biochem Behav 1998; 60: 387–93.
53. Huang W, Chen Y, Shohami E, et al. Neuroprotective effect of rasagiline, a selective monoamine oxidase-B inhibitor, against closed head injury in the mouse. Eur J Pharmacol 1999; 366: 127–35.
54. Buys YM, Trope GE, Tatton WG. (–)-Deprenyl increases the survival of rat retinal ganglion cells after optic nerve crush. Curr Eye Res 1995; 14: 119–26.
55. Hobbenaghi R, Tiraihi T. Neuroprotective effect of deprenyl in sensory neurons of axotomized dorsal root ganglion. Clin Neuropharmacol 2003; 26: 263–9.
56. Tatton WG. Selegiline can mediate neuronal rescue rather than neuronal protection. Mov Disord 1993; 8:S20–30.
57. Abu-Raya S, Blaugrund E, Trembovler V, et al. Rasagiline, a monoamine oxidase-B inhibitor, protects NGF-differentiated PC12 cells against oxygen-glucose deprivation. J Neurosci Res 1999; 58: 456–63.
58. Shahani N, Gourie-Devi M, Nalini A, et al. (–)-Deprenyl alleviates the degenerative changes induced in the neonatal rat spinal cord by CSF from amyotrophic lateral sclerosis patients. Amyotroph Lateral Scler Other Motor Neuron Disord 2004; 5: 172–9.
59. Kupsch A, Sautter J, Gotz ME, et al. Monoamine oxidase-inhibition and MPTP-induced neurotoxicity in the non-human primate: Comparison of rasagiline (TVP 1012) with selegiline. J Neural Transm 2001; 108: 985–1009.
60. Cohen G, Pasik P, Cohen B, et al. Pargyline and deprenyl prevent the neurotoxicity of 1-methyl-4-phenyl-1,2,3,6-tetrahydropyridine (MPTP) in monkeys. Eur J Pharmacol 1984; 106: 209–10.
61. Benakis A. Pharmacokinetic Study in Man of 14 C Jumex. Study Report, Data on File. Framous Group Ltd Research Centre, 1981.

62. Szoko E, Kalasz H, Kerecsen L, et al. Binding of (–) deprenyl to serum proteins. Pol J Pharmacol Pharm 1984; 36: 413–21.
63. Ahola R, Haapalinna A, Heinonen E, et al. Protection by L-deprenyl of intact peripheral sympathetic neurons exposed to neurotoxin 6-hydroxy-dopamine (6-OHDA). New Trends Clin Neuropharamcol 1994; 7: 287.
64. Fowler JS, MacGregor RR, Wolf AP, et al. Mapping human brain monoamine oxidase A and B with 11C-labeled suicide inactivators and PET. Science 1987; 23: 481–5.
65. Yoshida T, Yamada Y, Yamamoto T, et al. Metabolism of deprenyl, a selective monoamine oxidase (MAO) B inhibitor in rat: relationship of metabolism to MAO-B inhibitory potency. Xenobiotica 1986; 16: 129–36.
66. Knoll J. R-(–)-deprenyl (Selegiline, Movergan) facilitates the activity of the nigrostriatal dopaminergic neuron. J Neural Transm Suppl 1987; 25: 45–66.
67. Heinonen EH, Lammintausta R. A review of the pharmacology of selegiline. Acta Neurol Scand Suppl 1991; 84: 44–59.
68. Borbe HO, Neibich G, Nickel B. Kinetic evaluation of MAO-B activity following oral administration of selegiline and desmethyl-selegiline in the rat. J Neural Transm Suppl 1990; 32: 131–7.
69. Knoll J. The possible mechanism of action of (–)deprenyl in Parkinson's disease. J Neural Transm 1978; 43: 177–98.
70. Bronzetti E, Felici L, Ferrante F, et al. Effect of ethylcholine mustard aziridinium (AF64A) and of the monoamine oxidase-B-inhibitor L-deprenyl on the morphology of the rat hippocampus. Int J Tissue React 1992; 14: 175–81.
71. Richard IH, Kurlan R, Tanner C, et al. Serotonin syndrome and the combined use of deprenyl and an antidepressant in Parkinson's disease. Neurology 1997; 48: 1070–7.
72. Zornberg GL, Bodkin JA, Cohen BM. Severe adverse interaction between pethidine and selegiline. Lancet 1991; 337: 246.
73. Parkinson Study Group. Effects of tocopherol and deprenyl on the progression of disability in early Parkinson's disease. N Engl J Med 1993; 328: 176–83.
74. Tetrud JW, Langston JW. The effect of deprenyl (selegiline) on the natural history of Parkinson's disease. Science 1989; 245: 519–22.
75. Palhagen S, Heinonen EH, Hagglund J, et al. Selegiline delays the onset of disability in de novo parkinsonian patients. Neurology 1998; 51: 520–5.
76. Myllylä VV, Sotaniemi KA, Vuorinen JA, et al. Selegiline in de novo parkinsonian patients: the Finnish study. Mov Disord 1993; 8: 41–4.
77. Parkinson Study Group. Impact of deprenyl and tocopherol treatment on Parkinson's disease in DATATOP patients requiring levodopa. Ann Neurol 1996; 39: 37–45.
78. Parkinson Study Group. Impact of deprenyl and tocopherol treatment on Parkinson's disease in DATATOP subjects not requiring levodopa. Ann Neurol 1996; 39: 29–36.
79. Shoulson I, Oakes D, Fahn S, et al. Impact of sustained deprenyl (selegiline) in levodopa-treated Parkinson's disease: a randomized placebo-controlled extension of the deprenyl and tocopherol antioxidative therapy of parkinsonism trial. Ann Neurol 2002; 51: 604–12.
80. Palhagen S, Heinonen E, Hagglund J, et al. Selegiline slows the progression of the symptoms of Parkinson disease. Neurology 2006; 66: 1200–6.
81. Allain H, Cougnard J, Neukirch HC. Selgiline in de novo parkinsonian patients: the French selegiline multicenter trial (FSMT). Acta Neurol Scand 1991; 84: 73–8.
82. Olanow CW, Hauser RA, Gauger L, et al. The effect of deprenyl and levodopa on the progression of Parkinson's disease. Ann Neurol 1995; 38: 771–7.
83. Sivertsen B, Dupont E, Mikkelsen B, et al. Selegiline and levodopa in early or moderately advanced Parkinson's disease: A double-blind controlled short- and long-term study. Acta Neurol Scand 1989; 80: 147–52.
84. Heinonen EH, Rinne UK. Selegiline in the treatment of Parkinson's disease. Acta Neurol Scand 1989; 80: 103–11.
85. Lees AJ. Current controversies in the use of selegiline hydrochloride. J Neural Transm Suppl 1987; 25: 157–62.
86. Golbe LI, Lieberman AN, Muenter MD, et al. Deprenyl in the treatment of symptom fluctuations in advanced Parkinson's disease. Clin Neuropharmacol 1988; 11: 45–55.

87. Lees AJ; Parkinson's Disease Research Group of the United Kingdom. Comparison of therapeutic effects and mortality data of levodopa and levodopa combined with selegiline in patients with early mild Parkinson's disease. BMJ 1995; 311: 1602–7.
88. Olanow CW, Fahn S, Langston JW, et al. Selegiline and mortality: A point of view. Ann Neurol 1996; 40: 841–5.
89. Katzenschlager R, Head J, Schrag A, et al. Fourteen-year final report of the randomized PDRG-UK trial comparing three initial treatments in PD. Neurology 2008; 71: 474–80.
90. Parkinson Study Group. Mortality in DATATOP: a multicenter trial in early Parkinson's disease. Ann Neurol 1998; 43: 318–25.
91. Marras C, McDermott MP, Rochon PA, et al. Survival in Parkinson disease: thirteen-year follow-up of the DATATOP cohort. Neurology 2005; 64: 87–93.
92. Seager H. Drug-delivery products and the Zydis fast-dissolving dosage form. J Pharm Pharmacol 1998; 50: 375–82.
93. Clarke A, Brewer F, Johnson ES, et al. A new formulation of selegiline: improved bioavailability and selectivity for MAO-B inhibition. J Neural Transm 2003; 110: 1241–55.
94. Clarke A, Johnson ES, Mallard N, et al. A new low-dose formulation of selegiline: clinical efficacy, patient preference and selectivity for MAO-B inhibition. J Neural Transm 2003; 110: 1257–71.
95. Waters CH, Sethi KD, Hauser RA, et al. Zydis selegiline reduces off time in Parkinson's disease patients with motor fluctuations: a 3-month, randomized, placebo-controlled study. Mov Disord 2004; 19: 426–32.
96. Ondo WG, Sethi KD, Kricorian G. Selegiline orally disintegrating tablets in patients with Parkinson disease and "wearing off" symptoms. Clin Neuropharmacol 2007; 30: 295–300.
97. Ondo WG. Pooled analysis of two identical phase 3 studies of a novel selegiline preparation as adjunctive therapy for Parkinson's disease. Mov Disord 2006; 21:S126.
98. Lew MF, Pahwa R, Leehey M, et al. Safety and efficacy of newly formulated selegiline orally disintegrating tablets as an adjunct to levodopa in the management of 'off' episodes in patients with Parkinson's disease. Curr Med Res Opin 2007; 23: 741–50.
99. Thebault JJ, Guillaume M, Levy R. Tolerability, safety, pharmacodynamics, and pharmacokinetics of rasagiline: a potent, selective, and irreversible monoamine oxidase type B inhibitor. Pharmacotherapy 2004; 24: 1295–305.
100. Parkinson Study Group. A controlled trial of rasagiline in early Parkinson's disease: the TEMPO study. Arch Neurol 2002; 59: 1937–43.
101. Parkinson Study Group. A controlled, randomized, delayed-start study of rasagiline in early Parkinson disease. Arch Neurol 2004; 61: 561–6.
102. Hauser RA, Lew MF, Hurtig HI, et al. Long-term outcome of early versus delayed rasagiline treatment in early Parkinson's disease. Mov Disord 2009; 24: 564–73.
103. Olanow CW, Rascol O, Hauser R, et al. A double-blind, delayed-start trial of rasagiline in Parkinson's disease. N Engl J Med 2009; 361: 1268–78.
104. Rascol O, Fitzer-Attas CJ, Hauser R, et al. A double-blind, delayed start trial of rasagiline in Parkinson's disease (the ADAGIO study): prespecified and post-hoc analyses of the need for additional therapies, changes in UPDRS scores, and non-motor outcome. Lancet Neurol 2011; 10: 415–23.
105. Parkinson's Study Group. A randomized placebo-controlled trial of rasagiline in levodopa-treated patients with Parkinson disease and motor fluctuations: the PRESTO study. Arch Neurol 2005; 62: 241–8.
106. Rascol O, Brooks DJ, Melamed E, et al. Rasagiline as an adjunct to levodopa in patients with Parkinson's disease and motor fluctuations (LARGO, Lasting effect in Adjunct therapy with Rasagiline Given Once daily, study): a randomised, double-blind, parallel-group trial. Lancet 2005; 365: 947–54.
107. Giladi N, Rascol O, Brooks DJ, et al. Rasagiline treatment can improve freezing of gait in advanced Parkinson's Disease: A prospective randomized, double blind, placebo and entacapone controlled study. Neurology 2004; 62:A329–30.
108. Stocchi F, Rabey JM. Effect of rasagiline as adjunct therapy to levodopa on severity of OFF in Parkinson's disease. Eur J Neurol 2011; 18: 1373–8.

109. Wilson RE, Seeberger LC, Silver D, et al. Rasagiline: time to onset of antiparkinson effect is similar when used as a monotherapy or adjunct treatment. Neurologist 2011; 17: 318–24.
110. Parkinson Study Group. Tyramine challenge to assess the safety of rasagiline monotherapy in a placebo-controlled multicenter trial for early Parkinson's disease (the TEMPO study). Neurology 2001; 56:A345.
111. Goetz C, Schwid SR, Eberly SW, et al. Safety of rasagiline in elderly patients with Parkinson disease. Neurology 2006; 66: 1427–9.
112. Fernandes C, Reddy P, Kessel B. Rasagiline-induced serotonin syndrome. Mov Disord 2011; 26: 766–7.
113. Fasano A, Di Matteo A. Reversible Pisa syndrome in patients with Parkinson's disease on rasagiline therapy. Mov Disord 2011; 26: 2578–80.

Ronald F. Pfeiffer

The introduction of levodopa therapy for Parkinson's disease (PD), initially by Birkmayer et al. (1) in 1961, followed by Barbeau et al. (2) in 1962, and in its ultimately successful form by Cotzias et al. (3) in 1967, still represents the defining landmark in the treatment of PD. This dramatic advance did not materialize out of thin air. It was preceded by methodical basic laboratory research in the late 1950s and early 1960s, which formed a groundwork documenting the presence of striatal dopamine deficiency in PD (4–8) and paved the road for the application of this knowledge in the clinical arena.

These developments took place against a broader backdrop in which both the role of catecholamines and their metabolic pathways in the body and brain were being unraveled (9). As part of this panorama, Axelrod in 1957 first suggested that one of the metabolic pathways for catecholamines might be via O-methylation (9–11), and in the same year, Shaw et al. (12) proposed that catechol-O-methyltransferase (COMT) might be important in the inactivation of dihydroxyphenylalanine (DOPA) and dopamine. By 1964, the metabolic pathways for DOPA and dopamine had been delineated and the involved enzymes were identified. Aromatic amino acid decarboxylase (AAAD) and COMT were identified as being responsible for converting DOPA to dopamine and 3-O-methyldopa (3-OMD), respectively, whereas monoamine oxidase (MAO) and COMT were documented to convert dopamine to 3,4-dihydroxyphenylacetic acid (DOPAC) and 3-methoxytyramine (3-MT), respectively. As early as 1964, it was suggested that agents inhibiting COMT might potentiate the effects of DOPA (13).

COMT is present throughout the body, with highest concentrations in the liver, kidneys, gastrointestinal (GI) tract, spleen, and lungs (14–17). It is also present in the brain, where it resides primarily in non-neuronal cells, such as glia. There is little COMT in neurons and none has been identified in nigrostriatal dopaminergic neurons (18). COMT exists in a soluble form within the cytoplasm in most tissues, but membrane-bound COMT accounts for 70% of the total enzyme present in the brain (19). A number of substrates are acted upon by COMT, including catecholamines such as epinephrine, norepinephrine, and dopamine and their hydroxylated metabolites, but all known substrates have a catechol configuration (11). COMT mediates the transfer of a methyl group from S-adenosylmethionine to a hydroxyl group on the catechol molecule. Its actions, especially in peripheral structures such as the intestinal mucosa, seem to be primarily directed toward protecting the body by inactivating biologically active or toxic catechol compounds (11,18–20). Both levodopa and dopamine are examples of such biologically active compounds.

The COMT gene has been identified on chromosome 22q11 (21). Several polymorphisms and haplotypes of the COMT gene have been identified and studied, most notably the Val158Met polymorphism, which may impact cognitive function and behavior (22,23). The clinical relevance of this and other polymorphisms with regard to PD is uncertain (24).

Recognition of the limited bioavailability of orally administered levodopa in the treatment of PD, with perhaps only 1% of it actually reaching the brain because of extensive peripheral metabolism by both AAAD and COMT (18,25), fueled the search for drugs that might inhibit the two enzymes and improve the therapeutic efficacy of levodopa. This led to the introduction of two inhibitors of AAAD, carbidopa and benserazide, as adjunctive agents administered concomitantly with levodopa to PD patients (26,27). Administering levodopa in conjunction with an AAAD inhibitor remains the standard today. However, the use of these agents only expands the amount of levodopa reaching the brain to an estimated 10% of an administered dose, primarily because blocking AAAD simply shunts levodopa into the COMT metabolic pathway, with increased peripheral formation of 3-OMD (25).

FIRST-GENERATION COMT INHIBITORS

During the 1960s and 1970s, a number of COMT inhibitors were identified and studied. Pyrogallol (1,2,3-trihydroxybenzene) was, perhaps, the first COMT inhibitor to be identified (28,29), but its short duration of action, toxicity (methemoglobinemia and renal impairment), and probable lack of COMT specificity precluded its clinical use (11). The list of additional "first-generation" COMT inhibitors that were studied and subsequently abandoned as potential therapeutic agents is quite long. Catechol itself, adnamine and noradnamine, various flavonoids, tropolone and its derivatives, 8-hydroxyquinolines, S-adenosylhomocysteine, sulfhydryl binding agents, pyrones and pyridones, papaveroline, methylspinazarin, 2-hydroxylated estrogens, and 3-mercaptotyramine represent only a partial listing of such compounds (11). Even the two agents that are primarily recognized as inhibitors of AAAD, carbidopa and benserazide, have some modest COMT-inhibiting properties, although not enough to be clinically relevant (11).

Several of these early COMT inhibitors did undergo pilot testing in humans. N-butyl gallate (GPA 1714), a derivative of gallic acid, was found to be effective in alleviating signs and symptoms of PD when administered to 10 patients (30). The dose of levodopa was reduced by an average of 29% and the drug was also noted to alleviate nausea and vomiting. No significant adverse effects were noted in this initial study, but testing was eventually abandoned because of its toxicity (31). Another compound, 3,4-dihydroxy-2-methylpropiophenone (U-0521), demonstrated a significant COMT inhibition in animal studies, but when it was administered orally to a single human in progressively increasing doses, it demonstrated no effect on erythrocyte COMT activity (31).

SECOND-GENERATION COMT INHIBITORS

Little attention was devoted to COMT inhibitors for the treatment of PD during the mid-1980s, but the 1990s ushered in renewed interest in the potential clinical usefulness of these compounds. This renewed attention was prompted by the development of a "second generation" of COMT inhibitors, substances that were more potent, more selective, and less toxic than their predecessors. Several nitrocatechol compounds, eventually bearing the names nitecapone, entacapone, tolcapone, and nebicapone, became the focus of laboratory, and clinical study.

NITECAPONE

Nitecapone (OR 462) was demonstrated to be well-tolerated and modestly effective when administered to mice, rats, and monkeys (32–34). Its actions were confined to the periphery because it did not cross the blood–brain barrier (35), and its primary action appeared to be in the intestinal mucosa (36,37). In subsequent human studies, it was noted to "slightly but significantly" increase the relative bioavailability of levodopa and to reduce plasma 3-OMD (38), but it eventually ceded its place in clinical PD development to entacapone (OR 611), which was judged the more effective compound.

ENTACAPONE

Entacapone is readily absorbed across the intestinal mucosa and does not seem to be significantly affected by first-pass metabolism in the liver. The bioavailability of an oral dose of entacapone ranges from 30% to 46% (18,39–42). It is highly (98%) protein bound and metabolized via glucuronidation. Most reports place the elimination half-life of entacapone between 0.4 and 0.7 hours (18,39–41). Entacapone does not cross the blood–brain barrier to any significant extent and appears to exert its action exclusively in the periphery (43), although some inhibition of striatal COMT activity following entacapone administration in rats has been described (43,44). When administered to humans, the inhibition of COMT activity by entacapone is dose dependent. Soluble COMT is reduced by 82% with an entacapone dose of 800 mg, the maximum amount that has been administered (45). In multiple dose studies, 100 mg of entacapone, given four to six times daily with levodopa, reduced COMT activity by 25% compared with placebo, 200 mg produced a 33% reduction, and 400 mg generated a 32% diminution in COMT activity (40).

Entacapone also has a dose-related effect on both levodopa and 3-OMD pharmacokinetics. In the same group of patients noted earlier, the elimination half-life $(T_{1/2})$ of levodopa was prolonged by 23%, 26%, and 48% at entacapone doses of 100, 200, and 400 mg, respectively; the area under the levodopa plasma curve (AUC) was increased by 17%, 27%, and 37%, respectively (40). Investigators in two earlier studies, however, had noted a leveling off of the levodopa AUC increase between entacapone doses of 200 and 400 mg and suggested that this might be due to interference in carbidopa absorption by entacapone at a higher dose (46,47). In other studies utilizing an entacapone dose of 200 mg, increases in the levodopa AUC have ranged between 23% and 48%, and prolongation of the levodopa $T_{1/2}$ has hovered around 40% (18). Despite these rather dramatic alterations, no significant increase in either the time to reach the maximum plasma levodopa concentration (T_{max}) or the maximum plasma levodopa concentration itself (C_{max}) has been reported in most instances following concomitant administration of levodopa and entacapone. The T_{max} remains between 30 and 60 minutes (18,36,48–51). Nutt, however, notes that the absence of an effect on the levodopa T_{max} and C_{max} is true only for the initial dose of the day and that some modest progressive elevation of the levodopa C_{max} develops with repeated doses during the day (52). This does not carry over to the next day, however, and progressive escalation of COMT inhibition does not occur (18,48). Consistent with these findings, Nord et al. (53) reported an increase in the C_{max} for levodopa in both blood and cerebrospinal fluid (CSF) when entacapone was added to levodopa being infused intravenously; this was especially evident when carbidopa was also administered. Concomitant with these changes in levodopa pharmacokinetics, entacapone also induces a significant reduction in the plasma AUC of 3-OMD, reflecting reduced COMT-mediated peripheral metabolism of levodopa to 3-OMD (18,40,42). It was predicted that the clinical correlate of these pharmacokinetic alterations would be an extended efficacy of a levodopa dose, due to the combination of the prolonged $T_{1/2}$ and increased AUC of levodopa and the reduced AUC of 3-OMD, possibly without an increase in levodopa-related toxicity, in light of the absence of change in levodopa C_{max}. Subsequent full-scale clinical trials have largely validated these predictions and confirmed the safety and efficacy of entacapone.

The Safety and Efficacy of Entacapone Study Assessing Wearing-Off (SEE-SAW), a double-blind, placebo-controlled trial, evaluated the safety and efficacy of entacapone over a six-month period in 205 PD patients on levodopa with motor fluctuations (54,55). A significant 5% increase in "on" time per day (approximately 1 hour) was documented in patients receiving entacapone, compared with placebo. Motor function, as measured by the Unified Parkinson's Disease Rating Scale (UPDRS) (56), improved slightly in the entacapone-treated group, whereas it deteriorated in the placebo group during the six-month trial. The average daily levodopa dosage diminished by 12% (from 791 to 700 mg/day) in the entacapone-treated group, but did not change in the placebo group. Adverse effects were generally mild and manageable, consisting primarily of symptoms consistent with enhanced dopaminergic activity, such as dyskinesia, nausea and dizziness. Dyskinesia was reported as an adverse effect by 53% (55/103) of patients on entacapone, compared with 32% (33/102) of individuals on placebo. Yellow/orange discoloration of the urine also occurred in 37% of those receiving entacapone, but diarrhea was infrequent (7%).

A second, large multicenter study, the NOMECOMT Study, had a trial design very similar to the SEESAW Study and very similar results (53,55,57). This trial (also six months in duration) included 171 PD patients on levodopa who were experiencing motor fluctuations. In the entacapone-treated group, the mean "on" time increased by 1.4 hours, compared with an increase of 0.2 hours in the placebo group. This relative increase of 13% in the treatment group was significant. Average daily levodopa dosage diminished by 12% in the entacapone group, compared with a 2% increase in the placebo group. Adverse effects in this study were similar to those in the SEESAW study, except that worsening of dyskinesia was reported by only 8.2% of entacapone-treated participants (vs 1.2% of those on placebo), whereas diarrhea was reported by 20%. An open-label three-year extension of this study demonstrated a sustained benefit of entacapone (58).

Subsequent studies have augmented the findings of the SEESAW and NOMECOMT studies. Two additional large multicenter trials have investigated the safety and efficacy of entacapone in PD patients (59,60). In an open-label study of eight weeks duration, 489 patients were administered entacapone in conjunction with each dose of levodopa up to a maximum of 10 doses per day (59). Some reduction in "off" time was experienced by approximately 41% of patients, and quality of life, as measured by the PDQ-39, was also improved. In a double-blind study of 301 PD patients, most of whom were experiencing motor fluctuations, a significant improvement in both motor function and activities of daily living was documented with entacapone compared with placebo (60). However, in another double-blind study, a trend toward improvement was noted, but significance was not achieved (61).

Long-term benefit from entacapone beyond the positive results reported in the relatively short-term initial randomized, placebo-controlled trials has also been documented. In a retrospective, pooled analysis of three Phase III trials, Nissinen et al. (62) reported that subjects in whom entacapone was added to the treatment regimen earlier showed less functional decline than individuals in whom entacapone was added six months later; this benefit remained evident for up to five years.

Concerns that the efficacy of entacapone might be reduced when used in conjunction with controlled-release levodopa preparations, because of a potential "mismatch" in absorption and metabolism of the two drugs, led several groups of investigators to address the issue (47,60,63–66). The effect of entacapone was, for the most part, found to be comparable between the standard and controlled-release levodopa preparations.

Variations on the timing of administration of entacapone relative to carbidopa/levodopa dosing also have been studied. Delaying entacapone administration until 30 or 90 minutes after levodopa administration did not produce any alteration in levodopa pharmacokinetics compared with concomitant administration (65). In another clinical study, simultaneous administration of a combination of immediate-release and controlled release carbidopa/levodopa preparations in conjunction with entacapone provided prolongation of duration of levodopa efficacy, presumably because the half-life differences of the two levodopa preparations provided for prolonged elevation of plasma levodopa levels (67). In a single-day study, bimodal administration of entacapone, in which two doses of 200 mg were administered, the first simultaneously with carbidopa/levodopa (either as immediate-release or controlled-release) and the second 1 hour later, improved the response to levodopa, compared with subjects receiving only a single dose of entacapone (68). In a randomized, open-label trial, Destée et al. (69) compared the addition of entacapone to increased fractionation of carbidopa/levodopa dosage in patients who were experiencing wearing off. Although the group receiving entacapone displayed a trend toward reduced levodopa dosage, reduced dyskinesia, and reduced "off" time, the differences were not significant.

With the extended availability of entacapone as a therapeutic agent in PD, it has become clear that not all patients derive benefit from the addition of entacapone to their treatment regimen. The reason for this is not clear, but striking variations between individuals in the maximum peak plasma concentration (a 4.2-fold interindividual difference) and in the time to reach peak plasma concentration have been documented in patients with PD, possibly related to delayed gastric emptying (70).

In a study that compared rasagiline, entacapone, and placebo, both rasagiline and entacapone reduced "off" time by similar amounts (1.18 and 1.20 hours respectively), compared with a 0.4-hour reduction for placebo (71). A post-marketing surveillance study of 464 patients taking entacapone reported an approximate 57% reduction in mean "off" time. In this trial, diarrhea was the most frequently reported adverse event, occurring in approximately 8% of individuals (72). Two large open-label studies of 899 and 479 patients recorded improvement in both patient perception of quality of life and physician perception of global improvement (73,74). In another postmarketing report, Parashos et al. found that in their clinical practice the most common reason for discontinuation of entacapone was not the occurrence of adverse effects, but rather lack of efficacy (75). Actual aggravation of parkinsonism (worsening of symptoms) was the next most frequent reason for discontinuing the drug.

The mechanism of the diarrhea that can develop with entacapone administration is uncertain, but in an experiment performed on freshly isolated rat distal colon, entacapone stimulated cAMP-dependent chloride secretion (76). Although hepatic toxicity has primarily been associated with tolcapone, at least one report has described entacapone-induced hepatotoxicity (77). Excessive daytime sleepiness, including "sleep attacks," has also been described with entacapone (78).

Drug interactions are not a prominent problem with entacapone, although the capability of entacapone to chelate iron in the GI tract has been noted (79) and it has been suggested that an interval of 2–3 hours be allowed between entacapone and iron ingestion (18). Although animal studies have suggested that COMT inhibition may increase apomorphine bioavailability (80), such an effect has not been demonstrated in humans, even when administered a double dose of 400 mg of entacapone (81).

Levodopa may increase plasma homocysteine levels in individuals with PD (82–86). The clinical significance, if any, of this elevation is uncertain. Elevated homocysteine has been reported as a risk factor for vascular disease (87,88), dementia (89), and depression (90); whether this holds true for the modest elevations of homocysteine seen in levodopa-treated PD patients is less clear. Some investigators have reported that entacapone is able to prevent the levodopa-induced rise in homocysteine (91–94). Nevrly et al. (95), in a prospective study, confirmed that plasma homocysteine levels are higher in PD patients receiving levodopa, but they did not find that entacapone reduced the elevated levels; nevertheless, in a subsequent report they suggested that entacapone may protect against hyperhomocysteinemia in PD (96).

LEVODOPA/CARBIDOPA/ENTACAPONE (STALEVO)

The efficacy of entacapone in prolonging the effect of levodopa, along with the recognition that it must be administered with each dose of levodopa, prompted the creation of a preparation combining levodopa, carbidopa, and entacapone (LCE) into a single tablet. Several clinical trials have demonstrated the bioequivalence of this combination drug (Stalevo) to the administration of carbidopa/levodopa (or benserazide/levodopa) and entacapone as separate medications (97,98). Patients perceive both the reduction in the number of pills enabled by LCE and the smaller size of the LCE tablets to be desirable conveniences (99,100). Switching from a regimen of carbidopa/levodopa alone to one of LCE not only reduces wearing off (101), but also produces improvement in quality of life measures (102). Superior bioavailability of 200 mg of levodopa given as LCE, compared with 200 mg given as controlled release carbidopa/levodopa, at bedtime also has been demonstrated (103). In contrast, LeWitt et al. (104) suggested that, because the pharmacokinetic profiles of LCE and controlled release carbidopa/levodopa are similar, some individuals may benefit from an initial dose of immediate release carbidopa/levodopa along with their first morning dose of LCE in order to hasten their "on" time.

Using a sophisticated mathematical modeling process that accounts for both individual and societal benefits, Findley et al. concluded that LCE is cost-effective when compared with treatment with carbidopa/levodopa alone (105). Delea et al. utilized a large health insurance claims database to carry out a retrospective historical cohort study that demonstrated that satisfactory adherence to LCE treatment (both when entacapone was combined into LCE and when it was administered separately with carbidopa/levodopa) resulted in significant reductions in all-cause hospitalizations and costs for patients with PD (106). In an earlier report, also using a large health insurance claims database, they showed that patient adherence to an LCE regimen was superior to one in which carbidopa/levodopa and entacapone were administered as separate tablets (107).

TOLCAPONE

Tolcapone (Ro 40-7592), similar to entacapone, is rapidly absorbed after oral administration; in contrast to entacapone, it reaches T_{max} in approximately 1.5 to 2 hours (18,108,109). The bioavailability of an oral dose is about 60% (110). Tolcapone is very highly (99.9%) protein bound (111). Metabolism of tolcapone is primarily, but not exclusively, via glucuronidation (112) because both methylation and oxidation also occur (113). The elimination $T_{1/2}$ of tolcapone is between 2 and 3 hours, which is distinctly longer than that of entacapone (108). At doses above 200 mg three times a day (TID), some accumulation of tolcapone can occur, but this appears to be of no real practical significance because levels, even at doses of 800 mg TID, remain well below those associated with toxicity in animals (108).

Unlike entacapone, tolcapone is sufficiently lipophilic to cross the blood–brain barrier, at least to some degree (114). Tolcapone-induced inhibition of COMT within the brain has been demonstrated in animal experiments (113,115). In primates, in which administered tolcapone doses were within the therapeutic range, COMT activity within the cerebellum was reduced by 60% (116). It has been less convincingly demonstrated that similar central COMT inhibition takes place in humans receiving tolcapone in clinically relevant doses. However, fluorodopa positron emission tomography (PET) studies have provided some evidence that such central COMT inhibition does, indeed, take place with tolcapone doses of 200 mg (117). Tolcapone also has been identified in the CSF of patients with PD 1–4 hours after oral intake of 200 mg of tolcapone in concentrations sufficient to reduce CSF COMT activity by 75% (118). Inhibition of COMT within both peripheral and central nervous system (CNS) structures provides some theoretical advantages over peripheral inhibition alone because, in addition to the peripheral levodopa-sparing capability, concomitant central COMT inhibition would not only reduce metabolism of levodopa to 3-OMD within the striatum, but also would block one route of the metabolism of dopamine itself.

Single-dose studies demonstrated tolcapone to be a noticeably more potent COMT inhibitor than entacapone. At a dose of 200 mg, tolcapone increases the levodopa AUC by 50–100%, prolongs the levodopa $T_{1/2}$ by 60–80%, and reduces the AUC of 3-OMD by 64% (18,52,119,120). No appreciable increase in the levodopa C_{max} or T_{max} is evident at this dose of tolcapone, although some delay in the T_{max} develops at higher doses (119).

Several double-blind, placebo-controlled clinical trials have confirmed the efficacy of tolcapone in reducing motor fluctuations in individuals with PD (121–124). In each of these multicenter trials, which varied in length from six weeks to six months, significant increases in "on" time and reductions in "off" time were documented in the tolcapone-treated groups, compared with the placebo groups. Reduction in both total daily levodopa dosage and number of levodopa doses taken was often evident in the tolcapone-treated groups.

In these four multicenter studies, in which 517 patients (out of 745 enrolled) received tolcapone in various doses ranging from 50 to 400 mg TID, adverse effects were generally mild and most often dopaminergic in character (121–124). In the three studies in which the treatment groups consisted of placebo versus 100 mg versus 200 mg each TID, dyskinesia was reported as an adverse event in 19–21%, 37–62%, and 53–66%, respectively (122–124). Tolcapone has been compared favorably with two dopamine agonists, bromocriptine and pergolide, in clinical trials (125,126), although these trials were open-label and possibly underpowered (127).

Diarrhea, at times unresponsive to medication and of sufficient severity to warrant drug discontinuation, was reported in a relatively small percentage of individuals receiving tolcapone, possibly in a dose-related pattern (52,123,124). The mechanism of the diarrhea is uncertain, although tolcapone has been noted to trigger intestinal fluid and electrolyte secretion, albeit not actual diarrhea, in dogs (18,128). As with entacapone, yellow/orange urine discoloration also occurred in some individuals.

In the initial multicenter trials, elevation of liver transaminase levels occurred in a small number of individuals, but all were clinically asymptomatic and the laboratory abnormalities sometimes returned to normal, despite continued treatment. In all clinical trials of tolcapone, the reported incidence of transaminase elevations greater than three times the upper limit of normal was approximately 1% at a dose of 100 mg TID and 3% at a dose of 200 mg TID (129). However, following introduction of tolcapone into routine clinical use, three cases of fulminant hepatic failure with fatal outcome occurred, which led regulatory agencies in Europe and Canada to withdraw tolcapone from the market and the Food and Drug Administration in the United States to severely limit its use to situations where other drugs had not provided sufficient benefit (130). No further deaths have been reported and these restrictions now have been relaxed. Tolcapone can once again be used in Europe, with appropriate monitoring of liver function, in persons with symptom fluctuations receiving levodopa who cannot tolerate or have not responded to other COMT inhibitors (131). A report from the Quality Standards Subcommittee of the American Academy of Neurology also provides similar guidelines for tolcapone use (132). Baseline liver function tests must be normal and the monitoring of liver function must be performed on a regular basis (every two to four weeks for the first six months and thereafter as clinically necessary) in patients receiving tolcapone (132). In an analysis of aspartate aminotransferase (AST) and alanine aminotransferase (ALT) levels in 11,883 blood samples taken from individuals on tolcapone as part of this monitoring process, less than 1% (15/1725) of patients had elevations of AST or ALT greater than twice the upper limit of normal; in most instances, the elevations were transient (133).

The mechanism of tolcapone-induced hepatotoxicity is not entirely clear. Uncoupling of oxidative phosphorylation in mitochondria (131,134,135), perhaps mediated by oxidation of tolcapone metabolites to reactive intermediates (136), has been suggested. Tolcapone also may provoke cellular damage by a mechanism independent of its effects on oxidative phosphorylation, perhaps by opening the mitochondrial permeability transition pore, with consequent apoptotic cell death (135).

Despite the small, but present, risk of hepatotoxicity, recent reviews have confirmed a definite place for tolcapone in the treatment of PD. Tolcapone appears to be more effective than entacapone and, therefore, may be useful in individuals with motor fluctuations in whom entacapone is ineffective or not tolerated (137,138); it also may be appropriate to consider a trial of tolcapone before other more invasive infusion or surgical approaches are considered (139,140).

NEBICAPONE

Nebicapone (BIA 3-202) is the latest COMT inhibitor to undergo testing for use in PD. Like entacapone and tolcapone, it is a nitrocatechol compound and a reversible COMT inhibitor that acts primarily in the periphery and increases levodopa bio-availability (141). In a small, short-duration pilot clinical trial involving 19 PD patients, it increased the AUC of levodopa, reduced the AUC of 3-OMD and reduced "off" time (142). In a subsequent large, multicenter clinical trial that enrolled 298 subjects and in which the double-blind treatment phase was eight weeks, a dose-dependent reduction in "off" time was documented (143). However, some eleva-tions in liver function tests developed in four of 46 patients on the highest dose of nebicapone (150 mg), prompting concern regarding the safety of the drug, a concern also voiced by others (144,145). Therefore, the prospect for further development of this compound is uncertain.

CURRENT STATUS OF COMT INHIBITORS

Two COMT inhibitors are currently available for use as adjunctive therapy in PD, to be used in conjunction with levodopa and an AADC inhibitor in patients who have developed motor fluctuations with end-of-dose wearing-off. Tolcapone is the more potent of the two and, with its longer $T_{1/2,}$ can be given on a TID basis. Its potential to produce hepatic failure has limited its use to individuals in whom enta-capone has been ineffective or not tolerated (146). Because of the tolcapone-related safety issues, clinical use of COMT inhibition has largely centered on entacapone, despite its lesser relative potency. Because of its short $T_{1/2}$, entacapone must be administered with each dose of levodopa. At first glance this seems inconvenient, but since it really does not entail any more frequent dosing than that already being employed for the levodopa, the inconvenience is more perceived than real. The additional 1–2 hours of "on" time per day a COMT inhibitor typically affords to a fluctuating patient can be very welcome. A cost-effectiveness analysis of entaca-pone concluded that the additional drug costs when entacapone is employed are offset by reductions in other costs and improvement (6%) in "quality-adjusted life years" (147). Another study in Finland also concluded that entacapone (and the MAO-B inhibitor rasagiline) is cost-effective when used in conjunction with levodopa compared with levodopa alone and provides slightly over five months of quality-adjusted life years (148). Findley et al. (105) reached similar conclusions with regard to the triple combination, LCE.

   Although it is clear that COMT inhibitors provide quantifiable improvement in function for PD patients with motor fluctuations, their potential benefit in stable PD patients who have not yet developed motor fluctuations has received much less attention. Two clinical trials have addressed this question with tolcapone (149,150). In the larger of the two trials (149), a significant improvement in both the activities of daily living and the motor sections of the UPDRS were documented. Improvement was most evident in more severely affected patients. Fewer patients in the tolcapone-treated group developed motor fluctuations during the duration of the trial, which extended to a maximum of 12 months for some participants (average 8.5 months). Adverse events were similar to those encountered in earlier trials described in the previous sections. The second, smaller, trial actually did not examine nonfluctuating PD patients, but rather evaluated individuals who had previously experienced wearing-off with levodopa, which had been successfully controlled by levodopa dosage adjustment (150). A greater reduction of levodopa dosage was achieved in the tolcapone-treated group, but this was not significant. A single tolcapone trial in levodopa-untreated patients demonstrated no clinical benefit (151).

In a double-blind study involving 300 patients, 128 of whom were not experiencing motor fluctuations, entacapone produced improvement in both the fluctuating and the nonfluctuating groups (152). In the group without motor fluctuations, a significant improvement in UPDRS activities of daily living was evident in patients receiving entacapone, compared with those receiving placebo, although no difference in motor scores was found. A larger increase in levodopa dosage in the placebo group also occurred. In another double-blind, placebo-controlled study involving a total of 750 levodopa-treated subjects who were not experiencing motor fluctuations, entacapone did not produce improvement in UPDRS motor scores, but significant improvement was documented in some quality of life measures (153). Fung et al. (154) also reported improvement in quality-of-life measures in individuals with no, or minimal, motor fluctuations in whom entacapone was added to carbidopa/levodopa, compared with carbidopa/levodopa alone; they noted further that improvement occurred predominantly in the nonmotor rather than the motor domains of the quality-of-life measures.

The pathogenesis of motor fluctuations in individuals with PD receiving levodopa has been the subject of much speculation, but little certainty, over the years. Both peripheral and central mechanisms have been hypothesized. Both are likely active, but the predominant mechanisms driving the pathogenic process in most individuals probably are within the CNS and may involve both presynaptic and postsynaptic mechanisms. Evidence has accumulated that with PD progression the dwindling number of surviving nigrostriatal dopaminergic neurons are unable to maintain the normal synaptic atmosphere of constant dopaminergic stimulation; instead the environment becomes one in which dopamine receptor stimulation is intermittent, characterized by pulses of dopaminergic stimulation coincident with levodopa administration. This pulsatile stimulation may, in turn, incite a cascade of changes within the postsynaptic striatal spiny neurons that produces sensitization of glutamate receptors and altered motor responses (155,156).

If this is correct, providing and maintaining a synaptic environment of more constant dopaminergic stimulation from the beginning of treatment might forestall the development of the postsynaptic alterations and delay or prevent the appearance of motor fluctuations. This has led to the proposal that a COMT inhibitor, such as entacapone, be administered along with levodopa and carbidopa right from the initiation of therapy (157,158). Consonant with this, Jenner et al. reported that in marmosets with 1-methyl-4-phenyl-1,2,3,6-tetrahydropyridine–induced parkinsonism, initiation of treatment with frequent doses of levodopa combined with entacapone resulted in less frequent and less severe dyskinesia than that which developed in animals treated with comparable doses of levodopa alone (159). Several large clinical trials have been undertaken in an effort to determine whether the same pattern emerges in humans.

In the FIRST-STEP study, 423 subjects with early PD were randomized to either LCE or carbidopa/levodopa given TID and followed for 39 weeks (160). In this study, LCE provided greater clinical benefit than carbidopa/levodopa without increasing the development of dyskinesia, although other adverse effects, such as nausea and diarrhea, were more frequent with LCE. In contrast, in the STRIDE-PD study, in which 747 patients with early PD were enrolled and assigned to either LCE or carbidopa/levodopa taken four times daily at dosage intervals of 3.5 hours for up to 134 weeks, patients in the LCE group developed dyskinesia earlier and more frequently than individuals receiving only carbidopa/levodopa (161). In addition to the fact that individuals in the LCE group received a greater equivalent dose of levodopa during the STRIDE-PD trial (162), it is likely that in neither the STRIDE-PD nor the FIRST-STEP protocols was medication given frequently enough to actually achieve constant stimulation of dopamine receptors. There currently is no proven indication for the administration of entacapone (or tolcapone) right from the outset of dopaminergic therapy, and the role of COMT inhibitors remains that of adjunctive therapy to carbidopa/levodopa in individuals who have begun to experience end-of-dose wearing-off.

REFERENCES

1. Birkmayer W, Hornykiewicz O. Der 1-3,4 Dioxyphenylalanin (=DOPA): Effekt bei der Parkinson-Akinese. Wien Klin Wochenschr 1961; 73: 787–8.
2. Barbeau A, Sourkes TL, Murphy CF. Les catecholamines dans la maladie de Parkinson. In: de Ajuriaguerra J, ed. Monoamines et Systeme Nerveaux Central. Geneva: Gerog, 1962: 247–62.
3. Cotzias GC, Van Woert MH, Schiffer LM. Aromatic amino acids and modification of parkinsonism. N Engl J Med 1967; 276: 374–9.
4. Carlsson A, Lindquist M, Magnusson T. 3,4-dihydroxyphenylalanine and 5-hydroxy-tryptophan as reserpine antagonists. Nature 1957; 180: 200.
5. Bertler A, Rosengren E. Occurrence and distribution of catecholamines in brain. Acta Physiol Scand 1959; 47: 350–61.
6. Ehringer H, Hornykiewicz O. Verteilung von Noradrenalin und Dopamin (3-Hydroxy-tyramin) im Gehirn des Menschen und ihr Verhalten bei Erkrankungen des extrapyra-midalen systems. Wien Klin Wochenschr 1960; 38: 1236–9.
7. Anden NE, Carlsson A, Dahlstrom A, et al. Demonstration and mapping of nigroneo-striatal dopamine neurons. Life Sci 1964; 3: 523–30.
8. Poirier LJ, Sourkes TL. Influence of the substantia nigra on the catecholamine content of the striatum. Brain 1965; 88: 181–92.
9. Axelrod J. Catecholamine neurotransmitters, psychoactive drugs, and biological clocks. The 1981 Harvey Cushing oration. J Neurosurg 1981; 55: 669–77.
10. Axelrod J. The O-methylation of epinephrine and other catechols in vitro and in vivo. Science 1957; 126: 1657–60.
11. Guldberg HC, Marsden CA. Catechol-O-methyl transferase: pharmacological aspects and physiological role. Pharmacol Rev 1975; 27: 135–206.
12. Shaw KNF, McMillan A, Armstrong MD. The metabolism of 3,4-dihydroxyphenylala-nine. J Biol Chem 1957; 226: 255–66.
13. Carlsson A. Functional significance of drug-induced changes in brain monoamine lev-els. In: Himwich HE, Himwich WA, eds. Biogenic Amines (Progress in Brain Research, Vol 8). Amsterdam: Elsevier, 1964: 9–27.
14. Nissinen E, Tuominen R, Perhoniemi V, et al. Catechol-O-methyltransferase activity in human and rat small intestine. Life Sci 1988; 42: 2609–14.
15. Schultz E, Nissinen E. Inhibition of rat liver and duodenum soluble catechol-O-methyltransferase by a tight-binding inhibitor OR-462. Biochem Pharmacol 1989; 38: 3953–6.

16. Mannisto PT, Ulmanen I, Lundstrom K, et al. Characteristics of catechol-O-methyl-transferase (COMT) and properties of selective COMT inhibitors. Prog Drug Res 1992; 39: 291–350.
17. Ding YS, Gatley SJ, Fowler JS, et al. Mapping catechol-O-methyltransferase in vivo: initial studies with [18F]Ro41-0960. Life Sci 1996; 58: 195–208.
18. Teravainen H, Rinne U, Gordin A. Catechol-O-methyltransferase inhibitors in Parkinson's disease. In: Calne D, Calne S, eds. Parkinson's Disease (Advances in Neurology, Vol 86). Philadelphia: Lippincott Williams Wilkins, 2001: 311–25.
19. Tai CH, Wu RM. Catechol-O-methyltransferase and Parkinson's disease. Acta Med Okayama 2002; 56: 1–6.
20. Huotari M, Gogos JA, Karayiorgou M, et al. Brain catecholamine metabolism in catechol-O-methyltransferase (COMT)-deficient mice. Eur J Neurosci 2002; 15: 246–56.
21. Grossman MH, Emanuel BS, Budarf ML. Chromosomal mapping of the human catechol-O-methyltransferase gene to 22q11.1-q11.2. Genomics 1992; 12: 822–5.
22. Tunbridge EM. The catechol-O-methyltransferase gene: its regulation and polymorphisms. Int Rev Neurobiol 2010; 95: 7–27.
23. Dickinson D, Elevåg B. Genes, cognition and brain through a COMT lens. Neuroscience 2009; 164: 72–87.
24. Lee MS, Kim HS, Cho EK, et al. COMT genotype and effectiveness of entacapone in patients with fluctuating Parkinson's disease. Neurology 2002; 58: 564–7.
25. Olanow CW, Schapira AHV, Rascol O. Continuous dopamine-receptor stimulation in early Parkinson's disease. Trends Neurosci 2000; 23: S117–26.
26. Rinne UK, Sonninen V, Siirtola T. Treatment of parkinsonian patients with levodopa and extracerebral decarboxylase inhibitor, Ro 4-4602. In: Calne D, ed. Progress in the Treatment of Parkinsonism (Advances in Neurology, Vol 3). New York: Raven Press, 1973: 59–71.
27. Porter CC. Inhibitors of aromatic amino acid decarboxylase – their biochemistry. In: Yahr MD, ed. Treatment of Parkinsonism – The Role of Dopa Decarboxylase Inhibitors (Advances in Neurology, Vol 2). New York: Raven Press, 1973: 37–58.
28. Bacq ZM, Gosselin L, Dresse A, et al. Inhibition of O-methyltransferase by catechol and sensitization to epinephrine. Science 1959; 130: 453–4.
29. Axelrod J, LaRoche MJ. Inhibitor of O-methylation of epinephrine and norepinephrine in vitro and in vivo. Science 1959; 130: 800.
30. Ericsson AD. Potentiation of the L-Dopa effect in man by the use of catechol-O-methyl-transferase inhibitors. J Neurol Sci 1971; 14: 193–7.
31. Reches A, Fahn S. Catechol-O-methyltransferase and Parkinson's disease. In: Hassler RG, Christ JF, eds. Parkinson-Specific Motor and Mental Disorders (Advances in Neurology, Vol 40). New York: Raven Press, 1984: 171–9.
32. Linden IB, Nissinen E, Etemadzadeh E, et al. Favorable effect of catechol-O-methyltransferase inhibition by OR-462 in experimental models of Parkinson's disease. J Pharmacol Exp Ther 1988; 247: 289–93.
33. Tornwall M, Mannisto PT. Acute toxicity of three new selective COMT inhibitors in mice with special emphasis on interactions with drugs increasing catecholaminergic neurotransmission. Pharmacol Toxicol 1991; 69: 64–70.
34. Cedarbaum JM, Leger G, Reches A, et al. Effect of nitecapone (OR-462) on the pharmacokinetics of levodopa and 3-O-methyldopa formation in cynomolgus monkeys. Clin Neuropharmacol 1990; 13: 544–52.
35. Marcocci L, Maguire JJ, Packer L. Nitecapone: a nitric oxide radical scavenger. Biochem Mol Biol Int 1994; 34: 531–41.
36. Nissinen E, Linden IB, Schultz E, et al. Inhibition of catechol-O-methyltransferase activity by two novel disubstituted catechols in the rat. Eur J Pharmacol 1988; 153: 263–9.
37. Schultz E, Tarpila S, Backstrom AC, et al. Inhibition of human erythrocyte and gastroduodenal catechol-O-methyltransferase activity by nitecapone. Eur J Clin Pharmacol 1991; 40: 577–80.
38. Kaakkola S, Gordin A, Jarvinen M, et al. Effect of a novel catechol-O-methyltransferase inhibitor, nitecapone, on the metabolism of L-Dopa in healthy volunteers. Clin Neuropharmacol 1990; 13: 436–47.

39. Najib J. Entacapone: a catechol-O-methyltransferase inhibitor for the adjunctive treatment of Parkinson's disease. Clin Ther 2001; 23: 802–32.
40. Heikkinen H, Nutt JG, LeWitt PA, et al. The effects of different repeated doses of entacapone on the pharmacokinetics of L-Dopa and on the clinical response to L-Dopa in Parkinson's disease. Clin Neuropharmacol 2001; 24: 150–7.
41. Keranen T, Gordin A, Karlsson M, et al. Inhibition of soluble catechol-O-methyltransferase and single-dose pharmacokinetics after oral and intravenous administration of entacapone. Eur J Clin Pharmacol 1994; 46: 151–7.
42. Keranen T, Gordin A, Harjola V-P, et al. The effect of catechol-O-methyl transferase inhibition by entacapone on the pharmacokinetics and metabolism of levodopa in healthy volunteers. Clin Neuropharmacol 1993; 16: 145–56.
43. Nissinen E, Linden I-B, Schultz E, et al. Biochemical and pharmacological properties of a peripherally acting catechol-O-methyltransferase inhibitor entacapone. Naunyn Schmiedebergs Arch Pharmacol 1992; 346: 262–6.
44. Brannan T, Prikhojan A, Yahr MD. Peripheral and central inhibitors of catechol-O-methyl transferase: effects on liver and brain COMT activity and L-DOPA metabolism. J Neural Transm 1997; 104: 77–87.
45. Keranen T, Gordin A, Karlsson M, et al. Effect of the novel catechol-O-methyltransferase inhibitor OR-611 in healthy volunteers. Neurology 1991; 41(Suppl): 213.
46. Ruottinen HM, Rinne UK. A double-blind pharmacokinetic and clinical dose-response study of entacapone as an adjuvant to levodopa therapy in advanced Parkinson's disease. Clin Neuropharmacol 1996; 19: 283–96.
47. Ahtila S, Kaakkola S, Gordin A, et al. Effect of entacapone, a COMT inhibitor, on the pharmacokinetics and metabolism of levodopa after administration of controlled-release levodopa-carbidopa in volunteers. Clin Neuropharmacol 1995; 18: 46–57.
48. Rouru J, Gordin A, Huupponen R, et al. Pharmacokinetics of oral entacapone after frequent multiple dosing and effects on levodopa disposition. Eur J Clin Pharmacol 1999; 55: 461–7.
49. Heikkinen H, Saraheimo M, Antila S, et al. Pharmacokinetics of entacapone, a peripherally acting catechol-O-methyltransferase inhibitor, in man. A study using a stable isotope technique. Eur J Clin Pharmacol 2001; 56: 821–6.
50. Kaakkola S, Teravainen H, Ahtila S, et al. Effect of entacapone, a COMT inhibitor, on clinical disability and levodopa metabolism in parkinsonian patients. Neurology 1994; 44: 77–80.
51. Schapira AHV, Obeso JA, Olanow CW. The place of COMT inhibitors in the armamentarium of drugs for the treatment of Parkinson's disease. Neurology 2000; 55: S65–8.
52. Nutt JG. Effect of COMT inhibition on the pharmacokinetics and pharmacodynamics of levodopa in parkinsonian patients. Neurology 2000; 55: S33–7.
53. Nord M, Zsigmond P, Kullman A, et al. The effect of peripheral enzyme inhibitors on levodopa concentrations in blood and CSF. Mov Disord 2010; 25: 363–7.
54. Parkinson Study Group. Entacapone improves motor fluctuations in levodopa-treated Parkinson's disease patients. Ann Neurol 1997; 42: 747–55.
55. Kieburtz K, Hubble J. Benefits of COMT inhibitors in levodopa-treated parkinsonian patients: results of clinical trials. Neurology 2000; 55: S42–5.
56. Fahn S, Elton RL. Members of the UPDRS Development Committee. Unified Parkinson's disease rating scale. In: Fahn S, Marsden CD, Goldstein M, Calne DB, eds. Recent Developments in Parkinson's Disease. Vol. 2 New York: McMillan, 1987: 153–63.
57. Rinne UK, Larsen JP, Siden A, et al. Entacapone enhances the response to levodopa in parkinsonian patients with motor fluctuations. Nomecomt Study Group. Neurology 1998; 51: 1309–14.
58. Larsen JP, Worm-Petersen J, Siden A, et al. The tolerability and efficacy of entacapone over 3 years in patients with Parkinson's disease. Eur J Neurol 2003; 10: 137–46.
59. Durif F, Devaux I, Pere JJ, et al. Efficacy and tolerability of entacapone as adjunctive therapy to levodopa in patients with Parkinson's disease and end-of-dose deterioration in daily medical practice: an open, multicenter study. Eur Neurol 2001; 45: 111–18.
60. Poewe WH, Deuschl G, Gordin A, et al. Efficacy and safety of entacapone in Parkinson's disease patients with suboptimal levodopa response: a 6-month randomized

placebo-controlled double-blind study in Germany and Austria (Celomen Study). Acta Neurol Scand 2002; 105: 245–55.

61. Fenelon G, Gimenez-Roldan S, Montastruc JL, et al. Efficacy and tolerability of entacapone in patients with Parkinson's disease treated with levodopa plus a dopamine agonist and experiencing wearing-off motor fluctuations. A randomized, double-blind, multicenter study. J Neural Transm 2003; 110: 239–51.

62. Nissinen H, Kuoppamäki M, Leinonen M, et al. Early versus delayed initiation of entacapone in levodopa-treated patients with Parkinson's disease: a long-term, retrospective analysis. Eur J Neurol 2009; 16: 1305–11.

63. Piccini P, Brooks DJ, Korpela K, et al. The catechol-O-methyltransferase (COMT) inhibitor entacapone enhances the pharmacokinetic and clinical response to Sinemet CR in Parkinson's disease. J Neurol Neurosurg Psychiatry 2000; 68: 589–94.

64. Stocchi F, Barbato L, Nordera G, et al. Entacapone improves the pharmacokinetic and therapeutic response of controlled release levodopa/carbidopa in Parkinson's patients. J Neural Transm 2004; 111: 173–80.

65. Brusa L, Pierantozzi M, Bassi A, et al. Temporal administration of entacapone with slow release L-dopa: pharmacokinetic profile and clinical outcome. Neurol Sci 2004; 25: 53–6.

66. Paija O, Laine K, Kultalahti E-R, et al. Entacapone increases levodopa exposure and reduces plasma levodopa variability when used with Sinemet CR. Clin Neuropharmacol 2005; 28: 115–19.

67. Iansek R, Danoudis M. A single-blind cross over study investigating the efficacy of standard and controlled-release levodopa in combination with entacapone in the treatment of end-of-dose effect in people with Parkinson's disease. Parkinsonism Relat Disord 2011; 17: 533–6.

68. Bet L, Bareggi SR, Pacei F, et al. Bimodal administration of entacapone in Parkinson's disease patients improves motor control. Eur J Neurol 2008; 15: 268–73.

69. Destée A, Rérat K, Bourdeix I. Is there a difference between levodopa/dopa-decarboxylase inhibitor and entacapone and levodopa/dopa-decarboxylase inhibitor dose fractionation strategies in Parkinson's disease patients experiencing symptom re-emergence due to wearing-off? The Honeymoon Study. Eur Neurol 2009; 61: 69–75.

70. Nagai M, Kubo M, Nishikawa N, et al. Fluctuation in plasma entacapone concentrations in accordance with variable plasma levodopa concentrations. Parkinsonism Relat Disord 2010; 16: 697–9.

71. Rascol O, Brooks DJ, Melamed E, et al. Rasagiline as an adjunct to levodopa in patients with Parkinson's disease and motor fluctuations (LARGO, Lasting effect in Adjunct therapy with Rasagiline Given Once daily, study): a randomised, double-blind, parallel-group trial. Lancet 2005; 365: 947–54.

72. Kupsch A, Trottenberg T, Bremen D. Levodopa therapy with entacapone in daily clinical practice: results of a post-marketing surveillance study. Curr Med Res Opin 2004; 20: 115–20.

73. Gershanik O, Emre M, Bernhard G, et al. Efficacy and safety of levodopa with entacapone in Parkinson's disease patients suboptimally controlled with levodopa alone, in daily clinical practice: an international, multicenter, open-label study. Prog Neuropsychopharmacol Biol Psychiatry 2003; 27: 963–71.

74. Onofrj M, Thomas A, Vingerhoets F, et al. Combining entacapone with levodopa/DDCI improves clinical status and quality of life in Parkinson's disease (PD) patients experiencing wearing-off, regardless of the dosing frequency: results of a large multicenter open-label study. J Neural Transm 2004; 111: 1053–63.

75. Parashos SA, Wielinski CL, Kern JA. Frequency, reasons, and risk factors of entacapone discontinuation in Parkinson disease. Clin Neuropharmacol 2004; 27: 119–23.

76. Li LS, Zheng LF, Xu JD, et al. Entacapone promotes cAMP-dependent colonic Cl(-) secretion in rats. Neurogastroenterol Motil 2011; 23: 657–e277.

77. Fisher A, Croft-Baker J, Davis M, et al. Entacapone-induced hepatotoxicity and hepatic dysfunction. Mov Disord 2002; 17: 1362–5.

78. Bares M, Kanovsky P, Rektor I. Excessive daytime sleepiness and "sleep attacks" induced by entacapone. Fundam Clin Pharmacol 2003; 17: 113–16.

79. Orama M, Tilus P, Taskinen J, et al. Iron (III)-chelating properties of the novel catechol-O-methyltransferase inhibitor entacapone in aqueous solution. J Pharm Sci 1997; 86: 827–31.
80. Coudoré F, Durif F, Duroux E, et al. Effect of tolcapone on plasma and striatal apomorphine disposition in rats. Neuroreport 1997; 8: 877–80.
81. Zijlmans JCM, Debilly B, Rascol O, et al. Safety of entacapone and apomorphine coadministration in levodopa-treated Parkinson's disease patients: pharmacokinetic and pharmacodynamic results of a multicenter, double-blind, placebo-controlled, crossover study. Mov Disord 2004; 19: 1006–11.
82. O'Suilleabhain PE, Bottiglieri T, Dewey RB Jr, et al. Modest increase in plasma homocysteine follows levodopa initiation in Parkinson's disease. Mov Disord 2004; 19: 1403–8.
83. Miller JW, Selhub J, Nadeau MR, et al. Effect of L-dopa on plasma homocysteine in PD patients: relationship to B-vitamin status. Neurology 2003; 60: 1125–9.
84. Muller T, Werne B, Fowler B, et al. Nigral endothelial dysfunction, homocysteine, and Parkinson's disease. Lancet 1999; 354: 126–7.
85. Rogers JD, Sanchez-Saffon A, Frol AB, et al. Elevated plasma homocysteine levels in patients treated with levodopa: association with vascular disease. Arch Neurol 2003; 60: 59–64.
86. Yasui K, Nakaso K, Kowa H, et al. Levodopa-induced hyperhomocysteinaemia in Parkinson's disease. Acta Neurol Scand 2003; 108: 66–7.
87. Bots ML, Launer LJ, Lindemans J, et al. Homocysteine, atherosclerosis and prevalent cardiovascular disease in the elderly: the Rotterdam Study. J Intern Med 1997; 242: 339–47.
88. Bostom AG, Rosenberg IH, Silbershatz H, et al. Nonfasting plasma total homocysteine levels and stroke incidence in elderly persons: the Framingham Study. Ann Intern Med 1999; 131: 352–5.
89. Seshadri S, Beiser A, Selhub J, et al. Plasma homocysteine as a risk factor for dementia and Alzheimer's disease. N Engl J Med 2002; 346: 476–83.
90. Tiemeier H, van Tuijl HR, Hofman A, et al. Vitamin B12, folate, and homocysteine in depression: the Rotterdam Study. Am J Psychiatry 2002; 159: 2099–101.
91. Valkovič P, Benetin J, Blažíček P, et al. Reduced plasma homocysteine levels in levodopa/entacapone treated Parkinson patients. Parkinsonism Relat Disord 2005; 11: 253–6.
92. Lamberti P, Zoccolella S, Iliceto G, et al. Effects of levodopa and COMT inhibitors on plasma homocysteine in Parkinson's disease patients. Mov Disord 2005; 20: 69–72.
93. Zoccolella S, Lamberti P, Armenise E, et al. Plasma homocysteine levels in Parkinson's disease: role of antiparkinsonian medications. Parkinsonism Relat Disord 2005; 11: 131–3.
94. Müller T, Muhlack S. Peripheral COMT inhibition prevents levodopa associated homocysteine increase. J Neural Transm 2009; 116: 1253–6.
95. Nevrly M, Kanovsky P, Vranova H. Effect of levodopa and entacapone treatment on plasma homocysteine levels in Parkinson's disease patients. Parkinsonism Relat Disord 2009; 15: 477–8.
96. Nevrly M, Kanovsky P, Vranova H, et al. Effect of entacapone on plasma homocysteine levels in Parkinson's disease patients. Neurol Sci 2010; 31: 565–9.
97. Brooks DJ, Agid Y, Eggert K, et al. Treatment of end-of-dose wearing-off in Parkinson's disease: Stalevo® (levodopa/carbidopa/entacapone) and levodopa/DDCI given in combination with Comtess®/Comtan® (entacapone) provide equivalent improvements in symptom control superior to that of traditional levodopa/DDCI treatment. Eur Neurol 2005; 53: 197–202.
98. Koller W, Guarnieri M, Hubble J, et al. An open-label evaluation of the tolerability and safety of Stalevo (carbidopa, levodopa and entacapone) in Parkinson's disease patients experiencing wearing-off. J Neural Transm 2005; 112: 221–30.
99. Silver DE. Clinical experience with the novel levodopa formulation entacapone + levodopa + carbidopa (Stalevo®). Expert Rev Neurother 2004; 4: 589–99.

100. Hauser RA. Levodopa/carbidopa/entacapone (Stalevo). Neurology 2004; 62: S64–71.
101. Eggert K, Skogar O, Amar K, et al. Direct switch from levodopa/benserazide or levodopa/carbidopa to levodopa/carbidopa/entacapone in Parkinson's disease patients with wearing-off: efficacy, safety and feasibility – an open-label, 6-week study. J Neural Transm 2010; 117: 333–42.
102. Lew MF, Somogyi M, McCague K, et al. Immediate versus delayed switch from levodopa/carbidopa to levodopa/carbidopa/entacapone: effects on motor function and quality of life in patients with Parkinson's disease with end-of-dose wearing off. Int J Neurosci 2011; 121: 605–13.
103. Kuoppamäki M, Sauramo A, Korpela K, et al. Night-time bioavailability of levodopa/carbidopa/entacapone is higher compared to controlled-release levodopa/carbidopa. Int J Clin Pharmacol Ther 2010; 48: 756–60.
104. LeWitt PA, Jennings D, Lyons KE, et al. Pharmacokinetic-pharmacodynamic crossover comparison of two levodopa extension strategies. Mov Disord 2009; 24: 1319–24.
105. Findley LJ, Lees A, Apajasalo M, et al. Cost-effectiveness of levodopa/carbidopa/entacapone (Stalevo) compared to standard care in UK Parkinson's disease patients with wearing-off. Curr Med Res Opin 2005; 21: 1005–14.
106. Delea TE, Thomas SK, Hagiwara M. The association between adherence to levodopa/carbidopa/entacapone therapy and healthcare utilization and costs among patients with Parkinson's disease: a retrospective claims-based analysis. CNS Drugs 2011; 25: 53–66.
107. Delea TE, Thomas SK, Hagiwara M, et al. Adherence with levodopa/carbidopa/entacapone versus levodopa/carbidopa and entacapone as separate tablets in patients with Parkinson's disease. Curr Med Res Opin 2010; 26: 1543–52.
108. Jorga KM. Pharmacokinetics, pharmacodynamics, and tolerability of tolcapone: a review of early studies in volunteers. Neurology 1998; 50: S31–8.
109. Dingemanse J, Jorga K, Zurcher G, et al. Pharmacokinetic-pharmacodynamic interaction between the COMT inhibitor tolcapone and single-dose levodopa. Br J Clin Pharmacol 1995; 40: 253–62.
110. Jorga KM, Fotteler B, Heizmann P, et al. Pharmacokinetics and pharmacodynamics after oral and intravenous administration of tolcapone, a novel adjunct to Parkinson's disease therapy. Eur J Clin Pharmacol 1998; 54: 443–7.
111. Dingemanse J. Issues important for rational COMT inhibition. Neurology 2000; 55: S24–7.
112. Jorga K, Fotteler B, Heizmann P, et al. Metabolism and excretion of tolcapone, a novel inhibitor of catechol-O-methyltransferase. Br J Clin Pharmacol 1999; 48: 513–20.
113. Da Prada M, Borgulya J, Napolitano A, et al. Improved therapy of Parkinson's disease with tolcapone, a central and peripheral COMT inhibitor with an S-adenosyl-L-methionine-sparing effect. Clin Neuropharmacol 1994; 17: S26–37.
114. Dingemanse J. Catechol-O-methyltransferase inhibitors: clinical potential in the treatment of Parkinson's disease. Drug Dev Res 1997; 42: 1–25.
115. Zurcher G, Dingemanse J, Da Prada M. Potent COMT inhibition by Ro 40-7592 in the periphery and in the brain. Preclinical and clinical findings. In: Narabayashi H, Nagatsu T, Yanagisawa N, Mizuno Y, eds. Parkinson's Disease. From Basic Research to Treatment (Advances in Neurology, Vol 60). New York: Raven Press, 1993: 641–7.
116. Thiffault C, Langston JW, Di Monte DA. Cerebrospinal fluid 3,4-dihydroxyphenylacetic acid level after tolcapone administration as an indicator of nigrostriatal degeneration. Exp Neurol 2003; 183: 173–9.
117. Ceravolo R, Piccini P, Bailey DL, et al. 18F-dopa PET evidence that tolcapone acts as a central COMT inhibitor in Parkinson's disease. Synapse 2002; 43: 201–7.
118. Russ H, Muller T, Woitalla D, et al. Detection of tolcapone in the cerebrospinal fluid of parkinsonian subjects. Naunyn Schmiedebergs Arch Pharmacol 1999; 360: 719–20.
119. Sedek G, Jorga K, Schmitt M, et al. Effect of tolcapone on plasma levodopa concentrations after coadministration with levodopa/carbidopa to healthy volunteers. Clin Neuropharmacol 1997; 20: 531–41.
120. Kurth MC, Adler CH. COMT inhibition: a new treatment strategy for Parkinson's disease. Neurology 1998; 50: S3–S14.

121. Kurth MC, Adler CH, St. Hilaire M, et al. Tolcapone improves motor function and reduces levodopa requirement in patients with Parkinson's disease experiencing motor fluctuations: a multicenter, double-blind, randomized, placebo-controlled trial. Tolcapone Fluctuator Study Group I. Neurology 1997; 48: 81–7.

122. Adler CH, Singer C, O'Brien C, et al. Randomized, placebo-controlled study of tolcapone in patients with fluctuating Parkinson's disease treated with levodopa-carbidopa. Tolcapone Fluctuator Study Group III. Arch Neurol 1998; 55: 1089–95.

123. Rajput AH, Martin W, Saint-Hilaire M-H, et al. Tolcapone improves motor function in parkinsonian patients with the "wearing-off" phenomenon: a double-blind, placebo-controlled, multicenter trial. Neurology 1997; 49: 1066–71.

124. Baas H, Beiske AG, Ghika J, et al. Catechol-O-methyltransferase inhibition with tolcapone reduces the "wearing-off" phenomenon and levodopa requirements in fluctuating parkinsonian patients. J Neurol Neurosurg Psychiatry 1997; 63: 421–8.

125. Koller W, Lees A, Doder M, et al. Randomized trial of tolcapone versus pergolide as add-on to levodopa therapy in Parkinson's disease patients with motor fluctuations. Mov Disord 2001; 16: 858–66.

126. Tolcapone Study Group. Efficacy and tolerability of tolcapone compared with bromocriptine in levodopa-treated parkinsonian patients. Mov Disord 1999; 14: 38–44.

127. Deane KH, Spieker S, Clarke CE. Catechol-O-methyltransferase inhibitors versus active comparators for levodopa-induced complications in Parkinson's disease. Cochrane Database Syst Rev 2004; 4: CD004553.

128. Larsen KR, Dajani EZ, Dajani NE, et al. Effects of tolcapone, a catechol-O-methyltransferase inhibitor, and Sinemet on intestinal electrolyte and fluid transport in conscious dogs. Dig Dis Sci 1998; 43: 1806–13.

129. Watkins P. COMT inhibitors and liver toxicity. Neurology 2000; 55: S51–2.

130. Benabou R, Waters C. Hepatotoxic profile of catechol-O-methyltransferase inhibitors in Parkinson's disease. Expert Opin Drug Saf 2003; 2: 263–7.

131. Borges N. Tolcapone in Parkinson's disease: liver toxicity and clinical efficacy. Expert Opin Drug Saf 2005; 4: 69–73.

132. Pahwa R, Factor SA, Lyons KE, et al. Practice Parameter: treatment of Parkinson disease with motor fluctuations and dyskinesia (an evidence-based review). Report of the Quality Standards Subcommittee of the American Academy of Neurology. Neurology 2006; 66: 983–95.

133. Lew MF, Kricorian G. Results from a 2-year centralized tolcapone liver enzyme monitoring program. Clin Neuropharmacol 2007; 30: 281–6.

134. Nissinen E, Kaheinen P, Penttila KE, et al. Entacapone, a novel catechol-O-methyltransferase inhibitor for Parkinson's disease, does not impair mitochondrial energy production. Eur J Pharmacol 1997; 340: 287–94.

135. Korlipara LVP, Cooper JM, Schapira AHV. Differences in toxicity of the catechol-O-methyl transferase inhibitor, tolcapone and entacapone to cultured human neuroblastoma cells. Neuropharmacology 2004; 46: 562–9.

136. Smith KS, Smith PL, Heady TN, et al. In vitro metabolism of tolcapone to reactive intermediates: relevance to tolcapone liver toxicity. Chem Res Toxicol 2003; 16: 123–8.

137. Lees AJ. Evidence-based efficacy comparison of tolcapone and entacapone as adjunctive therapy in Parkinson's disease. CNS Neurosci Ther 2008; 14: 83–93.

138. Truong DD. Tolcapone: review of its pharmacology and use as adjunctive therapy in patients with Parkinson's disease. Clin Interv Aging 2009; 4: 109–13.

139. Canesi M, Zecchinelli AL, Pezzoli G, et al. Clinical experience of tolcapone in advanced Parkinson's disease. Neurol Sci 2008; 29: S380–2.

140. Antonini A, Abbruzzese G, Barone P, et al. COMT inhibition with tolcapone in the treatment algorithm of patients with Parkinson's disease (PD): relevance for motor and non-motor features. Neuropsychiatr Dis Treat 2008; 4: 1–9.

141. Bonifácio MJ, Palma PN, Almeida L, et al. Catechol-O-methyltransferase and its inhibitors in Parkinson's disease. CNS Drug Rev 2007; 13: 352–79.

142. Ferreira JJ, Almeida L, Cunha L, et al. Effects of nebicapone on levodopa pharmacokinetics, catechol-O-methyltransferase activity, and motor fluctuations in patients with Parkinson's disease. Clin Neuropharmacol 2008; 31: 2–18.

143. Ferreira JJ, Rascol O, Poewe W, et al. A double-blind, randomized, placebo and active-controlled study of nebicapone for the treatment of motor fluctuations in Parkinson's disease. CNS Neurosci Ther 2010; 16: 337–47.
144. Kaakkola S. Problems with the present inhibitors and a relevance of new and improved COMT inhibitors in Parkinson's disease. Int Rev Neurobiol 2010; 95: 207–25.
145. Haasio K. Toxicology and safety of COMT inhibitors. Int Rev Neurobiol 2010; 95: 163–89.
146. Keating GM, Lyseng-Williamson KA. Tolcapone: a review of its use in the management of Parkinson's disease. CNS Drugs 2005; 19: 165–84.
147. Nuijten MJ, van Iperen P, Palmer C, et al. Cost-effectiveness analysis of entacapone in Parkinson's disease: a Markov process analysis. Value Health 2001; 4: 316–28.
148. Hudry J, Rinne JO, Keranen T, et al. Cost utility model of rasagiline in the treatment of advanced Parkinson's disease in Finland. Ann Pharmacother 2006; 40: 651–7.
149. Waters CH, Kurth M, Bailey P, et al. Tolcapone in stable Parkinson's disease: efficacy and safety of long-term treatment. The Tolcapone Stable Study Group. Neurology 1997; 49: 665–71.
150. Dupont E, Burgunder J-M, Findley LJ, et al. Tolcapone added to levodopa in stable parkinsonian patients: a double-blind placebo- controlled study. Tolcapone in Parkinson's Disease Study Group II (TIPS II). Mov Disord 1997; 12: 928–34.
151. Hauser RA, Molho E, Shale H, et al. A pilot evaluation of the tolerability, safety, and efficacy of tolcapone alone and in combination with oral selegiline in untreated Parkinson's disease patients. Tolcapone De Novo Study Group. Mov Disord 1998; 13: 643–7.
152. Brooks DJ, Sagar H; and the UK-Irish Entacapone Study Group. Entacapone is beneficial in both fluctuating and non-fluctuating patients with Parkinson's disease: a randomised, placebo-controlled, double blind, six month study. J Neurol Neurosurg Psychiatry 2003; 74: 1071–9.
153. Olanow CW, Kieburtz K, Stern M, et al. Double-blind, placebo-controlled study of entacapone in levodopa-treated patients with stable Parkinson disease. Arch Neurol 2004; 61: 1563–8.
154. Fung VSC, Herawati L, Wan Y, et al. Quality of life in early Parkinson's disease treated with levodopa/carbidopa/entacapone. Mov Disord 2009; 24: 25–31.
155. Chase TN. Levodopa therapy: consequences of the nonphysiologic replacement of dopamine. Neurology 1998; 50: S17–25.
156. Chase TN, Oh JD. Striatal dopamine- and glutamate-mediated dysregulation in experimental parkinsonism. Trends Neurosci 2000; 23: S86–91.
157. Olanow CW, Obeso JA. Pulsatile stimulation of dopamine receptors and levodopa-induced motor complications in Parkinson's disease. Implications for the early use of COMT inhibitors. Neurology 2000; 55: S72–7.
158. Olanow CW, Stocchi F. COMT inhibitors in Parkinson's disease: can they prevent and/or reverse levodopa-induced motor complications? Neurology 2004; 62: S72–81.
159. Smith LA, Jackson MJ, Al-Barghouthy G, et al. Multiple small doses of levodopa plus entacapone produce continuous dopaminergic stimulation and reduce dyskinesia induction in MPTP-treated drug-naïve primates. Mov Disord 2005; 20: 306–14.
160. Hauser RA, Panisset M, Abbruzzese G, et al. Double-blind trial of levodopa/carbidopa/entacapone versus levodopa/carbidopa in early Parkinson's disease. Mov Disord 2009; 24: 541–50.
161. Stocchi F, Rascol O, Kieburtz K, et al. Initiating levodopa/carbidopa therapy with and without entacapone in early Parkinson disease: the STRIDE-PD study. Ann Neurol 2010; 68: 18–27.
162. Sampaio C, Ferreira JJ. Parkinson disease: adjunctive entacapone therapy increases risk of dyskinesia. Nat Rev Neurol 2010; 6: 590–1.

23

Investigational pharmacological treatments

Fernando L. Pagan and Jill Giordano Farmer

INTRODUCTION

Levodopa remains the most effective treatment for Parkinson's disease (PD) since its introduction in clinical practice in 1967. Over the last decade the management of PD has evolved, as our understanding of the disease increases. Particular interest in the nonmotor symptoms has lead clinical research to look for more effective motor management strategies that will minimize or improve motor complications, while not adversely affecting the nonmotor aspects of the disease. Newer treatments aim to improve motor and nonmotor symptoms and unique treatments are aimed at improving nonmotor symptoms without worsening motor symptoms.

Some of the most effective treatments can now be delivered more efficiently to further enhance the quality of life for PD patients with potentially fewer motor fluctuations. The newer formulations allow for more continuous dopaminergic stimulation, which has been at the forefront of PD pharmacological research over the past two decades. Novel agents for treating PD without directly addressing the dopamine deficiency are also being introduced to help alleviate motor and nonmotor symptoms, whereas others may potentially slow down the progression of the disease.

NEW DOPAMINERGIC AGENTS
Levodopa Formulations

The mainstay of PD treatment is the replacement of dopamine with the use of levodopa, which provides robust relief of motor symptoms and has been shown to be neuroprotective at low doses in animal studies. However, one third of patients on levodopa therapy will develop motor fluctuations after 3–5 years of use, and most patients taking levodopa for 10–12 years will have motor fluctuations (1,2). It is postulated that motor fluctuations are related to the short half-life of levodopa. As dopamine neurons are lost, patients become increasingly sensitive to levodopa plasma levels for relief of their symptoms and require more medication, which then leads to more side effects (3,4). To help prevent motor fluctuations, new formulations and ways of administering levodopa are being developed with a focus on maintaining a sustained plasma level of the medication. By preventing fluctuations in the plasma levels, these new treatments should in turn minimize fluctuations in the patients' motor symptoms.

Levodopa Carbidopa Intestinal Gel

One such advancement is Levodopa Carbidopa Intestinal Gel (LCIG) known as Duodopa®. This is an aqueous suspension containing 20 mg/mL levodopa and 5 mg/mL carbidopa. It is administered through a percutaneous double lumen endoscopic gastrostomy tube that can deliver the LCIG directly into the jejunum (5).

It is usually infused for 16 hours during the day, but can be infused for over an entire 24-hour period. In a large multicenter study conducted in France, a mean daily levodopa dose of 1388 mg showed a greater than 90% improvement in motor fluctuations, quality of life, and autonomy (1). In some patients it also reduced other side effects, such as hallucinations, perhaps because of the removal of other medications, such as dopamine agonists (5). While LCIG infusion has previously been thought of as a last line therapy, earlier consideration and implementation of this treatment warrants consideration, especially in patients where deep brain stimulation is contraindicated or no longer functioning or for whom oral medications are not adequate. Although the research is encouraging and indicates improvement in motor, nonmotor, and quality-of-life parameters, studies have also shown technical problems with the device in up to 70% of patients (6).

IPX066

IPX066 is a novel extended release formulation of carbidopa/levodopa (3). Current controlled release formulations of levodopa often have the problem of a slow onset of symptom relief and sometimes have to be administered along with an immediate release formulation. IPX066 would in essence mimic a rapid-acting immediate release formulation and then maintain plasma levels like a controlled release formulation. IPX066 is an extended release oral formulation of carbidopa/levodopa in a 1:4 ratio designed to rapidly attain and maintain therapeutic levodopa concentrations for a prolonged duration (3). A multicenter study compared IPX066 and immediate release carbidopa/levodopa and found a reduction in the overall frequency of levodopa dosing (5.4 times daily to 3.5 times) and amount of levodopa used (2054.4 mg reduced to 787.3 mg daily) with a more sustained levodopa plasma concentration with IPX066. The initial absorption rate for IPX066 and carbidopa/levodopa immediate release is similar, reaching 50% peak dose in 45 minutes, but with IPX066 the plasma concentrations were sustained above the peak dose for 4 hours, which resulted in less fluctuation in measured samples (3). The medication was well tolerated by study participants. The proposed brand name for IPX066 is Rytary and has an anticipated FDA approval date of January 2013.

XP21279

XP21279 is another formulation of sustained release levodopa, which takes advantage of an alternative method of absorption. While levodopa is absorbed through the jejunum, XP21279 is absorbed throughout the entire GI tract, which allows for a longer absorption time and therefore a more sustained plasma level of medication. Phase I trials demonstrated significantly less variability in levodopa concentration when compared with immediate release carbidopa/levodopa and a greater than 30% reduction of mean "off" time. The ratio of maximum concentration of levodopa to concentration of levodopa at 12 hours was 4.2 compared with 39.7 with carbidopa/levodopa immediate release. The smaller ratio would predict reduced fluctuations in plasma levels at twice a day dosing. The study also showed that with the larger area of absorption there was complete conversion to L-dopa in the blood samples measured during the study (7,8).

New Dopamine Agonists

Apomorphine pumps are currently standard of care in Europe, but are not available in the United States. A multicenter trial in Spain found an improvement in motor fluctuations in advanced PD patients with continuous subcutaneous apomorphine infusion, although a small study of four patients comparing apomorphine and LCIG showed a better response in symptomatic control and reduced motor fluctuations with LCIG (9,10).

Pardoprunox

Pardoprunox is a partial dopamine agonist and its safety and efficacy were studied in two randomized double-blind trials, Rembrandt and Vermeer. Partial dopamine agonists may help improve dopamine secretion without causing overstimulation, which often leads to side effects that can limit current dopamine agonist use in certain patients. Pardopronux is partial agonist and full 5HT-1A agonist and in animal models showed antiparkinsonian potential as both a monotherapy in early PD and adjunctive therapy in moderate-to-severe PD. The dose ranged from 6 to 42 mg/day in both studies. Rembrandt compared different dosing levels of pardoprunox to placebo, whereas Vermeer compared different dosing levels of pardoprunox to both placebo and pramipexole. In both the studies, patients taking pardoprunox demonstrated a significant (20%) reduction in Unified Parkinson's Disease Rating Scale (UPDRS) scores compared with placebo or pramipexole. The most noted side effects were somnolence, nausea, and dizziness and they were dose related. No minimum effective dose was established; however, both studies suggested that the 12–24 mg/day doses were higher than therapeutically required as this range had the highest dropout rate due to adverse effects (11).

An additional study looked at the use of pardoprunox specifically as adjunctive therapy to levodopa. It revealed increased ON time and decreased OFF time without worsening dyskinesia, but it also had a high dropout rate at levels of 12–42 mg/day due to side effects (12). Interestingly the articles do not comment on impulse control disorders that can be seen with current dopamine agonists and if this is less prevalent in patients on partial dopamine agonist therapy.

MONOAMINE OXIDASE INHIBITORS
Safinamide

Safinamide is an alpha-aminoamide and is being developed as a novel treatment due to its dual mechanisms of action (13,14). It is a highly selective, reversible monoamine oxidase inhibitor as well as a sodium and N-type calcium channel blocker. The first mechanism reduces the breakdown of dopamine and the creation of free radicals and the second inhibits the release of glutamate (14). The inhibition of glutamate may potentially have antidyskinetic effects (15). In a phase III multicenter trial, safinamide was compared at 40 mg, 70 mg, and in combination with dopamine agonists over 12 weeks. The results showed the most robust response in the patients at the 1 mg/kg dose or 70 mg in combination with a dopamine agonist (14). There was a reduction in the motor UPDRS score of 4.7 points. The specific dopamine agonist used did not appear to make a difference in response. The hypothesized mechanism of action is a summation of the two mechanisms of action of safinamide in combination with the mechanism of the dopamine agonists. In this way the action of endogenous dopamine is maximized through stimulation of the D1 receptors, while the agonist maximizes the D2 receptor responses (14). Another double-blind, randomized, placebo-controlled trial compared 100 and 200 mg doses of safinamide in combination with a dopamine agonist over 24 weeks and found a significant improvement in UPDRS scores of 6 points at the 100 mg dose. There was no significant difference between the 200 mg dose and placebo. Both studies show safinamide was well tolerated as monotherapy or adjunctive therapy and not only improved motor function, but reduced patient OFF time (13,15).

ADENOSINE A$_{2A}$ RECEPTOR ANTAGONISTS

As the drugs discussed above demonstrate, most PD medications focus on the dopaminergic system. Innovative research is being conducted to investigate novel targets of the dopaminergic pathways that do not utilize the neurotransmitter dopamine and in theory would not lead to the dopaminergic side effects that can be troublesome for so many patients. One such target is the A2 adenosine GABAergic receptor, which is selectively located in the basal ganglia comingling with the D2 receptors providing the excitatory and inhibitory balance of the indirect pathway (4,16). The indirect pathway promotes movement through negative inhibition via dopamine and the D2 receptors. As dopamine is lost, so is this negative inhibition, and the excitatory properties of adenosine go unchecked. An antagonist to this receptor would mimic a dopaminergic state (16).

Istradefylline

Istradefylline was the first selective A$_{2A}$ antagonist investigated (17). The A$_{2A}$ receptor is found in the caudate nucleus, globus pallidus, nucleus accumbens, and olfactory tubercles and plays an excitatory role in the indirect pathway for movement (4). Animal models with nonhuman primates treated with 1-methyl-4-phenyl-1, 2, 3, 6-tetrahydropyridine (MPTP) showed promising results with istradefylline monotherapy producing an improvement in motor function without inducing dyskinesia. In primates treated with levodopa and the addition of istradefylline, there was a potentiated and prolonged effect of a single dose of levodopa (18). Phase IIb/III studies were completed in humans looking at varying doses from 10 to 60 mg per day as monotherapy and as adjunctive therapy to levodopa. The monotherapy study did not show statistically significant improvement in motor function, but some of the studies examining istradefylline as an adjunct to levodopa did show improvement (6). In the studies examining the addition of istradefylline to levodopa, doses of 40 mg/day were found to consistently reduce OFF time of patients by over 1 hour across multiple studies and was well tolerated (17,19–21). In addition, UPDRS motor scores were improved by as much as 6 points with 40 mg/day in some studies, whereas the motor response was not as robust in other studies (21). Another endpoint was the development of dyskinesia. Istradefylline did induce dyskinesia; however, the dyskinesia were described as nonbothersome by the study participants across the different studies. The studies did not comment on the prolonged effect of levodopa when using istradefylline as seen in primate models and if this could lead to an overall lowering of levodopa dose in human patients (18).

Preladenant

Preladenant is a potent selective competitive antagonist of the A$_{2A}$ receptor, which is ubiquitous in the brain and the components of the indirect pathway (4). It has been studied in animal models and primates treated with MPTP and haloperidol and in both populations a dose-dependent improvement in motor function without associated dyskinesia was seen with levodopa at doses ranging from 1 to 12 mg/kg/day (16).

Multicenter, phase II trials conducted in human subjects revealed similarly promising results. In these trials patients received 1, 2, 5, or 10 mg oral twice daily dosing, and motor function, nonmotor symptoms, and dyskinesia were evaluated. The 5 and 10 mg doses showed an improvement in dyskinesia as well as some nonmotor symptoms such as motivation/initiative (5 and 10 mg) and thought process and depression (10 mg) after 12 weeks. The 5 and 10 mg dose also showed a reduction in mean daily OFF time of 1–2 hours (4).

TREATMENTS TARGETING DYSKINESIA
Another such target is the glutamatergic receptors responsible for the excitatory input to the basal ganglia. Overactivity of this pathway has been linked to the pathophysiology of levodopa-induced dyskinesia (22). Blocking one specific receptor, the mGluR5 receptor, has been shown to decrease dyskinesia without worsening motor function.

ADS-5102
Amantadine predates levodopa as a treatment for PD, but it does not have the robust motor response and comes with its own host of side effects. It is still used today as early monotherapy to help with mild symptoms or adjunctive therapy to help with tremor or dyskinesia. ADS-5102 is an extended release formulation of amantadine with a pharmacokinetic profile designed to overcome the dose-limiting side effects associated with immediate release forms of amantadine while offering potential for enhanced efficacy. The extended release form will offer a slower initial rate of rise of plasma level of the drug reducing the central nervous system (CNS) side effects while maintaining a constant state during the day, which is when dyskinesia are most troublesome. According to data from the manufacturer's website, phase I trials showed a reduction in CNS side effects and improvement in dyskinesia (23). Currently a phase II/III trial is being conducted called the Extended Release Amantadine Safety and Efficacy Study in Levodopa-induced Dyskinesias (EASED) to build upon the phase I results (24).

ADX48621
ADX48621 (dipraglurant) is an mGluR5 negative allosteric modulator and currently in Phase IIa clinical trials for PD (25). Allosteric modulators are an emerging class of small molecule drugs that have the potential to be even more specific than conventional orthosteric biological drugs. Dipraglurant is using this more specific targeting to block the glutamate receptor 5 and in turn potentially reduce levodopa-induced dyskinesia. In animal studies, primates who were rendered dyskinetic by levodopa showed an increase in the density of the mGluR5 receptor, and rodents where mGluR5 was blocked showed a decrease in dyskinesia (26,27). In preclinical testing, dipraglurant showed reduction in levodopa-induced dyskinesia, chorea, and dystonia, and was possibly neuroprotective (28).

AFQ056
AFQ056 is a novel subtype selective inhibitor of mGluR5. The development of dyskinesia has been linked to increased glutamatergic signaling in the basal ganglia from the striatum. By inhibiting this receptor, there is a reduction in postsynaptic excitability and the potentiation of N-methyl-D-aspartic acid (NMDA). Reduction

and downregulation of this transmission have been shown to alleviate dyskinesia (27). Medications with similar mechanisms of action of blocking NMDA receptors, such as amantadine, have been used throughout the course of PD treatment for their antiglutamatergic effect, but are often limited by their cognitive and psychiatric side effects (22). Alternative ways of achieving this effect in the glutamatergic pathway have led to investigations of AFQ056.

A review of two multicenter, double-blind, placebo-controlled trials of AFQ056 conducted in patients on levodopa therapy with dyskinesia support these data. In both studies the medication was titrated over 16 days to 150 mg twice a day in patients only taking levodopa. The medication was given 1 hour prior to their levodopa dose and 1.5 hours before a meal. The second study continued to 20 days and on days 17–20 the drug was gradually tapered (27). Overall, both studies showed a significant reduction in dyskinesia when measured by the Abnormal Involuntary Movement Scale (AIMS) and the Lang–Fahn Activities of Daily Living Dyskinesia scale without any increase in motor symptoms measured by the motor section of the UPDRS. The medication was generally well tolerated with the highest reported adverse effect being dizziness as well as worsening dyskinesia when the medication was lowered and stopped. Some patients also showed improved symptoms even at doses lower than 150 mg twice a day (14).

NOVEL AGENTS WITH UNIQUE MECHANISMS OF ACTION

The agents discussed below are either medications that are established for other diseases, such as hypertension and diabetes, or experimental therapies looking at modifying the disease process on a cellular level. Whether an established treatment revisited and focused through the lens of neurodegenerative disease or a truly novel gene therapy, what all the agents have in common is they are being looked at not for symptomatic control of PD but as potential neuroprotective and neuro-restorative treatments, which the current treatment paradigm is lacking.

Isradipine

Isradipine is a dyhydropyridine and an established antihypertensive agent, which blocks L-type calcium channels. Animal studies have shown that elevations of intracellular Ca^{2+} can be deleterious and there is a high density of these channels in the substantia nigra pars compacta. Influx of Ca^{2+} can increase mitochondrial oxidant stress in the substantia nigra pars compacta (29). Blocking L-type Ca channels by systemic administration of dyhydropryidines showed a protective effect to substantia nigra pars compacta neurons with both acute and chronic challenges of MPTP as well as intrastriatal 6-hydroxydopamine (6-OHDA). When mice were injected with 6-OHDA without the co-administration of isradipine, the striatal fiber density was decreased by 90% and the dopaminergic neurons in the substantia nigra pars compacta by 75% within 25 days when compared with the mice that had been given doses of isradipine (30). Studies have shown that the type of dyhydropyridine administered makes a difference. For example, nifedipine does not have the bioavailability or the selectivity of isradipine. Isradipine has a more than 40-fold affinity for the Cav1.3 subtype of the L-type Ca^{2+}, which is the specific subtype localized to the substantia nigra. Neuroprotection was dose dependent and the amount measured in the brain tissue (between 13 and 15 nM) was in the range approved for treatment of hypertension (30).

Because of this potential for neuroprotection, studies are being conducted to monitor the safety and tolerability of isradipine in early PD patients. The biggest concern with this medication is the potential to worsen any fluctuations in blood pressure that may already be present in early PD. An open-label dose escalation study found that after 12 weeks of slow titration by 5 mg each week up to a dose of 20 mg, most patients felt adverse effects above 10 mg. The most common adverse effect was leg edema and dizziness; precipitous drops in blood pressure were not seen. The doses of 10 mg or below were best tolerated and consistent with recommended dosing for antihypertensive treatment, which would allow for appropriate penetration across the blood–brain barrier (31).

PYM50028

PYM50028 is a novel, orally active nonpeptide neurotrophic factor inducer. It has been shown to increase striatal levels of brain-derived neurotrophic factor (BDNF) and glial cell line-derived neurotrophic factor (GDNF). BDNF and GDNF are of interest because previous studies have shown that they can be neuroprotective to dopaminergic neurons as their receptors are expressed in the cell bodies of the substantia nigra and in the regions targeted by those neurons. In animal studies, direct administration of these factors have shown neuronal protection, but administration to human brain tissue has been challenging. Studies in transplanted neural progenitor cells, intrastriatal grafting, and intrathecal administration have not been successful or due to their surgical nature not applicable to some patients.

PYM50028 is orally administered and when tested in both in vivo and in vitro models at 10 mg/kg/day for 60 days, an increase in GDNF by 297% and in BDNF by 511% was obtained. The in vitro tests of mesencephalic neurons were pretreated for 24 hours with PYM50028 and when exposed to 1-methyl-4-phenylpyridinium (MPP+) there was only a neuronal loss of 4% as compared with 45% in the untreated specimen. In the in vivo test, mice treated with MPTP and oral PYM50028, dopamine transporter (DAT) binding was restored to 94% and not significantly different from the non-MPTP lesioned mice. The study also showed that when there was a delay in administering PYM50028, a restorative effect on the dopamine neurons was still seen (32). The mechanism of PYM50028 is unknown. In addition to its oral administration, it is also unique in that it has been shown to decrease damage to both cell body and terminal regions of the dopaminergic neurons on the nigrostriatal pathway. Evidence suggests that it may not only be protective but may potentially reverse early neuronal damage (32).

Pioglitazone

Pioglitazone, trade name Actos®, is a peroxisome proliferator-activated receptor (PPAR) agonist used in diabetic patients to increase insulin sensitization and modulate glucose (33). It is now being looked at through a new lens to see if it can play a role in a neurodegenerative disease such as PD by modulating neuroinflammation and oxidation toxicity. Excitotoxicity, oxidative phosphorylation, neuroinflammation, and the production of reactive oxygen species are important cell death mediators and such oxidative stress has been linked to dopaminergic neuronal death (34). The idea of anti-inflammatory use for possible neuroprotection in PD is not new and studies have looked into Cox-2 inhibitors and ibuprofen. Studies have looked at PPAR-γ and shown an anti-inflammatory and antioxidative effect, which is promising given the high density of this receptor in the striatum, substantia nigra pars compacta, cortex, and hippocampus (34). In vitro studies of MPTP model brains have also shown a decrease in dopaminergic neuronal damage theoretically linked to the mechanism of decreasing nitric oxide synthase expression and microglia inactivation. Doses of 5, 15, and 30 mg/kg of pioglitazone were tested in rat models and benefits were seen at the 30 mg/kg dose after one administration. Chronic use over 22 days did not produce the same benefits. Studies have also looked at potential cognitive benefits, but results have been inconclusive (34,35). Studies in MPTP-treated rhesus monkeys showed similar neuroprotective results at an orally administered 5 mg/kg dose (33). Animal studies have prompted a phase II clinical trial, Pioglitazone in Early Parkinson's Disease (FS-ZONE). Newly diagnosed PD patients are randomized to placebo or drug at doses of 15 and 45 mg over a 44-week period looking at attenuating clinical decline (36).

Gene Therapies
Both AAV2-GAD and AAV2-NTN gene therapies utilize a vector gene delivery system with adeno-associated virus (AAV2). AAV2 has advantages over other vectors in that it is nonpathogenic to humans, it is not associated with any disease or clinical symptoms, it is stripped of its own genes and cannot replicate, it does not enter the host chromosome and does not induce an inflammatory response (37). The potential of gene therapies lie in their potential for restoring degenerating dopaminergic neurons. They may also be a treatment option for advanced PD patients for whom traditional oral medical therapy has failed or produced limiting side effects and surgical therapies are not appropriate (38). The challenge of gene therapy is transferring the success seen in early animal models to the PD patient.

AAV2-GAD
Gene therapy with AAV2-GAD has been studied in animal models and humans. It is the only gene therapy that has substantiated the results of prior open-label trials and animal models through a recent randomized, double-blind, sham surgery study of 45 patients (23 sham surgery/22 gene therapy). Gene therapy consisting of insertion of glutamic acid decarboxylase (GAD) into the subthalamic nucleus provides the rate-limiting enzyme for GABA production. GABA is the neurotransmitter that inhibits the subthalamic nucleus in the normal state, and as dopaminergic neurons degenerate and the striato-pallidal circuitry is disrupted, the disinhibition of the subthalamic nucleus leads to the symptoms of PD. Treatments that reestablish that inhibition can help with some parkinsonian symptoms (38). In animal models, two isoforms of GAD were found to be beneficial. GAD67 improved motor function and GAD65 was found to be neuroprotective and a combination of the two was surgically infused into the bilateral subthalamic nucleus of PD patients with a motor UPDRS score of 25 or higher. The surgery consisted of creating a burr hole and inserting a catheter to the target of the STN. Once in place, the gene therapy was infused once over the course of 2.5 hours. At the end of six months the AAV2-GAD-treated patients showed an improvement of 8.1 points on their UPDRS motor score and an improvement in on–off fluctuations, with no changes to their medication regimens. There were no changes seen in cognition, activities of daily living, or dyskinesia (38).

AAV2-NTN
AAV2-NTN, also called CERE-120 or neurturin (NTN), has been studied extensively in rodent and nonhuman primate models and has shown promise for preserving

motor function and being neuroprotective. A double-blind, randomized, sham surgery study was not able to reproduce these initial findings and further examination of the differences between primate and human brains may lead to redesigned future studies. Neurotrophic factors can potentially stop or slow the degenerative process and alter the natural course of disease progression. Neurons in the substantia nigra pars compacta are exquisitely sensitive to GDNF and its naturally occurring analogue NTN, which have been shown to enhance dopaminergeic neuron survival and function in animal models of PD (37). NTN was ultimately chosen over GDNF for its ease of administration through just a stereotaxic injection in a single surgical setting without the need for chronically implanted catheters. In five MPTP-treated monkeys monitored over 10 months, all but one showed complete recovery of motor performance and on pathology showed enhancement and increased density of striatal tyrosine hydroxylase immunoreactive nigral neurons indicating a restorative effect to dopaminergic neurons (37). The one primate who did not have as robust a response was found to have poorly localized injections, which further supports the results of specific targeted areas of the caudate, putamen, and substantia nigra.

The results of the animal models and an open-label safety trial were the foundation for a multicenter, randomized, sham surgery trial, which unfortunately did not show the same results at 12 months, but at 18 months the AAV2-NTN-treated group was associated with a modest but significant benefit in motor score and secondary endpoints, such as dyskinesia and a timed motor test (39). Further examinations of the nuances between primate and human anatomy and pathophysiology of PD give plausible explanations to the discrepancies. Most notably, retrograde transport of the gene therapy seems to be impaired in human patients and not in primates, which allowed for the gene therapy to reach the targeted areas of the putamen and then substantia nigra effectively in the primates. This impaired retrograde transport may be the result of a number of factors. One may be the significant lack of dopaminergic neurons in advanced PD. Another may be that several gene mutations linked to PD (parkin, PINK1, DJ-1, and LRRK) are known to impair mitochondrial energy function, and axonal transport is highly energy dependent. Additionally, some α-synuclein mutations have been associated with impaired axonal transport. This suggests that targeting only the striatal terminal fields is insufficient for achieving clinical benefits (40). Further studies will look at targeting both degenerating cell bodies directly as well as their terminal field (i.e., the substantia nigra and the striatum).

TREATMENT FOR NONMOTOR SYMPTOMS

Droxidopa has been used for the treatment of neurogenic orthostatic hypotension in the setting of congenital dopamine beta hydroxylase deficiency with symptomatic improvement. Orthostatic hypotension is caused by a deficiency in norepinephrine, which is a product of the dopamine metabolic pathway. Levodopa is broken down by aromatic-L-amino acid decarboxylase into dopamine, which is then broken down by dopamine-beta-hydroxylase (the rate-limiting step) into norepinephrine. Droxidopa is unique in that it is analogous to levodopa with the addition of a hydroxyl group that allows it to bypass the rate-limiting step and be broken down by aromatic-L-amino acid decarboxylase directly into norepinephrine (41).

Orthostatic hypotension is a problem in many parkinsonian disorders and droxidopa studies looked at symptomatic relief in patients with multiple system atrophy (MSA). Doses ranging from 200 to 1200 mg were used based on patient tolerance and orthostatic blood pressures. Results showed an increase in supine and standing blood pressure as well as an increase in circulating norepinephrine as early as 1 hour after the dose was administered, and lasting 6 hours without significant change in heart rate. There was clear symptomatic improvement in orthostasis, with less lightheadedness and a reported overall feeling of being able to stand longer. Actual differences in blood pressure were not provided.

The concern for PD patients in taking droxidopa is the use of carbidopa, which as an inhibitor of aromatic-L-amino acid decarboxylase, could inactivate the droxidopa. A study looked at administering droxidopa along with carbidopa 200 mg, which resulted in no effect on blood pressure. Carbidopa at lower doses, such as the doses used in combination with levodopa, do not have the same effect on the medication, and therefore this may be an option for treating neurogenic orthostatic hypotension in PD patients (41).

CONCLUSION

Research into innovative treatments for PD is flourishing. There are novel therapies, surgeries and drug delivery systems being investigated and some are very near approval for the practical care for our patients. Research continues to investigate treatments for symptomatic relief, but even more exciting is the research investigating possible disease modifying therapies. Continued collaboration of academic, private, and government resources will help propel this forward thinking momentum and one day lead to a cure.

ACKNOWLEGMENTS

We thank Dr. Nicole Dietz and Dr. Ishita Gambhir for reviewing this manuscript with the same discerning eye and thoughtful attention to detail they bring to patient care.

REFERENCES

1. Devos D; French DUODOPA Study Group. Patient profile, indications, efficacy and safety of duodenal levodopa infusion in advanced Parkinson's disease. Mov Disord 2009; 24: 993–1000.
2. Fahn S, Oakes D, Shoulson I, et al. Levodopa and the progression of Parkinson's disease. N Engl J Med 2004; 351: 2498–508.
3. Hauser RA, Ellenbogen AL, Metman LV, et al. Crossover comparison of IPX066 and a standard levodopa formulation in advanced Parkinson's disease. Mov Disord 2011; 26: 2246–52.
4. Hauser RA, Cantillon M, Pourcher E, et al. Preladenant in patients with Parkinson's disease and motor fluctuations: a phase 2, double-blind, randomised trial. Lancet Neurol 2011; 10: 221–9.
5. Klostermann F, Jugel C, Marzinzik F. Jejunal levodopa infusion in long-term DBS patients with Parkinson's disease. Mov Disord 2011; 26: 2298–9.
6. Fernandez HH, Odin P. Levodopa-carbidopa intestinal gel for treatment of advanced Parkinson's disease. Curr Med Res Opin 2011; 27: 907–19.
7. Xenoport announces positive results of a phase 1 clinical trial. [Available from: http://www.drugs.com/clinical_trials/xenoport-announces-positive-results-phase-1-clinical-trial-xp21279-3559.html]

8. Hauser RA. Future treatments for Parkinson's disease surfing the PD pipeline. Int J Neurosci 2011; 121: 53–62.
9. Nyholm D, Constantinescu R, Holmberg B, Dizdar N, Askmark H. Comparison of apomorphine and levodopa infusions in four patients with Parkinson's disease with symptom fluctuations. Acta Neurol Scand 2009; 119: 345–8.
10. Garcia Ruiz PJ, Sesar Ignacio A, Ares Pensado B, et al. Efficacy of long-term continuous subcutaneous apomorphine infusion in advanced Parkinson's disease with motor fluctuations: a multicenter study. Mov Disord 2008; 23: 1130–6.
11. Sampaio C, Bronzova J, Hauser RA, et al. Pardoprunox in early Parkinson's disease: results from 2 large, randomized double-blind trials. Mov Disord 2011; 26: 1464–76.
12. Rascol O, Bronzova J, Hauser RA, et al. Pardoprunox as adjunct therapy to levodopa in patients with Parkinson's disease experiencing motor fluctuations: Results of a double-blind, randomized, placebo-controlled, trial. Parkinsonism Relat Disord 2012; 18: 370–6.
13. Stocchi F, Borgohain R, Onofrj M, et al. A randomized, double-blind, placebo-controlled trial of safinamide as add-on therapy in early Parkinson's disease patients. Mov Disord 2011; 27: 106–12.
14. Stocchi F, Arnold G, Onofrj M, et al. Improvement of motor function in early Parkinson disease by safinamide. Neurology 2004; 63: 746–8.
15. Schapira AH. Safinamide in the treatment of Parkinson's disease. Expert Opin Pharmacother 2010; 11: 2261–8.
16. Hodgson RA, Bedard PJ, Varty GB, et al. Preladenant, a selective A(2A) receptor antagonist, is active in primate models of movement disorders. Exp Neurol 2010; 225: 384–90.
17. Factor S, Mark MH, Watts R, et al. A long-term study of istradefylline in subjects with fluctuating Parkinson's disease. Parkinsonism Relat Disord 2010; 16: 423–6.
18. Pourcher E, Fernandez HH, Stacy M, et al. Istradefylline for Parkinson's disease patients experiencing motor fluctuations: results of the KW-6002-US-018 study. Parkinsonism Relat Disord 2011; 18: 178–84.
19. LeWitt PA, Guttman M, Tetrud JW, et al. Adenosine A2A receptor antagonist istradefylline (KW-6002) reduces "off" time in Parkinson's disease: a double-blind, randomized, multicenter clinical trial (6002-US-005). Ann Neurol 2008; 63: 295–302.
20. Hauser RA, Shulman LM, Trugman JM, et al. Study of istradefylline in patients with Parkinson's disease on levodopa with motor fluctuations. Mov Disord 2008; 23: 2177–85.
21. Mizuno Y, Hasegawa K, Kondo T, Kuno S, Yamamoto M; Japanese Istradefylline Study Group. Clinical efficacy of istradefylline (KW-6002) in Parkinson's disease: a randomized, controlled study. Mov Disord 2010; 25: 1437–43.
22. Gregoire L, Morin N, Ouattara B, et al. The acute antiparkinsonian and antidyskinetic effect of AFQ056, a novel metabotropic glutamate receptor type 5 antagonist, in L-Dopa-treated parkinsonian monkeys. Parkinsonism Relat Disord 2011; 17: 270–6.
23. Adamas pharmaceuticals. [Available from: http://www.adamaspharma.com/products/parkinsonsdisease.html]
24. Extended release Amantadine safety and efficacy in Levodopa-induced Dyskinesias. [Available from: http://www.pdtrials.org/en/browse/all/view/320]
25. Study of ADX48621 for the treatment of Levodopa-Induced Dyskinesia in people with Parkinson's disease. [Available from: http://www.pdtrials.org/en/browse/all/view/321]
26. Addex pharmaceuticals. [Available from: http://www.addespharma.com/key-indications/dipraglurant/]
27. Berg D, Godau J, Trenkwalder C, et al. AFQ056 treatment of levodopa-induced dyskinesias: results of 2 randomized controlled trials. Mov Disord 2011; 26: 1243–50.
28. Addex pharmaceuticals. [Available from: http://www.addespharma.com]
29. Chan CS, Gertler TS, Surmeier DJ. A molecular basis for the increased vulnerability of substantia nigra dopamine neurons in aging and Parkinson's disease. Mov Disord 2010; 25: S63–70.
30. Ilijic E, Guzman JN, Surmeier DJ. The L-type channel antagonist isradipine is neuroprotective in a mouse model of Parkinson's disease. Neurobiol Dis 2011; 43: 364–71.
31. Simuni T, Borushko E, Avram MJ, et al. Tolerability of isradipine in early Parkinson's disease: a pilot dose escalation study. Mov Disord 2010; 25: 2863–6.

32. Visanji NP, Orsi A, Johnston TH, et al. PYM50028, a novel, orally active, nonpeptide neurotrophic factor inducer, prevents and reverses neuronal damage induced by MPP+ in mesencephalic neurons and by MPTP in a mouse model of Parkinson's disease. FASEB J 2008; 22: 2488–97.

33. Swanson CR, Joers V, Bondarenko V, et al. The PPAR-gamma agonist pioglitazone modulates inflammation and induces neuroprotection in parkinsonian monkeys. J Neuroinflammation 2011; 8: 91.

34. Barbiero JK, Santiago RM, Lima MM, et al. Acute but not chronic administration of pioglitazone promoted behavioral and neurochemical protective effects in the MPTP model of Parkinson's disease. Behav Brain Res 2011; 216: 186–92.

35. Kumar P, Kaundal RK, More S, Sharma SS. Beneficial effects of pioglitazone on cognitive impairment in MPTP model of Parkinson's disease. Behav Brain Res 2009; 197: 398–403.

36. Pioglitazone in early Parkinson's disease. [Available from: http://www.pdtrials.org/en/browse/all/view/317]

37. Kordower JH, Herzog CD, Dass B, et al. Delivery of neurturin by AAV2 (CERE-120)-mediated gene transfer provides structural and functional neuroprotection and neurorestoration in MPTP-treated monkeys. Ann Neurol 2006; 60: 706–15.

38. LeWitt PA, Rezai AR, Leehey MA, et al. AAV2-GAD gene therapy for advanced Parkinson's disease: a double-blind, sham-surgery controlled, randomised trial. Lancet Neurol 2011; 10: 309–19.

39. Marks WJ Jr, Bartus RT, Siffert J, et al. Gene delivery of AAV2-neurturin for Parkinson's disease: a double-blind, randomised, controlled trial. Lancet Neurol 2010; 9: 1164–72.

40. Bartus RT, Herzog CD, Chu Y, et al. Bioactivity of AAV2-neurturin gene therapy (CERE-120): differences between Parkinson's disease and nonhuman primate brains. Mov Disord 2011; 26: 27–36.

41. Kaufmann H. L-dihydroxyphenylserine (Droxidopa): a new therapy for neurogenic orthostatic hypotension: the US experience. Clin Auton Res 2008; 18: 19–24.

24

Deep brain stimulation

Kelly E. Lyons, Jules M. Nazzaro, and Rajesh Pahwa

Stereotactic surgeries for movement disorders were introduced in the late 1940s (1–3) but were not widely accepted due to significant morbidity, mortality, and limited knowledge of the appropriate target for symptomatic benefit. With advancements in pharmacological therapy, particularly the availability of levodopa, these surgeries were rarely performed for Parkinson's disease (PD) until the late 1980s (4). Based on the limitations of drug treatments for PD, and a better understanding of the physiology and circuitry of the basal ganglia there has been a marked increase in surgical therapies for PD. In addition, advances in surgical techniques, neuroimaging and improved electrophysiological recordings allow stereotactic procedures to be done more accurately leading to reduced morbidity. Deep brain stimulation (DBS) has largely replaced ablative surgery as the preferred surgical treatment for PD. There are currently three potential brain targets for the treatment of PD: the ventral intermediate (Vim) nucleus of the thalamus, the globus pallidus interna (GPi), and the subthalamic nucleus (STN).

HISTORY

There is an extensive neurosurgical history regarding stereotactic ablative procedures for PD (5,6). Prior to DBS, the lesioning procedures, thalamotomy and pallidotomy, were performed as the surgical treatment of choice for PD. Using the Hassler thalamic nomenclature (7,8), lesions for PD were initially directed to the ventral lateral thalamic nuclei and focused on the ventral oralis anterior (Voa), ventral oralis posterior (Vop), and the Vim (9). Ultimately, the thalamic procedure of choice for parkinsonian tremor was radiofrequency lesioning within the Vim and significant and lasting tremor control was reported in the majority of PD patients (10). Vim thalamotomy, however, resulted in little benefit for parkinsonian signs and symptoms other than tremor, did not treat drug-induced dyskinesia and did not lower dopaminergic medication requirements (11). Furthermore, only unilateral procedures were recommended, as bilateral Vim thalamotomy was associated with significant permanent morbidity, particularly with regard to speech, swallowing, and balance (12).

In order to treat all of the cardinal symptoms of PD as well as motor fluctuations and dyskinesia, attention turned to other basal ganglia sites. Pallidotomy, directed to the GPi, became the surgical treatment of choice for PD and was associated with lasting improvements in drug-induced dyskinesia as well as significant improvements in bradykinesia, rigidity, and tremor (13–15). However, the benefits were primarily contralateral to the lesion, and bilateral pallidotomy was rarely performed given the risk of significant lasting neurological morbidity with bilateral procedures.

A primary limitation of ablative surgery is that the surgical lesions are irreversible and permanent neurological deficits with both unilateral and bilateral thalamotomy and pallidotomy procedures were reported in many patients (16–18). Lesioning of other sites, such as the STN, is rarely performed given the risk of hemiballism (19,20). In the course of stereotactic surgeries, to help ensure therapeutic efficacy and safety during ablative procedures, many neurosurgeons obtained anatomic definition using stimulation prior to lesion creation. During thalamotomy, it was noted that stimulation above 100 Hz within the Vim resulted in tremor relief (4). These observations led investigators to implant stimulating electrodes in the Vim for tremor control rather than lesioning the area (4,21,22). Subsequently, stimulating electrodes were implanted within the GPi and STN and were found to improve the cardinal symptoms of PD, including tremor, bradykinesia, and rigidity, as well as levodopa-induced motor fluctuations and dyskinesia (23,24). Stimulating electrodes afforded the option of adjusting stimulation parameters based on clinical response and adverse events. If the electrode placement is suboptimal in location, electrode revision is an option. Furthermore, operations in which stimulating electrodes were implanted within the GPi or STN, including bilateral procedures, were much better tolerated than ablative procedures. With these developments, bilateral DBS of the GPi and STN largely replaced pallidotomy as the most commonly performed surgical treatment for PD.

DEEP BRAIN STIMULATION HARDWARE

The Activa® Tremor Control and the Activa® Parkinson Control therapies (Medtronic, Minneapolis, Minnesota, U.S.A.) are approved in the United States, Europe, and multiple other countries for the treatment of PD. Libra® and LibraXP™ systems (St. Jude Medical, St. Paul, Minnesota, U.S.A.) have been approved in Europe, Australia, and other countries outside the United States for DBS in PD patients. The DBS therapies consist of a DBS lead, an implantable pulse generator (IPG) that is the power source for the system, and an extension wire that connects the DBS lead to the IPG. There are two DBS leads available in the United States. The intracranial end of both leads has four platinum–iridium contacts each of which is 1.5 mm in length. One lead has contacts that are separated by 1.5 mm (Model 3387, Medtronic, Minneapolis, Minnesota, U.S.A.) and the second lead has contacts that are separated by 0.5 mm (Model 3389, Medtronic, Minneapolis, Minnesota, U.S.A.). The DBS leads are connected to the IPG by an extension wire that is tunneled under the skin down the neck to the IPG, which is generally placed in the infraclavicular area. The DBS leads are implanted stereotactically while the patient is awake and the extension wire and IPG are implanted under general anesthesia.

There are two constant voltage IPGs available in the United States, the single-channel Soletra (Medtronic, Inc, Minneapolis, Minnesota, U.S.A.) and the dual-channel Kinetra (Medtronic, Inc, Minneapolis, Minnesota, U.S.A.). In the setting of a dual-channel IPG, one neurostimulator may be utilized to control the DBS leads for both sides of the body, instead of two separate single-channel neurostimulators, one for each side. The single-channel SC and the dual-channel PC IPG models (Medtronic, Inc, Minneapolis, Minnesota, U.S.A.) have become available and are largely replacing the respective earlier models. The new IPGs afford further programming and stimulation options including stimulation using constant current or constant voltage and options such as monopolar stimulation at two lead-contacts of the same lead or monopolar stimulation at one lead-contact and bipolar stimulation using two other lead-contacts along the same lead (interleaving). When using the interleaving method, stimulation is delivered in an alternating manner between the respective configurations. In addition, a dual-channel rechargeable (RC) IPG (Medtronic, Inc, Minneapolis, Minnesota, U.S.A.) is also available. The RC has the same programming options as the PC. Factors influencing which IPG to use include surgeon, neurologist, and patient preference; cost of the different models; the individual patient's stimulation requirements; and the ability to maintain a rechargeable unit. All of the neurostimulators can be programmed for monopolar or bipolar stimulation. Adjustable parameters include pulse width, amplitude, stimulation frequency, and the choice of active contacts. The patient can turn the stimulator on or off using a hand-held therapy controller, which also has a feature to tell the patient if the neurostimulator is on or off and a feature to change the stimulation settings based on preset programming parameters. The typical stimulation parameters are frequency of 135 to 185 Hz, pulse width of 60–120 microseconds and amplitude of 1–3.5 V.

ADVANTAGES AND DISADVANTAGES OF DBS
The advantages of DBS compared with those of ablative surgeries include no destructive lesion in the brain, the ability to adjust stimulation parameters to increase efficacy or reduce adverse effects, the performance of bilateral procedures with increased safety and reduced adverse effects, and the reversibility of the system to accommodate the potential use of future therapies. The disadvantages include cost of the system, time and effort involved in programming the system, repeat surgeries related to device complications, use of general anesthesia for IPG and extension wire implantation, and battery replacement every 3–6 years for the nonrechargeable models and approximately 9 years with the rechargeable model.

DEEP BRAIN STIMULATION OF THE THALAMUS
In 1997, the United States Food and Drug Administration (FDA) approved unilateral Vim DBS as adjuvant therapy in advanced PD and essential tremor patients for the treatment of contralateral upper extremity tremor. The therapy was approved in Europe, Canada, and other countries in 1995. Vim DBS has largely replaced thalamotomy as the preferred surgery for the treatment of medication-resistant tremor. There are multiple reports demonstrating a significant reduction in tremor in 63–95% of patients receiving thalamic DBS for parkinsonian tremor (22,25–27); however, currently it is rarely used for PD as the majority of the studies have reported that although tremor is markedly improved, other PD symptoms continue to progress and cause significant disability (12,28). Therefore, this procedure is restricted to PD patients whose primary disability is tremor.

Several studies have demonstrated long-term benefit in PD tremor with thalamic DBS. Pollak and colleagues reported 80 PD patients who had DBS of the thalamus for drug-resistant tremor (29). After up to seven years of follow-up (mean three years) global evaluations showed the best control for parkinsonian rest tremor and the least satisfactory control for action tremor. There was no dramatic effect on other symptoms such as bradykinesia, rigidity, or dyskinesia. Lyons et al. (28) reported the results of 12 PD patients with a mean follow-up of 40 months and a maximum follow-up of 66 months. Although tremor scores continued to be improved by 87% there was a worsening of Unified Parkinson's Disease Rating Scale (UPDRS) motor scores suggesting the worsening of other parkinsonian symptoms. Finally, Pahwa and colleagues (12) reported a multicenter trial of 19 PD patients who received thalamic DBS (11 unilateral, eight bilateral) and were followed up to five years after surgery. There was a mean improvement in tremor of 85% in the targeted limb for the unilaterally operated patients and for bilaterally operated patients there was a 100% improvement in tremor on the left side and 90% on the right side. However, there were no improvements in symptoms other than tremor in unilateral or bilateral implanted patients and in bilateral implanted patients, therapeutic efficacy was limited due to a high rate of adverse events particularly with regard to dysphagia, dysarthria, and incoordination. It was concluded that thalamic DBS has limited use in the surgical treatment of PD.

DEEP BRAIN STIMULATION OF THE GLOBUS PALLIDUS INTERNA

In 2002, the U.S. FDA approved bilateral GPi DBS as adjuvant therapy in advanced PD. The therapy was approved earlier in Europe, Canada, and other countries. Surgery targeting the internal segment of the globus pallidus has been shown to improve all of the cardinal features of PD, including bradykinesia, rigidity, and tremor as well as levodopa-induced dyskinesia. Due to concerns of complications related to speech, balance, and cognition with bilateral pallidal lesions, bilateral DBS of the GPi is preferred to pallidotomy. Multiple studies have reported the efficacy of GPi stimulation for PD (Table 24.1) (30–41).

Kumar et al. (30) reported 22 PD patients who were treated with either unilateral ($n = 5$) or bilateral ($n = 17$) GPi stimulation. Evaluations performed in the medication off/stimulation on state at six months reported a 32% improvement in UPDRS motor scores and a 40% improvement in UPDRS activities of daily living (ADL) scores compared with baseline medication off scores. There was also a 68% reduction in dyskinesia. The DBS for Parkinson's Disease Study Group reported a multinational, prospective study of bilateral GPi stimulation in PD (31). Forty-one patients were enrolled, electrodes were implanted in 38 patients, and 36 were reported at six months. In comparison to baseline, there was a significant improvement of 33% in UPDRS motor scores in the medication off/stimulation on state. More specifically, tremor was reduced by 59%, rigidity was reduced by 31%, bradykinesia was reduced by 26%, gait improved by 35%, and postural instability improved by 36%. The patients' diaries revealed that the percentage of on time without dyskinesia increased from 28% to 64% and daily off time was reduced from 37% to 24%. The mean daily dose in levodopa equivalents was unchanged between baseline and six months.

Several studies have examined the long-term benefits of DBS of the GPi (Table 24.1). Lyons and colleagues (36) reported nine patients (three unilateral, six bilateral) with a mean follow-up of 48.5 months (range, 25–81 months) after GPi DBS. There was a significant improvement in the UPDRS ADL scores of 21% and a 37% improvement in the UPDRS motor scores. Dyskinesia were reduced by 64% and there were no significant reductions in antiparkinsonian medications. Rodriguez-Oroz et al. (37) reported three- to four-year results of a subset of 20 patients in a the multicenter Deep Brain Stimulation Study Group study (31) who

TABLE 24.1   Selected Studies of Deep Brain Stimulation of the Globus Pallidus Interna

| Author | No. of Patients | Follow-Up (Months) | UPDRS Improvement[a] | | Dyskinesia[b] (%) |
			ADL (%)	Motor (%)	
Kumar et al. (30)	17 (B)/5 (U)	6	40	32	68
DBSPDSG (31)[c]	36 (B)	6	36	33	67
Rodriguez-Oroz et al. (37)[c]	20 (B)	12	32	43	72
	20 (B)	36–48	28	39	76
Moro et al. (41)[c]	16 (B)	60–72	37	36	75
Rodrigues et al. (39)	7 (B)/4 (U)	7	—	46 (B)/18 (U)	76
Volkmann et al. (32)	11 (B)	12	42	68	80
Loher et al. (33)	9 (U)	12	33	38	55
	10 (B)	12	34	41	71
Anderson et al. (34)	10 (B)	12	18	39	89
Follett et al. (40)	152 (B)	24	17	28	73
Ghika et al. (35)	6 (B)	24–30	68	50	65
Lyons et al. (36)	6 (B)/3 (U)	25–81	21	37	64
Volkmann et al. (38)	10 (B)	12	49	55	58
	9 (B)	36	26	49	63
	6 (B)	60	−1.5	23	64

[a]%Improvement from baseline medication off state to medication off/stimulation on at follow-up.
[b]%Reduction in dyskinesia from baseline.
[c]Patients from same cohort.
Abbreviations: UPDRS, Unified Parkinson's Disease Rating Scale; ADL, activities of daily living; DBSPDSG, Deep Brain Stimulation for Parkinson's Disease Study Group; B, bilateral; U, unilateral.

received bilateral GPi DBS. Significant improvements in UPDRS ADL and motor scores in the medication off/stimulation on condition compared with the baseline medication off state were maintained. More specifically, at the three- to four-year visit, there were significant improvements in tremor (85%), rigidity (38%), bradykinesia (30%), gait (28%), and dyskinesia (76%) compared with baseline and there was no significant worsening compared with the one-year visit. At this follow-up, levodopa equivalents were actually increased by 344 mg/day. Moro et al. (41) reported data from the five- to six-year follow-up of 16 of the 20 PD patients included in the Rodriguez-Oroz study (37). There was a 37% improvement in UPDRS ADL scores at five- to six-years with medication off/stimulation on compared with medication off at baseline and a 36% improvement in UPDRS motor scores. Tremor (66%) and rigidity (42%) scores were the only subscores of the UPDRS significantly improved at the five- to six-year follow-up compared with baseline. UPDRS ADL scores remained stable compared with the thee- to four-year follow-up. Dyskinesia remained significantly improved compared with baseline, and levodopa equivalence units were not changed compared with baseline.

In contrast, some studies have shown a loss of effect of GPi DBS over time. Ghika et al. (35) reported six PD patients with a minimum follow-up of 24 months after GPi DBS. The mean improvement in UPDRS motor scores in the medication off/stimulation on state compared with the baseline medication off condition was 50% and for UPDRS ADL scores it was 68%. Mean daily off time decreased from 40% to 10% and dyskinesia was reduced by 65%. Although the improvements persisted beyond two years after surgery, signs of decreased efficacy were seen after 12 months. Volkmann et al. (38) reported long-term outcomes of bilateral GPi DBS 12, 36, and 60 months after surgery (Table 24.1). UPDRS motor scores were significantly improved in the medication off/stimulation on condition compared with baseline by 55% at 12 months and 43% at 36 months. However, at 60 months there was a nonsignificant improvement of 23% compared with baseline. Similarly, for UPDRS ADL scores, at 12 months there was a significant improvement of 49% compared with baseline; however, a 26% improvement at 36 months was not significantly different from baseline and at 60 months there was a worsening of 1.5%. More specifically, at 12 months there was a significant improvement in bradykinesia, rigidity, tremor, and postural instability/gait, at 36 months there were significant improvements only in bradykinesia and postural instability/gait and by 60 months there was a significant improvement only in rigidity. In contrast, dyskinesia continued to be significantly improved throughout the five-year follow-up.

In summary, multiple studies have demonstrated the short-term benefits of GPi DBS in controlling the cardinal symptoms of PD and reducing dyskinesia. Results have been inconsistent regarding the long-term benefits in the cardinal symptoms of PD with GPi DBS. The majority of studies have shown continued significant improvement in the long term; however, the magnitude of benefit decreases in the majority of reports over time, which is likely confounded by continued disease progression and other comorbidities. There is, however, consensus regarding a significant and sustained reduction in levodopa-induced dyskinesia despite minimal if any reductions in antiparkinsonian medications. Further research is necessary to confirm the long-term benefits of GPi DBS.

DEEP BRAIN STIMULATION OF THE SUBTHALAMIC NUCLEUS

In 2002, the U.S. FDA approved bilateral STN DBS as adjuvant therapy in advanced PD. The therapy had been approved earlier in Europe, Canada, and other countries. Multiple reports have demonstrated the short-term benefits of STN DBS in controlling the cardinal features of PD and reducing dyskinesia and antiparkinsonian medications (31,40,42–49). One of the largest short-term studies was conducted by the Deep Brain Stimulation for Parkinson's Disease Study Group (31). This was a multicenter study in which 96 PD patients received bilateral STN DBS and 91 completed the six-month follow-up visit. In the medication off/stimulation on condition at six months compared with the baseline medication off condition there was a mean improvement of 44% in the UPDRS ADL scores and a 51% improvement in UPDRS motor scores. More specifically, tremor was improved by 79%, rigidity by 58%, bradykinesia by 42%, gait by 56%, and postural instability by 50%, all of which were significant improvements compared with baseline. According to patient diaries, there was a significant decrease in daily off time from 49% to 19%, a significant increase in on time without dyskinesia from 27% to 74% and a decrease in on time with dyskinesia from 23% to 7%. The Rush Dyskinesia Scale demonstrated a significant improvement in dyskinesia of 58% and antiparkinsonian medications were reduced an average of 37%.

Several studies have demonstrated the long-term benefits of STN DBS (Table 24.2) (37,50–60). Rodriguez-Oroz and colleagues (37) examined 49 PD patients, who received bilateral STN DBS as part of the original DBS for PD Study Group trial (31), three to four years after initial implant. They demonstrated a 43%

TABLE 24.2 Selected Studies of Bilateral Deep Brain Stimulation of the Subthalamic Nucleus

Author	No. of Patients	Follow-Up (Months)	UPDRS Improvement[a] ADL (%)	Motor (%)	Dyskinesia[b] (%)	Medications[b]
DBSPDSG (31)[c]	91	6	44	52	58	37
Rodriguez-Oroz	49	12	50	57	51	41
et al. (37)[c]	49	36–48	43	50	59	34
Moro et al. (41)[c]	35	60–72	49	51	83	30
Deuschl	71	6	39	41	54	49
et al. (68)						
Ostergaard	26	12	66	64	86	19
et al. (48)	22	48	55	42	90	29
Ostergaard						
et al. (56)						
Anderson	10	12	28	48	62	38
et al. (34)						
Follett et al. (40)	147	24	12	25	65	32
Kleiner-Fisman	25	24	26	39	66	42
et al. (53)						
Pahwa et al. (54)	19	28	27	28	Significant	57
Krause	24	30	17	44	70	30
et al. (51)						
Schupbach	32	24	57	69	86	63
et al. (50)	30	60	37	54	79	58
Krack et al. (55)	43	12	66	66	71	59
	42	36	51	59	71	63
	42	60	49	54	71	63
Piboolnurak	33	36	27	35	76	48
et al. (57)	17	60	22	35	76	40
Gervais-Bernard	23	12	57	61	85[d]	71
et al. (58)	23	60	38	55	60[d]	54
Kishore et al. (59)	45	12	48	51	73	38
	36	36	43	43	73	41
	29	60	38	39	66	48
Toft et al. (60)	131	12	—	53	—	49
	110	24	—	44	—	46
	89	36	—	37	—	46
	52	48	—	31	—	48
	32	60	—	26	—	47
Fasano	20	60	—	55	—	58
et al. (61)	20	96	—	39	—	60
Castrioto	18	12	33	43	50	46
et al. (62)	18	60	35	36	69	43
	18	120	24	23	63	36

[a]%Improvement from baseline medication off state to medication off/stimulation on at follow-up.
[b]%Reduction compared with baseline.
[c]Data from same cohort.
[d]Both motor fluctuations and dyskinesia.
Abbreviations: UPDRS, Unified Parkinson's Disease Rating Scale; ADL, activities of daily living; DBSPDSG, Deep Brain Stimulation for Parkinson's Disease Study Group.

improvement in UPDRS ADL scores and a 50% improvement in UPDRS motor scores in the medication off/stimulation on condition compared with the baseline medication off state. More specifically, there was an 87% improvement in tremor, a 59% improvement in rigidity, a 42% improvement in bradykinesia, a 41% improvement in gait, a 31% improvement in postural instability, a 59% reduction in dyskinesia, and a 34% reduction in levodopa at the three- to four-year follow-up compared with baseline. Compared with the one-year visit, at three to four years after implant there was a worsening in UPDRS ADL and motor scores, gait, postural instability, and speech in the medication off/stimulation on condition although other than speech which was never improved, they were all still significantly improved compared with the baseline medication off state. Moro et al. (41) reported the five- to six-year outcomes of 35 of these 49 patients. In these patients there was a 51% improvement in UPDRS motor scores with stimulation; however, this was a reduction in benefit compared with this group's scores at the three- to four-year follow-up. More specifically, compared with baseline there was an 81% improvement in tremor, 59% for rigidity, 31% for akinesia, 67% for postural instability, and 33% for gait. There was also a 49% improvement in UPDRS ADL scores compared with baseline.

Schüpbach et al. (50) examined 30 PD patients five years after STN DBS. They found that UPDRS ADL (37%) and motor scores (54%) as well as axial symptoms (43%) were significantly improved at five years in the medication off/stimulation on condition compared with the baseline medication off state. However, there was a significant worsening in each of these scores compared with the two-year assessment. Dyskinesia (79%) and levodopa equivalent dose (58%) were significantly reduced at five years and there were no significant changes in these variables throughout the five-year period. On the other hand, there was a significant worsening at five years in UPDRS mentation scores, Mattis Dementia Rating Scale scores and frontal scores compared with baseline. Similarly, Krack and colleagues (55) examined 42 PD patients 60 months after bilateral STN DBS. In the medication off/stimulation on condition compared with baseline there was a 54% improvement in UPDRS motor scores and a 49% improvement in UPDRS ADL scores. Significant improvements were seen for tremor (75%), rigidity (71%), akinesia (49%), postural instability (44%), gait (52%), writing (37%), and freezing (46%). Although significantly better than baseline, compared with the one-year visit, there was significant worsening in UPDRS motor and ADL scores, akinesia, gait, and freezing. However, there were sustained reductions in dyskinesia of 71% and daily levodopa equivalence dose of 63%.

Toft et al. (60) retrospectively reported 131 PD patients after STN DBS with an average follow-up of 3.3 years (range 1–7 years), including 32 with a five-year follow-up. At one year, there was a 53% improvement in UPDRS medication off/stimulation on motor scores compared with baseline medication off scores, whereas at 60 months this benefit had declined to 26%. They found that between one and five years after surgery, there was on average a worsening of 3.2 UPDRS motor points annually. On the other hand, reductions in levodopa equivalents were maintained over the course of the study.

Fasano and colleagues (61) reported 20 PD patients eight years after bilateral STN DBS. In the medication off/stimulation on condition, five years after surgery there was a significant improvement (55%) in UPDRS motor scores compared with baseline. Significant improvements were seen five years after surgery for resting tremor (93%), postural tremor (67%), bradykinesia (56%), rigidity (55%), gait (55%), and postural instability (41%). At eight years significant reductions were maintained in resting tremor (92%), postural tremor (48%), rigidity (46%), bradykinesia (34%), and gait (41%); however, postural instability worsened. Speech was not improved by the surgery and did not significantly change over the course of the study. Eight years after surgery, anxiety and depression scores did not significantly differ from baseline; however, verbal fluency was worsened as well as abstract reasoning, episodic memory, and executive function.

Castrioto et al. (62) examined 18 PD patients 10 years after bilateral STN DBS. They found that UPDRS motor scores (25%) as well as resting tremor (85%), action tremor (88%), and bradykinesia (23%) were significantly improved at 10 years in blinded assessments of the medication off/stimulation on condition compared with the medication off/stimulation off state. In unblinded assessments, UPDRS motor (23%), resting tremor (88%), action tremor (53%), and rigidity (41%) were significantly improved with medication off/stimulation on compared with preoperative baseline 10 years after surgery. However, there was a significant worsening in UPDRS motor score (23%) in comparison to the five-year assessment (36%). In the unblinded assessments, bradykinesia was significantly improved five years (30%) but not 10 years (8%) after surgery in the medication off/stimulation on state. Raising from a chair, posture, gait, axial signs, and postural stability were significantly improved one year but not five or 10 years after surgery. Levodopa equivalent dose was significantly reduced at 10 years (36%) and there were no significant changes following the one-year follow-up (46%). On the other hand, there was a significant worsening at 10 years in UPDRS ADL, freezing, speech, and falling scores compared with baseline. The authors concluded that stimulation-induced motor improvements were sustained long term, although initial benefit decreased in part due to progressive loss of benefit in axial signs.

One study has been reported using the St. Jude Medical constant-current DBS system (63) (all previously reported studies in the text and tables are based on data from Medtronic DBS systems). In this study, 136 PD patients were implanted with bilateral STN leads and randomized to either immediate stimulation ($n = 101$) or stimulation delayed for three months ($n = 35$). On time, as measured by patient diaries, was significantly more improved in the immediate stimulation group (4.3 hr/day) than in the group without active stimulation (1.8 hr/day). At three months, UPDRS motor scores were improved by 39%. Adverse events were comparable to those typically reported for DBS studies. Further research is necessary to examine the long-term outcomes using this DBS system.

In summary, STN DBS has consistently been shown to control the primary symptoms of PD, as well as dyskinesia while allowing a significant and long-term reduction in antiparkinsonian medications. The benefits of STN DBS have been reported in studies with follow-up durations ranging from six months to 10 years after surgery. Although there is some deterioration in benefit over time, this appears to be related to the natural progression of the disease, particularly the worsening of axial symptoms over time.

PREDICTORS OF OUTCOME AFTER STN DBS

Several studies have examined the factors predictive of a positive outcome after STN DBS (42,53,64–66). Charles et al. (64) examined 54 PD patients after bilateral

STN DBS and found that age and preoperative levodopa response were the strongest predictors of outcome. In a study of 41 PD patients who had STN DBS, Welter et al. (42) used regression analyses to identify age and disease duration as predictors of outcome. They found that patients 56 years or younger had a 71% improvement in UPDRS ADL and motor scores compared with improvements of 57% and 62% for those older than 56 years. Similarly, those with disease duration less than 16 years had significantly better responses to surgery than those with disease duration greater than 16 years. The authors concluded that in addition to age and disease duration, levodopa responsiveness was the strongest predictor of outcome after STN DBS. Kleiner-Fisman et al. (53) examined age, gender, disease duration, medication usage, dyskinesia, age of onset, and levodopa responsiveness in 25 PD patients who received bilateral STN DBS. Levodopa responsiveness was the only factor related to outcome. Jaggi and colleagues (65) examined 39 patients after STN DBS. They found that age, preoperative change in UPDRS motor scores with medication, and disease duration were the strongest predictors of outcome. Finally, Pahwa and colleagues (66) examined 45 patients after bilateral STN DBS and found that the preoperative change in UPDRS motor scores with medication was the strongest predictor of outcome. They found no relationship with age or disease duration. The American Academy of Neurology Practice Parameter: Treatment of Parkinson's disease with motor fluctuations and dyskinesia (an evidence-based review) (67) concluded that preoperative response to levodopa is probably predictive of postsurgical improvement and younger age and disease duration less than 16 years are possibly predictive of greater improvement after STN DBS. It was recommended that preoperative response to levodopa should be considered as a factor predictive of outcome after STN DBS, whereas age and disease duration may be considered as predictive factors.

DEEP BRAIN STIMULATION OF THE GLOBUS PALLIDUS INTERNA OR THE SUBTHALAMIC NUCLEUS?

There are few studies that have compared STN and GPI DBS outcomes in a controlled fashion. In a randomized, blinded study, Anderson and colleagues (34) compared 10 patients who received bilateral STN DBS with 10 patients who received bilateral GPi DBS 12 months after surgery. UPDRS scores were significantly improved for both groups; however, there were no significant differences between the STN and GPi DBS groups. More specifically, UPDRS motor scores were improved 48% with STN DBS and 39% with GPi DBS; UPDRS ADL scores were improved by 28% with STN DBS and 18% with GPi DBS; bradykinesia was improved by 44% with STN DBS and 33% with GPi DBS; tremor was improved 89% with STN DBS and 79% with GPi DBS; rigidity was improved 48% with STN DBS and 47% with GPi DBS; and axial symptoms were improved 44% with STN DBS and 40% for GPi DBS. In addition, dyskinesia was reduced by 62% with STN DBS and 89% with GPi DBS; however, there was a levodopa reduction of 38% with STN DBS and only 3% with GPi DBS. Although the sample size was small, this study suggests that cognitive and behavioral problems may be more common after STN DBS compared with GPi DBS. It was also suggested that follow-up care might be more difficult after STN DBS due to the medication adjustments during stimulation parameter optimization, which are generally not required after GPi DBS.

In a multicenter, randomized, blinded fashion, the Veterans Affairs Cooperative Studies Program (CSP) 468 Study (40) compared 147 PD patients with bilateral STN DBS and 152 PD patients with bilateral GPi DBS 24 months postsurgery. There were no differences between the two groups in stimulation on/medication off UPDRS motor scores compared with baseline medication off scores, which improved by 28% with GPi DBS and 25% with STN DBS. Similarly, there were no differences in UPDRS ADL scores with STN DBS improving by 12% and GPi by 17% compared with baseline. There were no differences between the two groups in PDQ-39 quality-of-life scores with both groups having improvements in subscores of mobility, ADLs, emotional wellbeing, stigma, cognition, and bodily discomfort as well as total score, communication subscores were slightly worsened in both groups and the social support score was slightly worsened after GPi and slightly better after STN, although these differences were not significant. There were no differences in patient-reported diaries of motor function with on time improving by 4.9 hr/day in the GPi group and 4 hours in the STN group, reductions in off time of 2.7 hours in the GPi group and 2.5 hours in the STN group and troublesome dyskinesia was decreased by 3.2 hours with GPi and 2.6 hours with STN. There was a minimal and similar worsening on all neurocognitive assessments in the GPi and STN groups, except for processing speed as measured by the visuomotor component of the digit symbol task, which was significantly more worsened after STN DBS compared with GPi DBS. There was a significant difference in the change in depression at 24 months, as measured by the Beck Depression Inventory, with a slight improvement after GPi DBS and a slight worsening after STN DBS. A significant difference was also seen in the reduction of levodopa equivalents at 24 months, with a reduction of 32% after STN DBS and 18% after GPi DBS. Stimulation amplitudes and pulse widths were lower on average after STN DBS compared with GPi DBS (3.16 V vs 3.95 V; 75.9 microseconds vs 95.7 microseconds, respectively). There were no significant differences between the STN and GPi groups in the frequency or type of serious adverse events. Infection occurred in 7.9% of the GPi group and 7.5% of the STN group, suicidal depression occurred in two patients (1.3%) after GPi DBS and in one patient (0.7%) after STN DBS, cerebral hemorrhage occurred in one patient (0.7%) after GPi DBS and in two patients (1.4%) after STN DBS, stroke occurred in no patients after GPi DBS but did occur in three patients (2%) after STN DBS and intracranial hemorrhage occurred in three patients (2%) after GPi DBS but in no patients after STN DBS. Moderate to severe adverse events occurring in at least 20% of patients in both groups included falls, gait disturbance, depression, balance disorder, speech problem, freezing, bradykinesia, motor dysfunction, dyskinesia, dystonia, and confused state. The majority of these events resolved. The authors concluded that motor function is similarly improved with bilateral STN or GPi DBS in patients with advanced PD and that choice of surgical target might take into consideration several factors, including nonmotor symptoms.

DEEP BRAIN STIMULATION VS BEST MEDICAL MANAGEMENT

Although many studies have shown the beneficial effects of STN and GPi stimulation, only a few studies have compared treatment with DBS to best medical management (68–70). Deuschl et al. (68) conducted a multicenter, unblinded, randomized-pairs study in which patients were enrolled in pairs with one receiving STN DBS within six weeks and the other receiving best medical management. After six months there was a significantly greater improvement in UPDRS motor (41% vs 1.7%), UPDRS ADL (39% vs −4.5%) and total PDQ-39 quality-of-life (24% vs −1.5%) scores in the STN DBS group compared with the best medical management group. In addition, dyskinesia were reduced by 54% with DBS, whereas they were increased by 2.4% with best medical management and levodopa equivalents were reduced by 49% with DBS and 10% with best medical management. Severe adverse events were more common with STN DBS (12.8%) versus best medical management (3.8%), which included three deaths in the STN DBS group and one in the best medical management group. Regarding total adverse events, they occurred in 50% of the STN DBS group and 64% of the medical group.

Weaver et al. (69) conducted a controlled trial of 255 PD patients randomized to either DBS (STN = 60 or GPi = 61) or best medical management (*n* = 134). The primary outcome was change in patient-reported on time after six months, which was significantly improved by 4.6 hr/day after DBS and unchanged in the best medical management group. Similarly, after DBS, off time was reduced by 2.4 hr/day and time with troublesome dyskinesia was reduced by 2.6 hr/day, whereas no changes were noted in the medical group. In the stimulation on/medication off condition, UPDRS motor scores were improved by 28.6%, UPDRS ADL scores were improved by 24%, levodopa equivalents were reduced by 23%, and PDQ-39 quality-of-life scores were improved by 17%, whereas there were essentially no changes in the medical group. There were however significantly more adverse events in the DBS group.

Williams et al. (70) reported the multicenter PD SURG trial in which subjects were randomized to either DBS (STN = 174; GPi = 4) or best medical management (*n* = 171). The primary outcome variable was change in PDQ-39 quality-of-life scores after one year. There was a significant improvement in PDQ-39 total scores of 13% with DBS and no change with best medical management. The subscales of mobility, ADLs and bodily discomfort were all significantly more improved with DBS compared with best medical management. UPDRS motor scores were significantly more improved with DBS (35.7%) compared with medical management (2.6%), as were UPDRS ADL scores (26% vs 3%). Off time and dyskinesia were also significantly more improved with DBS and there were no differences between the two groups in cognition as measured by the Dementia Rating Scale (DRS-II). There were significantly more adverse events in the DBS group.

In summary, the studies comparing DBS to best medical management have consistently demonstrated that motor function as measured by UPDRS motor and ADL scores as well as complications such as off time and dyskinesia were significantly more improved with DBS. In addition, PDQ-39 quality-of-life scores were also consistently improved with DBS compared with best medical management. On the other hand, there is significantly greater incidence of serious adverse events with DBS compared with best medical management. A further follow-up of the outcomes of the current studies are needed to see if these improvements are maintained long term.

PATIENT SELECTION FOR PALLIDAL AND SUBTHALAMIC DEEP BRAIN STIMULATION

The criteria for patient selection for DBS of the GPi and STN for PD are similar. The ideal candidate is a patient with idiopathic levodopa-responsive PD who has medication-resistant motor fluctuations and/or dyskinesia. It is recommended that patients undergo a levodopa challenge. Generally patients arrive at the clinic 12 hours after not taking any antiparkinsonian medications at which time they are evaluated with a complete UPDRS and other site-specific measures. After these evaluations either the regular dose of antiparkinsonian medication or at some sites a dose of levodopa 150% of the usual dose (without any other antiparkinsonian medication) is usually given and evaluations are repeated after the patient has reached the best medication on state. Usually a 30% or greater improvement in UPDRS motor scores between the medication off and on conditions is required to recommend surgery.

Patients older than 75 years are generally not considered candidates as they may have difficulty tolerating the procedure and the programming. Patients should have been tried on combinations of different antiparkinsonian medications and evaluated by a movement disorder specialist if possible before being recommended for surgery. Patients with disabling medication-resistant tremor or an inability to tolerate antiparkinsonian medications may also be candidates for STN or GPi DBS. There should be no evidence of dementia or significant cognitive, psychiatric, or behavioral abnormalities as these can worsen after surgery. To rule these out, patients should undergo neuropsychological screening. There should be no significant abnormalities on neuroimaging and no other medical conditions that might increase surgical risk. Finally, the patient should have an adequate support network and be able to attend multiple visits to the surgical site for programming.

ADVERSE EFFECTS OF DBS
Complications of DBS are similar for the three targets, VIM, GPi, and STN. Complications can be divided into those related to the surgical procedure, those associated with the DBS hardware and those associated with stimulation. The occurrence of these complications is related to the technique and experience of the neurosurgeon, accurate placement of the DBS leads, and appropriate patient selection and postsurgical management.

Surgical Complications
Surgical complications are those that occur within 30 days of surgery. These complications are typical of those seen with other intracranial stereotactic procedures and generally occur in less than 5% of the patients. These complications include hemorrhage, ischemic lesions, seizures, infections, and misplaced leads. Several studies have focused on the examination of surgical complications related to DBS. Beric et al. (71) reported 86 patients who received 149 DBS implants in the VIM nucleus of the thalamus, GPi or STN for PD, essential tremor, multiple sclerosis, or dystonia. In this cohort, 2.3% ($n = 2$) of the patients had a hemorrhage, 2.3% ($n = 2$) had seizures, 1.2% ($n = 1$) had a delayed hematoma two months after surgery, and 4.7% ($n = 4$) had postsurgical confusion. Umemura et al. (72) reported surgical complications in 109 patients receiving DBS of the VIM nucleus of the thalamus, GPi, STN, or anterior nucleus of the thalamus for either PD, essential tremor, epilepsy, or dystonia. They reported two deaths, one from a pulmonary embolus and the other from pneumonia. Other surgical complications included pulmonary embolism (1.8%; $n = 2$), subcortical hemorrhage (1.8%; $n = 2$), chronic subdural hematoma (1.8%; $n = 2$), venous infarction (0.9%; $n = 1$), seizure (0.9%; $n = 1$), infection (3.7%; $n = 4$), cerebral spinal fluid leak (0.9%; $n = 1$), and skin erosion on the scalp (0.9%; $n = 1$). In addition to

these complications, several patients had postoperative sterile seromas at the IPG and three had transient confusion. Finally, Lyons et al. (73) reported complications in 81 PD patients after 160 STN DBS procedures. In this series, 4.9% ($n = 4$) of the procedures were aborted due to adverse events in the operating room in three and inability to get a response in one. There were no deaths or permanent neurological deficits related to surgery. Surgical complications included hemorrhage in 1.2% ($n = 1$) of patients, seizure in 1.2% ($n = 1$), system infection in 2.5% ($n = 2$), IPG infection in 3.7% ($n = 3$), and misplaced leads in 12.5% ($n = 10$).

Hardware-Related Complications

Several reports have also focused on hardware complications related to DBS. Beric et al. (71) examined complications in 86 DBS patients and found electrode failure in 3.5% ($n = 3$), extension wire failure in 4.7% ($n = 4$), IPG malfunction in 1.2% ($n = 1$), and pain at the IPG in 1.2% ($n = 1$). Kondziolka and colleagues (74) examined hardware complications in 66 patients undergoing unilateral thalamic DBS for either essential tremor, parkinsonian tremor, multiple sclerosis, or other forms of tremor. There were a total of 23 hardware-related complications affecting 27% of the patients. Lead breakage occurred in 10 patients (15.2%), system infection in seven patients (10.6%), connector erosion in two patients (3.0%), and cranial lead migration, chronic subdural hematoma, defective IPG, and a defective connector each in one patient (1.5%, each). Oh et al. (75) reported hardware complications for 79 patients who received 124 DBS implants. DBS was done for PD, essential tremor, pain, epilepsy, dystonia, multiple sclerosis, and Huntington's disease and placed either in the STN, GPi, thalamus, or periventricular gray matter. In total, 20 patients (25.3%) had 26 hardware complications that involved 23 (18.5%) of the devices. More specifically, 5.1% ($n = 4$) had lead fractures, 5.1% ($n = 4$) had lead migrations, 3.8% ($n = 3$) had short circuits or open circuits, 15.2% ($n = 12$) had an infection or device erosion, 2.5% ($n = 2$) had an allergic reaction, and 1.3% ($n = 1$) had a cerebral spinal fluid leak. Similarly, Lyons and colleagues (73) reported hardware complications from 80 PD patients with 155 DBS implants in the STN. Hardware complications occurred in 26.2% ($n = 21$) of patients with 10% ($n = 8$) of patients having complications of the lead or extension wire that required additional neurosurgery and 18.8% ($n = 15$) of patients having IPG complications that required additional surgery in the subcutaneous tissue of the chest. More specifically, lead fractures occurred in 2.5% ($n = 2$), lead migrations in 6.3% ($n = 5$), extension wire fractures in 2.5% ($n = 2$), extension wire erosions in 1.3% ($n = 1$), and IPG malfunctions in 13.8% ($n = 11$). In this report, complications were reduced as the experience of the neurosurgeon was increased.

Stimulation Complications

Stimulation-related adverse effects depend on the exact location of the lead and the intensity of stimulation. The majority of stimulation-related adverse effects can be reduced by changing the active electrode contact or by reducing the stimulation intensity. These adverse effects include eyelid apraxia, double vision, dystonic posturing, dysarthria, dyskinesia, paresthesia, limb and facial muscle spasms, depression, mood changes, paresthesias, visual disturbances, and pain. Occasionally nonspecific sensations such as anxiety, panic, palpitations, and nausea can also occur. If these adverse effects persist this usually indicates that the electrode is not in the ideal position.

There has been some concern about an increase in suicide after DBS. Burkhard et al. (76) reported a suicide rate of 4.6% in patients with movement disorders and DBS. Risk factors in this report were history of severe depression and multiple successive DBS surgeries. There was no relationship found with the underlying condition, DBS target, stimulation parameters, or treatment adjustments. Benabid and colleagues (77) have also suggested that depression and suicide in patients after DBS are related to pre-existing conditions rather than the surgical procedure or subsequent stimulation.

CONCLUSIONS

DBS is an effective and relatively safe treatment for levodopa-responsive PD patients with medication-resistant motor fluctuations and dyskinesia. DBS of the thalamus clearly reduces parkinsonian tremor; however, bradykinesia, rigidity, and dyskinesia are not significantly affected. Therefore, VIM DBS is reserved for disabling tremor-predominant PD. DBS of the GPi and STN both significantly improve all of the cardinal symptoms of PD as well as dyskinesia. Although these benefits are reduced over time, they have been shown to be maintained for at least five years after GPi DBS and 10 years after STN DBS. DBS of the STN often results in a significant reduction in antiparkinsonian medication, whereas PD medications are generally not significantly reduced after GPi DBS. Currently, DBS of the STN is the most commonly performed surgical procedure for PD; however, a large, blinded, randomized study has demonstrated that motor function improvement is essentially the same for GPi and STN DBS. Several studies have also demonstrated that DBS (STN or GPi) significantly improves motor function and quality of life compared with best medical management. Finally, although DBS is a relatively safe procedure, patients should be counseled about the surgical and hardware complications that can occur and can require additional surgeries.

REFERENCES

1. Svennilson E, Torvik A, Lowe R, et al. Treatment of parkinsonism by stereotatic thermolesions in the pallidal region. A clinical evaluation of 81 cases. Acta Psychiatr Scand 1960; 35: 358–77.
2. Hassler R, Riechert T. Indications and localization of stereotactic brain operations. Nervenarzt 1954; 25: 441–7.
3. Fenelon F. Account of four years of practice of a personal intervention for Parkinson's disease. Rev Neurol (Paris) 1953; 89: 580–5.
4. Benabid AL, Pollak P, Louveau A, et al. Combined (thalamotomy and stimulation) stereotactic surgery of the VIM thalamic nucleus for bilateral Parkinson disease. Appl Neurophysiol 1987; 50: 344–6.
5. Speelman JD, Bosch DA. Resurgence of functional neurosurgery for Parkinson's disease: a historical perspective. Mov Disord 1998; 13: 582–8.
6. Ohye C, Maeda T, Narabayashi H. Physiologically defined VIM nucleus. Its special reference to control of tremor. Appl Neurophysiol 1976; 39: 285–95.
7. Hassler R. Anatomy of the thalamus. In: Schaltenbrand G, Baily P, eds. Introduction to Stereotaxis with an Atlas of the Human Brain. Stuttgart: Thieme, 1959: 230–90.
8. Hassler R. Architectonic organization of the thalamic nuclei. In: Schaltenbrand G, Walker AE, eds. Stereotaxy of Human Brain Anatomical, Physiological and Clinical Applications. New York: Thieme, 1982: 140–80.
9. Schaltenbrand G, Wahren W. Atlas for Stereotaxy of the Human Brain. New York: Thieme, 1977.

10. Burchiel KJ. Thalamotomy for movement disorders. Neurosurg Clin N Am 1995; 6: 55–71.
11. Krack P, Dostrovsky J, Ilinsky I, et al. Surgery of the motor thalamus: problems with the present nomenclatures. Mov Disord 2002; 17: S2–8.
12. Pahwa R, Lyons KE, Wilkinson SB, et al. Long-term evaluation of deep brain stimulation of the thalamus. J Neurosurg 2006; 104: 506–12.
13. Laitinen LV, Bergenheim AT, Hariz MI. Leksell's posteroventral pallidotomy in the treatment of Parkinson's disease. J Neurosurg 1992; 76: 53–61.
14. Dogali M, Fazzini E, Kolodny E, et al. Stereotactic ventral pallidotomy for Parkinson's disease. Neurology 1995; 45: 753–61.
15. Vitek JL, Bakay RA, Freeman A, et al. Randomized trial of pallidotomy versus medical therapy for Parkinson's disease. Ann Neurol 2003; 53: 558–69.
16. Jankovic J, Cardoso F, Grossman RG, et al. Outcome after stereotactic thalamotomy for parkinsonian, essential, and other types of tremor. Neurosurgery 1995; 37: 680–6; discussion 6–7.
17. Schuurman PR, Bosch DA, Bossuyt PM, et al. A comparison of continuous thalamic stimulation and thalamotomy for suppression of severe tremor. N Engl J Med 2000; 342: 461–8.
18. Lang AE, Lozano A, Montgomery EB, et al. Posteroventral medial pallidotomy in advanced Parkinson's disease. Adv Neurol 1999; 80: 575–83.
19. Carpenter MB, Whittier JR, Mettler FA. Analysis of choreoid hyperkinesia in the Rhesus monkey; surgical and pharmacological analysis of hyperkinesia resulting from lesions in the subthalamic nucleus of Luys. J Comp Neurol 1950; 92: 293–331.
20. Alvarez L, Macias R, Pavon N, et al. Therapeutic efficacy of unilateral subthalamotomy in Parkinson's disease: results in 89 patients followed for up to 36 months. J Neurol Neurosurg Psychiatry 2009; 80: 979–85.
21. Benabid AL, Pollak P, Seigneuret E, et al. Chronic VIM thalamic stimulation in Parkinson's disease, essential tremor and extra-pyramidal dyskinesias. Acta Neurochir Suppl (Wien) 1993; 58: 39–44.
22. Benabid AL, Pollak P, Gao D, et al. Chronic electrical stimulation of the ventralis intermedius nucleus of the thalamus as a treatment of movement disorders. J Neurosurg 1996; 84: 203–14.
23. Siegfried J, Lippitz B. Bilateral chronic electrostimulation of ventroposterolateral pallidum: a new therapeutic approach for alleviating all parkinsonian symptoms. Neurosurgery 1994; 35: 1126–9; discussion 9-30.
24. Pollak P, Benabid AL, Gross C, et al. Effects of the stimulation of the subthalamic nucleus in Parkinson disease. Rev Neurol (Paris) 1993; 149: 175–6.
25. Koller W, Pahwa R, Busenbark K, et al. High-frequency unilateral thalamic stimulation in the treatment of essential and parkinsonian tremor. Ann Neurol 1997; 42: 292–9.
26. Limousin P, Speelman JD, Gielen F, et al. Multicentre European study of thalamic stimulation in parkinsonian and essential tremor. J Neurol Neurosurg Psychiatry 1999; 66: 289–96.
27. Ondo W, Jankovic J, Schwartz K, et al. Unilateral thalamic deep brain stimulation for refractory essential tremor and Parkinson's disease tremor. Neurology 1998; 51: 1063–9.
28. Lyons KE, Koller WC, Wilkinson SB, et al. Long term safety and efficacy of unilateral deep brain stimulation of the thalamus for parkinsonian tremor. J Neurol Neurosurg Psychiatry 2001; 71: 682–4.
29. Pollak P, Benabid AL, Limousin P, et al. Chronic intracerebral stimulation in Parkinson's disease. Adv Neurol 1997; 74: 213–20.
30. Kumar R, Lang AE, Rodriguez-Oroz MC, et al. Deep brain stimulation of the globus pallidus pars interna in advanced Parkinson's disease. Neurology 2000; 55: S34–9.
31. The Deep-Brain Stimulation for Parkinson's Disease Study G. Deep-brain stimulation of the subthalamic nucleus or the pars interna of the globus pallidus in Parkinson's disease. N Engl J Med 2001; 345: 956–63.
32. Volkmann J, Allert N, Voges J, et al. Safety and efficacy of pallidal or subthalamic nucleus stimulation in advanced PD. Neurology 2001; 56: 548–51.
33. Loher TJ, Burgunder JM, Pohle T, et al. Long-term pallidal deep brain stimulation in patients with advanced Parkinson disease: 1-year follow-up study. J Neurosurg 2002; 96: 844–53.

34. Anderson VC, Burchiel KJ, Hogarth P, et al. Pallidal vs subthalamic nucleus deep brain stimulation in Parkinson disease. Arch Neurol 2005; 62: 554–60.
35. Ghika J, Villemure JG, Fankhauser H, et al. Efficiency and safety of bilateral contemporaneous pallidal stimulation (deep brain stimulation) in levodopa-responsive patients with Parkinson's disease with severe motor fluctuations: a 2-year follow-up review. J Neurosurg 1998; 89: 713–18.
36. Lyons KE, Wilkinson SB, Troster AI, et al. Long-term efficacy of globus pallidus stimulation for the treatment of Parkinson's disease. Stereotact Funct Neurosurg 2002; 79: 214–20.
37. Rodriguez-Oroz MC, Obeso JA, Lang AE, et al. Bilateral deep brain stimulation in Parkinson's disease: a multicentre study with 4 years follow-up. Brain 2005; 128: 2240–9.
38. Volkmann J, Allert N, Voges J, et al. Long-term results of bilateral pallidal stimulation in Parkinson's disease. Ann Neurol 2004; 55: 871–5.
39. Rodrigues JP, Walters SE, Watson P, et al. Globus pallidus stimulation in advanced Parkinson's disease. J Clin Neurosci 2007; 14: 208–15.
40. Follett KA, Weaver FM, Stern M, et al. Pallidal versus subthalamic deep-brain stimulation for Parkinson's disease. N Engl J Med 2010; 362: 2077–91.
41. Moro E, Lozano AM, Pollak P, et al. Long-term results of a multicenter study on subthalamic and pallidal stimulation in Parkinson's disease. Mov Disord 2010; 25: 578–86.
42. Welter ML, Houeto JL, Tezenas du Montcel S, et al. Clinical predictive factors of subthalamic stimulation in Parkinson's disease. Brain 2002; 125: 575–83.
43. Kumar R, Lozano AM, Kim YJ, et al. Double-blind evaluation of subthalamic nucleus deep brain stimulation in advanced Parkinson's disease. Neurology 1998; 51: 850–5.
44. Vesper J, Klostermann F, Stockhammer F, et al. Results of chronic subthalamic nucleus stimulation for Parkinson's disease: a 1-year follow-up study. Surg Neurol 2002; 57: 306–11; discussion 11-3.
45. Doshi PK, Chhaya NA, Bhatt MA. Bilateral subthalamic nucleus stimulation for Parkinson's disease. Neurol India 2003; 51: 43–8.
46. Limousin P, Krack P, Pollak P, et al. Electrical stimulation of the subthalamic nucleus in advanced Parkinson's disease. N Engl J Med 1998; 339: 1105–11.
47. Rodriguez-Oroz MC, Gorospe A, Guridi J, et al. Bilateral deep brain stimulation of the subthalamic nucleus in Parkinson's disease. Neurology 2000; 55: S45–51.
48. Ostergaard K, Sunde N, Dupont E. Effects of bilateral stimulation of the subthalamic nucleus in patients with severe Parkinson's disease and motor fluctuations. Mov Disord 2002; 17: 693–700.
49. Kleiner-Fisman G, Herzog J, Fisman DN, et al. Subthalamic nucleus deep brain stimulation: summary and meta-analysis of outcomes. Mov Disord 2006; 21: S290–304.
50. Schupbach WM, Chastan N, Welter ML, et al. Stimulation of the subthalamic nucleus in Parkinson's disease: a 5 year follow up. J Neurol Neurosurg Psychiatry 2005; 76: 1640–4.
51. Krause M, Fogel W, Mayer P, et al. Chronic inhibition of the subthalamic nucleus in Parkinson's disease. J Neurol Sci 2004; 219: 119–24.
52. Romito LM, Scerrati M, Contarino MF, et al. Bilateral high frequency subthalamic stimulation in Parkinson's disease: long-term neurological follow-up. J Neurosurg Sci 2003; 47: 119–28.
53. Kleiner-Fisman G, Fisman DN, Sime E, et al. Long-term follow up of bilateral deep brain stimulation of the subthalamic nucleus in patients with advanced Parkinson disease. J Neurosurg 2003; 99: 489–95.
54. Pahwa R, Wilkinson SB, Overman J, et al. Bilateral subthalamic stimulation in patients with Parkinson disease: long-term follow up. J Neurosurg 2003; 99: 71–7.
55. Krack P, Batir A, Van Blercom N, et al. Five-year follow-up of bilateral stimulation of the subthalamic nucleus in advanced Parkinson's disease. N Engl J Med 2003; 349: 1925–34.
56. Ostergaard K, Aa Sunde N. Evolution of Parkinson's disease during 4 years of bilateral deep brain stimulation of the subthalamic nucleus. Mov Disord 2006; 21: 624–31.
57. Piboolnurak P, Lang AE, Lozano AM, et al. Levodopa response in long-term bilateral subthalamic stimulation for Parkinson's disease. Mov Disord 2007; 22: 990–7.
58. Gervais-Bernard H, Xie-Brustolin J, Mertens P, et al. Bilateral subthalamic nucleus stimulation in advanced Parkinson's disease: five year follow-up. J Neurol 2009; 256: 225–33.

59. Kishore A, Rao R, Krishnan S, et al. Long-term stability of effects of subthalamic stimulation in Parkinson's disease: Indian experience. Mov Disord 2010; 25: 2438–44.
60. Toft M, Lilleeng B, Ramm-Pettersen J, et al. Long-term efficacy and mortality in Parkinson's disease patients treated with subthalamic stimulation. Mov Disord 2011; 26: 1931–4.
61. Fasano A, Romito LM, Daniele A, et al. Motor and cognitive outcome in patients with Parkinson's disease 8 years after subthalamic implants. Brain 2010; 133: 2664–76.
62. Castrioto A, Lozano AM, Poon YY, et al. Ten-year outcome of subthalamic stimulation in Parkinson disease: a blinded evaluation. Arch Neurol 2011; 68: 1550–6.
63. Okun MS, Gallo BV, Mandybur G, et al. Subthalamic deep brain stimulation with a constant-current device in Parkinson's disease: an open-label randomised controlled trial. Lancet Neurol 2012; 11: 140–9.
64. Charles PD, Van Blercom N, Krack P, et al. Predictors of effective bilateral subthalamic nucleus stimulation for PD. Neurology 2002; 59: 932–4.
65. Jaggi JL, Umemura A, Hurtig HI, et al. Bilateral stimulation of the subthalamic nucleus in Parkinson's disease: surgical efficacy and prediction of outcome. Stereotact Funct Neurosurg 2004; 82: 104–14.
66. Pahwa R, Wilkinson SB, Overman J, et al. Preoperative clinical predictors of response to bilateral subthalamic stimulation in patients with Parkinson's disease. Stereotact Funct Neurosurg 2005; 83: 80–3.
67. Pahwa R, Factor SA, Lyons KE, et al. Practice Parameter: treatment of Parkinson disease with motor fluctuations and dyskinesia (an evidence-based review): report of the Quality Standards Subcommittee of the American Academy of Neurology. Neurology 2006; 66: 983–95.
68. Deuschl G, Schade-Brittinger C, Krack P, et al. A randomized trial of deep-brain stimulation for Parkinson's disease. N Engl J Med 2006; 355: 896–908.
69. Weaver FM, Follett K, Stern M, et al. Bilateral deep brain stimulation vs best medical therapy for patients with advanced Parkinson disease: a randomized controlled trial. JAMA 2009; 301: 63–73.
70. Williams A, Gill S, Varma T, et al. Deep brain stimulation plus best medical therapy versus best medical therapy alone for advanced Parkinson's disease (PD SURG trial): a randomised, open-label trial. Lancet Neurol 2010; 9: 581–91.
71. Beric A, Kelly PJ, Rezai A, et al. Complications of deep brain stimulation surgery. Stereotact Funct Neurosurg 2001; 77: 73–8.
72. Umemura A, Jaggi JL, Hurtig HI, et al. Deep brain stimulation for movement disorders: morbidity and mortality in 109 patients. J Neurosurg 2003; 98: 779–84.
73. Lyons KE, Wilkinson SB, Overman J, et al. Surgical and hardware complications of subthalamic stimulation: a series of 160 procedures. Neurology 2004; 63: 612–16.
74. Kondziolka D, Whiting D, Germanwala A, et al. Hardware-related complications after placement of thalamic deep brain stimulator systems. Stereotact Funct Neurosurg 2002; 79: 228–33.
75. Oh MY, Abosch A, Kim SH, et al. Long-term hardware-related complications of deep brain stimulation. Neurosurgery 2002; 50: 1268–74; discussion 74-6.
76. Burkhard PR, Vingerhoets FJ, Berney A, et al. Suicide after successful deep brain stimulation for movement disorders. Neurology 2004; 63: 2170–2.
77. Benabid AL, Chabardes S, Seigneuret E. Deep-brain stimulation in Parkinson's disease: long-term efficacy and safety: what happened this year? Curr Opin Neurol 2005; 18: 623–30.

25 Investigational surgical therapies

Neil M. Issar and Joseph S. Neimat

INTRODUCTION

Over the past several decades, the surgical treatment of Parkinson's disease (PD) has undergone significant changes. Deep brain stimulation (DBS) has progressed from a novel or experimental procedure to an accepted and even anticipated therapy for PD patients in the later stages of disease. The therapy is now supported by several randomized studies demonstrating both superior motor performance and improved quality of life (1–4). The number of PD patients treated with DBS to date is estimated at greater than 100,000 (Medtronic, Inc, personal communication). The ultimate goal of surgical therapies is to reverse the underlying pathophysiology of PD and restore function to the extrapyramidal motor system.

Beyond current DBS strategies there has been increasing investigation into novel surgical therapies that might improve upon the capabilities of current surgical therapy. These therapies promise to provide more complete symptomatic control and perhaps to reverse elements of the PD degenerative pathology. The possibilities presented are among the most interesting and novel concepts in the field of PD today.

SHORTCOMINGS OF CURRENT SURGICAL THERAPIES

Despite the success of DBS therapy and the striking benefit it provides in treating advanced PD, DBS fails to treat many aspects of the disease. These include the prominent gait and balance issues that are inherent to PD and the gradual cognitive and emotional decline that is known to occur from extranigral neuronal attrition (5). The diffuse, multisystemic nature of these changes may require measures beyond focal electrical stimulation. Strategies being researched range from the application of DBS to a novel target area to more advanced cellular and genetic therapies that seek to address the primary pathology of PD.

DBS therapy is not without adverse effects, ranging from the psychiatric effects of mania or depression to effects of vocal hypophonia, weight gain, eyelid apraxia, increased libido, sialorrhea, decreased memory, dyskinesia, and dystonia. A review of reported studies noted adverse effects in 19% of patients receiving DBS of the subthalamic nucleus (STN) (6–10). Another issue is the possibly high suicide rate among patients having undergone DBS surgery. Reported suicide rates range from less than 1% to a single study that noted a rate of 4.3% in a cohort of 140 patients (11,12). These findings demonstrate the need to investigate and refine DBS therapy for PD. Advancements in the engineering of implant technology may make DBS therapy more efficacious while limiting adverse effects. The exploration of novel targets may also lead to stimulatory therapies that address some of the current shortcomings. It is hoped that some of these targets will yield similar or greater benefits while producing more limited adverse effects.

NEW STIMULATION SYSTEMS

Several investigators have suggested that more refined neural interface systems might improve upon the efficacy and tolerability of current brain stimulation technologies. The proposed systems typically make use of closed loop technology where information about the state of local neurons is recorded and stimulation is adjusted in a more physiologically appropriate manner. Some of the signals that have been explored to assess functional states within the basal ganglia include spectral band fluctuations within local field potential (LFP) measurements from implanted electrodes, electrochemical sensing via implanted carbon fiber probes, and more simple accelerometers contained within the implanted device (13–17). Several groups have developed implantable devices that record such signals and could potentially be used to modulate stimulation therapy (15,18). A collaboration between academia and industry has produced an implantable device that is being released for preclinical trials. This prototype device records LFP signals from standard DBS electrodes and also contains an accelerometer to assess movement symptomatology. These elements are contained within the body of a standard size pulse generator. Information gathered can be transmitted by telemetry and assessed by a clinician or used to directly modify stimulation via automated guidance of the device itself (15). Appropriate applications for such a device are currently being explored with preliminary results suggesting that closed-loop DBS may be superior in ameliorating PD and PD-like symptoms (19).

NOVEL STIMULATION TARGETS

The current surgical therapies are based on a model of basal ganglia function, which suggests that motor systems are regulated by the balanced activity of two separate circuits within the basal ganglia (20). This model was able to explain the effect of known ablative targets, such as the globus pallidus interna (GPi), STN, and thalamus. Although the initial model has been instructive, numerous anatomic studies have unveiled a far more complex connectivity in the basal ganglia than is accounted for in the model. It is clear now that there are dopaminergic projections to the pallidum and STN, as well as to the striatum. The thalamic centromedian and parafascicular nuclei form important "stabilizing" circuits with the pallidum and STN (21,22). The pedunculopontine nucleus (PPN) is considered to be a potentially important output nucleus, which receives projections from the STN (23). The zona incerta (ZI) has also been investigated as a potential target due to its widespread connections to the diencephalon and basal ganglia (24). These findings point to a more complex, internally regulating system, of which the traditionally described direct and indirect pathways tell only a part of the whole story (25–30). With this enhanced understanding of basal ganglia structure and complexity, several new surgical targets have been suggested.

Pedunculopontine Nucleus

The PPN is an important output target of the STN. It has also been implicated in the mediation of gait and posture, aspects of PD which are not well treated by DBS of the STN or GPi (27). In 2005 Mazzone and colleagues reported two patients, with PD causing significant gait disturbance, who underwent implantation of PPN DBS electrodes. They demonstrated the safety of the procedure and the ability of low-frequency intraoperative stimulation to improve selective elements of the

Unified Parkinson's Disease Rating Scale (UPDRS) motor scale (31). A study by Plaha and Gill also reported two patients who underwent PPN DBS implantation and had improvements in UPDRS motor scores and in additional measures of balance and gait (32). These preliminary reports served as the impetus for the first open and blinded studies, the results of which have been promising. In 2007 Stefani et al. reported a series of six patients who underwent bilateral DBS implantation of both the STN and PPN. Both STN and PPN DBS independently provided improvement in the patients' UPDRS motor scores of 54% and 32%, respectively. PPN DBS was found to be particularly effective in those whose response to STN-only DBS had deteriorated over time. Furthermore, combined DBS of both targets provided improvement greater than either target alone and showed the greatest efficacy in gait and postural measures as well as in activities of daily living (ADLs) (33). Moro et al. also reported a substantial reduction in falls in six advanced PD patients with significant gait and postural abnormalities treated with unilateral PPN DBS (34). In addition, Ferraye et al. reported the addition of bilateral PPN DBS in six patients whose severe freezing of gait, was unresponsive to STN DBS. At one-year follow-up, freezing episodes and related falls had decreased with PPN stimulation. A two-month double-blind assessment of gait measures, however, did not show significant improvement (35).

Some of the variance in reported benefit of stimulation may stem from disagreement on the location of the stimulating electrode. There has been some debate in the literature on the optimal location to be used to affect gait (36). A prospective study by Thevathasan and colleagues reported the use of a more caudal PPN target for the treatment of PD with prominent symptoms of axial freezing, postural instability, and falls. They reported significant improvement on the Gait and Falls Questionnaire maintained for two years, suggesting that the precise location of PPN stimulation is important to see benefit (37). Finally, Kahn and colleagues conducted a trial of seven patients whom they treated with bilateral stimulation both of the PPN and the caudal Zona Inserta (cZI). They were able to demonstrate a synergistic effect of stimulation at these two targets to improve a composite axial subscore from the UPDRS motor section (38).

As our knowledge of the subcortical circuitry underlying motor regulation improves, DBS may be tailored to the pathologies of individual patients. In addition, further controlled studies with longer follow-ups are needed to determine whether or not optimization of patient selection and/or targeting and setting of stimulation parameters might improve outcomes to transform DBS of the PPN from an experimental and adjunctive surgical approach to a viable surgical alternative.

Posterior Subthalamic Area

The posterior subthalamic area (PSA) is a region of dense white matter connections and interlaminar nuclei, which is positioned posterior to the STN nucleus and inferior to the ventral intermediate motor (VIM) nucleus of the thalamus. It is a site that was well described as a target for traditional lesional interventions (39,40). In the past decade it has seen increasing utilization in the DBS treatment of movement disorders. In these explorations it has also been referred to as the cZI and the prelemniscal radiations.

Within this PSA region, the ZI has reciprocal connections to the dorsal thalamus, and provides predominantly glutamatergic input to the substantia nigra and PPN (24). The region also represents an intersection between cerebellothalamic and pallidothalamic white matter tracts (41). It has been demonstrated that this region may be partly responsible for the generation of resting tremor in PD (42). This target-rich anatomy and the historical precedent for surgical intervention in this area have garnered the PSA increasing attention in recent years. Several groups have explored the PSA as a target in the treatment of PD. Each has demonstrated significant improvements (44–65%) in UPDRS motor scores with particularly significant improvement in tremor (43,44). A study by Plaha and colleagues in 2006 provided a direct comparison of cZI DBS and STN DBS in medically refractory PD patients and demonstrated that high frequency stimulation of the cZI resulted in greater improvement in contralateral motor scores (45).

Later studies by the same group combined cZI and PPN stimulation and proposed that combined stimulation uniquely benefited axial symptoms (46). The complicated anatomy of this region makes the precise mechanism of benefit difficult to ascertain. Microelectrode and stimulation mapping are also more difficult to interpret than the more established DBS targets. This may be one reason that the PSA has, until recently, been largely overlooked. Like any surgical target, the stimulation of the PSA is not without concerns. There have been case reports of bilateral stimulation of the ZI in PD patients causing severe irritability, psychomotor agitation, and progressive insomnia (47). Some reports of the surgery also demonstrated prolonged surgical recovery as a potential detractor to this target (44). Larger, randomized, controlled studies are needed to confirm the safety and efficacy of ZI DBS in the treatment of PD.

Motor Cortex Stimulation

Anecdotal evidence of tremor improvement in patients treated with stimulation of the motor cortex for chronic pain (48,49) led to the suggestion that stimulation of the motor cortex might be an effective means of treating patients with tremor-dominant PD. Canavero and colleagues first performed motor cortex stimulation (MCS) for PD and reported positive results in three patients (50–52). They demonstrated that a benefit comparable to STN DBS could be achieved with low-frequency, but not high-frequency stimulation. Since then, studies of larger cohorts of patients have shown that MCS may be less efficacious than STN DBS, with some benefit lost over time (53–56). It also appears to be less efficacious in PD than in essential tremor (56). At this time limitations of the therapy have decreased interest in the target's applicability.

Early Deep Brain Stimulation

Several groups have suggested the possibility of using early DBS to slow the pathologic progress of PD. Theoretically, glutamatergic projections from the STN to the substantia nigra pars compacta (SNc) represent an excitotoxic circuit. Thus, early dopaminergic loss causes increased STN activity, which, in turn, increases excitation and injury in the SNc. This process could have a similar toxic effect on other targets, including the GPi, substantia nigra pars reticulata (SNr), and PPN (27). This has been supported in rodent and primate models demonstrating that previous STN ablation or active STN stimulation has a protective effect on the SNc from mitochondrial toxins known to cause dopaminergic attrition (57,58). This concept remains controversial, as there is not clear evidence supporting neuroprotection in human DBS subjects. It is also not clear that STN DBS reduces glutamate output. Indeed, there is some evidence to the contrary. One study has demonstrated continued dopaminergic loss in the striatum of patients treated with STN DBS; in 30 patients, fluorodopa uptake decreased by 9–12% a year. This reduction is similar to known progression rates in unoperated patients (59). A multicenter trial is currently underway to assess the safety and utility of early DBS treatment. Early results indicate that perioperative adverse events in patients with early-stage PD (Hoehn and Yahr Stage II) are comparable to those reported for STN DBS in advanced PD (60). Neurophysiologic evidence from the same study has demonstrated that neuronal firing rates in the STN of these early PD patients is significantly lower than those encountered in a group of age-/sex-matched controls (28.7 Hz vs 36.3 Hz) (61). This finding supports the "rate" model of PD pathology. Outcomes from this phase I study are anticipated in the coming year.

INTRACEREBRAL DRUG INFUSION
Glial Cell Line-Derived Neurotrophic Factor

Glial cell line-derived neurotrophic factor (GDNF) was first identified in the early 1990s as a member of the transforming growth factor (TGF)-beta superfamily with potent effects on embryonic neuronal cultures and specifically on dopaminergic cell lines (62). It was subsequently found to be potently expressed in the developing rodent striatum (63). Its potential as a possible agent for the protection of dopaminergic projections was quickly recognized and there was investigation into the delivery of the agent in PD animal models.

Early studies showed that local GDNF administration was able to protect and restore dopaminergic cells in rodent models of PD (64,65). Shortly thereafter, trials in primates confirmed the ability of GDNF both to protect dopaminergic cells from degeneration and to improve functional assessments of motor behavior in 1-methyl-4-phenyl-1,2,3,6-tetrahydropyridine (MPTP)-treated rhesus monkeys (66,67). The success of these studies generated hope for the clinical utility of GDNF in patients with PD (68,69). Initial reports, however, were mixed, with some indicating improvement (70) and others indicating treatment futility (71). Yet, the preclinical evidence was sufficiently compelling to spur broader investigation.

The first, large, randomized trial of intraventricular GDNF was published in 2003. In this trial, 50 patients underwent placement of pumps and intraventricular catheters. The patients were randomized to receive either carrier alone or one of several concentrations of recombinant GDNF. At six to eight months, none of the GDNF groups had demonstrated improvements over placebo and several of the groups had worsened (72). Additionally, adverse effects were noted in all patients receiving GDNF; these included nausea, anorexia, and shock-like sensory symptoms resembling Lhermitte phenomena. It was suggested that the relative size of the human brain makes the transependymal diffusion of GDNF insufficient to create the necessary concentrations to produce an effect (73).

A series of trials evaluated the effects of intrastriatal microinfusion of GDNF. A phase I safety study reported that microinfusion in five Parkinsonian patients produced no significant adverse effects and improved UPDRS scores by 48%. Furthermore, positron emission tomography (PET) scanning demonstrated increased striatal dopamine uptake (73). Notable adverse effects also included anorexia, with significant weight loss, and Lhermitte's phenomenon. The results of this study were sufficient to begin a double-blind, placebo-controlled phase II study with 34 patients who underwent implantation of intraputaminal catheters and pumps and received either GDNF or saline carrier alone. At six months, the GDNF-treated patients failed to show significant changes in their off-medication UPDRS scores compared with placebo. Although there was a trend for more severely affected patients to derive improvement, this did not meet significance. Additionally, four of the patients developed anti-GDNF antibodies during or subsequent to the six-month period of study, raising concerns that autoimmune consequences might ensue (74). Despite the failure of clinical response in this study, PET imaging performed in treated patients did demonstrate an average increase of 23.1% in F-dopa uptake, compared with a decrease of 8.8% in placebo-treated patients (74). This objective sign of a treatment effect and the benefits demonstrated in previous open label studies raised the possibility that GDNF treatment may still hold promise, with the aforementioned trial failure perhaps due to inadequate diffusion of the molecule throughout the target region (75). Current hopes rest on cell- and viral-based gene therapy treatments, which may provide a more effective means of factor delivery.

Neurturin

Neurturin is a GDNF homologue (76) also expressed in the developing midbrain (77). It too has been demonstrated to exert potent trophic effects on dopaminergic neurons in vitro and in vivo (77). When injected into the substantia nigra of 6-hydroxydopamine (6-OHDA)-lesioned rats, neurturin significantly protected dopaminergic nigral cells, resulting in greater cell survival. These results were nearly identical to the effects of GDNF (77,78). Protective results have also been noted in rats treated with striatal neurturin injections preceding lesioning (78). Both studies correlated these results with behavioral improvements. Other members of this gene family have also been identified and tested for dopaminergic neuroprotection (79–81). It is possible that these agents may be considered for future clinical therapies. Like GDNF, gene therapy may represent the most effective means of delivery for these agents. Specific studies are examined below in the section "Gene Therapy."

FETAL TRANSPLANTATION

Among PD treatments, no therapy has raised greater hopes or stirred more controversy than fetal transplantation. Although clinical trial failures have curtailed interest in this therapy, it remains an area of considerable research and discussion. Understanding the work that has been done in this area may be instrumental in guiding future cellular restorative therapies, such as stem cell transplantation.

Rodent and primate models of PD have shown dramatic response to the transplantation of fetal cells (82–85). The demonstration of behavioral improvements (86–88) and histologic re-innervation of striatal regions by dopaminergic transplants (85) suggested that a successful treatment strategy had been identified. The first human cases of fetal transplantation for PD were reported in 1990 (89,90). Early anecdotal cases reported dramatic benefit and there was great anticipation that the procedure would see widespread application. Several of these studies were also able to corroborate observed clinical improvements with PET evidence of increased dopamine uptake or with histologic evidence of re-innervation by transplanted fetal cells (91). An open-label study demonstrated significant improvements in each of seven treated patients for 12–46 months following surgery. All seven patients demonstrated improvement in ADLs, and five had significant improvement in UPDRS motor scores. The group also demonstrated medication reductions by an average of 39% (92).

In 2001, a double-blind, sham-surgery, controlled study was published. Patients treated with fetal transplantation showed no significant difference in the primary outcome measure of subjective self-reported improvement. Neither the treated patients nor the sham-surgery controls reported any subjective benefit. Secondary objective measures, including UPDRS motor scores, were slightly more promising. Treated patients demonstrated an 18% improvement in UPDRS motor scores off medication, compared with no improvement in sham controls. The effect was more pronounced in the group of patients younger than 60 years, whose scores improved by 34%. No additional benefit was accrued in the on-medication state in any group. Notably, the study was performed without immunosuppression (93).

The negative results produced by this study after such promising early trials spurred a second double-blind, controlled trial by Olanow et al. in which 34 patients were randomized to sham surgery or to intraputaminal implantation with one or four grafts per side. Notably, solid mesencephalic grafts were used (as opposed to dissociated cell suspensions) and patients were kept on immunosuppression for a period of six months. Patients were then followed for a total of 24 months and the primary endpoint was objective change in the UPDRS motor score. Results demonstrated no significant improvement in either treatment group when compared with the placebo group. At six months, the treatment groups showed significant benefit compared with the controls; however, this effect was gradually lost over the subsequent six to nine months. This suggests that immunosuppression may have an important protective role in cellular therapies. Further subgroup analysis demonstrated that patients with less severe disease (UPDRS motor score < 49) did show significant improvement and that there was further significant benefit to treatment with multiple donors (94).

The blinded studies also demonstrated a significant incidence of graft-induced dyskinesia (GID), which persisted even after the withdrawal of antiparkinsonian medication. This troubling adverse effect was reported in 15% of patients in the study by Freed et al. (93) and in 58% of patients in the Olanow et al. study (94). The desire to re-establish fetal cell transplantation as a safe and effective treatment for PD has led to significant efforts to understand the mechanisms underlying GID. For example, several studies have elicited amphetamine-induced dyskinesia in grafted 6-OHDA-lesioned rats to serve as a model for the study of GID (95–97). Current hypotheses for the cause of GID include dysregulated dopamine release from serotonergic terminals (98), elevated serotonin–dopamine transporter ratio (99), serotonergic hyperinnervation of the striatum (99), and/or partial or incomplete dopaminergic re-innervation of the striatum (100). In addition, a few case reports have described patients suffering from off-medication graft-induced dyskinesia benefitting from subsequent GPi DBS (101,102).

The failure of double-blind studies to demonstrate consistent benefit has halted the application of fetal transplantation. However, the apparent success of individual patients and the evidence for substantive re-innervation as demonstrated by histology or by PET imaging have led investigators to identify several factors that may influence results and contribute to treatment success (103). First, the amount and age of transplanted tissue may be of importance. One group reported an optimal fetal age of 5.5–8 weeks for transplantation (104). Second, the handling of fetal tissue prior to implantation may also have a critical effect. This has been evidenced in part by the few patients who came to autopsy. These reports demonstrate significant variability in the extent of striatal re-innervation by transplanted neurons. One study demonstrated a single patient who had derived a significant benefit from his transplantation and was found at autopsy to have widespread and confluent striatal innervation with minimal inflammatory reaction (91). Contrasting histologic reports demonstrated far more limited survival from fetal transplants that were older or had undergone cryopreservation (105,106). Finally, several studies have examined the necessity of immunosuppression to allow cellular integration of the foreign transplants. The Olanow et al. study suggested that steroid suppression was beneficial up to six months and its withdrawal might account for the subsequent worsening of UPDRS motor scores in transplanted patients. Piccini et al. identified six patients who underwent steroid suppression for more than two years. In these patients, the withdrawal of steroids at an average of 29 months produced no rebound in UPDRS motor scores and no changes in striatal dopamine uptake on PET scanning (103).

These studies demonstrate the extremely tenuous nature of the technique. It may be that the failed transplantation trials resulted from technical sensitivities and not from a failure of principle. This observation provides hope that new cellular-based therapies may be effective if larger numbers of cells can be transplanted or greater cell survival can be achieved. A multicenter clinical trial is currently underway in which younger early PD patients with no or low levels of L-dopa-induced dyskinesia receive grafts of embryonic tissue dissected to minimize the inclusion of serotonergic neurons. They will also have long-term immunosuppression and will undergo a carefully considered panel of assessments at stages prior to and following transplantation (107).

STEM CELL THERAPY

Stem cell therapies provide significant promise for achieving cellular transplants of greater cell number and potential survivability. Stem cells are developmentally immature cells with several critical properties. (*i*) They are self-renewing or amplifiable in vitro. This ability to clonally expand large numbers of cells is a critical advantage for stem cell therapies. It allows transplants of much larger cell populations addressing one of the key failures of fetal mesenchymal transplants. (*ii*) They are pluripotent or multipotent, meaning that in the proper cellular niche they can differentiate into desired cell types. Pluripotent stem cells can differentiate into cells of any germ layer, whereas multipotent stem cells are restricted to the lineage of a single system.

The current stem cell technologies derive cells from four potential sources. These are embryonic stem (ES) cells, induced pluripotent stem (iPS) cells, mesenchymal stem cells (MSC), and neural progenitor cells (NPC) (108). The ES and iPS cells are the most pluripotent, accompanied with both the greatest potential for clonal expansion and differentiation as well as the greatest risk for tumor formation (109). MSC and NPC populations are more predictable but may possess less potent capacities for restoration. Once the population of stem cell has been chosen, strategies have segregated between cellular replacement therapies (where stem cells are implanted to replace lost dopaminergic cells) and cellular support therapies (where stem cells are modified to express neurotrophic factors that support endogenous cell survival).

Embryonic Stem Cells

ES cells from mouse, nonhuman primate, and humans (110) have been differentiated into dopaminergic neurons. In current research, human ES cells typically have been donated as excess material, following in vitro fertilization. Several studies have encouraged differentiation of stem cells into dopaminergic neurons through genetic manipulation and hormonal treatment, such as overexpression of the Nurr-1, Pitx3, or Lmx1a transcription factors; exposure to fibroblast growth factor (FGF) and Sonic Hedgehog; or inhibition of bone morphogenic protein (BMP) signaling by using the soluble factor Noggin (111–116). When implanted into animal models, these stem cell-derived neurons re-innervate the striatum and ameliorate some parkinsonian symptoms (117–119). One concern has been the development of teratomas in the brains of some (120) but not all animals (121). Another concern may be disease pathology affecting the cells derived from the transplanted cells, as has been observed in intrastriatal grafts of embryonic mesencephalic tissue more than a decade after they were implanted in PD patients (122).

Induced Pluripotent Stem Cells

The controversy over ES cell acquisition makes the more recently described potential of iPS cells more appealing. This process involves the dedifferentiation of autologous somatic cells, such as fibroblasts, into a pluripotent stem cell line with capabilities similar to those of ES cells (108,123). The autologous nature of these cells (similar to MSCs below) has the advantage of immunocompatability. On the other hand, any genetic predisposition toward PD would also be present in this cell group and might limit transplant longevity before these cells too exhibit degenerative features.

Mesenchymal Stem Cells

Genetic and hormonal manipulations of stem cells from bone marrow (124), retinal pigmented epithelial cells (125), adipose adult stromal tissue (126), and umbilical cord blood (127) have produced cells with neuronal characteristics. Bone marrow-derived cells have been induced in some experiments to produce dopamine. For example, Zou and colleagues injected adult bone marrow-derived stem cells containing the gene for tyrosine hydroxylase into 6-OHDA-lesioned rats. After 10 days, injected rats showed improved motor control and greater dopamine content in the SNc and striatum, indicating the ability of the transplanted cells to produce dopamine (128). However, conversion of these cell populations remains challenging. Some studies have suggested that the apparent conversion of stem cells to neurons may be due to cell fusion rather than differentiation (129). In addition, there is evidence that mesenchymal stem cells can be a source of tumor formation upon deposition in the brain (130). In light of their increased complexity and potential dangers, the use of non-neuronal stem cells to generate neurons for the treatment of PD remains controversial.

Neuronal Stem Cells

A significant conceptual shift in the past decade has come with the understanding that the adult brain does actively replenish its cells, generating multipotent stem cells in the subventricular zone and the subgranular region of the hippocampal dentate gyrus. Peripheral neuronal stem cells may also be harvested from the carotid body or other regions under investigation (131). Because these cells are committed to a neuronal phenotype differentiation to dopaminergic neurons they may be safer and more efficacious (132). Although dopaminergic neurons have been obtained from neuronal stem cell lines, particularly after treatment with FGF, GDNF, and other modulators of cell signaling (133), the dominant cell type produced is often not neuronal but astroglial (134). Such glial transplants might themselves be useful as they may express neuroreparative factors, including GDNF, and provide "homeostatic adjustments" to the microenvironment (135). In any case, encouraging results have been obtained in animal models transplanted with neuronal stem cells, including survival and migration of transplanted stem cells resulting in a functional impact, such as substantial behavioral improvement and significant restitution of motor function (136–138).

Stem cells provide a potential solution to the problems associated with the acquisition and transplantation of fetal dopaminergic neurons for the treatment of PD. However, the use of stem cells introduces additional complexity, as greater control of cellular growth and differentiation is required. The results, although preliminary, are encouraging, as stem cell transplantation has been demonstrated to produce functional improvements in animal models of PD. Human studies, however, must await the solution to the many technical and safety challenges.

GENE THERAPY FOR PD
Perhaps the most potent prospects for the future therapy of PD lie in gene therapy. Theoretically, the alteration or insertion of genetic material to correct or compensate diseased neurons should provide the most comprehensive and elegant therapy for a degenerative disease such as PD. A host of promising technologies are currently in various stages of clinical and preclinical trials (139).

Strategies of Gene Therapy
Ongoing research in gene therapy has segregated itself into several specific strategies of disease treatment. These include the viral transmission of enzymes in the dopamine synthesis pathway to restore local dopamine concentrations; the transmission of genes for neurotrophic factors such as GDNF and neurturin to support and protect remaining dopaminergic neurons; the delivery of genes, such as Parkin, designed to restore underlying genetic deficits; and the delivery of genes that alter the phenotypic function of local cells to perpetually rebalance the aberrant function of the basal ganglia. All share the advantage that, if they are effective, they could provide a single-intervention treatment for PD without the need for pump refilling, periodic replacement of a chronically implanted device hardware, or clinician adjustment of stimulation parameters to achieve desired effects, and without the potential ethical complications of cellular transplantation therapies.

Dopamine Synthesis Gene Therapy
One obvious strategy for treating PD is to confer a dopaminergic phenotype to cells within the striatum. This method should result in local production of levodopa or dopamine, thereby avoiding the variance and adverse effects of systemic drug delivery. To this end, several groups have designed therapies that deliver, via a viral carrier, genes in the dopamine biosynthetic pathway. The first reports in the early 1990s relied on the implantation of exogenously modified fibroblasts. These cells were harvested, amplified, and then genetically modified to produce enzymes such as tyrosine hydroxylase. Re-implantation resulted in an increase in striatal dopamine levels in rodent models (140–142).

Later studies accomplished the delivery of such genes directly to striatal cells with viral agents. A study by During et al. demonstrated that direct striatal transmission of tyrosine hydroxylase to rats by defective herpes simplex virus produced substantial increases in levodopa and dopamine (as measured by striatal microdialysis), and produced a 60% reduction in amphetamine-induced spinning behavior, which was maintained for a full year after treatment (143). Other studies demonstrated the adeno-associated virus (AAV) delivery of aromatic amino acid decarboxylase (AADC) in rat models of PD. Transfer of the AADC gene significantly increased dopamine production, from 5% to 50% in 6-OHDA-lesioned rats (144,145).

The generation and release of dopamine is a complex process. Dopamine synthesis requires tyrosine hydroxylase, guanine triphosphate cyclophydrolase I (GTP-CHI), and AADC (145–147). Moreover, production alone does not confer the machinery for transmitter packaging and organized release. For this reason, several researchers have adopted strategies designed to deliver multiple genes involved in dopamine production. Results suggest that the combined delivery of these genes is more effective than transduction with individual genes (148). One study additionally provided a vesicular monoamine transporter (VAT-2), enabling coordinated dopamine release and preventing elevated dopamine in the cytosol from inhibiting the action of tyrosine hydroxylase. This construct had a greater effect on rotational behavior of rats than constructs without the VAT-2 gene and produced local levels of dopamine that were similar to those measured in normal rats (149). The conference of multiple enzymes has been shown to decrease drug-induced dyskinesia by 85%. It is thought that the continuous release of dopamine conferred by gene transfer corrects the otherwise pulsatile delivery, even when medical therapies are ongoing (150).

Studies have been extended to primate models as well. An early study demonstrated the feasibility of transfecting tyrosine hydroxylase and AADC to produce dopamine in the primate striatum but showed no significant behavioral changes (151). Matsumura et al. demonstrated that AAV transmission of tyrosine hydroxylase, AADC, and GTP-CHI in primates produced substantial improvements in manual dexterity tasks and resulted in increased striatal dopamine levels relative to the untreated side (152). Later, Jarraya et al. treated MPTP-lesioned macaques with an equine infectious anemia virus (EIAV) transmitting the three genes, opting for EIAV instead of AAV due to the former's tricistronic capacity. This agent, termed ProSavin, produced long-term correction of motor deficits without producing dyskinesia, increased striatal dopamine, and reversed MPTP-induced signaling properties in the globus pallidus and STN compared with untreated and sham-treated MPTP-lesioned macaques. There was no evidence of tissue alteration, production of dopamine outside intended areas, inflammation beyond the injection area, or abnormal MRI signal (153). The ProSavin therapy is currently under evaluation in a clinical phase I/II trial. Most recently, a phase I open-label, dose-escalation study in 10 moderately advanced PD patients with motor fluctuations showed that bilateral putaminal infusions of AAV-AADC vector were well tolerated over four years. The results of this trial suggest that AAV-mediated gene transfer is likely permanent and it is not altered by the ongoing neurodegeneration of PD (154).

These techniques certainly hold great promise for the clinical treatment of PD by methods that are more physiologic and have potentially fewer adverse effects. Further clinical trials employing viral delivery of dopamine synthesis enzymes are ongoing.

Genetic Delivery of Neurotrophins

The second strategy relies on the neuroprotective effects of the neurotrophin GDNF or its close relative neurturin. These factors have previously been demonstrated to provide substantial preservation of dopaminergic inputs to striatum. Demonstrations of this effect in animal models and in clinical case reports represent a considerable body of evidence that the strategy is sound. Despite the negative trials of GDNF microinfusion by intraventricular administration (72,155) and by direct administration into the striatum (74), it is possible that local expression of GDNF provided by gene therapy would generate sufficient product to create benefit (156). Local production might also limit the adverse effects noted with exogenous delivery.

Numerous studies have demonstrated success of viral GDNF therapy in rats. Several viral vectors have been used to deliver GDNF to the striatum and SNc, including adenovirus, AAV, herpes virus, and lentiviruses. Of these, herpes viruses were noted to be problematic, providing only limited benefit and demonstrating significant toxicity related to purification methods (157). The other models have demonstrated the ability to generate stable and sufficient quantities of GDNF, to maintain or restore tyrosine hydroxylase activity, and, in several cases, to improve parkinsonian behavioral correlates (158,159).

Some studies have adopted more complex models to better approximate PD. In one study, Brizard et al. selected a rat model for progressive degeneration by injecting the SNc with a partial dose of 6-OHDA. This model is thought to more closely approximate the gradual degeneration of PD. They found that, four weeks after lesioning, addition of a lentiviral vector conferring GDNF production (lenti-GDNF) restored dopaminergic innervation of the striatum to near normal levels. This was accompanied by behavioral improvements in a task requiring paw-reaching to obtain food pellets (160). Similar studies have examined performance of complex motor selection tasks in rats pretreated with lenti-GDNF prior to 6-OHDA lesioning (161). These studies suggest similar treatment success in behavioral models more relevant to human disease.

Several other neurotrophins have been tested for their protective effect on nigrostriatal neurons. A study by Fjord-Larsen and colleagues demonstrated that in vivo lentiviral delivery of a modified neurturin construct produced neuroprotection of rat nigrostriatal projections. Tyrosine hydroxylase immunoreactive neurons were 91% of the unlesioned side. This was equivalent to the effect of lentiviral GDNF transduction (162).

GDNF delivery by lentivirus has been demonstrated in primates to produce stable transmission of the GDNF gene in both aged unlesioned monkeys and in young MPTP-lesioned monkeys. PET studies in the aged monkeys, who had received lentiviral GDNF administration to both the striatum and the substantia nigra, demonstrated that putaminal GDNF administration increased fluorodopa uptake by 37% on the treated side, with stable delivery of GDNF and migration from the injection site into the pallidum. Tyrosine hydroxylase immunoreactivity was also increased 39% and 44% in the caudate and putamen, respectively. The number of tyrosine hydroxylase-reactive cells in the substantia nigra increased 85% on the side of GDNF viral delivery. Young monkeys were treated with GDNF one week after unilateral administration of MPTP. Treatment with the lenti-GDNF showed significant increases in striatal fluorodopa uptake, averaging a threefold increase, compared with controls. The treated monkeys also showed significant improvements both in a clinical assessment with a modified clinical rating scale and in speed on a hand-reaching task (163).

Similarly, monkeys injected with AAV-neurturin to both striatum and substantia nigra following MPTP lesioning had 80–90% improvement in MPTP-induced motor impairments, as well as preserved nigral neurons and striatal dopaminergic innervations in contrast to controls. In an aged monkey model of nigrostriatal dopamine deficiency, striatal injection caused robust expression, increased fluorodopa uptake on the treated site, enhancement of tyrosine hydroxylase-positive fibers, and an increase in the number of tyrosine hydroxylase-positive cells (164). The expression of GDNF after viral delivery has been noted specifically to increase the number of tyrosine hydroxylase-expressing striatal cells by an average of sevenfold. This suggests that the addition of GDNF and GDNF-related neurotrophins may act to confer a dopaminergic phenotype to adult striatal cells, in addition to preserving dopaminergic nigral inputs onto the striatum (165).

An initial phase I, open-label study of this Cere-120 agent assessed various secondary measures of motor function and change in putaminal uptake of fluorodopa. There was a significant improvement in the off-medication UPDRS scores, but there was no change in fluorodopa uptake (166). A subsequent randomized phase II trial controlled by sham surgery enrolled 58 patients with advanced PD and focused on off-medication UPDRS motor scores between the treated and control groups at 12 months. The study failed to show a significant difference between the groups' scores (167). Issues that may have contributed to a lack of positive results include measuring the primary efficacy measure too early, inclusion of subjects whose PD was too advanced, and/or poor or inadequate target choice (168). Nonetheless, with GDNF and neurturin gene therapy established in rodent and primate models, the treatment modality holds considerable promise. New trials targeting both the striatum and substantia nigra, and using higher striatal doses and a later end point, have been initiated.

Gene Therapy to Alter Basal Ganglia Physiology

The manipulation of basal ganglia circuit function may be possible by the strategic placement of genes designed specifically to alter neuronal phenotype. Studies by Kaplitt et al. have used gene therapy to change the normal excitatory input of the STN-GPi projection to an inhibitory gamma-amino butyric acid (GABA)ergic projection. Rats with chemical lesions in the substantia nigra were treated with viral delivery of glutamic acid decarboxylase (GAD) via an AAV vector into the STN. They subsequently showed a reversal of SNr responses to STN stimulation with excitatory and inhibitory ratios changing from 83% and 6% to 17% and 78%, respectively. This was associated with a 65% decrease in amphetamine-induced rotational behavior (169). Another 6-OHDA rodent study confirmed changes in biochemical and physiologic properties of the STN-SNr projection and alleviated symptoms of PD (170). Similarly, macaques with MPTP-induced hemiparkinsonism were followed for one year after injection of AAV-GAD. The treatment was found to be safe, and gross motor function, tremor, and bradykinesia were all significantly improved (171).

A phase I, open-label, dose-escalation study found no intervention-related adverse events in 12 moderately advanced PD patients. In addition, there was no induction of autoantibodies against GAD, and there was significant improvement in off- and on-medication UPDRS scores after three months (172). A six-month phase II, double-blind, sham surgery-controlled, randomized trial found the only intervention-related adverse effects to be headache and nausea, and reported a significant difference in off-medication UPDRS score improvement between the treatment and control groups (173). While gene therapy to alter basal ganglia physiology may not provide neuroprotection or address PD symptoms outside the motor circuit, the results of the aforementioned trials support continued study of the therapy's safety and efficacy as a potential future alternative treatment.

Parkin Gene Therapy

The apparent success of gene therapy in conferring novel capabilities to nigral and striatal cells has led some researchers to question if the pathology underlying PD can be reversed in a more physiologic manner. Genetic analyses of PD families have demonstrated a number of genes linked to the disease. These mutations seem to share a role in intracellular housekeeping and the processing of intracellular protein residue. It is estimated that approximately 0.4–0.7% of patients diagnosed with idiopathic PD have Parkin mutations. This proportion dramatically increases to nearly 20% in cases of early-onset sporadic PD, and to almost 50% if there is evidence of familial transmission (174). In these patients, loss of Parkin's E3 ubiquitin ligase activity leads to degeneration of dopaminergic neurons (175,176).

Lo Bianco et al. have used lentiviral delivery to increase expression of the normal Parkin gene in the substantia nigra of rats that were also transfected with the human alpha-synuclein gene. Viral expression of alpha-synuclein is known to cause degeneration of dopaminergic nigral neurons in rats. The addition of a vector delivering a wild-type Parkin gene was found to have a substantial protective effect, reducing dopaminergic cell loss from 31% to 9%. Interestingly, this was accompanied by a 45% increase in alpha-synuclein inclusions, suggesting that Parkin exerts its neuroprotective effect by precipitating an otherwise soluble toxic synuclein compound (177). This has significant implications for the pathogenesis of the disease.

More recently, Imam et al. demonstrated that the loss of Parkin's ligase and cytoprotective activities were caused by tyrosine phosphorylation by the stress-signaling nonreceptor tyrosine kinase c-Abl. This suggests a potential neuroprotective therapy that could be used to halt the progress of PD, as they also showed a selective c-Abl inhibitor prevented tyrosine phosphorylation of Parkin and restored its E3 ligase and protective functions both in vitro and in vivo (178).

Other studies have examined the effect of chaperone heat-shock proteins (Hsp) in nigral protection. Hsp-70 has been shown to be a suppressor of alpha-synuclein toxicity in various cellular and Drosophila models of PD (179–181), whereas Hsp-104 reduced the formation of alpha-synuclein inclusions and prevented dopaminergic degeneration in a rat model (182). A study by Dong et al. used an AAV carrier to deliver Hsp-70 to the substantia nigra of MPTP-treated mice. They demonstrated that expression of the gene reduced nigral cell loss from 37% to 16% in control animals. It also was found to produce an increase in amphetamine-induced rotational behavior, indicating that behaviorally significant neuroprotection had occurred (183). The common strategy of providing or restoring protective factors in cells failing to process cellular waste is particularly appealing, as it targets and reverses what may be the central pathology of PD.

Intravenous Gene Delivery

Although the majority of gene therapy studies have relied on a surgical delivery of genetically altered cells or of viral vectors to transmit the desired genes, a novel line of research has experimented with engineered liposomes that are immunologically targeted to be taken up by neurons. Plasmid DNA containing the gene intended for transfer (such as tyrosine hydroxylase) is packaged in a 100-nm liposome. The structure is stabilized by the incorporation of several thousand polyethylene glycol residues. A percentage of these are conjugated to monoclonal antibodies that target either the insulin or transferrin receptors. The antibody targeting causes the liposomes to be selectively taken up in the brain. Association of the desired gene with a glial fibrillary acidic protein (GFAP) promoter further specifies the location of gene activity (184).

Genes packaged by this technique can be delivered by a simple intravenous administration. Pardridge et al. demonstrated the ability of this technique to deliver a desired gene specifically to the brain in both rodents and in rhesus monkeys (184). It has further been shown that the same intravenous delivery of the tyrosine hydroxylase gene and of GDNF can reverse rotational behavior in 6-OHDA-lesioned rats (184–188). Although studies are still quite preliminary, they offer the additional hope that the genetic modifications described earlier might eventually be delivered with decreased risk and discomfort to the patient. This might also allow a more measured and gradual titration of delivery to maximize therapeutic benefit and limit adverse effects.

SUMMARY

The future of PD treatment will be significantly influenced by the innovative therapeutic modalities described above. Evidence suggests that PD treatment is already undergoing a transmutation, as surgical therapies have accumulated Class 1 evidence and are firmly integrated in current treatment paradigms. We anticipate that the next decade will see a substantial maturation of stimulation therapies as new devices and targets enable more sensitive and effective treatments. Cellular transplantation and gene therapy will also begin to play a significant role as current phase I and II studies are followed by more conclusive trials. In time, the stimulatory interventions that have been so successful in the last decade may give way to strategies that can restore and, perhaps, eventually reverse the degenerative pathology of PD.

REFERENCES

1. Deuschl G, Schade-Brittinger C, Krack P, et al. A randomized trial of deep-brain stimulation for Parkinson's disease. N Engl J Med 2006; 355: 896–908.
2. Schupbach WM, Maltete D, Houeto JL, et al. Neurosurgery at an earlier stage of Parkinson's disease: a randomized, controlled trial. Neurology 2007; 68: 267–71.
3. Weaver FM, Follett K, Stern M, et al. Bilateral deep brain stimulation vs best medical therapy for patients with advanced Parkinson's disease: a randomized controlled trial. JAMA 2009; 301: 63–73.
4. Williams A, Gill S, Varma T, et al. Deep brain stimulation plus best medical therapy versus best medical therapy alone for advanced Parkinson's disease (PD SURG trial): a randomised, open-label trial. Lancet Neurol 2010; 9: 581–91.
5. Braak H, Del Tredici K, Rub U, et al. Staging of brain pathology related to sporadic Parkinson's disease. Neurobiol Aging 2003; 24: 197–211.
6. Santens P, De Letter M, Van Borsel J, et al. Lateralized effects of subthalamic nucleus stimulation on different aspects of speech in Parkinson's disease. Brain Lang 2003; 87: 253–8.
7. Saint-Cyr JA, Trepanier LL, Kumar R, et al. Neuropsychological consequences of chronic bilateral stimulation of the subthalamic nucleus in Parkinson's disease. Brain 2000; 123: 2091–108.

8. Gentil M, Garcia-Ruiz P, Pollak P, et al. Effect of bilateral deep-brain stimulation on oral control of patients with Parkinsonism. Eur Neurol 2000; 44: 147–52.

9. Hamani C, Richter E, Schwalb JM, et al. Bilateral subthalamic nucleus stimulation for parkinson's disease: a systematic review of the clinical literature. Neurosurgery 2005; 56: 1313–24.

10. Dromey C, Kumar R, Lang AE, et al. An investigation of the effects of subthalamic nucleus stimulation on acoustic measures of voice. Mov Disord 2000; 15: 1132–8.

11. Burkhard PR, Vingerhoets FJ, Berney A, et al. Suicide after successful deep brain stimulation for movement disorders. Neurology 2004; 63: 2170–2.

12. Kenney C, Simpson R, Hunter C, et al. Short-term and long-term safety of deep brain stimulation in the treatment of movement disorders. J Neurosurgery 2007; 106: 621–5.

13. Weinberger M, Hutchison WD, Lozano AM, et al. Increased gamma oscillatory activity in the subthalamic nucleus during tremor in Parkinson's disease patients. J Neurophysiol 2009; 101: 789–802.

14. Weinberger M, Mahant N, Hutchison WD, et al. Beta oscillatory activity in the subthalamic nucleus and its relation to dopaminergic response in Parkinson's disease. J Neurophysiol 2006; 96: 3248–56.

15. Rouse AG, Stanslaski SR, Cong P, et al. A chronic generalized bi-directional brain-machine interface. J Neural Eng 2011; 8: 036018.

16. Agnesi F, Tye SJ, Bledsoe JM, et al. Wireless instantaneous neurotransmitter concentration system-based amperometric detection of dopamine, adenosine, and glutamate for intraoperative neurochemical monitoring. J Neurosurg 2009; 111: 701–11.

17. Bledsoe JM, Kimble CJ, Covey DP, et al. Development of the wireless instantaneous neurotransmitter concentration system for intraoperative neurochemical monitoring using fast-scan cyclic voltammetry. J Neurosurg 2009; 111: 712–23.

18. Kimble CJ, Johnson DM, Winter BA, et al. Wireless Instantaneous Neurotransmitter Concentration Sensing System (WINCS) for intraoperative neurochemical monitoring. Conf Proc IEEE Eng Med Biol Soc 2009; 2009: 4856–9.

19. Rosin B, Slovik M, Mitelman R, et al. Closed-loop deep brain stimulation is superior in ameliorating parkinsonism. Neuron 2011; 72: 370–384.

20. Albin RL, Young AB, Penney JB. The functional anatomy of basal ganglia disorders. Trends Neurosci 1989; 12: 366–75.

21. Fénelon G, Francois C, Percheron G, et al. Topographic distribution of pallidal neurons projecting to the thalamus in macaques. Brain Res 1990; 520: 27–35.

22. Mengual E, de las Heras S, Erro E, et al. Thalamic interaction between the input and the output systems of the basal ganglia. J Chem Neuroanat 1999; 16: 187–200.

23. Hammond C, Rouzaire-Dubois B, Feger J, et al. Anatomical and electrophysiological studies on the reciprocal projections between the subthalamic nucleus and nucleus tegmenti pedunculopontinus in the rat. Neuroscience 1983; 9: 41–52.

24. Mitrofanis J. Some certainty for the "zone of uncertainty"? Exploring the function of the zona incerta. Neuroscience 2005; 130: 1–15.

25. Obeso JA, Rodriguez MC, DeLong MR. Basal ganglia pathophysiology. A critical review. Adv Neurol 1997; 74: 3–18.

26. Obeso JA, Rodriguez-Oroz MC, Rodriguez M, et al. Pathophysiology of the basal ganglia in Parkinson's disease. Trends Neurosci 2000; 23: S8–S19.

27. Pahapill PA, Lozano AM. The pedunculopontine nucleus and Parkinson's disease. Brain 2000; 123: 1767–83.

28. Mink JW, Thach WT. Basal ganglia motor control. I. Nonexclusive relation of pallidal discharge to five movement modes. J Neurophysiol 1991; 65: 273–300.

29. Mink JW, Thach WT. Basal ganglia motor control. II. Late pallidal timing relative to movement onset and inconsistent pallidal coding of movement parameters. J Neurophysiol 1991; 65: 301–29.

30. Mink JW, Thach WT. Basal ganglia motor control. III. Pallidal ablation: normal reaction time, muscle cocontraction, and slow movement. J Neurophysiol 1991; 65: 330–51.

31. Mazzone P, Lozano A, Stanzione P, et al. Implantation of human pedunculopontine nucleus: a safe and clinically relevant target in Parkinson's disease. Neuroreport 2005; 16: 1877–81.

32. Plaha P, Gill SS. Bilateral deep brain stimulation of the pedunculopontine nucleus for Parkinson's disease. Neuroreport 2005; 16: 1883–7.
33. Stefani A, Lozano AM, Peppe A, et al. Bilateral deep brain stimulation of the pedunculo-pontine and subthalamic nuclei in severe Parkinson's disease. Brain 2007; 130: 1596–607.
34. Moro E, Hamani C, Poon YY, et al. Unilateral pedunculopontine stimulation improves falls in Parkinson's disease. Brain 2010; 133: 215–24.
35. Ferraye MU, Debu B, Fraix V, et al. Effects of pedunculopontine nucleus area stimula-tion on gait disorders in Parkinson's disease. Brain 2010; 133: 205–14.
36. Zrinzo L, Zrinzo LV, Hariz M. The pedunculopontine and peripeduncular nuclei: a tale of two structures. Brain 2007; 130: e73; author reply e74.
37. Thevathasan W, Coyne TJ, Hyam JA, et al. Pedunculopontine nucleus stimulation improves gait freezing in Parkinson's disease. Neurosurgery 2011; 69: 1248–53; discus-sion 1254.
38. Khan S, Mooney L, Plaha P, et al. Outcomes from stimulation of the caudal zona incerta and pedunculopontine nucleus in patients with Parkinson's disease. Br J Neurosurg 2011; 25: 273–80.
39. Spiegel EA, Wycis HT, Szekely EG, et al. Campotomy in various extrapyramidal disor-ders. J Neurosurg 1963; 20: 871–84.
40. Velasco F, Jimenez F, Perez ML, et al. Electrical stimulation of the prelemniscal radia-tion in the treatment of Parkinson's disease: an old target revised with new techniques. Neurosurgery 2001; 49: 293–306; discussion 306–8.
41. Gallay MN, Jeanmonod D, Liu J, et al. Human pallidothalamic and cerebellothalamic tracts: anatomical basis for functional stereotactic neurosurgery. Brain Struct Funct 2008; 212: 443–63.
42. Plaha P, Filipovic S, Gill SS. Induction of parkinsonian resting tremor by stimulation of the caudal zona incerta nucleus: a clinical study. J Neurol Neurosurg Psychiatry 2008; 79: 514–21.
43. Kitagawa M, Murata J, Uesugi H, et al. Two-year follow-up of chronic stimulation of the posterior subthalamic white matter for tremor-dominant Parkinson's disease. Neu-rosurgery 2005; 56: 281–9; discussion 281–9.
44. Carrillo-Ruiz JD, Velasco F, Jimenez F, et al. Bilateral electrical stimulation of prelem-niscal radiations in the treatment of advanced Parkinson's disease. Neurosurgery 2008; 62: 347–57; discussion 357–9.
45. Plaha P, Ben-Shlomo Y, Patel NK, et al. Stimulation of the caudal zona incerta is supe-rior to stimulation of the subthalamic nucleus in improving contralateral parkinsonism. Brain 2006; 129: 1732–47.
46. Khan S, Gill SS, Mooney L, et al. Combined pedunculopontine-subthalamic stimulation in Parkinson's disease. Neurology 2012; 78: 1090–5.
47. Merello M, Cavanagh S, Perez-Lloret S, et al. Irritability, psychomotor agitation and progressive insomnia induced by bilateral stimulation of the area surrounding the dor-sal subthalamic nucleus (zona incerta) in Parkinson's disease patients. J Neurol 2009; 256: 2091–3.
48. Katayama Y, Fukaya C, Yamamoto T. Control of poststroke involuntary and voluntary movement disorders with deep brain or epidural cortical stimulation. Stereotact Funct Neurosurg 1997; 69: 73–9.
49. García-Larrea L, Peyron R, Mertens P, et al. Electrical stimulation of motor cortex for pain control: a combined PET-scan and electrophysiological study. Pain 1999; 83: 259–73.
50. Canavero S, Bonicalzi V. Cortical stimulation for Parkinsonism. Arch Neurol 2004; 61: 606.
51. Canavero S, Paolotti R. Extradural motor cortex stimulation for advanced Parkinson's disease: case report. Mov Disord 2000; 15: 169–71.
52. Canavero S, Paolotti R, Bonicalzi V, et al. Extradural motor cortex stimulation for advanced Parkinson's disease. J Neurosurg 2002; 97: 1208–11.
53. Arle JE, Apetauerova D, Zani J, et al. Motor cortex stimulation in patients with Parkin-son's disease: 12-month follow-up in 4 patients. J Neurosurg 2008; 109: 133–9.
54. Pagni CA, Albanese A, Bentivoglio A, et al. Results by motor cortex stimulation in treatment of focal dystonia, Parkinson's disease and post-ictal spasticity. In: Chiu W-T, Kao M-C,

Chiang Y-H, et al. eds. The Experience of the Italian Study Group of the Italian Neurosurgical Society Reconstructive Neurosurgery. Springer: Vienna, 2008: 13–21.

55. Gutiérrez JC, Seijo FJ, Alvarez Vega MA, et al. Therapeutic extradural cortical stimulation for Parkinson's disease: report of six cases and review of the literature. Clin Neurol Neurosurg 2009; 111: 703–7.

56. Moro E, Schwalb JM, Piboolnurak P, et al. Unilateral subdural motor cortex stimulation improves essential tremor but not Parkinson's disease. Brain 2011; 134: 2096–105.

57. Nakao N, Nakai E, Nakai K, et al. Ablation of the subthalamic nucleus supports the survival of nigral dopaminergic neurons after nigrostriatal lesions induced by the mitochondrial toxin 3-nitropropionic acid. Ann Neurol 1999; 45: 640–51.

58. Wallace BA, Ashkan K, Heise CE, et al. Survival of midbrain dopaminergic cells after lesion or deep brain stimulation of the subthalamic nucleus in MPTP-treated monkeys. Brain 2007; 130: 2129–45.

59. Hilker R, Portman AT, Voges J, et al. Disease progression continues in patients with advanced Parkinson's disease and effective subthalamic nucleus stimulation. J Neurol Neurosurg Psychiatry 2005; 76: 1217–21.

60. Kahn E, D'Haese PF, Dawant B, et al. Deep brain stimulation in early stage Parkinson's disease: operative experience from a prospective randomised clinical trial. J Neurol Neurosurg Psychiatry 2012; 83: 164–70.

61. Remple MS, Bradenham CH, Kao CC, et al. Subthalamic nucleus neuronal firing rate increases with Parkinson's disease progression. Mov Disord 2011; 26: 1657–62.

62. Lin L, Doherty DH, Lile JD, et al. GDNF: a glial cell line-derived neurotrophic factor for midbrain dopaminergic neurons. Science 1993; 260: 1130–2.

63. Scharr DG, et al. Regional and cell-specific expression of GDNF in rat brain. Exp Neurol 1993; 124: 368–71.

64. Beck KD, Valverde J, Alexi T, et al. Mesencephalic dopaminergic neurons protected by GDNF from axotomy-induced degeneration in the adult brain. Nature 1995; 373: 339–41.

65. Tomac A, Lindqvist E, Lin LF, et al. Protection and repair of the nigrostriatal dopaminergic system by GDNF in vivo. Nature 1995; 373: 335–9.

66. Gash DM, Zhang Z, Ovadia A, et al. Functional recovery in parkinsonian monkeys treated with GDNF. Nature 1996; 380: 252–5.

67. Olson L. Toward trophic treatment in parkinsonism: a primate step. Nat Med 1996; 2: 400–1.

68. Lapchak PA, Gash DM, Collins F, et al. Pharmacological activities of Glial Cell Line-Derived Neurotrophic Factor (GDNF): Preclinical development and application to the treatment of Parkinson's disease. Exp Neurol 1997; 145: 309–21.

69. Lapchak PA, Gash DM, Jiao S, et al. Glial Cell Line-Derived Neurotrophic Factor: A novel therapeutic approach to treat motor dysfunction in Parkinson's disease. Exp Neurol 1997; 144: 29–34.

70. Gill SS, et al. Intraparenchymal putaminal administration of glialderived neurotrophic factor in the treatment of advanced Parkinson's disease. Neurology 2002; 58:A241.

71. Kordower JH, Palfi S, Chen EY, et al. Clinicopathological findings following intraventricular glial-derived neurotrophic factor treatment in a patient with Parkinson's disease. Ann Neurol 1999; 46: 419–24.

72. Nutt JG, Burchiel KJ, Comella CL, et al. Randomized, double-blind trial of glial cell line-derived neurotrophic factor (GDNF) in PD. Neurology 2003; 60: 69–73.

73. Gill SS, Patel NK, Hotton GR, et al. Direct brain infusion of glial cell line-derived neurotrophic factor in Parkinson's disease. Nat Med 2003; 9: 589–95.

74. Lang AE, Gill S, Patel NK, et al. Randomized controlled trial of intraputamenal glial cell line–derived neurotrophic factor infusion in Parkinson's disease. Ann Neurol 2006; 59: 459–66.

75. Salvatore MF, Ai Y, Fischer B, et al. Point source concentration of GDNF may explain failure of phase II clinical trial. Exp Neurol 2006; 202: 497–505.

76. Kotzbauer PT, Lampe PA, Heuckeroth RO, et al. Neurturin, a relative of glial-cell-line-derived neurotrophic factor. Nature 1996; 384: 467–70.

77. Horger BA, Nishimura MC, Armanini MP, et al. Neurturin exerts potent actions on survival and function of midbrain dopaminergic neurons. J Neurosci 1998; 18: 4929–37.
78. Oiwa Y, Yoshimura R, Nakai K, et al. Dopaminergic neuroprotection and regeneration by neurturin assessed by using behavioral, biochemical and histochemical measurements in a model of progressive Parkinson's disease. Brain Res 2002; 947: 271–83.
79. Quartu M, Serra MP, Manca A, et al. Neurturin, persephin, and artemin in the human pre- and full-term newborn and adult hippocampus and fascia dentata. Brain Res 2005; 1041: 157–66.
80. Masure S, Geerts H, Cik M, et al. Enovin, a member of the Glial Cell-Line-Derived Neurotrophic Factor (GDNF) family with growth promoting activity on neuronal cells. Eur J Biochem 1999; 266: 892–902.
81. Baloh RH, Tansey MG, Lampe PA, et al. Artemin, a novel member of the GDNF ligand family, supports peripheral and central neurons and signals through the GFRα3–RET receptor complex. Neuron 1998; 21: 1291–302.
82. Clarke DJ, Brundin P, Strecker RE, et al. Human fetal dopamine neurons grafted in a rat model of Parkinson's disease: ultrastructural evidence for synapse formation using tyrosine hydroxylase immunocytochemistry. Exp Brain Res 1988; 73: 115–26.
83. Brundin P, Strecker RE, Widner H, et al. Human fetal dopamine neurons grafted in a rat model of Parkinson's disease: immunological aspects, spontaneous and drug-induced behaviour, and dopamine release. Exp Brain Res 1988; 70: 192–208.
84. Sladek JR, Collier TJ, Haber SN, et al. Reversal of Parkinsonism by fetal nerve cell transplants in primate brain. Ann N Y Acad Sci 1987; 495: 641–57.
85. Bankiewicz KS, Plunkett RJ, Jacobowitz DM, et al. The effect of fetal mesencephalon implants on primate MPTP-induced parkinsonism. J Neurosurg 1990; 72: 231–44.
86. Perlow M, Freed WJ, Hoffer BJ, et al. Brain grafts reduce motor abnormalities produced by destruction of nigrostriatal dopamine system. Science 1979; 204: 643–7.
87. Brundin P, Nilsson OG, Strecker RE, et al. Behavioural effects of human fetal dopamine neurons grafted in a rat model of Parkinson's disease. Exp Brain Res 1986; 65: 235–40.
88. Bankiewicz KS, et al. Chapter 63 Behavioral recovery from MPTP-induced parkinsonism in monkeys after intracerebral tissue implants is not related to CSF concentrations of dopamine metabolites. In: Dunnett SB, Richards SJ, eds. Progress in Brain Research. Elsevier, 1990: 561–71.
89. Freed CR, Breeze RE, Rosenberg NL, et al. Transplantation of human fetal dopamine cells for Parkinson's disease: results at 1 year. Arch Neurol 1990; 47: 505–12.
90. Lindvall O, Brundin P, Widner H, et al. Grafts of fetal dopamine neurons survive and improve motor function in Parkinson's disease. Science 1990; 247: 574–7.
91. Kordower JH, Freeman TB, Snow BJ, et al. Neuropathological evidence of graft survival and striatal reinnervation after the transplantation of fetal mesencephalic tissue in a patient with Parkinson's disease. N Engl J Med 1995; 332: 1118–24.
92. Freed CR, Breeze RE, Rosenberg NL, et al. Survival of implanted fetal dopamine cells and neurologic improvement 12 to 46 months after transplantation for Parkinson's disease. N Engl J Med 1992; 327: 1549–55.
93. Freed CR, Greene PE, Breeze RE, et al. Transplantation of embryonic dopamine neurons for severe Parkinson's disease. N Engl J Med 2001; 344: 710–19.
94. Olanow CW, Goetz CG, Kordower JH, et al. A double-blind controlled trial of bilateral fetal nigral transplantation in Parkinson's disease. Ann Neurol 2003; 54: 403–14.
95. Carlsson T, Winkler C, Lundblad M, et al. Graft placement and uneven pattern of reinnervation in the striatum is important for development of graft-induced dyskinesia. Neurobiol Dis 2006; 21: 657–68.
96. Lane EL, Winkler C, Brundin P, et al. The impact of graft size on the development of dyskinesia following intrastriatal grafting of embryonic dopamine neurons in the rat. Neurobiol Dis 2006; 22: 334–45.
97. Lane EL, Vercammen L, Cenci MA, et al. Priming for L-DOPA-induced abnormal involuntary movements increases the severity of amphetamine-induced dyskinesia in grafted rats. Exp Neurol 2009; 219: 355–8.
98. Lane EL. Clinical and experimental experiences of graft-induced dyskinesia. Int Rev Neurobiol 2011; 98: 173–86.

99. Politis M, Oertel WH, Wu K, et al. Graft-induced dyskinesias in Parkinson's disease: high striatal serotonin/dopamine transporter ratio. Mov Disord 2011; 26: 1997–2003.

100. Olanow CW, Gracies JM, Goetz CG, et al. Clinical pattern and risk factors for dyskinesias following fetal nigral transplantation in Parkinson's disease: A double blind video-based analysis. Mov Disord 2009; 24: 336–43.

101. Graff-Radford J, Foote KD, Rodriguez RL, et al. Deep brain stimulation of the internal segment of the globus pallidus in delayed runaway dyskinesia. Arch Neurol 2006; 63: 1181–4.

102. Herzog J, Pogarell O, Pinsker MO, et al. Deep brain stimulation in Parkinson's disease following fetal nigral transplantation. Mov Disord 2008; 23: 1293–6.

103. Piccini P, Pavese N, Hagell P, et al. Factors affecting the clinical outcome after neural transplantation in Parkinson's disease. Brain 2005; 128: 2977–86.

104. Olanow CW, Kordower JH, Freeman TB. Fetal nigral transplantation as a therapy for Parkinson's disease. Trends Neurosci 1996; 19: 102–9.

105. Redmond D, Naftolin F, Collier TJ, et al. Cryopreservation, culture, and transplantation of human fetal mesencephalic tissue into monkeys. Science 1988; 242: 768–71.

106. Redmond DE, Leranth C, Spencer DD, et al. Fetal neural graft survival. Lancet 1990; 336: 820–2.

107. Katsnelson A. Experimental therapies for Parkinson's disease: Why fake it? Nature 2011; 476: 142–4.

108. Lunn JS, Sakowski SA, Hur J, et al. Stem cell technology for neurodegenerative diseases. Ann Neurol 2011; 70: 353–61.

109. Snyder BJ, Olanow CW. Stem cell treatment for Parkinson's disease: an update for 2005. Curr Opin Neurol 2005; 18: 376–85.

110. Perrier AL, Tabar V, Barberi T, et al. Derivation of midbrain dopamine neurons from human embryonic stem cells. Proc Natl Acad Sci USA 2004; 101: 12543–8.

111. Torres EM, Monville C, Lowenstein PR, et al. Delivery of sonic hedgehog or glial derived neurotrophic factor to dopamine-rich grafts in a rat model of Parkinson's disease using adenoviral vectors: Increased yield of dopamine cells is dependent on embryonic donor age. Brain Res Bull 2005; 68: 31–41.

112. Friling S, Perlmann T, Ericson J, et al. Efficient production of mesencephalic dopamine neurons by Lmx1a expression in embryonic stem cells. Proc Natl Acad Sci USA 2009; 106: 7613–18.

113. Chung S, Hedlund E, Hwang M, et al. The homeodomain transcription factor Pitx3 facilitates differentiation of mouse embryonic stem cells into AHD2-expressing dopaminergic neurons. Mol Cell Neurosci 2005; 28: 241–52.

114. Sonntag K-C, Pruszak J, Yoshizaki T, et al. Enhanced yield of neuroepithelial precursors and midbrain-like dopaminergic neurons from human embryonic stem cells using the bone morphogenic protein antagonist noggin. Stem Cells 2007; 25: 411–18.

115. Smith JR, Vallier L, Lupo G, et al. Inhibition of activin/nodal signaling promotes specification of human embryonic stem cells into neuroectoderm. Dev Biol 2008; 313: 107–17.

116. Chambers SM, Fasano CA, Papapetrou EP, et al. Highly efficient neural conversion of human ES and iPS cells by dual inhibition of SMAD signaling. Nat Biotech 2009; 27: 275–80.

117. Björklund LM, Sánchez-Pernaute R, Chung S, et al. Embryonic stem cells develop into functional dopaminergic neurons after transplantation in a Parkinson rat model. Proc Natl Acad Sci USA 2002; 99: 2344–9.

118. Takagi Y, Takahashi J, Saiki H, et al. Dopaminergic neurons generated from monkey embryonic stem cells function in a Parkinson primate model. J Clin Invest 2005; 115: 102–9.

119. Yang D, Zhang ZJ, Oldenburg M, et al. Human embryonic stem cell-derived dopaminergic neurons reverse functional deficit in parkinsonian rats. Stem Cells 2008; 26: 55–63.

120. Brederlau A, Correia AS, Anisimov SV, et al. Transplantation of human embryonic stem cell-derived cells to a rat model of Parkinson's disease: effect of in vitro differentiation on graft survival and teratoma formation. Stem Cells 2006; 24: 1433–40.

121. Ben-Hur T, Idelson M, Khaner H, et al. Transplantation of human embryonic stem cell–derived neural progenitors improves behavioral deficit in Parkinsonian rats. Stem Cells 2004; 22: 1246–55.

122. Kordower JH, Chu Y, Hauser RA, et al. Lewy body-like pathology in long-term embryonic nigral transplants in Parkinson's disease. Nat Med 2008; 14: 504–6.

123. Toma JG, Akhavan M, Fernandes KJ, et al. Isolation of multipotent adult stem cells from the dermis of mammalian skin. Nat Cell Biol 2001; 3: 778–84.

124. Mezey É, Chandross KJ, Harta G, et al. Turning blood into brain: cells bearing neuronal antigens generated in vivo from bone marrow. Science 2000; 290: 1779–82.

125. Stover NP, Bakay RA, Subramanian T, et al. Intrastriatal implantation of human retinal pigment epithelial cells attached to microcarriers in advanced Parkinson's disease. Arch Neurol 2005; 62: 1833–7.

126. McCoy MK, Martinez TN, Ruhn KA, et al. Autologous transplants of Adipose-Derived Adult Stromal (ADAS) cells afford dopaminergic neuroprotection in a model of Parkinson's disease. Exp Neurol 2008; 210: 14–29.

127. Fu Y-S, Cheng YC, Lin MY, et al. Conversion of human umbilical cord mesenchymal stem cells in wharton's jelly to dopaminergic neurons in vitro: potential therapeutic application for parkinsonism. Stem Cells 2006; 24: 115–24.

128. Zou Z, Jiang X, Zhang W, et al. Efficacy of tyrosine hydroxylase gene modified neural stem cells derived from bone marrow on Parkinson's disease – a rat model study. Brain Res 2010; 1346: 279–86.

129. Terada N, Hamazaki T, Oka M, et al. Bone marrow cells adopt the phenotype of other cells by spontaneous cell fusion. Nature 2002; 416: 542–5.

130. Snyder EY. The risk of putting something where it does not belong: Mesenchymal stem cells produce masses in the brain. Exp Neurol 2011; 230: 75–7.

131. Lunn JS, Sakowski SA, Federici T, et al. Stem cell technology for the study and treatment of motor neuron diseases. Regen Med 2011; 6: 201–13.

132. Lorenz S, Viviane T, Ron M. Transplantation of Expanded Mesencephalic Precursors Leads to Recovery in Parkinsonian Rats. Nature Publishing Group, 1998.

133. Wang X, Lu Y, Zhang H, et al. Distinct efficacy of pre-differentiated versus intact fetal mesencephalon-derived human neural progenitor cells in alleviating rat model of Parkinson's disease. Int J Dev Neurosci 2004; 22: 175–83.

134. Redmond DE, Weiss S, Elsworth JD, et al. Cellular repair in the Parkinsonian nonhuman primate brain. Rejuvenation Res 2010; 13: 188–94.

135. Freeman MR. Sculpting the nervous system: Glial control of neuronal development. Curr Opin Neurobiol 2006; 16: 119–25.

136. Parati E, Bez A, Ponti D, et al. Neural stem cells. Biological features and therapeutic potential in Parkinson's disease. J Neurosurg Sci 2003; 47: 8–17.

137. Redmond DE Jr, Bjugstad KB, Teng YD, et al. Behavioral improvement in a primate Parkinson's model is associated with multiple homeostatic effects of human neural stem cells. Proc Natl Acad Sci USA 2007; 104: 12175–80.

138. O'Keeffe FE, Scott SA, Tyers P, et al. Induction of A9 dopaminergic neurons from neural stem cells improves motor function in an animal model of Parkinson's disease. Brain 2008; 131: 630–41.

139. Wakeman DR, Dodiya HB, Kordower JH. Cell transplantation and gene therapy in Parkinson's disease. Mt Sinai J Med 2011; 78: 126–58.

140. Horellou P, Brundin P, Kalen P, et al. In vivo release of DOPA and dopamine from genetically engineered cells grafted to the denervated rat striatum. Neuron 1990; 5: 393–402.

141. Horellou P, Marlier L, Privat A, et al. Behavioural effect of engineered cells that synthesize L-DOPA or dopamine after grafting into the rat neostriatum. Eur J Neurosci 1990; 2: 116–19.

142. Fisher LJ, Jinnah HA, Kale LC, et al. Survival and function of intrastriatally grafted primary fibroblasts genetically modified to produce l-dopa. Neuron 1991; 6: 371–80.

143. During MJ, Naegele JR, O'Malley KL, et al. Long-term behavioral recovery in parkinsonian rats by an HSV vector expressing tyrosine hydroxylase. Science 1994; 266: 1399–403.

144. Leff SE, Spratt SK, Snyder RO, et al. Long-term restoration of striatal l-aromatic amino acid decarboxylase activity using recombinant adeno-associated viral vector gene transfer in a rodent model of Parkinson's disease. Neuroscience 1999; 92: 185–96.

145. Sanchez-Pernaute R, Harvey-White J, Cunningham J, et al. Functional effect of adeno-associated virus mediated gene transfer of aromatic L-Amino acid decarboxylase into the Striatum of 6-OHDA-Lesioned rats. Mol Ther 2001; 4: 324–30.

146. Bencsics C, Wachtel SR, Milstien S, et al. Double transduction with GTP Cyclohydrolase I and Tyrosine Hydroxylase is necessary for spontaneous synthesis ofl-DOPA by primary fibroblasts. J Neurosci 1996; 16: 4449–56.

147. Kang U. Potential of gene therapy for Parkinson's disease: neurobiologic issues and new developments in gene transfer methodologies. Mov Disord 1998; 13: 59–72.

148. Fan D-S, Ogawa M, Fujimoto KI, et al. Behavioral recovery in 6-Hydroxydopamine-Lesioned rats by cotransduction of striatum with tyrosine hydroxylase and aromatic L-amino acid decarboxylase genes using two separate adeno-associated virus vectors. Hum Gene Ther 1998; 9: 2527–35.

149. Sun M, Li Z, Zhang Y, et al. Coexpression of tyrosine hydroxylase, GTP cyclohydrolase I, aromatic amino acid decarboxylase, and vesicular monoamine transporter 2 from a helper virus-free herpes simplex virus type 1 vector supports high-level, long-term biochemical and behavioral correction of a rat model of Parkinson's disease. Hum Gene Therapy 2005; 15: 1177–96.

150. Carlsson T, Winkler C, Burger C, et al. Reversal of dyskinesias in an animal model of Parkinson's disease by continuous l-DOPA delivery using rAAV vectors. Brain 2005; 128: 559–69.

151. During MJ, Samulski RJ, Elsworth JD, et al. In vivo expression of therapeutic human genes for dopamine production in the caudates of MPTP-treated monkeys using an AAV vector. Gene Ther 1998; 5: 820–7.

152. Muramatsu S, Fujimoto K, Ikeguchi K, et al. Behavioral recovery in a primate model of Parkinson's disease by triple transduction of striatal cells with adeno-associated viral vectors expressing dopamine-synthesizing enzymes. Hum Gene Ther 2002; 13: 345–54.

153. Jarraya B, Boulet S, Ralph GS, et al. Dopamine gene therapy for Parkinson's disease in a nonhuman primate without associated Dyskinesia. Sci Transl Med 2009; 1: 2ra4.

154. Mittermeyer G, Christine CW, Rosenbluth KH, et al. Long-term evaluation of a phase 1 study of AADC gene therapy for Parkinson's Disease. Hum Gene Ther 2012; 23: 377–81.

155. Kordower JH. In vivo gene delivery of glial cell line–derived neurotrophic factor for Parkinson's disease. Ann Neurol 2003; 53: S120–34.

156. Betchen SA, Kaplitt M. Future and current surgical therapies in Parkinson's disease. Curr Opin Neurol 2003; 16: 487–93.

157. Monville C, Torres E, Thomas E, et al. HSV vector-delivery of GDNF in a rat model of PD: partial efficacy obscured by vector toxicity. Brain Res 2004; 1024: 1–15.

158. Bensadoun J-C, Deglon N, Tseng JL, et al. Lentiviral vectors as a gene delivery system in the mouse midbrain: cellular and behavioral improvements in a 6-ohda model of parkinson's disease using GDNF. Exp Neurol 2000; 164: 15–24.

159. Rosenblad C, Grønborg M, Hansen C, et al. In Vivo protection of nigral dopamine neurons by lentiviral gene transfer of the novel GDNF-family member neublastin/artemin. Mol Cell Neurosci 2000; 15: 199–214.

160. Brizard M, Carcenac C, Bemelmans AP, et al. Functional reinnervation from remaining DA terminals induced by GDNF lentivirus in a rat model of early Parkinson's disease. Neurobiol Dis 2006; 21: 90–101.

161. Dowd E, Monville C, Torres EM, et al. Lentivector-mediated delivery of GDNF protects complex motor functions relevant to human Parkinsonism in a rat lesion model. Eur J Neurosci 2005; 22: 2587–95.

162. Fjord-Larsen L, Johansen JL, Kusk P, et al. Efficient in vivo protection of nigral dopaminergic neurons by lentiviral gene transfer of a modified Neurturin construct. Exp Neurol 2005; 195: 49–60.

163. Kordower JH, Emborg ME, Bloch J, et al. Neurodegeneration prevented by lentiviral vector delivery of GDNF in primate models of Parkinson's disease. Science 2000; 290: 767–73.

164. Herzog CD, Dass B, Holden JE, et al. Striatal delivery of CERE-120, an AAV2 vector encoding human neurturin, enhances activity of the dopaminergic nigrostriatal system in aged monkeys. Mov Disord 2007; 22: 1124–32.
165. Palfi S, Leventhal L, Chu Y, et al. Lentivirally delivered Glial Cell Line-Derived Neurotrophic factor increases the number of striatal dopaminergic neurons in primate models of Nigrostriatal degeneration. J Neurosci 2002; 22: 4942–54.
166. Marks WJ Jr, Ostrem JL, Starr PA, et al. Safety and tolerability of intraputaminal delivery of CERE-120 (adeno-associated virus serotype 2–neurturin) to patients with idiopathic Parkinson's disease: an open-label, phase I trial. Lancet Neurol 2008; 7: 400–8.
167. Marks WJ Jr, Bartus RT, Siffert J, et al. Gene delivery of AAV2-neurturin for Parkinson's disease: a double-blind, randomised, controlled trial. Lancet Neurol 2010; 9: 1164–72.
168. Witt J, Marks W. An update on gene therapy in Parkinson's disease. Curr Neurol Neurosci Rep 2011; 11: 362–70.
169. Luo J, Kaplitt MG, Fitzsimons HL, et al. Subthalamic GAD gene therapy in a Parkinson's disease rat model. Science 2002; 298: 425–9.
170. Lee B, Lee H, Nam YR, et al. Enhanced expression of glutamate decarboxylase 65 improves symptoms of rat parkinsonian models. Gene Ther 2005; 12: 1215–22.
171. Emborg ME, Carbon M, Holden JE, et al. Subthalamic glutamic acid decarboxylase gene therapy: changes in motor function and cortical metabolism. J Cereb Blood Flow Metab 2006; 27: 501–9.
172. Kaplitt MG, Feigin A, Tang C, et al. Safety and tolerability of gene therapy with an adeno-associated virus (AAV) borne GAD gene for Parkinson's disease: an open label, phase I trial. Lancet 2007; 369: 2097–105.
173. LeWitt PA, Rezai AR, Leehey MA, et al. AAV2-GAD gene therapy for advanced Parkinson's disease: a double-blind, sham-surgery controlled, randomised trial. Lancet Neurol 2011; 10: 309–19.
174. Dekker MCJ, Bonifati V, van Duijn CM. Parkinson's disease: piecing together a genetic jigsaw. Brain 2003; 126: 1722–33.
175. Ko HS, von Coelln R, Sriram SR, et al. Accumulation of the authentic parkin substrate Aminoacyl-tRNA synthetase cofactor, p38/JTV-1, leads to catecholaminergic cell death. J Neurosci 2005; 25: 7968–78.
176. Ko HS, Kim SW, Sriram SR, et al. Identification of far upstream element-binding protein-1 as an authentic parkin substrate. J Biol Chem 2006; 281: 16193–6.
177. Lo Bianco C, Schneider BL, Bauer M, et al. Lentiviral vector delivery of parkin prevents dopaminergic degeneration in an α-synuclein rat model of Parkinson's disease. Proc Natl Acad Sci USA 2004; 101: 17510–15.
178. Imam SZ, Zhou Q, Yamamoto A, et al. Novel regulation of parkin function through c-abl-mediated tyrosine phosphorylation: implications for Parkinson's disease. J Neurosci 2011; 31: 157–63.
179. Auluck PK, Chan HY, Trojanowski JQ, et al. Chaperone suppression of α-synuclein toxicity in a drosophila model for Parkinson's disease. Science 2002; 295: 865–8.
180. Ebrahimi-Fakhari D, Wahlster L, McLean PJ. Molecular chaperones in Parkinson's disease – present and future. J Parkinson's Dis 2011; 1: 299–320.
181. Labrador-Garrido A, Bertoncini CW, Roodveldt C. In: Rana AQ, ed. The Hsp70 Chaperone System in Parkinson's Disease, in Etiology and Pathophysiology of Parkinson's Disease. Vienna, Austria: InTech, 2011: 221–46.
182. Lo Bianco C, Shorter J, Régulier E, et al. Hsp104 antagonizes alpha-synuclein aggregation and reduces dopaminergic degeneration in a rat model of Parkinson's disease. J Clin Invest 2008; 118: 3087–97.
183. Dong Z, Wolfer DP, Lipp HP, et al. Hsp70 gene transfer by adeno-associated virus inhibits MPTP-induced Nigrostriatal degeneration in the mouse model of Parkinson's disease. Mol Ther 2005; 11: 80–8.
184. Pardridge WM. Tyrosine Hydroxylase replacement in experimental Parkinson's disease with transvascular gene therapy. NeuroRx 2005; 2: 129–38.

185. Pardridge WM. Blood-brain barrier drug targeting: the future of brain drug development. Mol Interv 2003; 3: 90–105; 51.
186. Zhang Y, Schlachetzki F, Zhang YF, Boado RJ, Pardridge WM. Normalization of striatal tyrosine hydroxylase and reversal of motor impairment in experimental parkinsonism with intravenous nonviral gene therapy and a brain-specific promoter. Hum Gene Ther 2004; 15: 339–50.
187. Xia C-F, Boado RJ, Zhang Y, et al. Intravenous glial-derived neurotrophic factor gene therapy of experimental Parkinson's disease with trojan horse liposomes and a tyrosine hydroxylase promoter. J Gene Med 2008; 10: 306–15.
188. Fu A, Zhou QH, Hui EK, et al. Intravenous treatment of experimental Parkinson's disease in the mouse with an IgG-GDNF fusion protein that penetrates the blood–brain barrier. Brain Res 2010; 1352: 208–13.

26

Physical and occupational therapy

Ingrid H.W.M. Sturkenboom, Samyra H.J. Keus,
Marten Munneke, and Bastiaan R. Bloem

INTRODUCTION

The current medical management is only partially effective in controlling the symptoms and signs of Parkinson's disease (PD). Particularly the motor and nonmotor impairments that occur late in the course of the disease, such as freezing or dementia, respond poorly to medication, and may even be caused by medication (1). Moreover, the current medical management mainly targets dopaminergic impairments and is therefore not effective for impairments that are largely related to nondopaminergic lesions in PD, such as impaired balance (2). Consequently, even patients with optimal medical management face mounting and varied problems in daily functioning (3,4).

INTERNATIONAL CLASSIFICATION OF FUNCTIONING, DISABILITY, AND HEALTH

The extent to which patients experience problems in daily functioning is not solely predicted by the severity of impairments. A patient with mild impairments can experience severe problems in daily life, whereas a severely affected patient may manage surprisingly well. This is because daily functioning is the outcome of the interaction between the health condition (PD) and contextual factors, which are made up of environmental factors (i.e., physical, social, and societal) and personal factors (e.g., coping strategies, preferences, and attitudes). For example, in a clinical situation patients may have sufficient confidence, muscle strength, joint mobility, physical capacity, and motor planning skills to walk independently. Still, they may be limited in walking around their garden at home. Narrow passages, created by their outdoor furniture and plants, may provoke them to freeze; an environmental factor. But also negative thinking, like "I do not like to exercise, I rather stay seated in my chair," may refrain them from exercising; a personal factor. This interaction is illustrated in the biopsychosocial model of the International Classification of Functioning, Disability, and Health (ICF) of the World Health Organization (Fig. 26.1) (5).

The ICF classification provides an interdisciplinary framework and terminology (names and codes) for the description of health and health-related problems. Important in the ICF framework is the recognition of the interdependency of health condition, functions, activities, participation, and contextual factors. In the Netherlands, national organizations of 19 different health care disciplines, collaborated in providing an overview of impairments in functions, limitations in activities, and restrictions in participation related to the impact of PD using the ICF classification (Tables 26.1 and 26.2).

In comprehensive patient-centered care, attention to all factors that influence the impact of disease is essential. Consequently, in addition to neurology, a wide

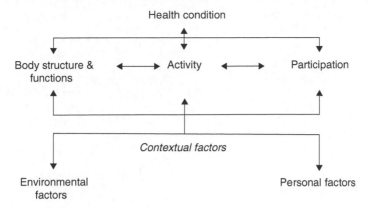

FIGURE 26.1   Model of International Classification of Functioning, Disability, and Health.

variety of health care disciplines can be involved in PD care (Fig. 26.2) (6). Physical therapy and occupational therapy are allied health care professions commonly involved to support patients to deal with the consequences of their disease in daily functioning. Although closely related, the focus of these professions is different. Referring to the ICF terminology (Fig. 26.1), the main focus of physical therapy is on mobility-related activity limitations, in which physical therapists also address contributing impairments in functions and contextual factors. The main focus of occupational therapy is on participation, in which occupational therapists also address contributing activity limitations and contextual factors. In this chapter we highlight the unique selling points, similarities, and options for collaboration of these two professions.

PHYSICAL THERAPY DOMAINS
In their aim to improve independence, safety, and wellbeing of patients through and during movement, physical therapists mainly focus on limitations in transfers, gait, balance, and manual activities, as well as reduced physical capacity (7,8). We next discuss the nature of these limitations as they can be seen in PD.

Gait
In most patients, limitations in gait start in early stages of the disease. Impairments include an asymmetrically reduced or absent arm swing, a stooped posture, an asymmetric step size, and difficulties turning around in the standing or recumbent positions. As the disease progresses, gait becomes slower and the typical parkinsonian gait develops with shuffling and short steps, a bilaterally reduced arm swing, and slow en bloc turns. These impairments form the so-called continuous gait disorder in PD (9). Additionally, patients can have an "episodic gait disorder," such as festination and freezing. This is experienced by 80% of patients with a disease duration longer than eight years (10). Although the prevalence of freezing increases with longer disease duration and greater severity, it can be present in early stages of PD. Most often freezing does not present as complete

TABLE 26.1   The Impact of Parkinson's Disease: Possible Impairments in Functions

b1: Mental functions	*b5: Functions of the digestive system*
• delirium (b110)	• impaired ingestion, e.g., drooling, vomiting,* and impaired swallowing (b510)
• dementia (b117)	• constipation* (b525)
• impairments in temperament and personality (b126)	• reduced weight maintenance (b530)
• impairments in energy and drive functions, e.g., reduced motivation and impulse control* (b130)	*b6: Genitourinary and reproductive functions*
• sleep impairments (b134)	• impaired urination, e.g., (urge)incontinence* (b620)
• reduced attention (b140)	• impaired sexual functions, e.g., impotence and increased sexual interest* (b640)
• reduced memory (b144)	*b7: Neuromusculoskeletal and movement-related functions*
• impairments in emotion, e.g., anxiety* (b152)	• reduced joint mobility* (b710)
• impairments in perceptual functions, e.g., reduced visuospatial perception and hallucinations* (b156)	• reduced muscle power* (b730)
• impairments in higher level cognitive functions, e.g., in planning, decision-making and mental flexibility (b164)	• impaired muscle tone functions, e.g., rigidityand dystonia (b735)
• impairments in mental functions of language, e.g., verbal perseveration (b167)	• reduced muscle endurance* (b740)
b2: Sensory functions and pain	• impaired motor reflex functions (b750), e.g., simultaneous contraction of antagonists
• seeing impairments, e.g., visual acuity* (b210)	• reduced postural responses (b755)
• dizziness* (b240)*	• reduced control of voluntary movements (b760), e.g., dysdiadochokinesia, reduced "motor set" causing starting problems and reduced or absence of internal cues causing problems in automated, sequential movements
• impairments in smell (b255)	• impaired involuntary movement functions (b765), e.g. bradykinesia, (resting) tremor and dyskinesia*
• proprioceptive function (b260)	• impairments in gait patterns, e.g., asymmetry, freezing, reduced step length, velocity, trunk rotation and arm swing (b770)
• tingling (b265)	• on/off periods* (b798)
• (central) pain (b280)	*b8: Functions of the skin and related structures*
b3: Voice and speech functions (b3)	• impairments in sweating and sebum production (b830)
• reduced pitch and loudness of voice (b310)	• impaired sensations related to the skin (pins and needles) (b840)
• impaired articulation (including dysarthria) (b320)	
• reduced fluency of speech (b330)	
b4: Functions of the cardiovascular and respiratory systems	
• impairments in blood pressure (e.g., orthostatic hypotension*) (b420)	
• reduced exercise tolerance* (b455)	

Note: Coding and terminology according to ICF classification.
*Secondary impairments (partly) due to primary impairments and medications.

akinesia, but rather as shuffling with small steps or trembling of the legs (11). Festination, characterized by rapid, small, shuffling steps can precede a freezing episode. However, festination can also occur without subsequent freezing of gait. When the center of gravity is displaced in a forward direction (trunk before feet) this leads to propulsion and tendency to fall forward; when center of gravity is displaced in backward direction this leads to retropulsion.

TABLE 26.2 The Impact of Parkinson's Disease: Possible Activity Limitations and Restrictions in Participation

Main Domain		Examples of Subdomains
d1	Learning and applying knowledge	Acquiring skills (d155), writing (d170), solving problems (d175) and making decisions (d177)
d2	General tasks and demands	Undertaking multiple tasks (d220), carrying out daily routine (230), handling stress and other psychological demands (d240)
d3	Communication	Speaking (d330), producing nonverbal messages (d335), writing messages (d345)
d4	Mobility	Changing and maintaining body position (d410-d429), carrying, moving and handling objects (d430-d449), walking and moving (d450-d469), moving around using transportation (d470-d489)
d5	Self-care	Self-care, e.g., washing oneself (d510), toileting (d530), dressing (d540), eating (d550) and drinking (d560)
d6	Domestic life	Shopping (d620), preparing meals (d630) and doing housework (d640)
d7	Interpersonal interactions and relationships	Basic interpersonal interactions (d710) and particular interpersonal relationships with strangers, formal persons, family, and husband or wife (d730-d779)
d8	Major life areas	Education (d810-839), work and employment (d840-d859) and economic life (d860-d879)
d9	Community, social and civic life	Recreation and leisure (d920), religion (d930), and political life (d950)

Note: Coding and terminology according to ICF classification.

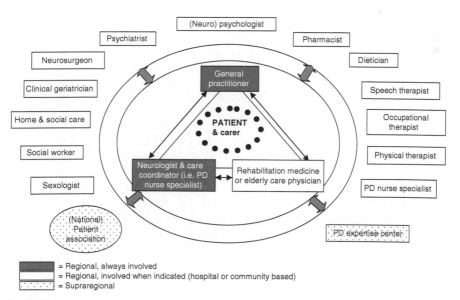

= Regional, always involved
= Regional, involved when indicated (hospital or community based)
= Supraregional

FIGURE 26.2 Organization of care in Parkinson's disease.

Balance and Falls

Although falls rarely occur at onset of the disease, eventually, most patients will eventually fall. Usually, five years after onset of the first impairments, postural instability develops. Falls emerge, on average, five years thereafter (12). However, even in the early stages, patients with PD may develop a fear to fall, which may lead to restrictions of daily activities and is a risk factor for future falls (13,14).

Most falls in persons with PD occur indoors, when turning, standing up, bending forward, or multitasking (15). The problems to maintain balance during multitasking, are a combination of decreased psychomotor speed and attentional flexibility (16). This is especially the case when multitasking concerns a combination of motor and mental tasks, for example, when walking and talking, or when rising from a sofa to answer the doorbell.

A stooped posture is often seen in PD, sometimes in severe forms i.e. camptocormia (17). It has been hypothesized that a stooped posture, apart from being a symptom of the disease itself, might in part also be a natural protective response to prevent backward falls (18).

Transfers

Activities such as rising from and sitting down on a chair, getting in or out of bed, and turning over in bed are complex composite movements and patients with PD often perform these activities poorly. A common problem in sit-to-stand transfers is that people with PD fail to lean forward far enough when standing up, and fall back into the chair. Likely factors that play a role are weak limb support against gravity and poor timing of velocity in forward movement of the trunk (19). Turning in bed is a complex movement, and is further complicated by the need to handle bedcovers. Moreover, turning in bed is usually performed at night when levodopa levels are low and visual guidance for performance is poor, further limiting this activity.

Manual Activities

Similar to transfers, most manual activities are complex movements, requiring a combination of sequentially executed submovements. In PD, the fluency, coordination, efficiency, and speed of reach and dexterous movements are often diminished. Impaired timing and integration of movement components play a role, as well as impaired regulation of the necessary force and impaired precision grip (20–22). In addition to these problems tremor can affect manual activities. A resting tremor generally disappears or diminishes when a movement is initiated. However, the tremor can re-emerge in isometric action of the muscles, for example, when holding an object for longer periods of time. In some patients, an action tremor can be observed affecting the entire track of a voluntary movement (23).

Physical Capacity

Physical capacity, which is a combination of muscle strength, endurance, and range of motion, is often reduced or at risk in PD. Patients with PD are inclined toward a sedentary lifestyle (24). This is related to mental impairments (e.g., depression, apathy, and dementia), limitations in mobility, fatigue, and personal factors (e.g., self-efficacy) (25). A sedentary lifestyle may "protect" patients from falling. However, an inverse linear relationship exists between volume of physical activity and multimorbidity, for example, pain, osteoporoses, depression, and cardiovascular diseases (24,25).

OCCUPATIONAL THERAPY DOMAINS

The primary role of occupational therapy in PD is to enable patients to engage in meaningful roles and activities in the home and community (26–28). This includes optimizing activity performance (i.e., independence, safety, amount of effort and time, routines) and satisfaction with activity performance and participation. Examples of activities that occupational therapy may address are shopping, putting on a coat, using the computer, gardening, and organizing the household. In early stages of PD, patients' goals in occupational therapy often include maintaining activities and prevention of giving up activities and roles. In later stages of PD goals will shift toward enabling an adapted involvement in valued activities. Depending on the needs of the caregivers, the role of occupational therapy extends to enabling caregivers to support and supervise the patient in daily activities while considering their own wellbeing (27).

Restrictions in Participation

Inevitably, PD results in changes in participation in meaningful activities and this can pertain to work, leisure, or community and social life (29–33). Patients who are employed often experience difficulties in their work due to PD and give up work early (31,32,34).Fatigue is associated with reduced participation in leisure activities (35). Patients with PD often give up activities that they can no longer perform the way they want, require too much time and effort, or are considered too dangerous by those close to them (33). For actual participation, not only the capacity to plan and perform activities is important, but also the patient's motivation, feeling of control, and level of acceptance; and the support from the social environment (29,33,36). For participation in work, support received from the employer also plays an important role (31).

Limitations in Activities

Limitations in walking, transfers, posture, balance and moving, and handling impact on complex daily activities such as self-care activities, housekeeping, leisure activities, work-related activities, or transport. In fact, movement-related limitations are often more apparent in complex daily activities as the high attention load and mental flexibility, that are required in these activities can further constrain motor performance (16). In patients with executive impairments, the planning and organizing of complex tasks and routines is difficult (37). This might become evident in activities such as managing medication, preparing a shopping list, or maintaining the household. Other nonmotor problems that may have an impact on daily activity performance are visual deficits (e.g., impaired contrast sensitivity) and visuospatial difficulties (38,39). A problem that we often observe in clinical practice is that many patients with PD fail to adjust their body position appropriately for the task. For example, when setting the table the patient does not take the final step to stand close to the table but instead reaches out far, resulting in increased effort and risk of falling. The attributing factors for this problem are not clear, but we hypothesize that difficulties in visuospatial planning may play a role in addition to motor problems.

Next to personal abilities, elements in the environmental context can be important contributors to limitations in activities. In the physical environment this can relate to the layout and available space, the height of furniture, the availability of supports and visual cues, or the quality of lighting.

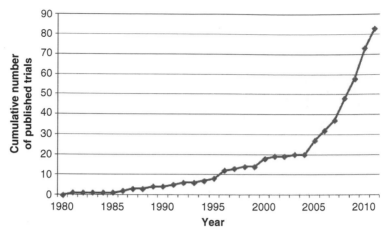

FIGURE 26.3 Cumulative number of controlled clinical trials on the efficacy or effectiveness of physical therapy in PD.

EVIDENCE-BASED CLINICAL GUIDELINES

Over the past decade, both the annual number and quality of controlled trials evaluating the effectiveness of physical therapy in PD have increased substantially. In 1981 the first controlled clinical trial was published (40). Since then, 82 trials have been published, of which more than 50% during the past four years (2008–2011) (Fig. 26.3) (41). In 2004, the first evidence-based physical therapy guidelines providing practice recommendations were developed (7,42). For these guidelines, all evidence related to physical therapy in PD (up to October 2003) was systematically gathered and evaluated. Evidence from research was supplemented with clinical expertise and patient values. Evidence was graded and translated into practice recommendations for both the diagnostic and therapeutic process, including outcome measures. Recommendations were arranged according to levels of evidence. The guidelines are still unique in its field and are currently being updated in a joint effort of 19 national physiotherapy associations throughout Europe, supported by the Association for Physiotherapists in Parkinson's Disease Europe (APPDE; www .APPDE.eu), the European Section of the World Confederation for Physical Therapy (EU-WCPT; www.physio-europe.org), and the European Parkinson's Disease Association (EPDA; www.EPDA.eu.com). These European guidelines will become available early 2013 and will be accessible for free at www.APPDE.eu.

With a similar structured approach, clinical guidelines for occupational and speech and language therapy were developed (published 2008), and have been adopted and translated by the National Parkinson Foundation (43,44). Referral, assessment, and interventions described in this chapter are based on these guidelines.

REFERRAL TO PHYSICAL OR OCCUPATIONAL THERAPY

Difficulties in daily activities, without loss of independent function can be present in early stages of PD (i.e., Unified Parkinson's Disease Rating Scale (UPDRS) < 20 and Hoehn & Yahr (HY) I–II) (4,45). This is specifically the case in patients with predominant symptoms of postural instability and gait difficulties (46). Therefore, timely referral to either discipline is recommended. From diagnosis onward,

TABLE 26.3 Referral Criteria Physical or Occupational Therapy

Physical Therapy	Occupational Therapy
Mobility-related impairments and limitations in: • gait (including freezing) • balance (including falls and fear of falls) • transfers • reaching and grasping • physical capacity (or risk for inactivity)	Patient: Limitations in activities and restrictions in participation related to: • self-care, domestic life, functional mobility • work (paid and unpaid) • leisure Caregiver: problems related to supporting the patient in daily activities

patients can be referred for intermittent periods of time for either prevention or management. Especially in the early stages of the disease, a consultation for information and advice may be sufficient. In the later stages, a trajectory of coaching and individual or group treatment may be required. Depending on the primary problem in daily functioning, a patient should be referred to either a physical or occupational therapist, or both. Referral criteria for both disciplines are provided in Table 26.3.

Information that should be provided with the referral includes: information on stage of disease (e.g., by providing scores on items of the UPDRS), relevant comorbidities, cognitive functioning, a history of any previously applied interventions for the problems, and an overview of medications.

ASSESSMENT

The initial aim of both the physical and occupational therapy assessment is to identify which problems in daily functioning are in the perception of the patient most important and relevant to address. For this, patient-centered tools are recommended, such as the Patient Specific Index for Parkinson's disease (47) (physical therapy) or the Canadian Occupational Performance Measure (48) (occupational therapy). This is followed by various assessments and tests to analyze which factors hinder or support movement-related activities (physical therapy) or engagement in activities and roles (occupational therapy). The assessments are used to design and evaluate the respective treatment plans collaboratively with the patient and the caregiver. In addition, the assessments may provide important information for medical management (e.g., effects of drug therapy, detection of signs for atypical parkinsonism) and multidisciplinary treatment plans. Similarly, the physical or occupational therapist may use relevant information from each other or other disciplines involved to get a comprehensive picture of the patient.

GENERAL TREATMENT CONSIDERATIONS

When delivering treatment, physical and occupational therapists need to consider several general principles.

Self-Management and Patient-Centeredness

A crucial point for behavioral interventions, such as physical and occupational therapy, is that the interventions fit with the needs, motivation, and abilities of the patient (and caregiver). Therefore a patient-centered approach is warranted (49,50). Due to the complexity of the disease and the wide scope of possible deficits and limitations to be addressed, it is important that the patient is empowered to make an informed choice of priorities and interventions (49). By promoting the patient (and caregiver) to self-reflect, prioritize, and apply problem-solving skills related to issues of activity performance and participation, self-management can be stimulated (51,52).

The instruction style used in therapy sessions has to fit with the needs and preference of the PD patient. A structured, graded approach allowing learning in a conscious and controlled manner and with sufficient repetition is generally recommended in PD patients (53,54).

Considering Fluctuations in Daily Functioning

Patients who use dopaminergic medication can experience fluctuations in the severity and type of motor and nonmotor impairments, and of activity limitations in the course of the day; the so-called *on–off* and wearing off states. These should be taken into account when planning treatment sessions. Interventions to increase physical capacity are recommended to be carried out during the *on* phase, as well as the learning of new strategies in activities. Once the patient is familiar with the strategies it is important to train their use in the moments the strategies are needed (the *off* state).

Advising and Training Caregivers

Involving the caregiver in the treatment and application of strategies is usually necessary, especially when the patient has cognitive impairments. The occupational therapy assessment can, however, also indicate specific needs of the caregiver in relation to supporting the patient in daily activities. In that case, therapists will (if applicable) educate the caregiver on the effects of PD in relation to activity performance; train specific skills needed to support the patient in activities; provide information about relevant aids and adaptations that may reduce the burden of care giving, and empower the caregiver to look for opportunities to maintain or reacquire a healthy balance in their own activities and care activities. For the latter, referral to other professionals or resources may be required. These types of interventions were found to be effective in trials on occupational therapy in dementia for improving perceived competence in care giving among caregivers and reducing the amount of care required (55,56). Aspects of disease associated with increased caregiver burden are similar in PD and dementia (57,58). Therefore, we expect that similar types of interventions can be effective for caregivers of PD patients.

Treatment Site

In patients with PD, learning of new skills is often task and context specific (59). Treatment focused on improving activities should therefore be provided within the context of functional tasks of everyday living, preferably at the patient's home. Treatment at home has the added benefits of enabling direct evaluation of the applicability of the strategies in normal daily functioning and of meeting and involving the caregiver in a more natural context. Specific exercises to improve physical capacity, gait, or balance can be performed in a clinic setting.

Interdisciplinary Collaboration

When collaborating in the care of patients, the most important issue is good communication in order to ensure a consistent and, patient-centered approach (60). Therapists need to be aware of each other's expertise and timely signal the need of involving other health professionals (61). When high-intensive interventions are applied, it may be necessary to sequence different interventions in time depending on the patient's priorities and capacities. Moreover, contradictive interventions or information should be avoided.

When physical and occupational therapists are both involved, communication topics for effective collaboration include the following:

- What has been assessed and what are the findings?
- What is the established main goal for treatment?
- How to continue with discipline unique assessment?
- Who will address what aspect of the main goal and when, and what intervention strategies will be used?
- What needs to be evaluated by the referring physician, and when?

The goal is to provide the best care and at the same time keep the strain on the person with PD to a minimum.

SPECIFIC TREATMENT STRATEGIES

To address the goals of patients with PD, physical and occupational therapists can apply a wide range of treatment strategies. The most important treatment strategies used are as follows:

1. Cueing strategies
2. Cognitive movement strategies
3. Exercise to increase physical capacity and balance (*physical therapy only*)
4. Optimizing day structure/routine (*occupational therapy only*)
5. Adjusting the patient's home environment (*mainly occupational therapy*)

In the guidelines, recommendations for strategies a, b, and c are supported by strong scientific evidence from two or more randomized, controlled clinical trials and therefore reach "level 2"-recommendation according to international criteria (41–43). Recommendations for strategies d and e are supported by evidence from related fields, as specific studies on the effectiveness of these strategies in PD are lacking.

Cueing Strategies

Patients who have difficulties with initiating or maintaining movement (e.g., gait) often report the use of simple tricks to partly overcome these difficulties. For example, patients may use the stripes of a zebra crossing to ease walking; a cueing strategy. The use of cueing strategies can be enhanced by physical and occupational therapists. They can assist patients to ascertain their best cueing modality, frequency, and timing for the situations in which they experience limitations in movement-related activities.

Replacing Internal Control

External cues are stimuli from the environment, that increase attention and automatic movements. Most likely, by using these cues, movements are controlled more directly from the cortex, with little or no involvement from the basal ganglia. In this way, cues may compensate for the reduced or even absent internal control that causes disturbance of automatic and repetitive movements.

The modalities of external cues are auditory, visual, and tactile or somatosensory. For therapeutic use, external cues are often divided into rhythmical recurring cues (to improve continuation of movement) and single on–off cues (to reduce initiation problems). Cues can be moving stimuli (e.g., light of a laser pen, a moving foot, and falling keys) or nonmoving stimuli (e.g., sound of a metronome, stripes on the floor, parallel lines for writing).

The effectiveness of cueing on gait (including turning) in PD has been well established, even in the patient's home environment, without increasing the risk for falls (41,62). In addition, cues enhance the performance of sit-to-stand (63) and reduce the interference caused by multiple tasks (64). Rhythmic auditory cues even seem to reduce interference effect of a dual task on gait (65). In upper limb activities, visual cues can improve handwriting (66) and self-vocalization or auditory cues can improve movement kinematics in reaching (67,68).

In addition to applying external cues, physical and occupational therapists can teach patients to use attentional strategies to improve movement-related activities (8,69). For example, patients can be taught to generate a mental image of the appropriate step length when walking. In combining mental strategies and external cues, patients can be asked to make "big steps" to the rhythm of the auditory cues, instead of taking "steps" to the rhythm (8). These cues, focusing on both temporal and spatial parameters of gait have been shown to improve walking speed and stride length in single and dual tasks, even in PD patients with mild cognitive impairment (70). Similar principles of mental strategies and combination strategies can be applied to functional manual activities, for example, when bringing food to the mouth, although the effects have not yet been ascertained.

Patient-Specific Cues

Not all patients benefit from using cues. As yet, there is no insight into which patients benefit and which do not. However, if a patient benefits from cues, this will be visible at the first try. The choice of cues is patient-specific and depends on the activity, the context, the underlying problem: initiation or continuation of movement, amplitude or speed of movement, and the response to cues. It is the role of therapists to explore patient's experiences in using cues (self-invented tricks) and explore and optimize the effectiveness of these. Other cues can be evaluated if required the possible effectiveness of several cues with their patients. This starts off with evaluation of, the patient's experiences in using cues (self-invented tricks). The quality and application of these self-invented cues can possibly be optimized. Even within a specific cueing modality variation can be explored. For example, using two-dimensional visual cues (by means of lines of colored sticky tape on the floor) or three-dimensional visual cues (by means of thin wooden sticks) may make a large difference in effectiveness. In rhythmic cues the optimal frequency needs to be explored, as this depends on the activity and context in which the cues are used. For example, the frequency of a rhythmic auditory cue will generally be lower for walking indoors (e.g., from the bathroom to the kitchen) than for walking outdoors (e.g., when walking to a shop). To determine the appropriate frequency, the number of steps needed to perform the 10-m walk test or the 6-minute walk test can be used as a baseline (42). The frequency of beats (steps per minute) can be increased or decreased in order to evaluate the effect on gait. Caution should be taken in freezers. Whereas increasing cueing frequencies above baseline values may have a gait-enhancing effect in nonfreezers, it may provoke freezing episodes in freezers (71).

Cognitive Movement Strategies

The therapist can teach patients to use cognitive movement strategies to improve the performance of complex movements, such as transfers and manual activities (7,42). With these strategies, complex, goal-directed movements, which can no longer be performed automatically, are broken down (reorganized) into simple movement components (8,72). These components need to be performed in a defined sequence and with conscious control. The intention is therefore not for the activity or the movement performance to become automatic. In using cognitive movement strategies the need for multitasking during complex, automatic activities is minimized. A possible neuroanatomical explanation for the success of cognitive movement strategies is that motor pathways are accessed via indirect projections involving the cerebellum, rather than the basal ganglia.

The selection and training of the cognitive movement strategy follows a structured stepwise approach and uses mental or motor imagery. Especially when combined with physical practice, motor imagery can have a positive effect on motor performance and skills (73). In short, the selection and training of the appropriate strategy entails the following steps:

1. The therapist observes the patient in performing the activity to analyze which components of the activity are limited.
2. The therapist supports the patient in reorganizing the activity and selecting the most optimal movement components and sequence. In general, this will be limited to four to six components.
3. The therapist summarizes the agreed sequence of components in key phrases, preferably supported by visuals.
4. The therapist physically guides the patient in the performance of the movement components.
5. The patient rehearses the key phrases aloud.
6. The patient uses motor imagery (mental training) of the appropriate movement components.
7. The patient carries out the components consecutively and consciously controlled.

The training should be tailored to the individual patient, for example, the order of steps can be changed, or the caregiver can be involved. The complexity of components that can be trained at the same time depends on the abilities of the patient. To obtain the optimal result, the training should be task specific and within the natural performance context.

Often, cognitive movement strategies are combined with the use of external cues (such as a visual anchor point when standing up). The training can be supplemented with exercises to increase physical capacity (e.g. muscle strength exercises of the lower extremities in order to improve rising from a chair).

Exercises to Increase Physical Capacity, Gait, and Balance

Physical therapists can advise or coach patients to do exercises in order to prevent or reduce impairments in physical capacity and balance. The therapist will coach patients toward a more active lifestyle, based on the patient's preferences and sports history. Movement-based leisure time activities with demonstrated effectiveness are Tai Chi, Nordic Walking, and dance (74–76). In middle and later stages, or for more cognitively impaired patients, therapists may offer patients functional exercises on land or in water, or resistance and treadmill training (77–79). For patients who are confined to a wheelchair or bed the main goal is to maintain vital functions. Exercises are then integrated in the daily routines and in collaboration with other care professionals (e.g., nurses).

The exercises to improve physical capacity can often be performed in classes for groups of patients. The social component of group exercise enables patients to support each other in attending the classes, increases the fun during exercise, and allows contacts with peers during a social gathering after class. However, in some patients individual treatment is preferred, for example, in patients with severe cognitive impairments.

Exercises to improve balance and physical capacity are supported by high levels of evidence, that is, supported by results from more than two randomized, controlled clinical trials (7,80).

Optimizing Day Structure and Routine

To increase satisfaction with activity patterns, the occupational therapist can coach the patient in careful planning of daily and weekly routines. Aspects such as medication effects, performance capacity (including speed of performance), and demands of the tasks and context need to be considered. Patients often have to re-evaluate personal standards and values and reset priorities. The effectiveness of interventions aimed at optimizing day structure and routines has not yet been studied in PD. However, the aspect of carefully planning daily routines is part of an energy conservation protocol, that has found to be effective in patients with chronic conditions suffering from fatigue (81,82).

The intervention of providing a structured daily or weekly activity plan may also benefit patients who have problems in initiating or planning/organizing activities. In that case, the activity plan offers an external prompt and overview of activities to be done.

Adjusting the Patient's Home Environment

Advising on environmental modification and the use of assistive devices and adaptations improves independence and safety in activity performance of elderly, community living patients (83,84). As movement-related limitations such as freezing and falls are partly influenced by constraints in the physical environment, we expect that assistive devices and environmental modifications enhance quality and safety of activity performance in PD. The range of possible adaptations is extensive, but commonly advised modifications and devices in PD include removal of obstacles, re-arranging furniture or working space, improving lighting conditions, optimizing height or support of furniture, assistive mobility devices, and grab rails. Structuring the environment and providing reminder-cues may be useful for patients with cognitive deficits.

The effectiveness of assistive mobility devices in PD has not yet been examined extensively (85). Standard and wheeled walkers may increase confidence and balance, but they also reduce walking velocity. Moreover, standard walkers may increase freezing (86). For manual activities, small to medium size handles and light weight utensils appear to be better than built-up handles and weighted utensils (87,88).

To ensure appropriate devices and modifications are selected, it is recommended that the beneficial effect of the modification is evaluated as well as acceptability for the patient. Training should ensure correct and safe use of the aids and adaptations.

ILLUSTRATIVE CASE STUDY

John is a 67-year-old man with a five-year history of idiopathic PD. In a consultation session with the neurologist he reports some difficulties with transfers and gait and is referred to physical therapy in an outpatient facility. The physical therapist evaluates, through structured interview using the Patient-Specific Index for Physiotherapy in Parkinson's Disease (89) and the Falls History Questionnaire, which limitations John perceives in activities in the domains of gait (including freezing), balance (including posture and falls), transfers, manual dexterity, and physical capacity. John reports no fall incidences, but reports to have difficulties in:

- getting out of bed (particularly during the night)
- getting up from the toilet
- getting up from a chair
- turning
- walking longer distances outdoors

The main activity he would like to address is getting out of bed and reaching the toilet in time at night. Currently his wife needs to assist him. To further analyze this problem, the physical therapist performs physical examinations on the domains of transfers and gait using the Modified Parkinson Activity Scale and the Timed Up and Go test (47,89). In addition, leg muscle strength is evaluated with the Five Times Sit-To-Stand test (79). Results from these examinations demonstrate:

- Bed transfer: independent, but moderately increased effort turning from back to side position in bed, lack of trunk flexion, and increased effort in standing up from the side of the bed.
- Transfer from low chair with no arms (similar to toilet): independent with some increased effort. Difficultly to control sitting down.
- Gait: speed reduced, no observed problems turning.
- Leg muscle strength: insufficient; the Five Times Sit-To-Stand Test took more than 20 seconds (79).

The results do not fully explain the level of difficulty at home and during the night. The physical therapist contacts the neurologist to check whether the medication regime at night could be an issue. Moreover, he suggests a referral to an occupational therapist for a joint home visit. During the home visit, the therapists observe performance of the full activity, the performance context (environment) and discuss usual routines with John and his wife. Important additional information gained from this visit:

- Routines: John usually wakes up twice in the night to go to the toilet and then prefers to sit down on the toilet to urinate. His wife assists her husband in getting out of bed, in turning him to sit down on the toilet, in standing up from the toilet, and in pulling up his pants and pajama trousers.
- Environmental context: the space around the bed and the toilet is very confined. The mattress is fairly soft and there is an over bed hoist. At night a small night light in the hall way is put on.

- Performance: John does not use the over bed hoist and when he tries, it does not facilitate getting from lying to sitting. In the toilet John turns clockwise (which is the long way around) and he sits down before he has positioned himself appropriately in front of the toilet. John has difficulty achieving sufficient active range of motion to reach to his back and pull up his pants. This appeared not to be a problem of reduced shoulder mobility or strength, but a problem of inadequate calibration of movement and power.

Following collaborative goal setting and information on possible strategies and interventions, a treatment plan is set up for the goal: "Within three weeks, I can independently go to the toilet at night." The physical therapist trains three times 30–45 minutes a week for three weeks performance of the bed and toilet transfers using a combination of *cognitive movement strategies* and *visual cues* (reaching toward an anchor point). The complex movements of the transfers are broken down in sequences of single steps. The training is graded starting with demonstration by the therapist, followed by John carrying out the transfers with instructions of the therapist, with instructions of his wife and finally with self-instructions. At the end of each session, functional exercises to improve muscle strength of the legs are rehearsed.

The occupational therapist advices on *environmental modifications* such as removing the over bed hoist, moving a cabinet to create more space around the bed and trying out a firmer and slightly higher mattress to ease bed mobility. The therapist also discusses possible options for suitable *visual cues* in the toilet area to aid both appropriate positioning and standing up. For appropriate positioning, a mirror in front of the toilet is chosen as a reference point and a line on the floor. For getting up, the mirror is used as a visual anchor point. Moreover, the occupational therapist discusses the importance of proper lighting in the bedroom, hallway, and toilet to allow better visuospatial feedback when moving around in the night. John and his wife choose the option of lights with a movement sensor for the bedroom and hallway. The light in the bedroom is placed on the night cupboard in a way that it can also be used as a visual cue when reaching over to turn on his side for getting up. Pulling up pants and trousers is practiced using principles of *cognitive movement strategies*, *focused attention* on big movement and *auditory cues* ("1,2,3...up"). Finally, the full activity of getting up and going to the toilet and handling clothes is practiced.

At the end of three weeks, the goal of going to the toilet independently at night is evaluated. John is now able to go to the toilet without assistance of his wife. Although his wife still wakes up when he gets up, she has peace of mind that he can manage.

In this case study, the physical therapist was referred to first and he identified the value of adding the expertise of the occupational therapist to work on a mobility-related goal of the patient together. The collaborative approach around that goal was successful as both disciplines focused on different aspects in the assessment and interventions, while being aware of each other's instructions and strategies used.

REFERENCES

1. Espay AJ, Fasano A, van Nuenen BF, et al. "On" state freezing of gait in Parkinson disease: a paradoxical levodopa-induced complication. Neurology 2012; 78: 454–7.
2. Fox SH, Brotchie JM, Lang AE. Non-dopaminergic treatments in development for Parkinson's disease. Lancet Neurol 2008; 7: 927–38.
3. Alves G, Wentzel-Larsen T, Aarsland D, et al. Progression of motor impairment and disability in Parkinson disease: a population-based study. Neurology 2005; 65: 1436–41.

4. Shulman LM, Gruber-Baldini AL, Anderson KE, et al. The evolution of disability in Parkinson disease. Mov Disord 2008; 23: 790–6.
5. World Health Organization (WHO). International Classification of Functioning, Disability and Health (ICF). [Available from: www who int/classifications/icf/en/index html 2007] [Cited February 22, 2012].
6. Keus SHJ, Oude Nijhuis LB, Nijkrake MJ, et al. Improving community healthcare for patients with Parkinsons disease: the dutch model. Parkinson's Disease 2012; 2012: Article ID 543426: 7; doi: 10.1155/2012/543426.
7. Keus SH, Bloem BR, Hendriks EJ, et al. Evidence-based analysis of physical therapy in Parkinson's disease with recommendations for practice and research. Mov Disord 2007; 22: 451–60.
8. Morris ME. Movement disorders in people with Parkinson disease: a model for physical therapy. Phys Ther 2000; 80: 578–97.
9. Hausdorff JM. Gait dynamics in Parkinson's disease: common and distinct behavior among stride length, gait variability, and fractal-like scaling. Chaos 2009; 19: 026113.
10. Macht M, Kaussner Y, Moller JC, et al. Predictors of freezing in Parkinson's disease: a survey of 6,620 patients. Mov Disord 2007; 22: 953–6.
11. Giladi N. Freezing of gait. Clinical overview. Adv Neurol 2001; 87: 191–7.
12. Wenning GK, Ebersbach G, Verny M, et al. Progression of falls in postmortem-confirmed parkinsonian disorders. Mov Disord 1999; 14: 947–50.
13. Mak MK, Pang MY. Fear of falling is independently associated with recurrent falls in patients with Parkinson's disease: a 1-year prospective study. J Neurol 2009; 256: 1689–95.
14. Rahman S, Griffin HJ, Quinn NP, et al. On the nature of fear of falling in Parkinson's disease. Behav Neurol 2011; 24: 219–28.
15. Bloem BR, Grimbergen YA, Cramer M, et al. Prospective assessment of falls in Parkinson's disease. J Neurol 2001; 248: 950–8.
16. Koerts J, Van Beilen M, Tucha O, et al. Executive functioning in daily life in Parkinson's disease: initiative, planning and multi-task performance. PLoS ONE 2011; 6: e29254.
17. Doherty KM, van de Warrenburg BP, Peralta MC, et al. Postural deformities in Parkinson's disease. Lancet Neurol 2011; 10: 538–49.
18. Bloem BR, Beckley DJ, Van Dijk JG, et al. Influence of dopaminergic medication on automatic postural responses and balance impairment in Parkinson's disease. Mov Disord 1996; 11: 509–21.
19. Mak MK, Yang F, Pai YC. Limb collapse, rather than instability, causes failure in sit-to-stand performance among patients with Parkinson's disease. Phys Ther 2011; 91: 381–91.
20. Fellows SJ, Noth J. Grip force abnormalities in de novo Parkinson disease. Mov Disord 2004; 19: 560–5.
21. Bertram CP, Lemay M, Stelmach GE. The effect of Parkinson's disease on the control of multi-segmental coordination. Brain Cogn 2005; 57: 16–20.
22. Fellows SJ, Noth J, Schwarz M. Precision grip and Parkinson's disease. Brain 1998; 121: 1771–84.
23. Baumann CR. Epidemiology, diagnosis and differential diagnosis in Parkinson's disease tremor. Parkinsonism Relat Disord 2012; 18: S90–2.
24. Van Nimwegen M, Speelman AD, Hofman-van Rossum EJ, et al. Physical inactivity in Parkinson's disease. J Neurol 2011; 258: 2214–21.
25. Ellis T, Cavanaugh JT, Earhart GM, et al. Factors associated with exercise behavior in people with Parkinson disease. Phys Ther 2011; 91: 1838–48.
26. Dixon L, Duncan D, Johnson P, et al. Occupational therapy for patients with Parkinson's disease. Cochrane Database Syst Rev 2007: CD002813.
27. Nijkrake MJ, Keus SHJ, Kalf JG, et al. Alllied health care interventions and complementary therapies in Parkinson's disease. Parkinsonism Relat Disord 2007; 13: S488–94.
28. Deane KHO, Ellis-Hill C, Dekker K, et al. A Delphi survey of best practice occupational therapy for Parkinson's disease in the United Kingdom. Br J Occup Ther 2003; 66: 247–54.
29. Benharoch J, Wiseman T. Participation in occupations: some experiences of patiënts with Parkinson's disease. Br J Occup Ther 2004; 67: 380–7.

30. Foster ER, Hershey T. Everyday executive function is associated with activity participation in Parkinson disease without dementia. OTJR (Thorofare N J) 2011; 31: 16–22.
31. Banks P, Lawrence M. The disability discrimination act, a necessary, but not sufficient safeguard for people with progressive conditions in the workplace? The experiences of younger people with Parkinson's disease. Disabil Rehabil 2006; 28: 13–24.
32. Schrag A, Banks P. Time of loss of employment in Parkinson's disease. Mov Disord 2006; 21: 1839–43.
33. Elliott SJ, Velde BP. Integration of occupation for individuals affected by Parkinson's disease. Phys Occup Ther Geriatr 2005; 24: 61–80.
34. Martikainen KK, Luukkaala TH, Marttila RJ. Parkinson's disease and working capacity. Mov Disord 2006; 21: 2187–91.
35. Garber CE, Friedman JH. Effects of fatigue on physical activity and function in patients with Parkinson's disease. Neurology 2003; 60: 1119–24.
36. Nijhof G. Uncertainty and lack of trust with Parkinson's disease. Eur J Pub Health 1996; 6: 58–63.
37. Cahn DA, Sullivan EV. Differential contributions of cognitive and motor component processes to physical and instrumental activities of daily living. Arch Clin Neuropsychol 1998; 13: 575–83.
38. Seichepine DR, Neargarder S, Miller IN, et al. Relation of Parkinson's disease subtypes to visual activities of daily living. J Int Neuropsychol Soc 2011; 17: 841–52.
39. Uc EY, Rizzo M, Anderson SW, et al. Visual dysfunction in Parkinson disease without dementia. Neurology 2005; 65: 1907–13.
40. Gibberd FB, Page NG, Spencer KM, et al. Controlled trial of physiotherapy and occupational therapy for Parkinson's disease. Br Med J (Clin Res Ed) 1981; 282: 1196.
41. Keus SH, Munneke M, Nijkrake MJ, et al. Physical therapy in Parkinson's disease: evolution and future challenges. Mov Disord 2009; 24: 1–14.
42. Keus SHJ, Hendriks HJM, Bloem BR, et al. KNGF Guidelines for physical therapy in Parkinson's disease. Ned Tijdschr Fysiother 2004; 114: 3. [Available from: www.appde.eu].
43. Sturkenboom IHWM, Thijssen MCE, Gons-van de Elsacker JJ, et al. Ergotherapie bij de ziekte van Parkinson, een richtlijn van Ergotherapie Nederland. Utrecht/Den Haag: Ergotherapie Nederland/Uitgeverij Lemma, 2008; English translation in publication as Sturkenboom IHWM, Thijssen MCE, Gons-van Elsacker JJ, et al. Guidelines for Occupational Therapy in Parkinson's Disease Rehabilitation. Nijmegen, NL/Miami, FL: ParkinsonNet/National Parkinson Foundation, 2012.
44. Kalf JG, Sturkenboom I, Thijssen M, et al. New guidelines in Parkinson's disease: occupational therapy and speech therapy. EPNN J 2008; 4: 12–15.
45. Schenkman M, Ellis T, Christiansen C, et al. Profile of functional limitations and task performance among people with early- and middle-stage Parkinson disease. Phys Ther 2011; 91: 1339–54.
46. Hariz GM, Forsgren L. Activities of daily living and quality of life in persons with newly diagnosed Parkinson's disease according to subtype of disease, and in comparison to healthy controls. Acta Neurol Scand 2011; 123: 20–7.
47. Nijkrake MJ, Keus SH, Quist-Anholts GW, et al. Evaluation of a patient-specific index as an outcome measure for physiotherapy in Parkinson's disease. Eur J Phys Rehabil Med 2009; 45: 507–12.
48. Law M, Baptiste S, Carswell A, et al. Canadian Occupational Performance Measure, 5th edn. Toronto: CAOT Publications, 2005.
49. Nisenzon AN, Robinson ME, Bowers D, et al. Measurement of patient-centered outcomes in Parkinson's disease: what do patients really want from their treatment? Parkinsonism Relat Disord 2011; 17: 89–94.
50. Grosset KA, Grosset DG. Patient-perceived involvement and satisfaction in Parkinson's disease: effect on therapy decisions and quality of life. Mov Disord 2005; 20: 616–19.
51. Lowenstein N, Tickle-Degnen L. Developing an occupational therapy home program for patients with Parkinson's disease. In: Trail M, Protas EJ, Lai JS, eds. Neurorehabilitation In Parkinson's Disease, An Evidence-Based Treatment Model. Thorofare: Slack Incorporated, 2008: 231–43.

52. Tickle-Degnen L, Ellis T, Saint-Hilaire MH, et al. Self-management rehabilitation and health-related quality of life in Parkinson's disease: a randomized controlled trial. Mov Disord 2010; 25: 194–204.
53. Krebs HI, Hogan N, Hening W, et al. Procedural motor learning in Parkinson's disease. Exp Brain Res 2001; 141: 425–37.
54. Siegert RJ, Taylor KD, Weatherall M, et al. Is implicit sequence learning impaired in Parkinson's disease? A meta-analysis. Neuropsychology 2006; 20: 490–5.
55. Gitlin LN, Winter L, Corcoran M, et al. Effects of the home environmental skill-building program on the caregiver-care recipient dyad: 6-month outcomes from the Philadelphia REACH initiative. Gerontologist 2003; 43: 532–46.
56. Graff MJ, Vernooij-Dassen MJ, Thijssen M, et al. Community based occupational therapy for patients with dementia and their care givers: randomised controlled trial. BMJ 2006; 333: 1196.
57. Aarsland D, Bronnick K, Ehrt U, et al. Neuropsychiatric symptoms in patients with Parkinson's disease and dementia: frequency, profile and associated care giver stress. J Neurol Neurosurg Psychiatry 2007; 78: 36–42.
58. Habermann B, Davis LL. Caring for family with Alzheimer's disease and Parkinson's disease: needs, challenges and satisfaction. J Gerontol Nurs 2005; 31: 49–54.
59. Nieuwboer A, De Weerdt W, Dom R, et al. The effect of a home physiotherapy program for persons with Parkinson's disease. J Rehabil Med 2001; 33: 266–72.
60. Van der Eijk M, Faber MJ, Al Shamma S, et al. Moving towards patient-centered healthcare for patients with Parkinson's disease. Parkinsonism Relat Disord 2011; 17: 360–4.
61. Wensing M, Van der Eijk M, Koetsenruijter J, et al. Connectedness of healthcare professionals involved in the treatment of patients with Parkinson's disease: a social networks study. Implement Sci 2011; 6: 67.
62. Lim I, Van Wegen E, De Goede C, et al. Effects of external rhythmical cueing on gait in patients with Parkinson's disease: a systematic review. Clin Rehabil 2005; 19: 695–713.
63. Mak MK, Hui-Chan CW. Cued task-specific training is better than exercise in improving sit-to-stand in patients with Parkinson's disease: a randomized controlled trial. Mov Disord 2008; 23: 501–9.
64. Baker K, Rochester L, Nieuwboer A. The immediate effect of attentional, auditory, and a combined cue strategy on gait during single and dual tasks in Parkinson's disease. Arch Phys Med Rehabil 2007; 88: 1593–600.
65. Rochester L, Hetherington V, Jones D, et al. The effect of external rhythmic cues (auditory and visual) on walking during a functional task in homes of people with Parkinson's disease. Arch Phys Med Rehabil 2005; 86: 999–1006.
66. Oliveira RM, Gurd JM, Nixon P, et al. Micrographia in Parkinson's disease: the effect of providing external cues. J Neurol Neurosurg Psychiatry 1997; 63: 429–33.
67. Ma HI, Trombly CA, Tickle-Degnen L, et al. Effect of one single auditory cue on movement kinematics in patients with Parkinson's disease. Am J Phys Med Rehabil 2004; 83: 530–6.
68. Maitra KK. Enhancement of reaching performance via self-speech in people with Parkinson's disease. Clin Rehabil 2007; 21: 418–24.
69. Baker K, Rochester L, Nieuwboer A. The effect of cues on gait variability-reducing the attentional cost of walking in people with Parkinson's disease. Parkinsonism Relat Disord 2008; 14: 314–20.
70. Rochester L, Burn DJ, Woods G, et al. Does auditory rhythmical cueing improve gait in people with Parkinson's disease and cognitive impairment? A feasibility study. Mov Disord 2009; 24: 839–45.
71. Willems AM, Nieuwboer A, Chavret F, et al. The use of rhythmic auditory cues to influence gait in patients with Parkinson's disease, the differential effect for freezers and non-freezers, an explorative study. Disabil Rehabil 2006; 28: 721–8.
72. Kamsma YPT, Brouwer WH, Lakke JPWF. Training of compensatory strategies for impaired gross motor skills in patients with Parkinson's disease. Physiotherapy Theory Pract 1995; 11: 209–29.

73. Tamir R, Dickstein R, Huberman M. Integration of motor imagery and physical practice in group treatment applied to subjects with Parkinson's disease. Neurorehabil Neural Repair 2007; 21: 68–75.
74. Hackney ME, Earhart GM. Tai Chi improves balance and mobility in people with Parkinson disease. Gait Posture 2008; 28: 456–60.
75. Hackney ME, Earhart GM. Effects of dance on movement control in Parkinson's disease: a comparison of argentine tango and American ballroom. J Rehabil Med 2009; 41: 475–81.
76. Reuter I, Mehnert S, Leone P, et al. Effects of a flexibility and relaxation programme, walking, and nordic walking on Parkinson's disease. J Aging Res 2011: 232473.
77. Dibble LE, Addison O, Papa E. The effects of exercise on balance in persons with Parkinson's disease: a systematic review across the disability spectrum. J Neurol Phys Ther 2009; 33: 14–26.
78. Vivas J, Arias P, Cudeiro J. Aquatic therapy versus conventional land-based therapy for Parkinson's disease: an open-label pilot study. Arch Phys Med Rehabil 2011; 92: 1202–10.
79. Duncan RP, Leddy AL, Earhart GM. Five times sit-to-stand test performance in Parkinson's disease. Arch Phys Med Rehabil 2011; 92: 1431–6.
80. Goodwin VA, Richards SH, Taylor RS, et al. The effectiveness of exercise interventions for people with Parkinson's disease: a systematic review and meta-analysis. Mov Disord 2008; 23: 631–40.
81. Mathiowetz VG, Finlayson ML, Matuska KM, et al. Randomized controlled trial of an energy conservation course for persons with multiple sclerosis. Mult Scler 2005; 11: 592–601.
82. Matuska K, Mathiowetz V, Finlayson M. Use and perceived effectiveness of energy conservation strategies for managing multiple sclerosis fatigue. Am J Occup Ther 2007; 61: 62–9.
83. Steultjens EM, Dekker J, Bouter LM, et al. Occupational therapy for community dwelling elderly people: a systematic review. Age Ageing 2004; 33: 453–60.
84. Gitlin LN, Winter L, Dennis MP, et al. A randomized trial of a multicomponent home intervention to reduce functional difficulties in older adults. J Am Geriatr Soc 2006; 54: 809–16.
85. Constantinescu R, Leonard C, Deeley C, et al. Assistive devices for gait in Parkinson's disease. Parkinsonism Relat Disord 2007; 13: 133–8.
86. Cubo E, Moore CG, Leurgans S, et al. Wheeled and standard walkers in Parkinson's disease patients with gait freezing. Parkinsonism Relat Disord 2003; 10: 9–14.
87. Ma HI, Hwang WJ, Chen-Sea MJ, et al. Handle size as a task constraint in spoon-use movement in patients with Parkinson's disease. Clin Rehabil 2008; 22: 520–8.
88. Ma HI, Hwang WJ, Tsai PL, et al. The effect of eating utensil weight on functional arm movement in people with Parkinson's disease: a controlled clinical trial. Clin Rehabil 2009; 23: 1086–92.
89. Keus SH, Nieuwboer A, Bloem BR, et al. Clinimetric analyses of the modified Parkinson activity scale. Parkinsonism Relat Disord 2008; 15: 263–9.

27

Voice, speech, and swallowing disorders

Shimon Sapir, Lorraine Olson Ramig, and Cynthia Fox

INTRODUCTION

Nearly 90% of individuals with Parkinson's disease (PD) develop voice and speech disorders during the course of their disease (1,2). These disorders are characterized by reduced voice volume (hypophonia); a breathy, hoarse, or harsh voice quality (dysphonia); imprecise consonant and vowel articulation due to reduced range of articulatory movements (hypokinetic articulation), and a tendency of these movements to decay and/or accelerate toward the end of a sentence; reduced voice pitch inflections (hypoprosodia, monotone); and rushed, dysfluent, hesitant, or stuttered-like speech (palilalia). These disorders, collectively termed hypokinetic dysarthria (3), may be among the first signs of PD (1,2,4–6). The hypokinetic dysarthria in individuals with PD typically results in reduced speech intelligibility. Reduced facial expression (hypomimia) is also common in individuals with PD. Together these symptoms can result in an individual with PD being interpreted as cold, withdrawn, unintelligent, and moody (7,8). These factors may also impair the ability to socialize, convey important medical information, interact with family members, and maintain employment (7).

Nearly 90% of individuals with PD will also develop swallowing disorders (dysphagia) at some point (9). Dysphagia symptoms in PD include difficulty with lingual motility, reduced initiation of swallow, difficulty with bolus formation, delayed pharyngeal response, and decreased pharyngeal contraction (9–11). These symptoms are often accompanied by weight loss and lack of enjoyment of eating. Aspiration pneumonia is not uncommon, especially in the later stages and can be a cause of death in PD (12). Dysphagia and abnormalities in tongue and esophageal motility have been shown to be present in early-stage PD (13–16).

Neuropharmacologic, neurosurgical, and neurostimulation approaches have been shown to be effective in improving motor function of PD, yet their impact on voice, speech, and swallowing remains unclear (17–23). Traditional speech treatment of hypokinetic dysarthria has focused on rate, articulation, prosodic pitch inflection, and speaking in a louder voice, with only modest, short-lived therapeutic results (24,25). Swallowing treatment has focused on behavioral changes and diet modifications (11). A speech and voice treatment approach, known as the Lee Silverman Voice Treatment (LSVT LOUD™), has generated the first short- and long-term efficacy data (10,26–29) for successfully treating voice and speech disorders in PD. Preliminary data for LSVT LOUD also has been shown to improve tongue strength and motility (30), swallowing (10), facial expression (31), and brain function (32,33) in individuals with PD.

SPEECH AND VOICE CHARACTERISTICS

Studies using acoustic, aerodynamic, videostroboscopic, electroglottographic, kinematic, electromyographic (EMG), and perceptual methods have documented disorders of laryngeal, respiratory, articulatory, and velopharyngeal functions in individuals with PD (5,34–38). The neural mechanisms underlying these disorders are unclear (39–42). Traditionally, they have been attributed to rigidity, bradykinesia, hypokinesia, and tremor secondary to dopamine deficiency, yet there is little evidence in support of these etiologic factors (23). Alternative explanations for the speech and voice disorders have been proposed, such as deficits in internal cueing, sensory gating, scaling of movement amplitude, attention to action (vocal vigilance), and self-regulation of vocal effort (4,22,23,37,43–45). These deficits have been hypothesized to be related to nondopaminergic or special dopaminergic mechanisms (46,47).

PERCEPTUAL AND PHONETIC CHARACTERISTICS OF VOICE AND SPEECH DISORDERS IN PD

Darley et al. (3) reported one of the first systematic descriptions of perceptual characteristics of speech and voice in individuals with PD (3,48,49). They identified reduced loudness, monopitch, monoloudness, reduced stress, breathy, hoarse voice quality, imprecise articulation and short rushes of speech as most characteristic of the speech and voice disorders in PD. They termed these symptoms hypokinetic dysarthria. Logemann et al. (2) used phonetic and perceptual analyses to characterize voice and speech abnormalities in 200 nonmedicated individuals with PD. Of these individuals, 89% were found to have voice quality problems, such as breathiness, hoarseness, roughness, and tremor, and 45% also had speech prosody or articulation problems. Ho and colleagues (1) used perceptual and phonetic methods to characterize voice and speech problems in 200 individuals with PD. They found that voice problems were first to occur, with other speech problems (prosody, articulation, and fluency) gradually appearing later as the disease advances. Sapir et al. (4) studied voice, prosody, fluency, and articulation abnormalities in 42 PD patients with speech problems. Of these individuals, 86% were found to have voice abnormalities, which tended to occur early in the course of the disease, and 45% had prosodic, fluency, and articulation abnormalities that tended to occur at later stages. However, other studies provide evidence for abnormal articulation and prosody at early stages of the disease (5,6,37,38,50).

ACOUSTIC MEASURES OF ABNORMAL VOICE AND SPEECH IN PD

Acoustic analyses of voice and speech in individuals with PD have confirmed the perceptual descriptions of hypokinetic dysarthria. Fox and Ramig (51) documented reduced vocal sound pressure level (vocSPL) by 2–4 dB (at 30 cm) on a number of speech tasks in 29 individuals with PD, compared with age- and gender-matched controls, which is equal to a 40% change in vocal loudness. Ho et al. (52) found vocSPL in PD to decay much faster than in neurologically normal speakers. They interpreted this fading as symptomatic of frontostriatal dysfunction. Rosen and colleagues (53) examined vocSPL decay in the phonation of persons with and without PD on various speech tasks. They found that vocSPL declined more rapidly in PD than in normal, age-matched speakers during syllable repetition (speech diadochokinesis). They also found that in some of the individuals with PD there were abnormally abrupt changes in vocSPL during conversation. However, during sustained vowel phonation vocSPL in individuals with PD did not show decay more than that of normal controls. Some early studies (54,55) did not confirm a reduction in voc-SPL, although the speech of individuals with PD was perceptually characterized by reduced loudness. The reasons for these discrepant findings are not clear. The presence or absence of vocal decay in parkinsonian speech is related, at least partially, to the specific speech task being performed (53), as well as to the severity of hypokinetic dysarthria (52).

Prosodic pitch inflection in speech, measured acoustically as fundamental frequency (F0) variability, or standard deviation from the mean F0 (SDF0) has been reported to be consistently lower in individuals with PD when compared with controls. These findings are consistent with the perceptual characterization of parkinsonian speech as monotone or monopitch (48,49). A reduction in maximum fundamental frequency range has also been observed in the dysarthric speech of individuals with PD, when compared with the normal speech of healthy speakers (56). Voice quality is measured in terms of jitter (random cycle-to-cycle variation in the periodicity of the voice waveform), shimmer (random cycle-to-cycle variation in the amplitude of the voice waveform), and harmonics-to-noise ratio. These are acoustic indices of short-term phonatory instability. Such instability has been documented in the speech of individuals with PD, consistent with various perceptual characteristics of disordered voice quality (e.g., hoarse, breathy, harsh) (57–59). Long-term phonatory instability, reflected mainly in rhythmic changes in F0, has also been documented in individuals with PD (58).

PHYSIOLOGIC MEASURES OF LARYNGEAL DYSFUNCTION IN PD

Disordered laryngeal function has been documented in a number of videoendoscopic and videostroboscopic studies. Hansen et al. (39) reported vocal fold bowing resulting in poor vocal fold closure in 94% of 32 individuals with PD, together with greater amplitude of vibration and laryngeal asymmetry. Smith et al. (60), using videostroboscopic observations, found that 57% of 21 individuals with PD had a form of incomplete vocal fold closure (bowing, anterior or posterior chink) on fiberoptic examination. Perez et al. (61) observed laryngeal tremor in 55% of 29 individuals with PD. The primary site of tremor was vertical laryngeal motion; however, the most striking stroboscopic findings in this study were abnormal vocal fold phase closure and phase asymmetry.

Additional data to support vocal fold closure problems in individuals with PD come from analyses of electroglottographic (EGG) signals. Gerratt et al. (62) reported abnormally large speed quotient and poorly defined closing period in individuals with PD. Blumin and colleagues (63) used videostroboscopy and fiberoptic endoscopic techniques, as well as a voice handicap index (VHI) questionnaire, to assess laryngeal function in 15 individuals with severe PD. Of these individuals, 13 (87%) had significant vocal fold bowing, and 14 (93%) self-reported significant voice handicap. These observations were consistent with slow vocal fold opening relative to the rate of closure and incomplete closure of the vocal folds.

EMG studies of the laryngeal muscles provided further information regarding laryngeal pathology in PD. Hirose and Joshita (64) studied EMG data from the thyroarytenoid (TA) muscles in an individual with PD who had limited vocal fold movement. They observed no reduction in the number of motor unit discharges and no pathologic discharge patterns. They did find loss of reciprocal suppression of the TA during inspiration and interpreted this finding as evidence of deterioration in the reciprocal adjustment of the antagonist muscles. Their finding is consistent with deficits in sensory gating characteristics of PD (64). Luschei et al. (65) studied single motor unit activity in the TA muscle in individuals with PD and found decreased firing rate in TA in males with PD. They interpreted these findings to suggest that PD affects rate and variability in motor unit activation (firing) in the laryngeal musculature. Baker et al. (36) found that absolute TA amplitudes during a loudness level task in individuals with PD were lower than young normal adults and normal aging adults. Gallena and colleagues (66) used TA EMG and nasoendoscopy to compare laryngeal physiology during speech of individuals with PD, with and without levodopa, and controls. Some patients were observed to have higher levels of laryngeal muscle activation, more vocal fold bowing, and greater impairment in voice onset and offset control without levodopa than with levodopa as well as in comparison to the controls. The seemingly conflicting reports of excessive and reduced TA activity may represent a common problem underlying laryngeal motor control, namely, a deficit in sensorimotor gating.

RESPIRATORY DYSFUNCTION IN PD
A number of studies have provided evidence, through various aerodynamic measurements, for disordered respiratory function in individuals with PD. These disorders include reduced vital capacity, reduced total amount of air expended during maximum phonation tasks, reduced intraoral air pressure during consonant/vowel productions, and abnormal airflow patterns (67–69). The origins of these airflow abnormalities are not clear but they may be related to variations in airflow resistance due to abnormal movements of the vocal folds and supralaryngeal area (69) or abnormal chest wall movements and respiratory muscle activation patterns (40,67,70).

Huber and Darling (71) measured VocSPL, syllables per breath group, speech rate, and lung volume parameters in individuals with PD and healthy controls as they performed two speech tasks, reading aloud and extemporaneous speech. They found that the individuals with PD produced shorter utterances compared with control participants. They also found that relationships between utterance length and lung volume initiation and inspiratory duration were weaker for individuals with PD than for healthy controls, more so for the extemporaneous speech task. They interpreted these findings to suggest that in individuals with PD, in comparison to healthy individuals, there is less consistent planning for utterance length.

ARTICULATORY AND VELOPHARYNGEAL DISORDERS:
ACOUSTIC AND KINEMATIC CORRELATES
OF ARTICULATORY ABNORMALITIES IN PD
Imprecise consonants and vowels may be present in 45% of individuals with PD and dysarthria (2,37). Logemann et al. (2) reported articulation problems in 45% of 200 unmedicated individuals with PD. They suggested that inadequate narrowing of the vocal tract due to hypokinetic articulatory movements may underlie problems with stops/p/,/b/, affricates/sh/,/ch/, and fricatives/s/,/f/.

Acoustic correlates of disordered articulation include problems with timing of vocal onsets and offsets (voicing during normally voiceless closure intervals of voiceless stops) (41) and spirantization (presence of fricative-like, aperiodic noise during stop closures), as well as problems with articulatory undershoot, reflected in vowel formant frequencies (37). Dysarthric speakers with PD showed longer voice onset times (VOTs) than normal (72). Such abnormal VOTs may reflect a problem with movement initiation (72), which may be related to deficits in internal cueing, timing, and/or sensory gating (4,73).

Sapir and colleagues introduced three acoustic metrics that have been shown to be highly sensitive to dysarthric vowel articulation associated with PD. These metrics include the F2i/F2u Ratio (37,38), the Formant Centralization Ratio (38), and the Vowel Articulation Index (74). Using these metrics, these researchers, along with others (5,6,50,75), have documented vowel articulation abnormalities (typified by vowel centralization) in individuals with PD, even at early stages of the disease. Rhythmic abnormalities in vowel articulation have also been documented by acoustic analysis of speech (76,77).

Kinematic analyses of jaw movements demonstrated disordered articulatory movements in individuals with PD (72,78–81). These individuals show a significant reduction in the size and peak velocity of jaw movements during speech when compared with neurologically healthy individuals without speech problems (72,81–83). Also, jaw movement of individuals with PD is approximately half the size of the jaw movements observed in nondisordered speakers. Although the reduction in range of movement has been attributed to rigidity of the articulatory muscles (84), it is more likely that these movement abnormalities are related to problems with sensorimotor gating, perception, and/or amplitude scaling of speech and non-speech movements (1,43,44,73). In contrast to range of movements, durations of movements in individuals with PD have been reported to be similar to those of healthy individuals (22). Yunusova et al. (85) used the X-ray microbeam to study jaw, lower lip, tongue blade, and tongue dorsum during production of selected English vowels in speakers with PD and dysarthria and healthy controls. They found that tongue movements in individuals with PD were more consistently different from healthy controls than jaw and lower lip movements. Wong et al. (86) used electromagnetic articulography to study tongue movement in individuals with PD and healthy controls during speech. They found abnormalities in tongue movements during the production of consonants.

EMG studies of the lip and jaw muscles in individuals with and without PD have provided some evidence for increased levels of tonic resting and background activity (34,35,87) as well as loss of reciprocity between agonist and antagonistic muscle groups in these individuals (34,35). These findings are consistent with evidence for abnormal sensorimotor gating in the orofacial and limb systems, which are presumably related to basal ganglia dysfunction (88,89). Whether these abnormal sensorimotor findings are indicative of excess rigidity in the speech musculature is not clear (78,80,81). Hunker et al. (82) found evidence to suggest a positive correlation between muscle stiffness and decrements in the range of lip movement. However, Connor and colleagues (80,81) found no evidence for excess rigidity in jaw muscles during speech movements, but they did find some abnormalities during nonspeech visually guided movements. They concluded that motor impairment in PD may be task dependent. Caligiuri (78) obtained measures of labial muscle rigidity and movement for 12 parkinsonian and nine age-matched control subjects. Displacement amplitude, peak instantaneous velocity, and movement time were evaluated during repetitive syllable productions. He reported that while mean displacement amplitudes and velocities were lower for the subjects with PD compared with the normal controls, there was no statistical relationship between labial rigidity and the degree of movement abnormality. He concluded that while rigidity may play a part in the overall disability, it does not sufficiently explain the labial articulatory difficulties associated with PD. He further argued that rigidity and bradykinesia probably represent independent pathophysiologic phenomena.

DISORDERED VERSUS COMPENSATED RATE OF SPEECH IN PD

Disordered rate of speech has been reported in some individuals with PD and rapid rate or short rushes of speech, have been reported in 6–13% of individuals with PD. Palilalia or stuttering-like speech dysfluencies have been observed in a small percent of individuals with parkinsonism (47,48). The discrepant findings of speech rate in parkinsonian speech (slow vs rapid) may be related to the presence or absence of compensatory mechanisms. For example, Caligiuri (79) found, using kinematic analyses, that lip movements were normal when individuals with PD spoke at a rate of 3–5 syllable/sec, but hypokinetic when the rate increased to 5–7 syllable/sec, which is the typical rate of conversational speech. Similarly, Acker-mann et al. (73) described a patient with akinetic-rigid PD who was instructed to synchronize labial diadochokinesis to sequences of periodic acoustic stimuli (2.5–6 Hz). This individual was able to synchronize his diadochokinesis to the stimulus rate up to 4 Hz, but when the stimulus rate exceeded 4 Hz, his diadochokinesis was uncontrollably produced at 8–9 Hz, indicating speech hastening. These findings suggest that some individuals with PD may slow down their speech to prevent the tendency for the articulator to uncontrollably accelerate and deteriorate beyond a certain rate (90).

RESONANCE PROBLEMS IN PD

Resonance problems are not common in PD, but when they are present, the voice often sounds like a fog horn. The acoustic and physiologic nature of this phenomenon is not clear, and perceptually, it is difficult to determine whether the voice is hypernasal or hyponasal. Aerodynamic and kinematic studies suggest that velopharyngeal movements may be reduced in some of these individuals (39,72,80). Abnormal tongue posture may also contribute to the resonance in parkinsonian speech. The abnormal resonance may also reflect motor symptoms not directly caused by PD, such as pharmacologically induced dystonic or dyskinetic movements of the velopharyngeal and/or tongue muscles.

SENSORIMOTOR AND PERCEPTUAL DEFICITS UNDERLYING MOTOR DYSFUNCTION IN PD

It has been suggested that the main function of the basal ganglia is to serve as an amplifier, by controlling the gain, through gating and scaling, of cortically generated movement patterns (91). Penny and colleagues (92,93) suggested that basal ganglia excitatory circuits inadequately activate cortical motor centers and as a result, motor-neuron pools are not provided with adequate facilitation, thus movements are small and slow. Berardelli et al. (94) suggested that the defect in motor cortex activation is due to a perceptual failure to select the muscle commands to match the external force and speed requirements. Maschke et al. (95) referred to this as a problem with kinesthesia and stated that when individuals with PD match their effort to their kinesthetic feedback, they will constantly underscale their movement. Thus, hypothetically, the neurophysiologic mechanisms underlying hypokinetic dysarthria in PD may be due, at least partially, to sensorimotor gating abnormalities and poor perception of one's own voice.

Sensory problems in PD have been recognized for years (96), and these problems may underlie some of the disorders of the speech system. Sensorimotor deficits in the orofacial system (88,89,97) and abnormal auditory, temporal, and perceptual processing of voice and speech (43,44,73,98) have been documented in PD (37,89) and have been implicated as important etiologic factors in hypokinetic dysarthria secondary to PD (99). Schneider and colleagues (89) found marked sensorimotor deficits in the orofacial and limb systems of individuals with PD. They observed that individuals with PD, compared with age-matched controls, showed greater deficits in tests of sensory function and sensorimotor integration. They suggested that individuals with PD might have complex deficits in the utilization of specific sensory inputs to organize and guide movements due to abnormal sensory gating or filtering associated with basal ganglia motor dysfunction. Caligiuri and colleagues (88) described abnormal orofacial reflexes in some but not all individuals with PD. Problems in sensory perception of effort have been identified as an important focus of successful speech and voice treatment for individuals with PD (100). It has been observed (51) that when individuals with PD are asked to produce loud speech they increased their otherwise underscaled soft speech to a level within normal limits but felt they were talking too loud. Thus, it appears that sensory kinesthesia problems may be a factor in the speech and voice disorder observed in individuals with PD.

Sensorimotor abnormalities associated with the phonatory system may also be present in individuals with PD. Hammer and Barlow (101) used clinical ratings of voice and disease severity, endoscopic assessment of laryngeal somatosensory function, and aerodynamic and acoustic assessment of respiratory and phonatory control in individuals with PD and healthy controls. They found sensory deficits associated with timing of phonatory onset, voice intensity, respiratory driving pressure, laryngeal resistance, lung volume expended per syllable, disease severity, and voice severity. They interpreted these findings to suggest that PD results in somatosensory abnormalities and airway sensorimotor disintegration. Laryngeal reflexes and other sensorimotor mechanisms have been shown to affect voice production and control in humans (102–105). Abnormal voice auditory feedback has also been documented in individuals with PD (106,107). These abnormalities may be mediated via the periaqueductal gray (PAG), as this area seems to play an important role in vocalization and in gating sensory information relevant to phonatory control (108). Recently, the PAG has been implicated in the voice abnormalities associated with PD (109). Whether the involvement of the PAG is part of the brain abnormalities or a compensatory system is not clear at this point. Collectively, the aforementioned findings suggest that phonatory abnormalities in PD are due, at least partially, to sensorimotor processing deficits, and these deficits may be mediated via bulbar and suprabulbar pathways.

Perception of one's own voice appears to be faulty in individuals with PD. Ho and colleagues (44) compared voice loudness perception in individuals with PD and hypophonic dysarthria with that of neurologically normal speakers. They found that, unlike the normal speakers, the PD patients overestimated the loudness of their speech during both reading and conversation. They interpreted these findings to suggest that either impaired speech production is driven by a basic perceptual fault, or that abnormal speech perception is a consequence of impaired mechanisms involved in the generation of soft speech. The latter explanation may be related to the phenomenon of central inhibitory influences of the vocal motor system, via feed forward mechanisms, on auditory cortical activity during self-produced vocalization. This phenomenon has been demonstrated in humans and animals (110–113) and has been argued to be defective in PD, thus interfering with self-monitoring and self-regulation of vocal loudness and effort (37).

Ho et al. (43) also examined the ability of individuals with PD and neurologically normal individuals to adjust their voice volume in response to two types of implicit cues, background noise and instantaneous auditory feedback. Control subjects demonstrated the Lombard effect by automatically speaking louder in the presence of background noise. They also decreased speech loudness in the presence of increasing levels of facilitative instantaneous auditory feedback. Subjects with PD demonstrated decreased overall speech loudness; they were less able than controls to appropriately increase loudness as background noise increased, and to decrease volume as auditory feedback increased. However, under explicit loudness instructions, the ability of subjects with PD to regulate loudness was similar to that of the normal controls, suggesting that individuals with PD have the capacity to speak with normal loudness, provided that they consciously attend to speaking loudly. The subjects with PD had overall speech loudness that was always lower than for control subjects, suggesting either a reduction of cortical motor input to the speech subsystems, or abnormal perception of their own voice via motor-to-sensory inhibitory mechanisms.

DISORDERED LANGUAGE AND COGNITIVE–LINGUISTIC FUNCTIONS

Although the main focus of the present chapter is on sensorimotor aspects of voice and speech disorders in PD, one should not lose sight of the fact that language processes may also be impaired in PD. Indeed, there is evidence for deficits in cognitive–linguistic functions in individuals with PD, as reflected in abnormal verbal fluency, semantic knowledge, semantic priming, high-level language comprehension, syntactic ambiguity, and so on, for example, see Refs (113,114). These abnormalities are found in individuals who are neither demented nor depressed. Whether these abnormalities are truly language-based or are secondary to cognitive impairment (attention, memory, executive function) is not clear.

SWALLOWING DISORDERS

Identification of swallowing disorders is extremely important in this population given the ramifications on nutrition and the ability to take oral medication appropriately. Silent aspiration may be observed and pneumonia can be a cause of death in advanced PD. Kalf et al. (115) conducted a systematic literature review regarding dysphagia in individuals with PD and healthy controls. They found that subjective dysphagia occurred in one third of community-dwelling individuals with PD. In contrast, objectively measured dysphagia rates were much higher, with 82% of patients being affected. Using objective methods to diagnose dysphagia, Volonté et al. (16) found that of 65 individuals with early-stage PD, 70% had oral-phase (facial, tongue, and palatal musculature) abnormalities.

Swallowing abnormalities have been reported in all stages of PD (116) and many individuals with PD have more than one type of swallowing dysfunction (9). Disorders in both oral and pharyngeal stages of swallowing have been observed (9,116). Sharkawi et al. (10) found abnormalities in the oral phase of swallowing in PD, the most predominant being reduced tongue control and strength and reduced oral transit times. Others have reported a rocking-like motion of the tongue during the oral phase (11). This motion seemed to occur when the individuals with PD were unable to lower the posterior portion of the tongue to propel the bolus into the pharynx. Inability or delayed ability to trigger the swallowing reflex has also been observed in this population (11). These disorders may limit the ability of the individual with PD to control the food or liquid bolus while in the oral cavity. These problems may lead to choking, penetration, or aspiration of the food or liquid. Reduced nutritional intake, lack of enjoyment in eating, and difficulty in taking medications appropriately can result from oral-phase swallowing dysfunction.

The specific neurophysiologic mechanisms underlying such dysphagic abnormalities in PD are not clear. Sensory gating and cueing deficits, which have been implicated in the hypokinetic dysarthria of individuals with PD, may also be etiologic factors in dysphagia during the oral phase. Pharyngeal stage dysfunction includes residue in the valleculae due to reduced tongue base retraction. Sharkawi et al. (10) reported this problem to be the most common disorder in the pharyngeal stage of swallowing. Blumin and colleagues (63) reported that 15 (100%) individuals with severe PD had some degree of pharyngeal residue of solids on videostroboscopy and fiberoptic endoscopic evaluation of swallowing. Aspiration may occur in these individuals as a result of the residue left in the pharynx after the swallow is complete (11). Leopold and Kagel (9) found several disorders of laryngeal movement during swallowing in PD. These included slow closure, incomplete closure, absent closure, and slowed or delayed laryngeal excursion (9). Increased pharyngeal transit time was also reported.

Silent aspiration has been observed in the later stages of PD and can be a contributory cause of death (12). Dysfunction in the pharyngeal stage of swallowing may also lead to choking, penetration, aspiration, reduced nutritional intake, or reduced ability to take medication orally. Again, sensory and internal cueing deficits may underlie these swallowing problems. It is unlikely that muscle rigidity is responsible for the dysphagia, since swallowing dysfunction occurs even when individuals with PD are considered optimally medicated. Referral for swallowing evaluation is extremely important at the first sign of problems even if this is early in the disease.

Dysphagia is not merely a sensorimotor disorder. As suggested by Leopold and Kagel (9), swallowing involves a five-stage process of ingestion: preoral (anticipatory), preparatory, lingual, pharyngeal, and esophageal. The first stage involves an interaction of preoral motor, cognitive, psychosocial, and somataesthetic elements engendered by the meal. If deficits in internal cueing, sensorimotor gating, scaling of movement amplitude, and self-regulation of effort affect swallowing, especially during the preoral, preparatory, and lingual stages, and if mealtime is a social event, swallowing and conversation may be performed simultaneously or alternatingly and might be especially problematic for individuals with PD creating a greater risk for dysphagia and aspiration.

EFFECT OF MEDICAL TREATMENTS FOR PD
ON SPEECH AND SWALLOWING

Although neuropharmacologic and neurosurgical approaches have had positive effects on the primary symptoms of PD, their effects on voice, speech, and swallowing have been inconsistent. Several studies have assessed the effects of levodopa and dopamine agonists on voice and speech functions in PD. Gallena and colleagues (66) studied the effects of levodopa on laryngeal function in six persons with early PD who were not receiving medication. They found that levodopa reduced excessive laryngeal muscle activity and vocal fold bowing and improved voice onset and offset control during speech in some patients. De Letter and colleagues (117) reported significant improvement in speech intelligibility with levodopa. Goberman et al. (118) examined the acoustic-phonatory characteristics of speech in nine individuals with PD and motor fluctuations before and after taking levodopa. They found that the voice F0 variability in vowels and mean F0 were higher, and intensity range was lower when on, compared with off medication. They also found that differences in speech between on and off medication were small, although in some individuals, phonation clearly improved. Jiang and colleagues (119) assessed the effects of levodopa on vocal function in 15 PD patients with tremor using airflow and EGG measures. The subjects were recorded as they sustained vowel phonation before and after taking medication. Speed quotient, acoustic shimmer, and extent of tremor derived from acoustic intensity contours were found to significantly decrease, and vocSPL tended to increase after medication, indicating improvement in vocal function with levodopa. Sanabria and colleagues (120) used acoustic measures to study the effects of levodopa treatment on vocal function in 20 individuals with PD before and after levodopa. When compared to premedication, postmedication voice F0 was significantly increased, and jitter, soft phonation index (noise parameter), and frequency tremor intensity index significantly decreased. Cahill et al. (121) studied the effects of levodopa on lip function in 16 patients with PD, using a computerized semiconductor lip pressure transducer. Lip pressures recorded during both speech and nonspeech tasks tended to improve after levodopa administration.

Although the above studies indicate improvement in phonatory and articulatory functions with levodopa, numerous studies (122,123) have failed to find significant improvement in voice and speech functions with levodopa or dopamine agonists. These negative findings have raised questions regarding the role of dopamine as the sole, or major, etiologic factor in hypokinetic dysarthria, and have raised the possibility that either nondopaminergic or special dopaminergic mechanisms may play an important etiologic role. Importantly, whereas at a group level studies failed to find significant effects of dopamine medication on speech (6,21,124), several of these studies nevertheless have shown that some individuals did show marked improvement with dopamine medication; see Refs (6,124). Why some individuals with PD seem to benefit from dopamine medication and others do not is not clear.

Future studies should assess the therapeutic role of such nondopaminergic mechanisms on parkinsonian speech. Interestingly, clonazepam (dosage 0.25–0.5 mg/day), a nondopaminergic agent, has been reported to significantly improve speech in 10 of 11 individuals with PD and hypokinetic dysarthria (125). More studies are needed to examine the role of nondopaminergic agents on speech in individuals with PD.

DEEP BRAIN STIMULATION

Many studies of deep brain stimulation (DBS) of the subthalamic nucleus (STN), globus pallidus internus (GPi), and ventral intermediate (Vim) nucleus of the thalamus have reported dysarthria and dysphagia as side effects (126–128). Several studies examined specific aspects of voice, speech, swallowing and related orofacial and respiratory-laryngeal functions associated with DBS treatment of PD. Santens and colleagues (129) found that left-brain stimulation had a profound negative effect on prosody, articulation, and intelligibility not seen with right-brain stimulation. With bilateral stimulation, no differences in speech characteristics were observed on and off stimulation. Wang and colleagues (130) also studied the effects of unilateral STN DBS on respiratory/phonatory subsystems of speech production in PD. Speech recordings were made in the medication off state at baseline and three months post-DBS with stimulation on and off, in six right-handed patients. Three patients who received left-brain STN DBS showed a significant decline in vocal intensity and vowel duration compared with baseline, which the authors attributed to microlesions of the dominant hemisphere for speech.

Some studies indicate improvement in voice and speech functions with DBS. Gentil and colleagues (131) assessed the effects of bilateral STN DBS on hypokinetic dysarthria using force measurements of the articulatory organs and acoustic analysis in 16 PD patients. They noted that STN DBS reduced reaction and movement time of the articulatory organs, increased maximal strength and precision of these organs, and improved respiratory and phonatory functions. Gentil and colleagues (132) also compared the effects of bilateral STN DBS versus Vim DBS on oral control in 14 individuals with PD. They used force transducers to sample ramp-and-hold force contractions generated by the upper lip, lower lip and tongue at 1- and 2-Newton target force levels, as well as maximal force. With STN stimulation, dynamic and static control of the articulatory organs improved greatly, whereas with Vim stimulation it worsened. In another study of 26 individuals with PD treated with bilateral STN DBS, Gentil and colleagues (133), using acoustic analysis of voice, found that stimulation resulted in longer duration of sustained vowels, shorter duration of sentences, words, and pauses, increased variability in voice F0 in sentences, and increased stability of voice F0 during sustained vowels. There was no difference in vocal intensity between the on- and off-stimulation conditions. Pinto and colleagues (134) assessed the impact of bilateral STN DBS on forces and control of the upper lip, lower lip, and tongue in 26 dysarthric individuals with PD before and after DBS surgery. They reported that with stimulation there was improvement in the maximal voluntary force, reaction time, movement time, precision of the peak force and the hold phase during an articulatory force task. They also reported that these beneficial effects of DBS on articulatory forces persisted up to five years.

Dromey and colleagues (135) studied the effects of bilateral STN DBS on acoustic measures of voice in seven individuals with PD. Acoustic recordings of voice were made before surgery in the medication off and medication on conditions and after surgery with and without stimulation in the medication on and off conditions. Six months after surgery, there were significant though small increases in vocSPL and F0 variability when on medication with DBS. Rousseaux and colleagues (136) studied the effects of bilateral STN DBS on speech parameters and intelligibility in seven dysarthric PD patients. Speech was evaluated before and three months after surgery with stimulation off and on, and with and without a suprathreshold levodopa dose. Modest beneficial effects were reported on several motor speech parameters, especially lip movements. Modulation of voice pitch and loudness improved mildly. Articulation was not affected and speech intelligibility was slightly reduced in the on-stimulation condition, especially when patients received levodopa. Marked negative effects on intelligibility were observed in two patients, due to increased facial and trunk dyskinesia.

In sum, DBS can result in a moderate benefit on the speech motor system during nonspeech tasks, and minimal therapeutic or adverse effects on voice and speech functions. Although the follow-up studies suggest deterioration in speech following DBS, it is not clear to what extent this deterioration is due to the DBS surgery, to voltage spread from the stimulating electrodes (137), and to the natural progression of PD.

Although DBS of the STN has been the main procedure to alleviate motor symptoms of PD, other studies have assessed DBS of other brain structures, namely, the region of the pallidofugal fibres and the caudal zona incerta (cZi), which lies dorsal/dorsomedial to the STN, and the region that is the junction between the dorsal border of the STN and the cZi. Plaha et al. (138) compared stimulation of each of these regions, to examine their effect on the contralateral Unified Parkinson's Disease Rating Scale (UPDRS) motor score (off medication/off stimulation versus off medication/on stimulation) measured at follow-up. They also measured the UPDRS motor subscores of tremor, bradykinesia, and rigidity. Overall, stimulation of the cZi region seemed to yield better results than STN DBS as far as the contralateral UPDRS score was concerned. For on- versus off-stimulation 12 months after surgery, mean voice intensity during reading changed significantly for both STN and cZi groups, but in different directions: The STN group showed an increase of 2.1 dB, whereas the cZi group showed a reduction of 1.15 dB. These results were consistent across individuals within the group (8 of 8 in the STN group, 7 of 8 in the cZi group). These findings suggest that the overall motor improvement with cZi DBS is at the cost of deterioration in vocal intensity. Interestingly, DBS did not affect vocal decay in either group. Karlsson et al. (139) compared the effects of STN DBS and cZi DBS on speech articulation diadochokinetic rate in individuals with PD. They had participants perform repetitive speech tasks using measurements of articulation rate and quality of the production of plosive consonants. They found that the STN DBS group increased articulation rate in the stimulation on condition on one speech task. The cZi DBS group decreased articulation rate in the stimulation on condition and showed a reduction in the production quality of consonants. They concluded that cZi DBS is more detrimental for extended articulatory movements than STN DBS. Thus, the two studies suggest that improvement in general motor function with cZi DBS is likely to be at the cost of speech motor functions.

TRANSCRANIAL AND EXTRADURAL BRAIN STIMULATION

Dias and colleagues (140) studied the effects of repetitive transcranial magnetic stimulation (rTMS) on vocal function in 30 individuals with PD. Stimulation of the primary motor cortex (M1)-mouth area induced a significant improvement in voice F0 and intensity. Stimulation of the left dorsolateral prefrontal cortex resulted in subjective improvement of voice-related quality of life, but not in objective measures of voice F0 and intensity. Murdoch et al. (141) applied high-frequency (5 Hz) rTMS to 10 active stimulation and 10 sham placebo patients with PD for 10 min/day (3000 pulses), for 10 days during speech production. Stimulation was applied to the primary motor cortex representing the mouth motor region. Speech outcome measures and lingual kinematic parameters were recorded at baseline and 1 week, 2 and 12 months poststimulation. Results showed positive, treatment-related, changes in the active rTMS group when compared with the sham placebo control group at 2 and 12 months poststimulation in maximum velocity of tongue movements, distance of tongue movements, speech intelligibility, and communication efficiency. Pagni and colleagues (142) studied the effects of extradural motor cortex stimulation in three individuals with PD. They reported that unilateral stimulation resulted in improvement in speech and swallowing. Overall, these findings are encouraging, but need to be explored further to ascertain the utility of brain stimulation.

ABLATIVE SURGERY
Pallidotomy

Ablative surgery for PD has been used extensively in the past, but it has been largely replaced by DBS. In general, ablative surgeries have yielded therapeutic effects on motor functions, but their effects on speech have been variable, minimal, or adverse. The effects of pallidotomy on speech have been assessed in several studies. Schulz and colleagues (143) assessed six PD patients after pallidotomy and found all six to have positive changes in at least one acoustic measure. In another study Schulz and colleagues (144) assessed changes in vocSPL following unilateral pallidotomy in 25 hypokinetic dysarthric individuals with PD. They found that mildly dysarthric individuals had significantly greater increases in vocSPL following pallidotomy, whereas moderately or severely dysarthric individuals had decreases in vocSPL. Uitti and colleagues (145) assessed 57 PD patients after pallidotomy and found that speech intelligibility was preserved, with a tendency to decline mildly in one-third of patients. Scott and colleagues (146) compared the effects of unilateral and bilateral pallidotomy three months postsurgery and reported a fall in speech diadochokinetic rates and self-perceived worsening of pre-existing dysarthria, hypophonia, and hypersalivation/drooling following bilateral pallidotomy.

Thalamotomy and Subthalamotomy

Nagulic and colleagues (147) used acoustic analyses to assess the effects of stereotactic thalamotomy in seven male patients with PD and found that the mean vocSPL during the initial segment of the speech signal and the voice F0 increased after thalamotomy. The voice formants F1 and F2 shifted to the higher energy and frequency regions. Parkin and colleagues (148) studied the effects of bilateral subthalamotomy for PD and reported speech disturbance as one of three major complications.

Farrell and colleagues (149) studied the effects of various neurosurgical procedures (pallidotomy, thalamotomy, DBS) on perceptual speech characteristics, speech intelligibility, and oromotor function in 22 individuals with PD. The surgical group was compared with a group of 16 participants with PD who did not undergo neurosurgery and 25 neurologically healthy individuals matched for age and sex. Results indicated that none of the neurosurgical interventions significantly changed perceptual speech dimensions or oromotor function, in spite of significant postoperative improvements in general motor function.

PERIPHERAL SURGERY FOR VOICE AND SWALLOWING PROBLEMS
Collagen Augmentation of Vocal Folds for Hypophonia
The effects of collagen augmentation of the vocal folds, via percutaneous injection and fiberoptic guidance, on phonation in hypophonic individuals with PD were reported in two studies. Berke and colleagues (150) assessed 35 hypophonic PD patients treated with collagen augmentation with a telephone survey and found that 75% expressed satisfaction with the improvement in their voice, compared with 16% who expressed dissatisfaction with the results of collagen augmentation. Kim and colleagues (151), using a telephone interview of 18 PD patients treated with this procedure, found that 11 patients (61%) considered their voice improved for at least two months. Of the seven patients (28%) that were not improved with this procedure, five were aphonic before and after the collagen injection. They concluded that although the majority of patients are likely to benefit from the procedure, patients with advanced neurologic disease with aphonia, difficulty with speech initiation, dysphagia, or ambulatory difficulty are less likely to respond to this procedure. Although these preliminary results are promising, more objective methods of voice evaluation are needed, as are long-term, controlled outcome studies. Remacle and Lawson (152), in their review of the literature, concluded that collagen injection for PD-related hypophonia and dysphonia is an effective temporary method of subjectively improving voice and speech in selected individuals with PD. They also noted that complications from the procedure are uncommon, but individuals with PD need to be advised that the results may not be stable and may be unpredictable.

Cricopharyngeal Myotomy for Swallowing
Born et al. (153) assessed the effects of cricopharyngeal myotomy in four patients with PD and dysphagia associated with cricopharyngeal dysfunction, diagnosed with radiologic and manometric methods. They reported positive results with sustained improvement in swallowing.

Hypotheses Regarding Neural Mechanisms Underlying Voice and Speech Disorders in PD
We have suggested that hypokinetic dysarthria, among other motor disorders in PD, may be related, at least partially, to abnormal nondopaminergic or special dopaminergic mechanisms, and that these abnormalities underlie several high-level processes that are important for the regulation and control of speech movements (22,23,45,47,123). We briefly discuss four such high-level processes. These include scaling movement amplitude, sensory processing, internal cueing, and attention to action (vocal vigilance).

Scaling Movement Amplitude
A major factor underlying hypokinetic dysarthria in PD is reduced amplitude of output (hypokinesia) and *abnormal scaling and maintenance of movement amplitude or force*. Reduced range (hypokinesia) of respiratory, laryngeal, and orofacial movements during speech sound production in individuals with PD, with the tendency of the amplitude of the movements to decay (become more hypokinetic) within and across utterances has been documented in various studies (41,52,53,72,79). This reduction in amplitude and force may manifest as a systematic reduction and decay of vocal loudness, pitch intonation, and precision of vowels, consonants, and other

sounds of speech (37,38,53,72,75,154) and may be attributed to the inability of individuals with PD to scale and/or maintain movement amplitude, force, or related parameters (91,155–159).

Sensory Processing

Another factor likely to underlie hypokinetic dysarthria is *abnormality in sensory processing*. Behavioral and physiologic studies of speech and nonspeech oral and head and neck functions in individuals with PD have documented sensory abnormalities, manifested as errors on tasks of kinesthesia (160–162), difficulties with orofacial perception, including decreased jaw proprioception, tactile localization on tongue, gums and teeth, and targeted and tracking head movements to perioral stimulation (89); problems utilizing proprioceptive information for normal movement (89,161); abnormal higher order processing of afferent information as demonstrated by abnormal reflex and voluntary motor responses to proprioceptive input (88,97,163,164); and abnormal sensory processing of speech in individuals with PD (41,43,44,98,165,166). Laryngeal sensorimotor deficits in PD have also been documented (101,167). These sensorimotor abnormalities may account, at least partially, for the deficits in scaling and maintaining speech movement amplitude.

One aspect of *sensory processing deficits* in individuals with PD is misperception of self-produced voice and vocal effort. Individuals with PD are often unaware of the magnitude of their reduced vocal loudness and will report, "my voice is fine, but my spouse needs a hearing aid" (99). This is similar to the inaccurate perception of body awareness and lack of self-corrections of smaller and slower movements in everyday living even in early PD (168). Furthermore, when individuals with PD and hypokinetic dysarthria are asked to produce "loud" speech (i.e., increase amplitude of motor output), they typically increase their speech to a normal conversational loudness level, yet they complain that this louder voice is "way too loud." This phenomenon has been documented by Ho and colleagues (44). These researchers found that although individuals with PD spoke with a softer voice than healthy controls, they nevertheless perceived their own speech to be louder than that judged by the healthy controls. In addition, individuals with PD overestimated the loudness of their speech during both reading and conversation. Furthermore, sensorimotor abnormalities in auditory–vocal feedback and feed forward mechanisms have been indirectly demonstrated in individuals with PD by behavioral (106) and neurophysiologic (169) methods. Finally, Ramig and colleagues have shown that addressing problems of sensory processing deficits is an important therapeutic goal for a successful treatment of hypokinetic dysarthria in individuals with PD (28,29,100).

Internal Cueing

A third factor underlying hypokinesia is *deficits in internal cueing*. One of the most striking characteristics of hypokinetic dysarthria in individuals with PD is the dramatic improvement in speech when these individuals are externally cued or instructed to speak loudly and/or clearly. The improvement in speech with external cueing is most likely a compensatory response to deficits in internal cueing (170). This conclusion is empirically supported by a series of experimental studies conducted by Ho and colleagues (43,44,165). It is also consistent with the phenomenon of micrographia (abnormally small handwriting) in individuals with PD, which tends to improve dramatically (although transiently) when these individuals are verbally instructed to "write big" or when they are provided with dots or lines on the paper, and asked to write so that the letters touch the dots or the lines (external cues) (171). The use of external cueing has also been shown to positively impact gait in PD, with long-term retention, when cueing strategies were systematically trained over several weeks time (172).

Attention to Action (Vocal Vigilance)
A fourth factor underlying hypokinetic dysarthria may be impairment in *self-monitoring and self-regulation* of speech motor output. There is evidence that attention to action is impaired in individuals with PD, and that this impairment may contribute to the abnormal control of movements in PD (173,174). By inference, impaired attention to action of the voice in individuals with PD may have an adverse effect on motor speech control, which may partially account for the hypokinetic dysarthria in these individuals (22). Importantly, it has been shown that attention to action in individuals with PD can be improved significantly by intensive training (166,175). As discussed below, the LSVT LOUD treatment regimen, which has been designed to train individuals with PD to pay attention to their speech output and to monitor the effort to produce this output, has been shown to be effective in the long-term maintenance of treatment outcome (4,28).

Behavioral Speech, Voice, and Swallowing Treatment for Parkinson's Disease
Although the incidence of speech and voice disorders in individuals with PD is extremely high, only 3–4% have been reported to receive speech treatment (176). One explanation for this is that carryover and long-term treatment outcomes have been disappointing and consequently the primary challenges in the treatment of hypokinetic dysarthria associated with PD. Clinicians have long been aware that when individuals with PD and dysarthria are receiving direct stimulation, prodding, or feedback from the speech clinician or an external cue (177,178), they are likely to show dramatic improvement in speech and voice production and overall intelligibility. However, maintaining these improvements without these external cues is extremely difficult for most of these individuals.

One explanation for the inability of individuals with PD to maximize and maintain treatment gains may be their deficits in internal cueing, attention to action (vocal vigilance), scaling amplitude of vocal output, and self-perception and self-regulation of vocal loudness and efforts (22,23,45,89,94). To maximize and maintain treatment effects, speech therapy of individuals with PD and dysarthria should address these deficits. Ramig et al. (26,27) documented that improving amplitude of vocal output and sensory perception of vocal loudness and effort, as obtained via the LSVT LOUD program, are key elements in successful speech treatment for individuals with PD. In addition, deficits in implicit or procedural learning (179) may underlie the challenges that individuals with PD have in maintaining long-term treatment effects and in learning to habituate newly acquired methods of speech production. Efforts to overcome these cognitive problems as part of treatment may also facilitate long-term outcome.

Intensive Voice Treatment for Parkinson's Disease
The unique aspects of the LSVT LOUD include the combination of (*i*) an exclusive target on increasing amplitude (loudness in the speech motor system), (*ii*) a focus

on sensory recalibration to help patients recognize that speech with increased amplitude is within normal limits, even if they feel "too loud," and (*iii*) training self-cueing and attention-to-action to facilitate long-term maintenance of treatment outcomes. In addition, the intensive mode of delivery is consistent with principles that drive activity-dependent neuroplasticity and motor learning (180–182). This approach is graphically represented in Figure 27.1. Treatment is administered four consecutive days a week (1-hour sessions) for one month. In addition, the LSVT LOUD is administered in a manner to maximize compliance and motivation from individuals with PD by assigning treatment activities that make an immediate impact on daily functional communication. The rationale for the concepts of the LSVT LOUD is graphically represented in Figure 27.2. The protocol for LSVT LOUD has been described in detail elsewhere (183).

Specifically, the LSVT LOUD uses high effort, but not strenuous, increased vocal loudness to encourage optimal vocal fold closure and maximum phonatory efficiency. Individuals with PD are taken through exercises on a daily basis, repeatedly practicing and emphasizing maximum duration loud phonations, maximum high and low pitch phonations, and speech exercises with increased vocal loudness. This scaled-up vocal loudness is then systematically trained into speech and conversation following a standardized hierarchy, with focus on monitoring the amount of effort required to sustain sufficient vocal loudness (sensory recalibration). No direct attention is given to speech rate, prosodic pitch inflection, or articulation.

The goal of the LSVT LOUD is to improve functional communication for at least 6–12 months without additional treatment. After 16 sessions of individual treatment, most individuals with PD will be able to maintain speech and voice changes for at least six months and sometimes for up to one (4) or two years (27,112) without additional speech treatment. Within the 16 initial sessions of treatment, individuals with PD establish a daily homework routine that they maintain on their own once treatment is over. All individuals with PD are encouraged to return for a reassessment at six months at which time some may benefit from a few tune-up sessions of LSVT LOUD. Further details of the LSVT LOUD have been described elsewhere (112).

Treatment data suggest that individuals with mild-to-moderate PD have the most positive treatment outcomes following the LSVT LOUD. Early administration of the LSVT LOUD or other intensive voice and speech treatment programs is also important since research shows that the most effective ways to induce neuroplasticity with behavioral treatment is to apply therapy before neurotoxicity and before the degenerative process is severe (181,182,184). Individuals with severe PD, severe depression, or severe dementia may have a poorer prognosis with LSVT LOUD; however, individuals with co-occurring mild-to-moderate depression and dementia can benefit from therapy (26). Because treatment focuses on voice, all individuals with PD must have a laryngeal examination before treatment to rule out any contraindications (e.g., vocal nodules, gastric reflux, laryngeal cancer). It is important to clarify that the goal of LSVT LOUD is to maximize phonatory efficiency. It is never the goal to teach a hyperfunctional voice quality (pressed, strained, too loud), but rather to improve vocal fold adduction for optimum loudness and quality and without undue strain. Indeed, several studies have demonstrated improvement in vocal efficiency and vocal quality due to LSVT LOUD, with no evidence for vocal abuse or impairment (45,60,185–188).

PRE-TREATMENT

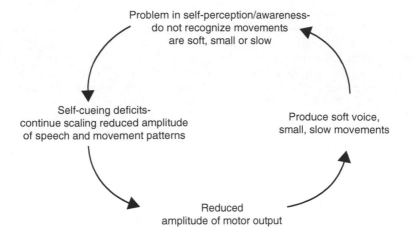

TREATMENT FOCUS – mode of delivery is intensive, high effort, salient

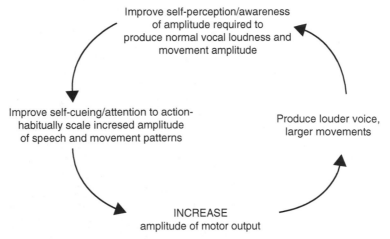

FIGURE 27.1 We hypothesize that pretreatment (*top*), individuals with Parkinson's disease have reduced amplitude of motor output, which results in soft voice and small movements. Due to problems in sensory self-perception they are not aware of the soft voice and small movements, or they do not recognize the extent of their soft voice and smaller movements. As a result, no error correction is made and individuals continue to program or self-cue reduced amplitude of motor output. They are "stuck" in a cycle of being soft and small. The focus in treatment (*bottom*) is on increasing the amplitude of motor output by having individuals with PD produce a louder voice and larger movements. Individuals are then taught that what feels/sounds/looks "too loud" or "too big" is within normal limits and has a positive impact on daily functional living. Therefore at the end of treatment, individuals habitually self-cue increased amplitude of motor output and have attention to action. Now they are in a cycle of a louder voice and bigger movements.

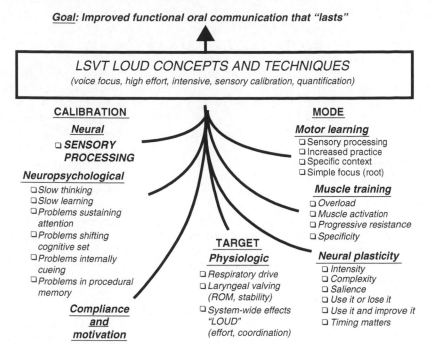

Goal: Improved functional oral communication that "lasts"

LSVT LOUD CONCEPTS AND TECHNIQUES
(voice focus, high effort, intensive, sensory calibration, quantification)

CALIBRATION

Neural
❏ **SENSORY PROCESSING**

Neuropsychological
❏ Slow thinking
❏ Slow learning
❏ Problems sustaining attention
❏ Problems shifting cognitive set
❏ Problems internally cueing
❏ Problems in procedural memory

Compliance and motivation

TARGET

Physiologic
❏ Respiratory drive
❏ Laryngeal valving (ROM, stability)
❏ System-wide effects "LOUD" (effort, coordination)

MODE

Motor learning
❏ Sensory processing
❏ Increased practice
❏ Specific context
❏ Simple focus (root)

Muscle training
❏ Overload
❏ Muscle activation
❏ Progressive resistance
❏ Specificity

Neural plasticity
❏ Intensity
❏ Complexity
❏ Salience
❏ Use it or lose it
❏ Use it and improve it
❏ Timing matters

FIGURE 27.2 This figure graphically summarizes the rationale underlying the five essential concepts and techniques of the LSVT LOUD from a neural, speech mechanism physiology, motor learning, muscle training, neuroplasticity, neuropsychological, and compliance perspective. The neural bases are the reduction in muscle activation and self-monitoring and consequent problem in programming an output target with adequate amplitude. The physiological basis is the focus on respiratory drive and laryngeal valving to generate a maximally efficient vocal source. "Loud" is used as the system trigger for improving effort and coordination across the speech mechanism. The LSVT LOUD is administered in a manner consistent with principles of motor learning in order to maximize treatment effectiveness. Emphasis on sensory processing, increased practice, practice within specific context and a simple "root" focus (e.g., "loud") are key elements of treatment. The neuropsychological aspects of Parkinson's disease: slow thinking, slow learning, problems sustaining attention, problems shifting cognitive set, problems internally cueing, and problems in procedural memory, are also taken into account with the LSVT LOUD. The LSVT LOUD is also administered in a way consistent with muscle training. Treatment technique overloads the muscles using progressive resistance in specific activities. The LSVT LOUD is designed to maximize patient compliance. From day 1 of treatment, activities are designed to maximize impact on daily functional communication. *Abbreviation*: LSVT LOUD, Lee Silverman Voice Treatment.

EFFECTIVENESS OF LSVT LOUD ON VOICE

LSVT LOUD was developed during the late 1980s. Initially, case studies, single subject designs, and nonrandomized studies were published (189). These studies provided the first evidence of successful treatment outcomes for individuals with PD and suggested that intensive treatment focusing on increasing phonatory effort and self-monitoring of such effort could improve vocal communication in individuals with PD. Based on those findings, a number of randomized and blinded studies were conducted. In one study, 45 individuals with PD were randomly assigned to one of two forms of treatment: respiratory effort treatment (RET) or (LSVT LOUD). Short- (26) and long-term (27,28,185) data have been reported from these studies. Only subjects who received the LSVT LOUD rated a significant decrease post-treatment on the impact of PD on their communication. Corresponding perceptual ratings by blinded raters (186) revealed only the male subjects who had the LSVT LOUD improved in ratings of breathiness and intonation. The acoustic findings were supported in studies at one-year (27) and two-year follow-up (28). Only those subjects in the LSVT LOUD group improved or maintained vocal SPL above pre-treatment levels. In addition, perceptual reports by patients and family members supported the positive impact of LSVT LOUD on functional daily communication. In another study (190) 29 individuals with PD were studied over six months. A half of the group received LSVT LOUD and the other half served as an untreated control group. In addition, neurologically healthy, age-matched controls were studied over this time period. Only subjects who received the LSVT LOUD demonstrated significant increases in variables such as vocSPL (related to loudness) and semitone standard deviation (related to intonation) at pre-, post-, and six-month follow-up.

Improvement in laryngeal function with LSVT LOUD has been documented physiologically. Smith et al. (60) found increases in vocal fold closure following treatment in individuals who received the LSVT LOUD, but not in individuals who received RET. These data were collected by clinicians not directly involved in the study and therefore support carryover of treatment effects. Importantly, laryngeal examination has shown no evidence of hyperfunctional laryngeal behaviors or vocal fold pathology induced by loud phonation training with LSVT LOUD. In fact, it has been shown that LSVT LOUD tends to decrease pretreatment hyper-functional behavior (false fold overclosure, anterior–posterior hyperfunction, laryngeal elevation) (187), increase subglottal air pressure and maximum flow declination rate (188), and reduce breathiness and hoarseness in individuals with PD (186). These findings reflect increased respiratory drive, improved vocal fold adduction, less abusive or strenuous voice use, and more efficient voice production after LSVT LOUD.

EFFECTS OF LSVT LOUD ON THE OROFACIAL SYSTEM

Not only does LSVT LOUD improve phonatory effort and vocal characteristics (loudness, pitch variability, vocal quality), it also improves speech articulation. Dromey (83) compared the effects of two treatment approaches, LSVT LOUD and exaggerated articulation during speech, and found that the LSVT LOUD was significantly more effective in improving speech articulation. Sapir et al. (37,38) used acoustic and perceptual analyses to assess the impact of LSVT LOUD on vowel articulation in dysarthric individuals with PD ($n = 14$). There was a significant improvement in both vowel acoustics (formants) and perceptual ratings (vowel goodness postrelative to pre-LSVT®), as well as in VocSPL, in the group receiving LSVT LOUD, but not in other individuals with PD ($n = 15$) or healthy age-matched controls ($n = 14$) who did not receive treatment. The improvement in vowel acoustics and ratings were interpreted as evidence for improvement in vowel articulation associated with LSVT LOUD. These findings are consistent with a previous perceptual study (4) documenting increased ratings of speech loudness and speech quality in individuals with PD receiving LSVT LOUD, but not in individuals with PD receiving RET.

The improvement in vowel articulation with LSVT LOUD in individuals with PD is consistent with Schulman (191) showing that as a speaker talks louder there are accompanying vocal tract and articulatory changes. These effects have been long lasting and treatment specific as documented in a 12-month follow-up study (185). LSVT LOUD has also been shown to improve facial expression (31), tongue strength and motility (30), and swallowing (10) in individuals with PD. Recently, individuals with PD and dysarthria post-STN DBS have been reported to respond favorably to LSVT LOUD, showing improvement in voice quality, loudness, prosody, articulatory function, or a combination of these (192). These findings are in contrast to findings by Tripoliti et al. (193) who found no significant improvement in speech with LSVT in individuals with STN DBS. The reasons for these discrepancies are not clear.

EFFECTS OF LSVT LOUD ON BRAIN ACTIVITY

Two brain imaging studies using O^{15} positron emisson tomography (PET) in a small number of individuals with PD have documented changes in brain function immediately following LSVT LOUD (32,33). The most recent study by Narayana et al. (33) examined the neural mechanisms underlying the effects of training increased vocal loudness in 10 individuals with PD and hypophonia. Cerebral blood flow during rest and reading conditions was measured by H_2 ^{15}O-PET. Z-score images were generated by contrasting reading with rest conditions for pre- and post-LSVT LOUD sessions, and neural activity was correlated with the corresponding change in vocal SPL (loudness). Narayana et al. hypothesized that brain activation patterns associated with LSVT LOUD training would reflect improved loudness, improved perception of self-generated voice output, and improved attention to action. Further it was hypothesized that these outcomes would likely be mediated via the right hemisphere, and involve speech motor and premotor cortical areas (re: loudness), the auditory cortices (re: recalibration of perception of self-produced loudness), and dorsolateral prefrontal cortex (re: attention to action). To a large extent, the results of the study are consistent with these hypotheses. These initial neural findings underlying LSVT LOUD outcomes are being further examined and verified in ongoing imaging studies as discussed in ongoing research.

SWALLOWING TREATMENT FOR PARKINSON'S DISEASE

Treatment of swallowing disorders in PD has not been well studied. Conventional techniques have included oral motor exercises to improve muscle strength, range of motion and coordination, and behavioral modifications such as effortful breathhold, chin positioning, double swallow, the Mendelsohn maneuver, swallow/cough, effortful swallow, and diet and liquid modifications (25,194). Effectiveness of these techniques varies and can be dependent on patient motivation and cooperation, family support, and the timeliness of the referral for a swallowing evaluation. Efficacy studies of the impact of behavioral treatment on dysphagia in PD are lacking (195). The effects of LSVT LOUD on swallowing dysfunction in individuals with PD have been studied by Sharkawi et al. (10). These researchers found that the LSVT LOUD reduced swallowing motility disorders by 51%. Some temporal measures of swallowing were also reduced, as was the amount of residue. This is the first study to find positive changes in both voice and swallowing function following intensive voice therapy alone without a therapy focusing on swallowing. A study by De Angelis and colleagues (196) documented improved voice, speech, and swallowing functions in individuals with PD participating in an intensive treatment with a schedule similar to that of the LSVT LOUD and with a clinical goal of improved glottic closure. These studies collectively point to the utility of intensive voice treatment for the reduction of swallowing dysfunction.

EFFECTS OF LSVT LOUD ON FACIAL EXPRESSION IN PD
Spielman and colleagues (31) examined the impact of LSVT LOUD on facial expression in individuals with PD. Videos of 44 individuals with PD before and after one month of either LSVT LOUD or RET were randomized and rated by trained raters, who judged each video clip for facial mobility and engagement. Overall, members of the LSVT LOUD group received more ratings of increased facial mobility and engagement following treatment relative to members of the RET group.

ADMINISTRATION OF LSVT LOUD BY ELECTRONIC DEVICES AND VIRTUAL CLINICIANS
Technology has been recently adapted to make LSVT LOUD available to individuals who are far away from the clinic, to improve practice at home, and to reduce cost of treatment and clinician time. Technology includes the use of tele-practice for delivery of speech treatment and a specialized software program that works with a standardized calibrated microphone to deliver LSVT LOUD treatment (197). The LSVT Companion® has been programmed to collect acoustic data and provide feedback as it guides the individual with PD through the LSVT LOUD exercises. Instead of the usual 16 treatment sessions of in-person clinician-delivered LSVT LOUD, only nine sessions are with a clinician, and the other seven are completed independently at home by the patient utilizing the LSVT COMPANION. Pilot studies have demonstrated marked and long-term (six-month follow-up) improvement in voice and speech with the COMPANION, with treatment outcome comparable to that obtained with the original in person clinician-administered LSVT LOUD (197). These findings support the feasibility of using state-of-the-art technology to administer speech treatment and keep records of patients' progress.

ACKNOWLEDGMENT
This work was supported in part by NIH-NIDCD R01 DC01150; P60 DC00976 and OE-NIDRR 8133G40108.

REFERENCES
1. Ho AK, Iansek R, Marigliani C, Bradshaw JL, Gates S. Speech impairment in a large sample of patients with Parkinson's disease. Behav Neurol 1998; 11: 131–7.
2. Logemann JA, Fisher HB, Boshes B, Blonsky ER. Frequency and coocurrence of vocal tract dysfunctions in the speech of a large sample of Parkinson patients. J Speech Hear Disord 1978; 43: 47–57.
3. Darley FL, Aronson AE, Brown JR. Motor Speech Disorders. Philadelphia: WB Saunders, 1975.

4. Sapir S, Ramig L, Hoyt P, et al. Phonatory-Respiratory effort (LSVT) vs. respiratory effort treatment for hypokinetic dysarthria: comparing speech loudness and quality before and 12 months after treatment. Folia Phoniatr (Basel) 2002; 54: 296–303.
5. Rusz J, Cmejla R, Ruzickova H, Ruzicka E. Quantitative acoustic measurements for characterization of speech and voice disorders in early untreated Parkinson's disease. J Acoust Soc Am 2011; 129: 350–67.
6. Skodda S, Visser W, Schlegel U. Short- and long-term dopaminergic effects on dysarthria in early Parkinson's disease. J Neural Transm 2010; 117: 197–205.
7. Miller N, Noble E, Jones D, Burn D. Life with communication changes in Parkinson's disease. Age Ageing 2006; 35: 235–9.
8. Pitcairn TK, Clemie S, Gray JM, Pentland B. Impressions of parkinsonian patients from their recorded voices. Br J Disord Commun 1990; 25: 85–92.
9. Leopold NA, Kagel MA. Laryngeal deglutition movement in Parkinson's disease. Neurology 1997; 48: 373–5.
10. Sharkawi AE, Ramig L, Logemann JA, et al. Swallowing and voice effects of Lee Silverman Voice Treatment (LSVT®): a pilot study. J Neurol Neurosurg Psychiatry 2002; 72: 31–6.
11. Logemann JA. Evaluation and Treatment of Swallowing Disorders. Texas: Pro-Ed, 1998.
12. Robbins J, Logemann JA, Kirshner H. Swallowing and speech production in Parkinson's disease. Ann Neurol 1986; 11: 283–7.
13. Bassotti G, Germani U, Pagliaricci S, et al. Esophageal manometric abnormalities in Parkinson's disease. Dysphagia 1998; 13: 28–31.
14. Sung HY, Kim JS, Lee KS, et al. The prevalence and patterns of pharyngoesophageal dysmotility in patients with early stage. Mov Disord 2010; 25: 2362–8.
15. Van Lieshout PH, Steele CM, Lang AE. Tongue control for swallowing in Parkinson's disease: effects of age, rate, and stimulus consistency. Mov Disord 2011; 26: 1725–9.
16. Volonté MA, Porta M, Comi G. Clinical assessment of dysphagia in early phases of Parkinson's disease. Neurol Sci 2002; 23: S121–2.
17. Larson K, Ramig LO, Scherer RC. Acoustic and glottographic voice analysis during drug-related fluctuations in Parkinson's disease. J Med Speech Lang Pathol 1994; 2: 211–26.
18. D'Alatri L, Paludetti G, Contarino MF, et al. Effects of bilateral subthalamic nucleus stimulation and medication on parkinsonian speech impairment. J Voice 2008; 22: 365–72.
19. Dromey C, Bjarnason S. A preliminary report on disordered speech with deep brain stimulation in individuals with Parkinson's disease. Parkinsons Dis 2011; 2011: 796205.
20. Klostermann F, Ehlen F, Vesper J, et al. Effects of subthalamic deep brain stimulation on dysarthrophonia in Parkinson's disease. J Neurol Neurosurg Psychiatry 2008; 79: 522–9.
21. Plowman-Prine EK, Okun MS, Sapienza CM, et al. Perceptual characteristics of Parkinsonian speech: a comparison of the pharmacological effects of levodopa across speech and non-speech motor systems. NeuroRehabilitation 2009; 24: 131–44.
22. Sapir S, Ramig L, Fox C. Speech and swallowing disorders in Parkinson disease. Curr Opin Otolaryngol Head Neck Surg 2008; 16: 205–10.
23. Sapir S, Ramig LO, Fox CM. Intensive voice treatment in Parkinson's disease: Lee Silverman voice treatment. Expert Rev Neurother 2011; 11: 815–30.
24. Yorkston KM. Treatment efficacy: dysarthria. J Speech Hear Res 1996; 39: S46–57.
25. Helm N. Management of palilalia with a pacing board. J Speech Hear Disord 1979; 44: 350–3.
26. Ramig LO, Countryman S, Thompson LL, Horii Y. Comparison of two forms of intensive speech treatment for Parkinson disease. J Speech Hear Res 1995; 38: 1232–51.
27. Ramig LO, Countryman S, O'Brien C, Hoehn M, Thompson L. Intensive speech treatment for patients with Parkinson's disease: short and long term comparison of two techniques. Neurology 1996; 47: 1496–504.
28. Ramig L, Sapir S, Countryman S, et al. Intensive voice treatment (LSVT®) for individuals with Parkinson's disease: a two year follow-up. J Neurol Neurosurg Psychiatry 2001; 71: 493–8.

29. Ramig L, Sapir S, Fox C, Countryman S. Changes in vocal intensity following intensive voice treatment (LSVT®) in individuals with Parkinson disease: A comparison with untreated patients and normal age-matched controls. Mov Disord 2001; 16: 79–83.

30. Ward E, Theodoros D, Murdoch B, et al. Changes in maximum capacity tongue function following the Lee Silverman voice treatment program. J Med Speech Lang Pathol 2000; 8: 331–5.

31. Spielman JL, Borod JC, Ramig LO. The effects of intensive voice treatment on facial expressiveness in Parkinson disease: preliminary data. Cogn Behav Neurol 2003; 16: 177–88.

32. Liotti M, Ramig LO, Vogel D, et al. Hypophonia in Parkinson's disease: neural correlates of voice treatment revealed by PET. Neurology 2003; 60: 432–40.

33. Narayana S, Fox PT, Zhang W, et al. Neural correlates of efficacy of voice therapy in Parkinson's disease identified by performance-correlation analysis. Hum Brain Mapp 2010; 31: 222–36.

34. Leanderson R, Meyerson BA, Persson A. Lip muscle function in Parkinsonian dysarthria. Acta Otolaryngol 1972; 74: 350–7.

35. Leanderson R, Meyerson BA. Persson, A. Effect of L-dopa on speech in Parkinsonism an EMG study of labial articulatory function. J Neurol Neurosurg Psychiatry 1971; 43: 679–81.

36. Baker KK, Ramig LO, Luschei ES, Smith ME. Thyroarytenoid muscle activity associated with hypophonia in Parkinson disease and aging. Neurology 1998; 51: 1592–8.

37. Sapir S, Spielman J, Ramig LO, et al. Effects of intensive voice treatment (LSVT®) on vowel articulation in dysarthric individuals with idiopathic Parkinson disease: acoustic and perceptual findings. J Speech Lang Hear Res 2007; 50: 899–912.

38. Sapir S, Ramig LO, Spielman JL, Fox C. Formant centralization ratio: a proposal for a new acoustic measure of dysarthric speech. J Speech Lang Hear Res 2010; 53: 114–25.

39. Hansen DG, Gerratt BR, Ward PH. Cinegraphic observations of laryngeal function in Parkinson's disease. Laryngoscope 1984; 94: 348–53.

40. Estenne M, Hubert M, Troyer AD. Respiratory-muscle involvement in Parkinson's disease. N Engl J Med 1984; 311: 1516–17.

41. Ackermann H, Ziegler W. Articulatory deficits in Parkinsonian dysarthria. J Neurol Neurosurg Psychiatry 1991; 54: 1093–8.

42. Hoodin RB, Gilbert HR. Nasal airflows in parkinsonian speakers. J Commun Disord 1989; 22: 169–80.

43. Ho AK, Bradshaw JL, Iansek R, Alfredson R. Speech volume regulation in Parkinson's disease: effects of implicit cues and explicit instructions. Neuropsychologia 1999a; 37: 1453–60.

44. Ho AK, Bradshaw JL, Iansek T. Volume perception in parkinsonian speech. Mov Disord 2000; 15: 1125–31.

45. Ramig LO, Fox C, Sapir S. Speech treatment for Parkinson's disease. Expert Rev Neurother 2008; 8: 297–309.

46. Goberman AM. Correlation between acoustic speech characteristics and non-speech motor performance in Parkinson disease. Med Sci Monit 2005; 11: CR109–16.

47. Sapir S, Pawlas A, Ramig L, et al. Voice and speech abnormalities in Parkinson disease: relation to severity of motor impairment, duration of disease, medication, depression, gender and age. J Med Speech Lang Pathol 2001; 9: 213–26.

48. Darley FL, Aronson AE, Brown JR. Clusters of deviant speech dimensions in the dysarthrias. J Speech Hear Res 1969; 12: 462–9.

49. Darley FL, Aronson A, Brown J. Differential diagnostic patterns of dysarthria. J Speech Hear Res 1969; 12: 246–69.

50. Skodda S, Grönheit W, Schlegel U. Impairment of vowel articulation as a possible marker of disease progression in Parkinson's disease. PLoS One 2012; 7: e32132.

51. Fox C, Ramig L. Vocal sound pressure level and self-perception of speech and voice in men and women with idiopathic Parkinson disease. Am J Speech Lang Pathol 1997; 2: 29–42.

52. Ho AK, Iansek R, Bradshaw JL. Motor instability in parkinsonian speech intensity. Neuropsychiatry Neuropsychol Behav Neurol 2001; 14: 109–16.

53. Rosen KM, Kent RD, Duffy JR. Task-based profile of vocal intensity decline in Parkinson's disease. Folia Phoniatr Logop 2005; 57: 28–37.
54. Stewart C, Winfield L, Hunt A, et al. Speech dysfunction in early Parkinson's disease. Mov Disord 1995; 10: 562–5.
55. Metter EJ, Hanson WR. Clinical and acoustical variability in hypokinetic dysarthria. J Commun Disord 1986; 19: 347–66.
56. King J, Ramig L, Lemke JH, et al. Parkinson's disease: longitudinal changes in acoustic parameters of phonation. J Med Speech Lang Pathol 1994; 2: 29–42.
57. Zwirner P, Murry T, Woodson GE. Phonatory function of neurologically impaired patients. J Commun Disord 1991; 24: 287–300.
58. Ramig L, Scherer RC, Titze IR, Ringel SP. Acoustic analysis of voices of patients with neurologic disease: rationale and preliminary data. Ann Otol Rhinol Laryngol 1988; 97: 164–72.
59. Little MA, McSharry PE, Hunter EJ, Spielman J, Ramig LO. Suitability of dysphonia measurements for telemonitoring of Parkinson's disease. IEEE Trans Biomed Eng 2009; 56: 1015.
60. Smith ME, Ramig LO, Dromey C, Perez KS, Samandari R. Intensive voice treatment in Parkinson's disese: laryngostroboscopic findings. J Voice 1995; 9: 453–9.
61. Perez KS, Ramig LO, Smith ME, Dromey C. The Parkinson larynx: tremor and videostroboscopic findings. J Voice 1996; 10: 354–61.
62. Gerratt BR, Hansen DG, Berke GS. Glottographic measures of laryngeal function in individuals with abnormal motor control. In: Baer T, Sasaki C, Harris K, eds. Laryngeal Function in Phonation and Respiration. Boston: College-Hill Press, 1987.
63. Blumin JH, Pcolinsky DE, Atkins JP. Laryngeal findings in advanced Parkinson's disease. Ann Otol Rhinol Laryngol 2004; 113: 253–8.
64. Hirose H, Joshita Y. Laryngeal behavior in patients with disorders of the central nervous system. In: Hirano M, Kirchner JA, Bless DM, eds. Neurolaryngology: Recent Advances. Boston: Little Brown, 1987.
65. Luschei ES, Ramig LO, Baker KL, Smith ME. Discharge characteristics of laryngeal single motor units during phonation in young and older adults and in persons with Parkinson disease. J Neurophysiol 1999; 81: 2131–9.
66. Gallena S, Smith PJ, Zeffiro T, Ludlow CL. Effects of levodopa on laryngeal muscle activity for voice onset and offset in Parkinson disease. J Speech Lang Hear Res 2001; 44: 1284–99.
67. Solomon NP, Hixon TJ. Speech breathing in Parkinson's disease. J Speech Hear Res 1993; 36: 294–310.
68. Schiffman PL. A "saw-tooth" pattern in Parkinson's disease. Chest 1985; 87: 24–126.
69. Vincken WG, Gauthier SG, Dollfuss RE, et al. Involvement of upper-airway muscles in extrapyramidal disorders, a cause of airflow limitation. N Engl J Med 1984; 311: 438–42.
70. Murdoch BE, Chenery HJ, Bowler S, Ingram JC. Respiratory function in Parkinson's subjects exhibiting a perceptible speech deficit: A kinematic and spirometric analysis. J Speech Hear Disord 1989; 54: 610–26.
71. Huber JE, Darling M. Effect of Parkinson's disease on the production of structured and unstructured speaking tasks: respiratory physiologic and linguistic considerations. J Speech Lang Hear Res 2011; 54: 33–46.
72. Forrest K, Weismer G, Turner G. Kinematic, acoustic and perceptual analysis of connected speech produced by Parkinsonian and normal geriatric adults. J Acoust Soc Am 1989; 85: 2608–22.
73. Ackermann H, Konczak J, Hertrich I. The temporal control of repetitive articulatory movements in Parkinson's disease. Brain Lang 1997; 56: 312–19.
74. Sapir S, Spielman J, Ramig L, Fox C. Acoustic metrics of dysarthric vowel articulation: differentiating individuals with and without Parkinson's disease. A paper presented at the 56th Annual Conference of the Israeli Association of Physical and Rehabilitation Medicine. Tel Aviv, Israel, 2005.
75. Skodda S, Visser W, Schlegel U. Vowel articulation in Parkinson's disease. J Voice 2011; 25: 467–72.
76. Liss JM, LeGendre S, Lotto AJ. Discriminating dysarthria type from envelope modulation spectra. J Speech Lang Hear Res 2010; 53: 1246–55.

77. Skodda S, Schlegel U. Speech rate and rhythm in Parkinson's disease. Mov Disord 2008; 23: 985–92.
78. Caligiuri MP. Labial kinematics during speech in patients with Parkinsonian rigidity. Brain 1987; 110: 1033–44.
79. Caligiuri MP. The influence of speaking rate on articulatory hypokinesia in Parkinsonian dysarthria. Brain Lang 1989; 36: 493–502.
80. Conner NP, Abbs JH. Task-dependent variations in Parkinsonian motor impairments. Brain 1991; 114: 321–32.
81. Conner NP, Abbs JH, Cole KJ, Gracco VL. Parkinsonian deficits in serial mulitarticulate movements for speech. Brain 1989; 112: 997–1009.
82. Hunker CJ, Abbs JH, Barlow SM. The relationship between Parkinsonian rigidity and hypokinesia in the orofacial system: quantitative analysis. Neurology 1982; 32: 749–54.
83. Dromey C. Articulatory kinematics in patients with Parkinson's disease using different speech treatment approaches. J Med Speech Lang Pathol 2001; 8: 155–61.
84. Gath I, Yair E. Analysis of vocal tract parameters in Parkinsonian speech. J Acoust Soc Am 1988; 84: 1628–34.
85. Yunusova Y, Weismer G, Westbury JR, Lindstrom MJ. Articulatory movements during vowels in speakers with dysarthria and healthy controls. J Speech Lang Hear Res 2008; 51: 596–611.
86. Wong MN, Murdoch BE, Whelan BM. Kinematic analysis of lingual function in dysarthric speakers with Parkinson's disease: an electromagnetic articulograph study. Int J Speech Lang Pathol 2010; 12: 414–25.
87. Netsell R, Daniel B, Celesia GG. Acceleration and weakness in Parkinsonian dysarthria. J Speech Hear Disord 1975; 40: 170–8.
88. Caligiuri MP, Abbs JH. Response properties of the perioral reflex in Parkinson's disease. Exp Neurol 1987; 98: 563–72.
89. Schneider JS, Diamond SG, Markham CH. Deficits in orofacial sensorimotor function in Parkinson's disease. Ann Neurol 1986; 19: 275–82.
90. Goberman AM, Elmer LW. Acoustic analysis of clear versus conversational speech in individuals with Parkinson disease. J Commun Disord 2005; 38: 215–30.
91. Desmurget M, Grafton S, Vindras P, Grea H, Turner RS. Basal ganglia network mediates the control of movement amplitude. Exp Brain Res 2003; 153: 197–209.
92. Albin RL, Young AB, Penny JB. The functional anatomy of basal ganglia disorders. Trends Neurosci 1989; 12: 366–75.
93. Penny JB, Young AB. Speculations on the functional anatomy of basal ganglia disorders. Annu Rev Neurosci 1983; 6: 73–94.
94. Berardelli A, Dick JP, Rothwell JC, Day BL, Marsden CD. Scaling of the size of the first agonist EMG burst during rapid wrist movements in patients with Parkinson's disease. J Neurol Neurosurg Psychiatry 1986; 49: 1273–9.
95. Maschke M, Gomez CM, Tuite PJ, Konczak J. Dysfunction of the basal ganglia, but not the cerebellum, impairs kinaesthesia. Brain 2003; 126: 2312–22.
96. Koller WC. Sensory symptoms in PD. Neurology 1984; 34: 957–9.
97. Diamond SG, Schneider JS, Markham CH. Oral sensorimotor defects in patients with Parkinson's disease. Adv Neurol 1987; 45: 335–8.
98. Graber S, Hertrich I, Daum I, Spieker S, Ackermann H. Speech perception deficits in Parkinson's disease: underestimation of time intervals compromises identification of durational phonetic contrasts. Brain Lang 2002; 82: 65–74.
99. Fox CM, Morrison CE, Ramig LO, Sapir S. Current perspectives on the Lee Silverman Voice Treatment (LSVT) for individuals with idiopathic Parkinson's disease. Am J Speech Lang Pathol 2002; 11: 111–23.
100. Ramig LO, Pawlas A, Countryman S. The Lee Silverman Voice Treatment (LSVT): A Practical Guide to Treating the Voice and Speech Disorders in Parkinson Disease. Iowa City, IA: National Center for Voice and Speech, 1995.
101. Hammer MJ, Barlow SM. Laryngeal somatosensory deficits in Parkinson's disease: implications for speech respiratory and phonatory control. Exp Brain Res 2010; 201: 401–9.

102. Larson KK, Sapir S. Orolaryngeal reflex responses to changes in affective state. J Speech Hear Res 1995; 38: 990–1000.
103. Larson CR, Altman KW, Liu H, Hain TC. Interactions between auditory and somatosensory feedback for voice F0 control. Exp Brain Res 2008; 187: 613–21.
104. Sapir S, McClean MD, Luschei ES. Effects of frequency-modulated auditory tones on the voice fundamental frequency in humans. J Acoust Soc Am 1983; 73: 1070–3.
105. Sapir S, Baker KK, Larson CR, Ramig LO. Short-latency changes in voice F0 and neck surface EMG induced by mechanical perturbations of the larynx during sustained vowel phonation. J Speech Lang Hear Res 2000; 43: 268–76.
106. Kiran S, Larson CR. Effect of duration of pitch-shifted feedback on vocal responses in patients with Parkinson's disease. J Speech Lang Hear Res 2001; 44: 975–87.
107. Liu H, Wang EQ, Metman LV, Larson CR. Vocal responses to perturbations in voice auditory feedback in individuals with Parkinson's disease. PLoS One 2012; 7: e33629.
108. Jürgens U. The neural control of vocalization in mammals: a review. J Voice 2009; 23: 1–10.
109. Rektorova I, Mikl M, Barrett J, et al. Functional neuroanatomy of vocalization in patients with Parkinson's disease. J Neurol Sci 2012; 313: 7–12.
110. Curio G, Neuloh G, Numminen J, Jousmaki V, Hari R. Speaking modifies voice-evoked activity in the human auditory cortex. Hum Brain Mapp 2000; 9: 183–91.
111. Numminen J, Curio G. Differential effects of overt, covert and replayed speech on vowel-evoked responses of the human auditory cortex. Neurosci Lett 1999; 27: 29–32.
112. Paus T, Perry DW, Zatorre RJ, Worsley KJ, Evans AC. Modulation of cerebral blood flow in the human auditory cortex during speech: role of motor-to-sensory discharges. Eur J Neurosci 1996; 8: 2236–46.
113. Arnott WL, Copland DA, Chenery HJ, et al. The influence of dopamine on automatic and controlled semantic activation in Parkinson's disease. Parkinsons Dis 2011; 2011: 157072.
114. Grossman M, Cooke A, DeVita C, et al. Grammatical and resource components of sentence processing in Parkinson's disease: an fMRI study. Neurology 2003; 60: 775–81.
115. Kalf JG, de Swart BJ, Bloem BR, Munneke M. Prevalence of oropharyngeal dysphagia in Parkinson's disease: a meta-analysis. Parkinsonism Relat Disord 2012; 18: 311–15.
116. Stroudley J, Walsh M. Radiographic assessment of dysphagia in Parkinson's disease. Br J Radiol 1991; 64: 890–3.
117. De Letter M, Santens P, Van Borsel J. The effects of levodopa on word intelligibility in Parkinson's disease. J Commun Disord 2005; 38: 187–96.
118. Goberman A, Coelho C, Robb M. Phonatory characteristics of parkinsonian speech before and after morning medication: the ON and OFF states. J Commun Disord 2002; 35: 217–39.
119. Jiang J, Lin E, Wang J, Hanson DG. Glottographic measures before and after levodopa treatment in Parkinson's disease. Laryngoscope 1999; 109: 1287–94.
120. Sanabria J, Ruiz PG, Gutierrez R, et al. The effect of levodopa on vocal function in Parkinson's disease. Clin Neuropharmacol 2001; 24: 99–102.
121. Cahill LM, Murdoch BE, Theodoros DG, et al. Effect of oral levodopa treatment on articulatory function in Parkinson's disease: preliminary results. Mot Contr 1998; 2: 161–72.
122. Kompoliti K, Wang QE, Goetz CG, Leurgans S, Raman R. Effects of central dopaminergic stimulation by apomorphine on speech in Parkinson's disease. Neurology 2000; 54: 458–62.
123. Trail M, Fox C, Ramig LO, et al. Speech treatment for Parkinson's disease. NeuroRehabilitation 2005; 20: 205–21.
124. Spencer KA, Morgan KW, Blond E. Dopaminergic medication effects on the speech of individuals with Parkinson's disease. J Med Speech Lang Pathol 2009; 17: 125–44.
125. Biary N, Pimental PA, Langenberg PW. A double-blind trial of clonazepan in the treatment of parkinsonian dysarthria. Neurology 1988; 38: 255–8.
126. Pahwa R, Lyons KE, Wilkinson SB, et al. Long-term evaluation of deep brain stimulation of the thalamus. J Neurosurg 2006; 104: 506–12.

127. Rodriguez-Oroz MC, Obeso JA, Lang AE, et al. Bilateral deep brain stimulation in Parkinson's disease: a multicentre study with 4 years follow-up. Brain 2005; 128: 2240–9.
128. Krack P, Batir A, Van Blercom N, et al. Five-year follow-up of bilateral stimulation of the subthalamic nucleus in advanced Parkinson's disease. N Engl J Med 2003; 349: 1925–34.
129. Santens P, De Letter M, Van Borsel J, De Reuck J, Caemaert J. Lateralized effects of subthalamic nucleus stimulation on different aspects of speech in Parkinson's disease. Brain Lang 2003; 87: 253–8.
130. Wang E, Verhagen Metman L, Bakay R, Arzbaecher J, Bernard B. The effect of unilateral electrostimulation of the subthalamic nucleus on respiratory/phonatory subsystems of speech production in Parkinson's disease-a preliminary report. Clin Linguist Phon 2003; 17: 283–9.
131. Gentil M, Pinto S, Pollak P, Benabid AL. Effect of bilateral stimulation of the subthalamic nucleus on parkinsonian dysarthria. Brain Lang 2003; 85: 190–6.
132. Gentil M, Garcia-Ruiz P, Pollak P, Benabid AL. Effect of bilateral deep-brain stimulation on oral control of patients with parkinsonism. Eur Neurol 2000; 44: 147–52.
133. Gentil M, Chauvin P, Pinto S, Pollak P, Benabid AL. Effect of bilateral stimulation of the subthalamic nucleus on parkinsonian voice. Brain Lang 2001; 78: 233–40.
134. Pinto S, Gentil M, Fraix V, Benabid AL, Pollak P. Bilateral subthalamic stimulation effects on oral force control in Parkinson's disease. J Neurol 2003; 250: 179–87.
135. Dromey C, Kumar R, Lang AE, Lozano AM. An investigation of the effects of subthalamic nucleus stimulation on acoustic measures of voice. Mov Disord 2000; 15: 1132–8.
136. Rousseaux M, Krystkowiak P, Kozlowski O, et al. Effects of subthalamic nucleus stimulation on parkinsonian dysarthria and speech intelligibility. J Neurol 2004; 251: 327–34.
137. Tornqvist AL, Schalen L, Rehncrona S. Effects of different electrical parameter settings on the intelligibility of speech in patients with Parkinson's disease treated with subthalamic deep brain stimulation. Mov Disord 2005; 20: 416–23.
138. Plaha P, Ben-Shlomo Y, Patel NK, Gill SS. Stimulation of the caudal zona incerta is superior to stimulation of the subthalamic nucleus in improving contralateral parkinsonism. Brain 2006; 129: 1732–47.
139. Karlsson F, Unger E, Wahlgren S, et al. Deep brain stimulation of caudal zona incerta and subthalamic nucleus in patients with Parkinson's disease: effects on diadochokinetic rate. Parkinsons Dis 2011; 2011: 605607.
140. Dias AE, Barbosa ER, Coracini K, et al. Effects of repetitive transcranial magnetic stimulation on voice and speech in Parkinson's disease. Acta Neurol Scand 2006; 113: 92–9.
141. Murdoch BE, Ng ML, Barwood CH. Treatment of articulatory dysfunction in Parkinson's disease using repetitive transcranial magnetic stimulation. Eur J Neurol 2012; 19: 340–7.
142. Pagni CA, Zeme S, Zenga F. Further experience with extradural motor cortex stimulation for treatment of advanced Parkinson's disease. Report of 3 new cases. J Neurosurg Sci 2003; 47: 189–93.
143. Schulz GM, Peterson T, Sapienza CM, Greer M, Friedman W. Voice and speech characteristics of persons with Parkinson's disease pre- and post-pallidotomy surgery: preliminary findings. J Speech Lang Hear Res 1999; 42: 1176–94.
144. Schulz GM, Greer M, Friedman W. Changes in vocal intensity in Parkinson's disease following pallidotomy surgery. J Voice 2000; 14: 589–606.
145. Uitti RJ, Wharen RE, Duffy JR, et al. Unilateral pallidotomy for Parkinson's disease: speech, motor, and neuropsychological outcome measurements. Parkinsonism Relat Disord 2000; 6: 133–43.
146. Scott R, Gregory R, Hines N, et al. Neuropsychological, neurological and functional outcome following pallidotomy for Parkinson's disease. A consecutive series of eight simultaneous bilateral and twelve unilateral procedures. Brain 1998; 121: 659–75.
147. Nagulic M, Davidovic J, Nagulic I. Parkinsonian voice acoustic analysis in real-time after stereotactic thalamotomy. Stereotact Funct Neurosurg 2005; 83: 115–21.

148. Parkin S, Nandi D, Giladi N, et al. Lesioning the subthalamic nucleus in the treatment of Parkinson's disease. Stereotact Funct Neurosurg 2001; 77: 68–72.
149. Farrell A, Theodoros D, Ward E, Hall B, Silburn P. Effects of neurosurgical management of Parkinson's disease on speech characteristics and oromotor function. J Speech Lang Hear Res 2005; 48: 5–20.
150. Berke GS, Gerratt B, Kreiman J, Jackson K. Treatment of Parkinson hypophonia with percutaneous collagen augmentation. Laryngoscope 1999; 109: 1295–9.
151. Kim SH, Kearney JJ, Atkins JP. Percutaneous laryngeal collagen augmentation for treatment of parkinsonian hypophonia. Otolaryngol Head Neck Surg 2002; 126: 653–6.
152. Remacle M, Lawson G. Results with collagen injection into the vocal folds for medialization. Curr Opin Otolaryngol Head Neck Surg 2007; 15: 148–52.
153. Born LJ, Harned RH, Rikkers LF, Pfeiffer RF, Quigley EM. Cricopharyngeal dysfunction in Parkinson's disease: role in dysphagia and response to myotomy. Mov Disord 1996; 11: 53–8.
154. Liss JM, Spitzer SM, Caviness JN, Adler C. The effects of familiarization on intelligibility and lexical segmentation in hypokinetic and ataxic dysarthria. J Acoust Soc Am 2002; 112: 3022–30.
155. Bartels AL, Leenders KL. Parkinson's disease: the syndrome, the pathogenesis and pathophysiology. Cortex 2009; 45: 915–21.
156. Demirci M, Grill S, McShane L, Hallet M. Impairment of kinesthesia in Parkinson's disease. Neurology 1995; 45: A218.
157. Desmurget M, Grafton ST, Vindras P, Gréa H, Turner RS. The basal ganglia network mediates the planning of movement amplitude. Eur J Neurosci 2004; 19: 2871–80.
158. Hallet M. Sensorimotor integration and mysterious sensory phenomena in movement disorders. In: Hallet M, ed. Motor Control. American Academy of Neurology, 1997.
159. Morris M, Iansek R, Matyas T, Summers J. Abnormalities in the stride length-cadence relation in parkinsonian gait. Mov Disord 1998; 13: 61–9.
160. Demirci M, Grill S, McShane L, Hallett M. A mismatch between kinesthetic and visual perception in Parkinson's disease. Ann Neurol 1997; 41: 781–8.
161. Jobst EE, Melnick ME, Byl NN, Dowling GA, Aminoff MJ. Sensory perception in Parkinson's disease. Arch Neurol 1997; 54: 450–4.
162. Klockgether T, Borutta M, Rapp H, Spieder S, Dichgans J. A defect of kinesthesia in Parkinson's disease. Brain 1997; 120: 460–5.
163. Rickards C, Cody FW. Proprioceptive control of wrist movements in Parkinson's disease. Brain 1997; 120: 977–90.
164. Schneider JS, Lidsky TI. Basal Ganglia and Behavior: Sensory Aspects of Motor Functioning. Toronto, Canada: Hans Huber, 1987.
165. Ho AK, Iansek R, Bradshaw JL. Regulations of parkinsonian speech volume: the effect of interlocuter distance. J Neurol Neurosurg Psychiatry 1999; 67: 199–202.
166. Solomon NP, Robin DA, Lorell DM, Rodnitzky RL, Luschei ES. Tongue function testing in Parkinson's disease: indicators of fatigue. In: Till JA, Yorkston KM, Beukelman R, eds. Motor Speech Disorders: Advances in Assessment and Treatment. Baltimore, MD: Paul H. Brooks, 1994: 147–60.
167. Hammer MJ. Design of a new somatosensory stimulus delivery device for measuring laryngeal mechanosensory detection thresholds in humans. IEEE Trans Biomed Eng 2009; 56: 1154–9.
168. Hirsch MA, Farley BG. Exercise and neuroplasticity in persons living with Parkinson's disease. Eur J Phys Rehabil Med 2009; 45: 215–29.
169. Liotti M, Vogel D, Sapir S, et al. Abnormal auditory gating in Parkinson's disease before & after LSVT. Paper presented at the Annual Meeting of the American Speech. Language and Hearing Association, Washington DC, USA, 2000.
170. Cunnington R, Iansek R, Bradshaw JL. Movement-related potentials in Parkinson's disease: external cues and attentional strategies. Mov Disord 1999; 14: 63–8.
171. Oliveira RM, Gurd JM, Nixon P, Marshall JC, Passingham RE. Micrographia in Parkinson's disease: the effect of providing external cues. J Neurol Neurosurg Psychiatry 1997; 63: 429–33.

172. Rochester L, Rafferty D, Dotchin C, et al. The effect of cueing therapy on single and dual-task gait in a drug naïve population of people with Parkinson's disease in northern Tanzania. Mov Disord 2010; 25: 906–11.
173. Bohnen NI, Kaufer DI, Hendrickson R, et al. Cognitive correlates of cortical cholinergic denervation in Parkinson's disease and Parkinsonian dementia. J Neurol 2006; 253: 242–7.
174. Rowe J, Stephan KE, Friston K, et al. Attention to action in Parkinson's disease: impaired effective connectivity among frontal cortical regions. Brain 2002; 125: 276–89.
175. Morris ME, Iansek R, Matyas TA, Summers JJ. Stride length regulation in Parkinson's disease. Normalization strategies and underlying mechanisms. Brain 1996; 119: 551–68.
176. Hartelius L, Svensson P. Speech and swallowing symptoms associated with Parkinson's disease and multiple sclerosis: a survey. Folia Phoniatr Logop 1994; 46: 9–17.
177. Scott S, Caird FL. Speech therapy for Parkinson's disease. J Neurol Neurosurg Psychiatry 1983; 46: 140–4.
178. Rubow RT, Swift E. A microcomputer-based wearable biofeedback device to improve transfer of treatment in Parkinsonian dysarthria. J Speech Hear Disord 1985; 50: 178–85.
179. McNamara P, Obler LK, Au R, et al. Speech monitoring skills in Alzheimer's disease, Parkinson's disease and normal aging. Brain Lang 1992; 42: 38–51.
180. Kleim JA, Jones TA. Principles of experience-dependent neural plasticity: implications for rehabilitation after brain damage. J Speech Lang Hear Res 2008; 51: S225–39.
181. Fisher B, Petzinger GM, Nixon K, et al. Exercise-induced behavioral recovery and neuroplasticity in the 1-methyl-4-phenyl-1,2,3,6-tetrahydropyridine-lesioned mouse basal ganglia. J Neurosci Res 2004; 77: 378–90.
182. Tillerson J, Cohen AD, Philhower J, et al. Forced limb-use effects on the behavioral and neurochemical effects of 6-hydroxydopamine. J Neurosci 2001; 21: 4427–35.
183. Fox C, Ebersbach G, Ramig L, Sapir S. LSVT LOUD and LSVT BIG: behavioral treatment programs for speech and body movement in Parkinson disease. Parkinson's Dis 2012; 2012: 391946.
184. Tillerson J, Caudle WM, Reveron ME, Miller GW. Exercise induces behavioral recovery and attenuates neurochemical deficits in rodent models of Parkinson's disease. Neuroscience 2003; 119: 899–911.
185. Dromey C, Ramig LO, Johnson A. Phonatory and articulatory changes associated with increased vocal intensity in Parkinson disease: a case study. J Speech Hear Res 1995; 38: 751–63.
186. Baumgartner C, Sapir S, Ramig LO. Voice quality changes following phonatory-respiratory effort treatment (LSVT®) versus respiratory effort treatment for individuals with Parkinson disease. J Voice 2001; 15: 105–14.
187. Countryman S, Ramig LO. Effects of intensive voice therapy on speech deficits associated with bilateral thalamotomy in Parkinson's disease: a case study. J Med Speech Lang Pathol 1993; 1: 233–49.
188. Ramig LO, Bonitati C, Lemke J, et al. Voice treatment for patients with Parkinson disease: Development of an approach and preliminary efficacy data. J Med Speech Lang Pathol 1994; 2: 191–209.
189. Ramig LO, Dromey C. Aerodynamic mechanisms underlying treatment-related changes in SPL in patients with Parkinson disease. J Speech Hear Res 1996; 39: 798–807.
190. Schulman R. Articulatory dynamics of loud and normal speech. J Acoust Soc Am 1989; 85: 295–312.
191. Ramig LO, Sapir S, Fox C, Countryman S. Changes in vocal intensity following intensive voice treatment (LSVT®) in individuals with Parkinson disease: A comparison with untreated patients and with normal age-matched controls. Mov Disord 2001; 16: 79–83.
192. Spielman J, Mahler L, Halpern A, et al. Intensive voice treatment (LSVT®LOUD) for Parkinson's disease following deep brain stimulation of the subthalamic nucleus. J Commun Disord 2011; 44: 688–700.

193. Tripoliti E, Strong L, Hickey F, et al. Treatment of dysarthria following subthalamic nucleus deep brain stimulation for Parkinson's disease. Mov Disord 2011; 26: 2434–6.
194. Yorkston KM, Miller RM, Strand EA. Management of Speech and Swallowing in Degenerative Diseases. Communication Skill Builders, 1997.
195. Deane KH, Whurr R, Clarke CE, et al. Non-pharmacological therapies for dysphagia in Parkinson's disease. Cochrane Database Syst Rev 2001; 1: CD002816.
196. De Angelis EC, Mourao LF, Ferraz HB, et al. Effect of voice rehabilitation on oral communication of Parkinson's disease patients. Acta Neurol Scand 1997; 96: 199–205.
197. Halpern AE, Ramig LO, Matos CE, et al. Innovative technology for the assisted delivery of intensive voice treatment (LSVT(R)LOUD) for Parkinson's disease. Am J Speech Lang Pathol. 2012; 21: 354–67.

28 Complementary and alternative medicine in Parkinson's disease

Louis C.S. Tan and Kulthida Methawasin

INTRODUCTION

Parkinson's disease (PD) is a neurodegenerative disorder that results from the progressive loss of dopaminergic neurons. Although there are effective treatments for the motor symptoms of PD, these medications can have side effects. Some of these side effects are short-term but others have long-term implications, such as the occurrence of motor complications associated with the use of levodopa. In some parts of the world, access to PD medications is limited either because medications are not available or because medications are expensive and often not affordable. In addition, there are many nonmotor complications, such as sensory disturbances, sleep problems, autonomic symptoms, and mood disorders, for which few effective therapies are available. As a result of these factors and the chronic, debilitating nature of PD, patients often turn to the complementary and alternative medicine (CAM) in the search for therapies that would alleviate their condition. In the United States, the number of individuals using alternative medicine increased from 34% in 1990 to 42% in 1997, making it one of the fastest growing industries in health care (1).

DEFINITION OF COMPLEMENTARY AND ALTERNATIVE MEDICINE

CAM refers to a group of clinical activities or therapies that are outside the realm of conventional medical practice. The therapeutic goal of CAM is to stimulate the body's natural self-healing and self-regulating abilities (2). The aims of CAM practitioners are varied and include the desire to treat the patient as a whole, to satisfy the needs of the patient and to diversify the conceptual framework of medicine (3). By convention, when patients use such therapies in addition to conventional medical treatment, these therapies are considered a form of complementary medicine. However, when patients use such therapies alone as an alternative to conventional medicine, these therapies are considered a form of alternative medicine. Conventional medicine is based on disease-orientated management and supported by clinical trial research. However, many modalities of CAM have not been subjected to same rigor of scientific investigations due to the scarcity of proper clinical trials and the difficulties in designing good clinical studies. This is in part related to the problems with adequate blinding required to conduct good clinical trials and the selection of suitable placebos for CAM therapies. Despite these issues, the use of CAM is common across the world and gaining popularity in many countries.

PREVALENCE OF COMPLEMENTARY AND ALTERNATIVE MEDICINE USE IN PARKINSON'S DISEASE

To the best of our knowledge, there have been five studies on the use of CAM published in countries ranging from the United States, United Kingdom, Singapore, Argentina, and Korea. The results of these studies are summarized in Table 28.1. The prevalence of CAM use among PD patients ranges from 26% to 76% with higher figures found in the two Asian studies (Singapore and Korea) where the most common forms of CAM used were traditional, oriental medicine. Across the different studies and regions of the world, the use of vitamins and supplements, massage therapy, and acupuncture therapy were the most common. The factors associated with CAM use included younger-onset diagnosis of PD, higher baseline Unified Parkinson's Disease Rating Scale (UPDRS) motor score, female gender, middle age, and longer duration of PD. These factors suggest that patients with a higher disease burden are more likely to seek CAM use. The associated factors also provide a possible profile of PD patients likely to seek CAM use; however, this profile may vary from one country to another.

CLASSIFICATION OF COMPLEMENTARY AND ALTERNATIVE MEDICINE

Based on the use of CAM by PD patients, we have divided the different modalities and therapies of CAM into three main categories. These categories are

a. Medicinal therapies
b. Manipulative and touch therapies
c. Mind and emotional therapies.

Table 28.2 is a listing of all commonly used CAM under these three categories, although this list is not exhaustive. The therapies that have been reported in PD have been indicated in the table. Of these, the more common therapeutic modalities used in PD are reviewed in the following sections of the chapter. A brief description of each modality is provided together with its postulated mechanism of action. Where possible, a review of the clinical studies undertaken is also given. Exercise and exercise-related therapies, such as yoga, "tai-chi," and "qi-gong" (the latter two are traditional Chinese forms of martial arts), are not covered in this chapter as exercise and rehabilitation have been covered in previous sections of the book and they are considered an integral part of conventional therapy for PD.

Medicinal Therapies
Nutritional Therapy
Ketogenic Diets
A ketogenic diet contains high fatty acids that are converted to the ketone bodies, β-hydroxybutyrate, acetoacetate, and acetone in the body. When combined with low carbohydrate food, it is believed to have protective effects in PD. This hypothesis is based on animal studies, which showed that β-hydroxybutyrate in ketogenic diets protected dopamine neurons against degeneration induced by 1-methyl-4-phenyl-1,2,3,6-tetrahydropyridine (MPTP) in animal models of PD (9). A prospective population study has shown that eating a high-fat diet decreased the risk of developing PD (10) and an open-labeled study revealed improvement in UPDRS scores in PD patients (11).

TABLE 28.1 Complementary and Alternative Medicine Uses in Parkinson's Disease in Five Different Countries

Data	USA (4)	UK (5)	Singapore (6)	Argentina (7)	Korea (8)
Year of publication	1999	2001	2004	2005	2006
Number of PD patients recruited	201	80	159	300	123
Use of CAM for PD symptoms (%)	40	39	61	26	76
The top five of CAM used (%)[a]	1. Vitamins and supplements (59) 2. Massage (14) 3. Acupuncture (10) 4. Relaxation technique (8) 5. Magnets (5)	1. Massage (16)[b] 2. Aromatherapy (14) 3. Reflexology (7) 4. Acupuncture (7) 5. Conductive education (7) and spiritualism (7)	1. Traditional medicine (28) 2. Acupuncture (25) 3. Vitamins and supplement (18) 4. Massage (15) 5. Reflexology (8)	1. Acupuncture (49) 2. Yoga (49) 3. Homeopathy (42) 4. Massage (38) 5. Reiki (18)	1. Oriental medicine including acupuncture (77) 2. Traditional food (45) 3. Vitamins and supplements (32) 4. Korean traditional therapies (7) 5. Massage (7)
Factors associated with the use of CAM	Younger age of PD onset	Younger age of PD diagnosis	Higher baseline UPDRS motor score	Female gender and 50–69 years age group	Longer duration of PD

[a]Patients may use more than one CAM.
[b]42% were classified as using "other CAM" such as tai chi, yoga, herbs, gingko, homeopathy, TENS, cord liver oil, chiropractic, reiki.

TABLE 28.2 Classification of Complementary and Alternative Medicines

Medicinal Therapies	Manipulative and Touch Therapies	Mind and Emotional Therapies
Used in Parkinson's disease	*Used in Parkinson's disease*	*Used in Parkinson's disease*
Ayurveda	Acupressure	Art therapy
Chinese herbal medicine	Acupuncture	Biofeedback
Homeopathy	Alexander technique	Light therapy
Magnetic therapy	Aromatherapy	Meditation
Nutritional therapies	Chiropractic	Music therapy
	Massage	Psychotherapy and
Others	Osteopathy	counseling
Anthroposophical medicine	Reflexology	Relaxation technique
Bach flower remedies	Reiki	
Biochemic tissue salts	Trager therapy	*Others*
Clinical ecology		Autogenic training
Crystal therapy	*Others*	Biorhythms
Hydrotherapy	Aston patterning	Color therapy
Naturopathy	Craniosacral therapy	Feng shui
Orthomolecular therapy	Feldenkrais method	Flotation therapy
Western herbalism	Hellerwork	Geomancy
	Rolfing	Hypnotherapy
	Therapeutic touch	Sound therapy
		Visualization

Dietary Supplements

A prevalence study of CAM in the USA found that 63% of PD patients took nutritional supplements together with prescribed medications. However, only half of these patients consulted their physicians about their use of supplements. Vitamins were the most commonly used, with vitamin E topping the list, followed by vitamin C, vitamin B12, vitamin B complex, and vitamin B6. The most commonly used mineral supplement in that study was calcium (12). Many of the supplements used by patients are based on hypotheses that are not supported by clinical trials. The review of dietary supplements in PD will focus on vitamin E and Coenzyme Q10.

Vitamin E   Several studies have attempted to prove the benefit of vitamin E as a neuroprotective agent in PD. Some of these studies were positive while others have had negative results (13,14). The largest clinical trial with Vitamin E was the DATATOP study. This was a double-blind, multicenter, placebo-controlled clinical trial, which concluded that alpha-tocopherol did not delay the time to initiation of levodopa in PD patients (15). Although some epidemiological studies continue to suggest the usefulness of vitamin E in reducing the risk for developing PD (16–18), an evidence-based review of neuroprotective strategies and alternative therapies for PD by the American Academy of Neurology recommended that treatment with 2000 units of vitamin E should not be considered for neuroprotection in PD (19).

Coenzyme Q10   Coenzyme Q10 (CoQ10) is a natural substance of the human body that participates in aerobic cellular respiration as an essential cofactor of the electron transport chain. It is also an important antioxidant (20). Many PD patients use

CoQ10 as it theoretically promotes antioxidant activity that may improve clinical symptoms of PD or slow down the progression of PD. A placebo-controlled, multi-center, dose-ranging trial of CoQ10 in 80 patients with early PD after a follow-up of 16 months revealed that 1200 mg/day of CoQ10 treatment resulted in significantly less deterioration of motor function, as measured by the UPDRS, when compared with placebo (21). To confirm these effects in a larger clinical trial, the Parkinson Study Group embarked on a study that focused on the effects of CoQ10 at 1200 and 2400 mg daily on reducing the progression of early PD. This study was however halted in May 2011 as a mid-study analysis suggested that there was no improvement in the CoQ10-treated individuals in comparison to those who received placebo treatment (22).

Ayurveda

Ayurveda is the holistic healing system that originates in India. It encourages physical, mental, emotional, and spiritual wellbeing so as to maintain the balance of three doshas or vital energies. The key principle of this practice is the belief in the existence of five elements—ether, air, fire, water, and earth that form the basic structures of life. These elements continuously change and interact with each other. The doshas are a simple way to describe the function of these elements. In the human body, the levels of doshas are affected by various factors in daily life, such as food, time, and emotion, and they fluctuate continuously. The imbalances of doshas are due to the disruption of "prana" that flows throughout the body and the malfunction of "agni," the body digestive fire, resulting in the production of "ama," toxic substances (23).

The term "Kampavata" in Ayurveda is analogous to PD. There are 35 different formulations used to treat "Kampavala." The major constituent of these formulations is *Macuna pruriens* that is now known to contain levodopa. The first clinical trial of *M. pruriens* in the treatment of PD was conducted in 1978 (24). In 1999, Nagashayana and colleagues reported a clinical trial that evaluated two forms of Ayurvedic treatment. The eliminative treatment included oleation, sudation, purgation, enema, and errhines by Ayurveda drugs and the palliative treatment consisted of oral administration of dried seeds and roots of *M. pruriens*, *Hyoscyamus reticulatus*, *Withania somnifera*, and *Sida cordifolia* in milk. This study included 18 PD patients with five patients undergoing only palliative treatment and 13 patients undergoing both eliminative and palliative treatments. The results showed greater improvement of tremor, bradykinesia, stiffness, and cramp-like pain in the group receiving both treatments. Individuals who underwent both treatments showed improvement in activities of daily living (ADL) and motor examination, whereas those who underwent palliative treatment alone did not have a response. Pharmacological analysis of the herbal formulations revealed that approximately 200 mg of levodopa was present in each dose administered. The authors suggested that proper Ayurveda treatment appeared to be effective to treat PD and the eliminative treatment might be helpful in clearing gastrointestinal contents so that patients could better absorb Ayurveda drugs (25).

Basic science studies on *M. pruriens* have suggested that this herb may have antiparkinsonian effects due to components other than levodopa (26–29). Further clinical studies have also found that this herb is as efficacious as levodopa in the treatment of PD and have suggested that it may have greater bioavailability than standard levodopa (30,31).

Despite the efficacy of *M. pruriens* in the treatment of PD and the presence of levodopa as its main ingredient, some clinicians have concerns with its use primarily because it is difficult to ensure its purity or quantify the amount of levodopa present in the herb or powder formulation.

Chinese Herbal Medicine

The list of Chinese herbs and other natural materials in the treatment of PD was first recorded in the *"Shennong's Classic of Material Medica,"* the oldest pharmaceutical book of China since the Warring States Period. Today, some of these herbs are still being used and a number have been subjected to rigorous pharmacological research. There have been an increasing number of studies on Chinese herbs and herbal extracts in both animal models and clinical trials to understand the potential of Chinese herbs in retarding the degeneration of dopaminergic neurons, promoting neuronal survival and growth, and enhancing the functional recovery of damaged brain (32).

Various combinations of herbs are used to treat PD in traditional Chinese medicine (TCM). A systematic review of the efficacy, safety, and clinical applicability of herbal medicines in 2006 included nine studies. Of these, seven studies were performed in China on TCM. All studies declared their research methodology as randomized trials but only two studies reported methods of randomization and blinding to both assessors and participants. These studies had different interventions and outcome measurements. The herbs included in the review were cannabis plant extracts, *M. pruriens*, Zhiyinxifeng granules, Kanli decoction, Bhushen Pingchan decoction, Lemaikeli, tailor-made Chinese herbal decoction, and Wuling capsule. Zhiyinxifeng granules showed the same efficacy as levodopa treatment in the improvement of the Webster score, whereas the Kanli decoction demonstrated superior efficacy to levodopa. Only cannabis plant extracts had no effect on either dyskinesia or improvement of motor and nonmotor symptoms. As an adjunctive therapy, the combination of herbal medicines and levodopa exhibited significantly better outcomes in motor function and emotion when compared with the use of either herbal medicine or conventional treatments alone. No major adverse effects were reported from the use of these herbs. This review was unable to provide an indepth analysis of the data as a result of methodological flaws and significant heterogeneity across the different studies, and as such could not formulate any conclusions as to the efficacy or safety of the various herbal medicines (33).

Since the time of this systematic review, there have been at least two clinical trials on Chinese herbal medicine that have been published in English. One study evaluated the efficacy of the adjunctive use of the Chinese herbal formula, "Jia Wei Liu Jun Zi Tang" (JWLJZT) to stable doses of PD medications in a prospective, randomized, double-blind, placebo-controlled study with 22 patients in the treatment group and 25 patients in the control group. This herbal formulation consisted of 11 different herbs in granules and is believed to enhance "qi" in the spleen and stomach. This study did not show a significant improvement in the primary outcome measure, the PDQ-39 score (PD-specific health-related quality-of-life score), although there were improvements in the PDQ-39 communications scores and better scores in the UPDRS part IV, other complications section, in the treatment group (34).

The second paper evaluated the effects of the Chinese herbal medication, Zeng-xiao An-shen Zhi-chan 2 (ZAZ2), as add-on therapy to patients who were on stable PD medications. This herb contained 14 kinds of Chinese herbs in a soluble granule. One hundred and fifteen patients with PD were recruited, randomized, and evaluated in a double-blind fashion. The authors concluded that ZAZ2 improved ADLs in PD patients and that the herb was a potentially suitable drug for long-term use (35).

There have also been three other randomized, double-blind, controlled studies on TCM that were published in Chinese (36–38).

Green Tea and Other Plant Polyphenols

Green tea is a well-known herb and very popular in Eastern Asia, especially Japan, Korea, and China. Green tea contains polyphenols, in particular catechins, the most abundant of which is epigallocatechin gallate (EGCG). The antioxidant activities of plant polyphenols may be attributed to their iron-binding affinities that decrease the production of hydroxyl radicals. These plants therefore offer hope of a new strategy to prevent and treat neurodegenerative diseases.

Studies of catechins as an iron chelating agent to decrease neuronal damage in PD have provided mixed results. In the MPTP mouse model of PD, a study showed that EGCG and VK-28 (an iron chelator in the clioquinol group) prevented the accumulation of iron in the substantia nigra pars compacta (39), but this finding could not be replicated in the 6-hydroxydopamine (6-OHDA) rat model of PD (40). In the PC12 cell model of PD, EGCG and epicatechin gallate exhibited protective effects against 6-OHDA-induced cell death (41). We await the results of a clinical trial on green tea extracts being conducted in China, as this will provide the necessary evidence to support its use in PD.

There are also other plant sources of polyphenols. These include cranberry polyphenols, *Scutellaria baicalensis* Georgi (a flowering plant used in TCM) (42), and curcumin (found in Indian spice, turmeric) (43,44). These plants have strong chelating actions. For example, the flavonol quercetin of cranberry polyphenols has been shown to inhibit the Fenton reaction in an in vitro study (45), affect the stability of iron in an in vivo study (46) and remove intracellular iron in the mouse model of PD (47).

Other Herbs with Bioactive Agents in Parkinson's Disease

Other than *M. pruriens* of Ayurveda and the Chinese herbs used in TCM, there are several other plants that have exhibited neuroprotective effects in animal experiments or are thought to have therapeutic benefits in PD.

The *Vicia faba*, the Broad bean or Field bean that is native to North Africa and Southwest Asia has been found to increase plasma levels of levodopa that have been correlated with improvements in the motor function of PD patients in a small clinical trial (48).

Ginkgo biloba leaf extract that is known to protect hippocampal neurons damaged by nitric oxide or beta-amyloid-induced peptides has also been found to have neuroprotective effects in the rat model of PD (49).

Ginseng is a slow growing plant that belongs to the genus *Panax* of the family Araliaceae and is typically found in North America and East Asia because of their cool climates. It is most commonly used in Korea and may be found in their traditional medicines, tea, food, and cosmetic products as it is widely thought to promote body energy and good health. Ginsenoside is one of the active ingredients in Ginseng that is thought to have neuroprotective effects in neurons. In vitro studies have found that Ginsenoside Rg1 could suppress intracellular oxidative stress and prevent PC12 cells from dopamine-induced apoptosis (50) as well as protect the substantia nigra against MPTP-induced neuronal damage by blocking the Jun amino-terminal kinases signaling cascade (51,52). Another active ingredient of Ginseng, G115, has been found to inhibit tyrosine hydroxylase-positive cell loss in the substantia nigra of the MPTP-induced mouse model of PD with resultant improvement in motor function (53).

Homeopathy

Homeopathy is a medical system based on the theory that "like cures like." A poison that causes symptoms of illness in a healthy person can treat the same symptoms in someone who is ill. It is a popular form of complementary therapy in some parts of the world. Homeopathic practitioners treat patients with highly serially diluted substances that are believed to cause healthy people to exhibit symptoms that are similar to those exhibited by patients so as to stimulate the vital force necessary to fight the illness. For example, belladonna has been used to treat scarlet fever based on the principle that the symptoms of belladonna poisoning are similar to the symptoms of scarlet fever (54). Homeopathy has been used in many medical illnesses, such as rheumatoid arthritis (55), cancer (56), and atopic eczema (57), as well as for psychiatric conditions such as depression and anxiety (58), but systematic reviews have not found homeopathy to be efficacious. Although there have been no clinical trials conducted on the use of homeopathy in PD patients, its use is common in PD as shown by the study from Argentina, which revealed that 42% of patients have utilized it as a form of CAM (7).

Despite the laboratory evidence supporting the benefits of these nonconventional medicinal therapies in PD, most of them have not been adequately studied in nonhuman primates or humans. There is a need to translate these basic science findings into properly designed clinical trials so that more clinical evidence to support the use of these herbs and medications may be obtained.

Manipulative and Touch Therapies

Traditional Chinese Medicine

By definition, TCM refers to an ancient system of healing that focuses on an individual's pattern of symptoms rather than a specific disease entity. In Chinese philosophy, the concept of *yin* and *yang* is used to describe how polar opposites or seemingly contrary forces are interconnected and interdependent in the natural world, and how they give rise to each other in turn. The opposites need to work cooperatively so that they may be balanced in the human body. This is the underlying concept of TCM and a central principle for the different forms of Chinese martial arts and exercise.

TCM beliefs are also based on the concept that the body contains a network of channels carrying life energy called *"qi."* According to the TCM viewpoint, PD is caused by the deficiency of *yin* in the liver, spleen, and kidney, with the consequent formation of mucous that obstructs *"qi,"* which in turn leads to malnutrition of the muscles (24). TCM originated in China but its practice has become widespread around the world.

For PD, the various modalities of TCM that are used alone or in combination include Chinese herbal medicines, acupuncture, and other treatments, such as cupping therapy (59). This section will focus on manipulative and touch therapies.

Acupuncture

Acupuncture is an element of TCM that is practiced not only in China and other Asian countries, but also in many Western countries. This therapy treats patients by inserting and manipulating solid, thin needles in the body. Traditional Chinese practitioners use acupuncture to adjust the flow of "*qi*." It is believed that the application of acupuncture to specific points on the body called acupuncture points can activate the flow of "*qi*" that enables a patient to remain in a healthy balance. The acupuncture points are connected by channels named "meridians" (60).

In basic neuroscience, animal experiments have demonstrated that acupuncture exerts a neuroprotective effect (61,62). Studies have shown that stimulation at a frequency of 100 Hz in electro-acupuncture operated at *the baihui* and *dazhui* acupuncture points significantly increased the survival of dopaminergic neurons in the substantia nigra of the medial forebrain bundle of transected parkinsonian rats (63,64). Similarly, stimulation at the *renzhong* and *chengjiang* points also increased dopamine levels in the striatum (65). Electro-acupuncture also improved behavioral abnormalities, prevented degeneration of dopaminergic neurons, and increased striatal dopamine in the MPTP-lesioned mice (66).

Based on these findings, scientists have proposed that electro-acupuncture might activate and increase the amount of tyrosine hydroxylase, enhance reuptake of dopamine at the presynaptic terminals, suppress cellular reactive oxygen species, and increase the synthesis and release of neurotrophins. Two systematic reviews have been conducted to evaluate the beneficial effects of acupuncture in PD. Both had similar conclusions.

In one review, 11 randomized controlled trials (RCT) that compared electro- or needle acupuncture with placebo acupuncture, conventional drugs alone, and no treatment were reviewed. Three randomized, controlled trials assessed the effectiveness of acupuncture on the UPDRS compared with placebo acupuncture. The meta-analysis of these studies showed no significant effect. Another six randomized, controlled trials compared acupuncture plus conventional drugs to treatment with drugs only. A meta-analysis of two of these studies suggested a positive effect of scalp acupuncture. Two further randomized, controlled trials tested acupuncture versus no treatment. The meta-analysis of these studies also suggested beneficial effects of acupuncture. However, the results of the latter two trials failed to adequately control for nonspecific effects. This systematic review concluded that the evidence for the effectiveness of acupuncture in PD was not convincing as the number and quality of trials as well as their total sample size was too low to draw any firm conclusions (67).

Another systematic review of 10 randomized, controlled trials conducted to evaluate the efficacy and safety of acupuncture for idiopathic PD concluded that acupuncture, as an adjuvant therapy with standard medications, was potentially effective. However, the results were limited by the methodological flaws, unknowns in concealment of allocation, number of dropouts, and blinding methods in the studies. Both systematic reviews concluded that large, well-designed, placebo-controlled trials with rigorous methods of randomization and adequately concealed allocation, as well as intention-to-treat data analysis were needed (68).

Acupuncture appears to be an appropriate CAM that may enhance the effectiveness of conventional therapies and possibly offer psychological support to PD patients. However, its research methodology needs to be refined so that better clinical trials may be designed to evaluate its efficacy for both motor and nonmotor symptoms of PD patients. In addition, mechanistic models for acupuncture effects that have been investigated experimentally have focused on the effects of acupuncture needle stimulation on the nervous system, muscles, and connective tissue. These mechanistic models are not mutually exclusive. Repeated testing, expanding, and perhaps merging of such models will potentially lead to an incremental understanding of the effects of manual and electrical stimulation of acupuncture needles that is solidly rooted in physiology (69).

Cupping Therapy

Cupping therapy is an ancient technique that applies a local suction device to the skin and is based on the concept that increased blood flow can promote spontaneous healing. The suction is created by using fire and cups. Cupping doctors use fire to heat the air inside the cup and the rim of the cup is then applied to skin to form an airtight seal. As the air inside the cups becomes cooled, it contracts and results in a partial vacuum state so that the cup will pull skin and soft tissue inward and draw blood to that area. Sometimes, mechanical devices such as hand and electronic pumps are used.

Cupping therapy is currently performed to relieve pain, promote relaxation, and enhance strength. However, it can leave temporarily painful bruises and/or burns on the skin. As cupping is less popular than acupuncture, there are no studies on the sole use of cupping therapy in PD patients. One report on cupping therapy combined with acupuncture demonstrated an efficacy rate of 89.66% based on the Webster scale (70). However, there are limited clinical data available on cupping therapy.

Massage

Therapeutic massage is the manipulation of superficial and deeper layers of muscle and connective tissue that can be done manually with or without mechanical instruments. As the skin is the body's largest sensory organ, stimulation by massage releases endorphins that relieve pain and discomfort. This is thought to augment healthy living and enhance self-esteem. In addition, this manipulation is thought to promote the circulatory and immune systems of the body. The main uses of massage are to relieve stress-related conditions, to treat muscle and joint disorders, to relieve pain, to lower blood pressure, to relax mood and emotion, and to resolve digestive disorders such as constipation. Although, it has no curative effects, the feeling of wellbeing may be experienced with a resultant decrease in the levels of cortisol, epinephrine, and other stress hormones.

The basic techniques of massage include stroking or effleurage, which is a gentle action; kneading or petrissage that alternates between stretching and relaxing muscles; friction or frottage that applies deep pressure to release tension in the muscles around the spine and shoulders; and hacking where the therapist uses relaxed hands to give short, sharp taps to the body. Massage methods are many and varied depending on culture, religion, and country.

As massage is a totally human-involved procedure, it is difficult to perform a double-blind, controlled study. Its beneficial effects are subjective in nature and may be the consequence of relaxation and reduction of anxiety (24). An observational study of therapeutic massage using the PDQ-39, the Measure Yourself Medical Outcome Profile, and the Medication Change Questionnaire on seven patients showed improvement in the measures of self-confidence, wellbeing, walking, and

ADLs (71). A single-blind, controlled, perspective study of neuromuscular therapy (NMT), a widely accepted form of massage therapy, in 36 idiopathic PD patients with moderately advanced stage and stable medications compared the effects of NMT to music relaxation. The results from this study suggested that NMT could improve motor and selected nonmotor symptoms, such as mood and anxiety, in PD and that the effect was more durable for motor symptoms (72).

Chiropractic

Chiropractics are concerned with the diagnosis, treatment, and prevention of spine, joint, and muscle disorders by manual therapy, exercises, and lifestyle counseling. It has been widely used to successfully treat back problems, headache, and sports injuries. The key concept is that the body is similar to a machine and the most important mechanical structure is the spine, which connects the brain to the body, so that, if the skeletal structure works well, the natural healing process will be freely autonomous and result in the harmonization of all body system functions. On the other hand, the distortion of the spine results in functional deterioration of other body systems.

Although chiropractics are utilized by many patients in the United States, Canada, and Australia, the literature supporting the use of chiropractic management in PD consists only of case reports (73,74).

Reflexology

Reflexology has been defined as a natural healing art based on the principle that there are reflexes in the feet, hands, and ears and their referred areas that correspond to every part, gland, and organ of the body. Through application of pressure on these reflexes without the use of tools, creams, or lotions, the feet being the primary area of application, reflexology relieves tension, improves circulation, and helps promote the natural function of the related areas of the body (75). Reflexologists believe that there are granular accumulations of waste products concentrated in the form of uric acid and calcium crystals around reflex points. Reflexology breaks down these crystals to free the energy flow, open nerve pathways, and increase blood supply to flush away these toxins (76).

Although this therapy is widely used in many countries, a systematic review of randomized, controlled trials to evaluate the evidence and effectiveness of reflexology for treating medical conditions such as asthma, dementia, headache, and cancer revealed that the available evidence did not support any benefit of reflexology for any of these conditions (77). PD patients in many countries also use reflexology as a CAM without much scientific basis. There is only a small study, which suggested that reflexology may limit deterioration and maintain the wellbeing of PD patients (78).

Aromatherapy

Aromatherapy is a form of CAM that uses volatile plant materials, known as essential oils, and other aromatic compounds for the purpose of altering a person's mind, mood, cognitive function or health. It initially became popular as a beauty treatment, and its medicinal and therapeutic potential has recently been appreciated.

The basic mechanism offered to explain its purported effects is the influence of aroma on the brain, especially the limbic system through the olfactory system (79). Although aromatherapists often claim precise knowledge of the synergy between the body and aromatic oils, the efficacy of aromatherapy in PD remains unproven.

Reiki

Reiki is a form of Japanese spiritual healing. Through the use of this technique, practitioners believe that they can transfer universal energy (i.e., reiki) in the form of *"ki"* through their palms. This is thought to enable self-healing and the achievement of a state of equilibrium. Reiki practitioners draw on "reiki energy" and channel it to areas of need in the body. They borrow terminology from physics, claiming that reiki acts at an atomic level, causing the body's molecules to vibrate with higher intensity to dissolve energy blockages that lead to disharmony and disease.

There are two main branches of reiki, commonly referred to as Traditional Japanese Reiki and Western Reiki. The primary difference is that the Western form uses systematic hand-placements over different parts of the body rather than relying on an intuitive sense of hand-positions, which is commonly used in Japanese Reiki (80).

A systematic review of randomized clinical trials concluded that the evidence is insufficient to suggest that reiki is an effective treatment for any medical condition (81). Although reiki is commonly used in PD patients in some countries, no clinical studies in PD have been performed.

Alexander Technique

The Alexander technique aims to resolve postural problems, improve body movements and reduce muscle strain. This technique focuses on relearning basic movements such as how to stand, sit, and walk correctly and to be aware of wrong patterns of movements in daily life that can inflict stresses on the body. After a series of sessions, patients should gradually change their posture and movement in routine activities and develop new patterns of action that are more physically coordinated and less harmful to anatomical structures (82).

In PD patients, postural instability, gait difficulty, and reduced functional abilities are significant impairments, especially in the moderate stages of the disease. Two studies have evaluated the effectiveness of the Alexander technique in PD. A preliminary study to evaluate the effect of the Alexander technique on the management of disability and depressed mood in PD patients reported significant improvements in depression, positive body concept, and performance of daily activities (83). In a randomized, controlled study, the Alexander technique was conducted for 93 PD patients who were divided into a treatment group and a control group who received massage. The results showed significant improvement of the Self-Assessment PD Disability Scale and the Attitudes to Self Scale in the Alexander technique group. Patients in the treatment group were also less depressed (84). The results of these studies suggest that the Alexander technique may be useful to improve mood and disability. However, more studies are needed to investigate its effects on motor function and posture.

Trager Therapy

Trager therapy or Trager Psychophysical Integration was developed by Dr. Milton Trager in the United States and is aimed to be a gentle treatment to help patients to re-integrate the body and mind. This manipulation is a mind–body approach to movement education that is not concerned with the movement of particular muscles and joints, but uses the perception of motion in one's muscles and joints to create positive feelings. The light touch technique such as rocking and stretching helps the body to enter a state of profound relaxation, which is thought to facilitate the release of deep-seated patterns of physical and mental tension created unconsciously by past traumas and experiences. When the body becomes more relaxed, physical mobility is also improved.

The Trager approach can either be administered to patients who passively receive the movement therapy while lying on a padded table or patients may be taught to actively discover the free and proper movement by themselves called Mentastics. In PD patients, gentle stimulation can improve the coordination patterns required for fine motor movements (85).

Although there are a number of medical centers that use the Trager therapy as a CAM for PD, there is limited research data available. A pilot study attempted to quantify the changes of evoked stretch responses, which are electromyographic bursts when a subject's hand is passively flexed and extended, before and after Trager therapy. The results showed a reduction in evoked stretch responses lasting up to 11 minutes after therapy suggesting that Trager therapy may benefit rigidity in PD patients and that an objective evaluation of such therapy was possible (86).

Osteopathy
Osteopathy is a U.S.-originated holistic approach where practitioners use gentle touch and/or high-velocity manipulation to restore mobility and balance of the body and enhance the ability of self-healing. It is commonly used in patients with bone, joint, and muscular diseases. In contrast to chiropractics that mainly focuses on realignment of joints, osteopathy focuses on the soft tissue treatment. There are four principles of osteopathy:

1. The body is an integrated unit of mind, body, and spirit.
2. The body has self-regulatory mechanisms that can defend, repair, and remodel itself.
3. Body structures and their functions are interrelated.
4. Rational therapy is based on consideration of the first three principles.

The classification of osteopathic methods can be categorized as active or passive and direct or indirect in nature (87).

The main aim of this therapy is to improve locomotion and wellbeing. Although this manipulative therapy has no direct effect on the imbalance and rigidity caused by degeneration of dopaminergic neurons in PD, its effects in relieving pain and muscle spasms may be helpful to promote circulatory and lymphatic function. Only one study of osteopathy in PD patients has been performed to evaluate the effectiveness of this therapy on gait. The results showed a significant increase in stride length, cadence, and the maximum velocity of upper and lower extremities after osteopathy treatment. However, it was not clear how long these changes would last in treated patients (88).

Mind and Emotional Therapy
The concept of the mind is understood in different ways by different traditions, but the most widely accepted definition of the mind is that it is a state of human potential constituted by conscious experience, intelligent thought, and occasionally, subconscious experience. Common attributes of the mind include perception, reason,

imagination, memory, emotion, attention, and a capacity for communication. In 1637, Descartes, the French philosopher articulated the view that the body was a form of machine that was indivisible from the mind. In conventional medicine, the mind and body are considered to be intricately interconnected so that doctors should not only be concerned with treating a particular illness, but instead the whole person.

Among PD patients, many forms of mind and emotional therapy have been used as CAMs. Some of these modalities have been scientifically studied to evaluate the efficacy for motor or nonmotor symptoms of PD. However, most of these studies have been pilot studies or small controlled trials.

Psychotherapy

Psychotherapy is a general term referring to any form of therapeutic interaction or treatment contract between a trained professional and a client, patient, family, couple, or group where the problems addressed are psychological in nature. The process always includes counseling. Whether treating mental and emotional disorders or promoting self-awareness, psychotherapy, and counseling offer the opportunity for individuals to understand and resolve difficult thoughts, feelings, and situations by talking about them with a skilled listener. Psychotherapists employ a range of techniques based on experiential relationship building, dialogue, communication, and behavior change that are designed to improve the mental health of a client or patient, or to improve group relationships (such as in a family).

In addition to motor problems, PD patients often have neuropsychiatric problems that require therapeutic intervention. In clinical practice, psychotherapy and counseling play an important role as nonpharmacological treatments to resolve these problems. These nonpharmacological therapies are often used alongside specific psychiatric medications to manage the emotional disturbances and behavioral problems that afflict PD patients. Some examples of such a therapeutic approach include the management of depression (89), psychosis (90), and pathological gambling (91). Despite the common use of psychotherapy by doctors and patients, there are a few studies that have evaluated the effectiveness of such therapy for depression and other neuropsychiatric symptoms in PD patients.

A controlled trial evaluated the effectiveness of group psychotherapy in improving the quality of life and reducing the symptoms of anxiety and depression in 16 PD patients who were randomized into an experimental and control group. This study concluded that there were positive changes in depression, anxiety, and quality of life in patients in the psychotherapy group compared with the control group (92).

In another randomized, controlled trial on the use of cognitive–behavioral therapy (CBT) for the management of depression in PD, CBT was compared with clinical monitoring. This study found CBT to be associated with significant improvements in all clinician-rated and self-reported measures of depression. The CBT group also reported greater improvements in quality of life, coping, and anxiety as well as less motor decline (93).

Music Therapy

Music and dance are activities that people commonly participate in for relaxation and exercise. These activities are considered to be alternative forms of the nonverbal communication that enable individuals to express their feelings and emotions.

Music therapy (MT) has been developed in medicine to help patients with mental illnesses, psychological disorders, pain relief, and in terminal illnesses since the 1940s. During MT, the therapist may work with individuals or groups using active or passive forms of therapy. Active MT involves the improvisation of music by therapists and patients, who play an active part by using instruments and their own voices to obtain a motor or emotional response. Passive MT involves the use of music to calm a patient, so that they may enter a state of mental relaxation.

A randomized, controlled, single-blinded study evaluated 32 PD patients who received weekly sessions of either MT or physical therapy for three months. This study found that patients who received MT had significant improvements in motor function (especially bradykinesia), emotional functions, ADLs, and quality of life. The authors proposed that MT be included in PD rehabilitation programs (94).

Theater Therapy

Although music therapy revealed positive effects on motor symptoms, nonmotor symptoms and the quality of life in patients with PD, these changes were not persistent. The motor and emotional improvements in the study above disappeared two months after completion of MT. Theater therapy (TT), which shares some features with active music therapy, could have a more lasting effect than MT. This is because TT is thought to be more intensive in nature and requires patients to control their bodies and minds to represent their character's emotions during their performances.

A randomized, controlled, single-blinded study was performed on 20 PD patients for three years. Patients were randomly assigned to either an active theater program or to physiotherapy (control group). Patients who received TT had significant improvements in most of the nonmotor clinical scales used in the study (i.e., PDQ-39, Schwab and England scale, Hamilton depression scale), and to a lesser extent, the UPDRS motor scale. The authors suggested that TT is a valid CAM for PD (95).

Bright Light Therapy

Medical science has come to recognize the important role light plays in the regulation of the body's biological clock, which controls sleep, hormone production, and other functions. Bright light therapy (BLT) has been mainly used to treat skin conditions such as psoriasis and is proposed to be the treatment of choice for seasonal affective disorders, depression, insomnia, and sleep disturbances. Generally, a practitioner of BLT will place a patient under a fluorescent full spectrum or bright white light for up to an hour a day, depending on a patient's condition.

When light enters the eyes, it stimulates nerve impulses to the hypothalamus. These nerve impulses travel to the pineal gland, which regulates hormonal balance, including serotonin and melatonin. Release of melatonin is inhibited by retinal exposure to light and stimulated in the darkness. Melatonin controls sleep pattern by working as a chronological pacemaker and signaling the environment light/dark cycle to the brain. In PD patients, fluorodopa PET studies revealed pineal dysfunction and disturbance of melatonin secretion patterns (96). In addition, higher levels of melatonin were found in PD patients compared with healthy controls, and their levels returned to normal after stimulation of the internal globus pallidus (97). A number of observations indicate that melatonin might be unfavorable in PD due to its suppression of dopamine release in the striatum (98,99). In the rat model of PD, pinealectomy or constant light resulted in improvement of PD symptoms as a result of reduced melatonin release (100). These studies suggest that increased melatonin levels worsen PD symptoms, and light therapy with resultant reduction of melatonin levels alleviates the symptoms of PD.

To test the above hypothesis, a randomized, placebo-controlled, double-blind study in 36 PD patients who received BLT for 15 days in the morning, 30 minutes daily was conducted. Illuminance was 7.500 lux in the active treatment group and 950 lux in the placebo group. Although group differences were small, BLT led to significant improvements in tremor; UPDRS mentation, ADLs, and other complications scores; and depression in the active treatment group, but not in the placebo group. BLT was very well tolerated. Follow-up studies in more advanced patient populations employing longer treatment durations are warranted (101).

Relaxation Therapy

Relaxation therapy is any method, procedure, or activity that enables a person to attain a state of enhanced calmness or to reduce levels of anxiety, stress, or anger. Relaxation techniques are often employed as a component of stress management programs. It can decrease muscle tension, lower blood pressure, and slow down heart and respiratory rates. The various relaxation techniques available include breathing exercises, meditation, biofeedback, and Yoga. Visualization is another form of relaxation therapy where patients imagine positive images and outcomes to specific situations. This technique may be performed by patients alone or assisted by a practitioner and is known as relaxation-guided imagery (RGI).

In a pilot study, 20 PD patients with moderate-to-severe tremor participated in sessions where different relaxation techniques were implemented. Tremor was objectively monitored using an accelerometer. RGI dramatically decreased tremor in all 20 patients. In 15 patients, RGI completely abolished tremor for 1–13 minutes. Patients on RGI reported improvements lasting 2–14 hours. Relaxing music significantly reduced tremor, but to a smaller degree than RGI, while self-relaxation had no significant effect on tremor. This study suggested that RGI can supplement conventional medical treatments for tremor in patients with PD (102).

CONCLUSION

The use of CAM is widespread in PD as it is a neurodegenerative disease for which there is currently no cure. Many patients and caregivers turn to CAM in the hope of finding ways to retard the disease progression, avoid or minimize the use of medications, or to augment the effects of conventional therapy. Unfortunately many CAM are not backed with the scientific evidence that is necessary for physicians to comfortably endorse or recommend their use. For medicinal therapies, there is a need for well-designed clinical trials to evaluate their effectiveness. In the areas of manipulative, touch, mind, and emotional therapies, there are additional challenges in the design of clinical trials. This is because of the difficulty in ensuring adequate blinding of patients to the treatment received, and the selection of suitable controls for such studies. Innovative solutions to overcome these challenges are needed.

In addition to these challenges, there is also the issue of the placebo effect that exists in PD. Studies have found that a positive response is seen in up to 50%

of PD patients who receive placebo treatment. The response is more pronounced with invasive procedures and advanced disease. This effect is thought to occur through dopamine pathways that mediate reward (103). It is therefore not surprising that many patients report benefit after having undergone CAM. Some physicians are of the view that as long as patients find a benefit in CAM and if the therapy does not result in any major side effects, then patients should be encouraged to continue receiving the therapy. Such a view should be balanced against the cost of the CAM, and the possible noncompliance to conventional proven medications and therapies.

As physicians and healthcare professionals, we should keep the channels of communication open with our patients and caregivers with regard to the use of CAM. Patients and caregivers should not fear discussing the use of CAM with healthcare professionals. In addition, we need to keep an open mind to the use of CAM, and not be judgmental in our approach. It is useful to bear in mind that a lack of evidence does not equate to a lack of benefit to patients. Ultimately, our goal is to holistically manage our patients and to maximize their function in the areas of the body, mind, and soul.

REFERENCES

1. Eisenberg DM, Davis RB, Ettner SL, et al. Trends in alternative medicine use in the United States, 1990–1997: results of a follow-up national survey. JAMA 1998; 280: 1569–75.
2. Ernest E. The role of complementary and alternative medicine. BMJ 2000; 321: 1133–5.
3. Woodham A, Peters D, Pietroni P. What is complementary medicine? In: Benson C, Beresford T, Weil C, Graville N, Chakraverty M, Martin A, eds. Encyclopedia of Natural Healing. London: A Dorling Kindersley Book, 2000: 11–13.
4. Rajendran PR, Thompson RE, Reich SG. The use of alternative therapies by patients with Parkinson's disease. Neurology 2001; 57: 790–4.
5. Ferry P, Johnson M, Wallis P. Use of complementary therapies and non-prescribed medication in patients with Parkinson's disease. Postgrad Med J 2002; 78: 612–14.
6. Tan LC, Lau PN, Jamora RD, et al. Use of complementary therapies in patients with Parkinson's disease in Singapore. Mov Disord 2006; 21: 86–9.
7. Pecci C, Rivas MJ, Moretti CM, et al. Use of complementary and alternative therapies in outpatients with Parkinson's disease in Argentina. Mov Disord 2010; 25: 2094–8.
8. Kim SR, Lee TY, Kim MS, et al. Use of complementary and alternative medicine by Korean patients with Parkinson's disease. Clin Neurol Neurosurg 2009; 111: 156–60.
9. Gasior M, Rogawski MA, Hartman AL. Neuroprotective and disease-modifying effects of the ketogenic diet. Behav Pharmacol 2006; 17: 431–9.
10. de Lau LM, Bornebroek M, Witteman JC, et al. Dietary fatty acids and the risk of Parkinson disease: the Rotterdam study. Neurology 2005; 64: 2040–5.
11. Vanitallie TB, Nonas C, Di Rocco A, et al. Treatment of Parkinson disease with diet-induced hyperketonemia: a feasibility study. Neurology 2005; 64: 728–30.
12. Wolfrath SC, Borenstein AR, Schwartz S, et al. Use of nutritional supplements in Parkinson's disease patients. Mov Disord 2006; 21: 1098–101.
13. Férnandez-Calle P, Molina JA, Jiménez-Jiménez FJ, et al. Serum levels of alpha-tocopherol (vitamin E) in Parkinson's disease. Neurology 1992; 42: 1064–6.
14. Morens DM, Grandinetti A, Waslien CI, et al. Case-control study of idiopathic Parkinson's disease and dietary vitamin E intake. Neurology 1996; 46: 1270–4.
15. Shoulson I, Oakes D, Fahn S, et al. Parkinson Study Group. Impact of sustained deprenyl (selegiline) in levodopa-treated Parkinson's disease: a randomized placebo-controlled extension of the deprenyl and tocopherol antioxidative therapy of parkinsonism trial. Ann Neurol 2002; 51: 604–12.
16. Fahn S. A pilot trial of high-dose alpha-tocopherol and ascorbate in early Parkinson's disease. Ann Neurol 1992; 32(Suppl): S128–32.

17. de Rijk MC, Breteler MM, den Breeijen JH, et al. Dietary antioxidants and Parkinson disease. The Rotterdam Study. Arch Neurol 1997; 54: 762–5.
18. Etminan M, Gill SS, Samii A. Intake of vitamin E, vitamin C, and carotenoids and the risk of Parkinson's disease: a meta-analysis. Lancet Neurol 2005; 4: 362–5.
19. Suchowersky O, Gronseth G, Perlmutter J, et al. Quality Standards Subcommittee of the American Academy of Neurology. Practice parameter: neuroprotective strategies and alternative therapies for Parkinson disease (an evidence-based review): report of the quality standards Subcommittee of the American Academy of Neurology. Neurology 2006; 66: 976–82.
20. Mitsumoto Y. Mitochondrial nutrition as a strategy for Neuroprotection in Parkinson's disease-research focus in the department of alternative medicine and experimental therapeutics at Hokuriku University. eCAM 2007; 4: 263–5.
21. Shults CW, Oakes D, Kieburtz K, et al. Effects of coenzyme Q10 in early Parkinson disease: evidence of slowing of the functional decline. Arch Neurol 2002; 59: 1541–50.
22. [Available from: http://www.parkinson-study-group.org/parkinson-research/clinical-trials-in-progess]
23. Woodham A, Peters D, Moothy NS. Ayurveda. In: Benson C, Beresford T, Weil C, Graville N, Chakraverty M, Martin A, eds. Encyclopedia of Natural Healing. London: A Dorling Kindersley Book, 2000: 144–7.
24. Manyam BV, Sánchez-Ramos JR. Traditional and complementary therapies in Parkinson's disease. Adv Neurol 1999; 80: 565–74.
25. Nagashayana N, Sankarankutty P, Nampoothiri MR, et al. Association of L-DOPA with recovery following Ayurveda medication in Parkinson's disease. J Neurol Sci 2001; 184: 89–92.
26. Manyam BV, Dhanasekaran M, Hare TA. Effect of antiparkinson drug HP-200 (Mucuna pruriens) on the central monoaminergic neurotransmitters. Phytother Res 2004; 18: 97–101.
27. Tharakan B, Dhanasekaran M, Mize-Berge J. Anti-Parkinson botanical Mucuna pruriens prevents levodopa induced plasmid and genomic DNA damage. Phytother Res 2007; 21: 1124–6.
28. Dhanasekaran M, Tharakan B, Manyam BV. AntiParkinson's drug–Mucuna pruriens shows antioxidant and metal chelating activity. Phytother Res 2008; 22: 6–11.
29. Lieu CA, Kunselman AR, Manyam BV. A water extract of Mucuna pruriens provides long-term amelioration of parkinsonism with reduced risk for dyskinesias. Parkinsonism Relat Disord 2010; 16: 458–65.
30. Parkinson's Disease Study Group. An alternative medicine treatment for Parkinson's disease: results of a multicenter clinical trial. HP-200 in Parkinson's Disease Study Group. J Altern Complement Med 1995; 1: 249–55.
31. Katzenschlager R, Evans A, Manson A, et al. Mucuna pruriens in Parkinson's disease: a double blind clinical and pharmacological study. J Neurol Neurosurg Psychiatry 2004; 75: 1672–7.
32. Chen LW, Wang YQ, Wei LC, et al. Chinese herbs and herbal extracts for neuroprotection of dopaminergic neurons and potential therapeutic treatment of Parkinson's disease. CNS Neurol Disord Drug Targets 2007; 6: 273–81.
33. Chung V, Liu L, Bian Z, et al. Efficacy and safety of herbal medicines for idiopathic Parkinson's disease: a systematic review. Mov Disord 2006; 21: 1709–15.
34. Kum WF, Durairajan SS, Bian ZX, et al. Treatment of idiopathic Parkinson's disease with traditional chinese herbal medicine: a randomized placebo-controlled pilot clinical study. Evid Based Complement Alternat Med 2011; 2011: 724353.
35. Pan W, Kwak S, Liu Y, et al. Traditional chinese medicine improves activities of daily living in Parkinson's disease. Parkinsons Dis 2011; 2011: 789506.
36. Zhao GH, Meng QG, Yu XD, et al. A multi-centered randomized double-blinded controlled clinical study on efficacy of gulling pa'an capsule in treating Parkinson's disease [in Chinese]. Chin J Integr Tradit West Med 2009; 29: 590–4.
37. Yang MH, Li M, Dou YQ, et al. Effects of bushen huoxue granule on motor function in patients with parkinson's disease: a multicenter, randomized, double-blind and placebo-controlled trial [in Chinese]. J Chin Integr Med 2010; 8: 231–7.

38. Yuan CX, Zhi HP, Chen SZ, et al. Clinical multicenter randomized controlled study on treatment of Parkinson's disease with shudi pingchan decoction and western medicine [in Chinese]. Shanghai J Tradit Chin Med 2010; 44: 3–6.
39. Mandel S, Maor G, Youdim MBH. Iron and a-synuclein in the substantia nigra of MPTP-treated mice. Effect of neuroprotective drugs R-apomorphine and green tea polyphenol (−)-epigallocatechin-3-gallate. J Mol Neurosci 2004; 24: 401–16.
40. Datla KP, Zbarsky V, Rai D, et al. Short-term supplementation with plant extracts rich in flavonoids protect nigrostriatal dopaminergic neurons in a rat model of Parkinson's disease. J Am Coll Nut 2007; 26: 341–9.
41. Nie G, Cao Y, Zhao B. Protective effects of green tea polyphenols and their major component, (-)-epigallocatechin-3-gallate (EGCG), on 6-hydroxydopamine-induced apoptosis in PC12 cells. Redox Rep 2002; 7: 171–7.
42. Perez CA, Wei Y, Guo M. Iron-binding and anti-Fenton properties of baicalein and baicalin. J Inorg Biochem 2009; 103: 326–32.
43. Zbarsky V, Datla KP, Parkar S, et al. Neuroprotective properties of the natural phenolic antioxidants curcumin and naringenin but not quercetin and fisetin in a 6-OHDA model of Parkinson's disease. Free Radical Res 2005; 39: 1119–25.
44. Srichairatanakool S, Thephinlap C, Phisalaphong C, et al. Curcumin contributes to in vitro removal of non-transferrin bound iron by deferiprone and desferrioxamine in thalassemic plasma. Med Chem 2007; 3: 469–74.
45. Lopes GKB, Schulman HM, Hermes-Lima M. Polyphenol tannic acid inhibits hydroxyl radical formation from Fenton reaction by complexing ferrous ions. Biochim Biophys Acta 1999; 1472: 142–52.
46. Ramassamy C. Emerging role of polyphenolic compounds in the treatment of neurodegenerative diseases: a review of their intracellular targets. Eur J Pharmacol 2006; 545: 51–64.
47. Triantafyllou A, Liakos P, Tsakalof A, et al. The flavonoid quercetin induces hypoxiainducible factor-1a (HIF-1a) and inhibits cell proliferation by depleting intracellular iron. Free Radical Res 2007; 41: 342–56.
48. Rabey JM, Vered Y, Shabtai H, et al. Broad bean (Vicia faba) consumption and Parkinson's disease. Adv Neurol 1993; 60: 681–4.
49. Yang SF, Wu Q, Sun AS, et al. Protective effect and mechanism of Ginkgo biloba leaf extracts for Parkinson disease induced by 1-methyl-4-phenyl-1,2,3,6-tetrahydropyridine. Acta Pharmacol Sin 2001; 22: 1089–93.
50. Chen XC, Zhu YG, Zhu LA, et al. Ginsenoside Rg1 attenuates dopamine-induced apoptosis in PC12 cells by suppressing oxidative stress. Eur J Pharmacol 2003; 473: 1–7.
51. Chen XC, Chen Y, Zhu YG, et al. Protective effect of ginsenoside Rg1 on MPTP-induced apoptosis in mouse substantia nigra neurons and its mechanisms. Acta Pharmacol Sin 2002; 23: 829–34.
52. Chen XC, Zhou YC, Chen Y, et al. Ginsenoside Rg1 reduces MPTP-induced substantia nigra neuron loss by suppressing oxidative stress. Acta Pharmacol Sin 2005; 26: 56–62.
53. Van Kampen J, Robertson H, Hagg T, et al. Neuroprotective actions of the ginseng extract G115 in two rodent models of Parkinson's disease. Exp Neurol 2003; 184: 521–9.
54. Woodham A, Peters D, Geddes N. Homeopathy. In: Benson C, Beresford T, Weil C, Graville N, Chakraverty M, Martin A, eds. Encyclopedia of Natural Healing. London: A Dorling Kindersley Book, 2000: 126–30.
55. Ernst E. Musculoskeletal conditions and complementary/alternative medicine. Best Pract Res Clin Rheumatol 2004; 18: 539–56.
56. Frenkel M. Homeopathy in cancer care. Altern Ther Health Med 2010; 16: 12–16.
57. Simonart T, Kabagabo C, De Maertelaer V. Homoeopathic remedies in dermatology: a systematic review of controlled clinical trials. Br J Dermatol 2011; 165: 897–905.
58. Davidson JR, Crawford C, Ives JA, et al. Homeopathic treatments in psychiatry: a systematic review of randomized placebo-controlled studies. J Clin Psychiatry 2011; 72: 795–805.
59. Wang Y, Lin XM, Zheng GQ. Traditional Chinese medicine for Parkinson's disease in China and beyond. J Altern Complement Med 2011; 17: 385–8.

60. Shulman LM, Wen X, Weiner WJ, et al. Acupuncture Therapy for the Symptoms of Parkinson's Disease. Mov Disord 2002; 17: 799–802.

61. Wang X, Liang XB, Li FQ, et al. Therapeutic strategies for Parkinson's disease: the ancient meets the future–traditional Chinese herbal medicine, electroacupuncture, gene therapy and stem cells. Neurochem Res 2008; 33: 1956–63.

62. Joh TH, Park HJ, Kim SN, et al. Recent development of acupuncture on Parkinson's disease. Neurol Res 2010; 32: 5–9.

63. Liang XB, Liu XY, Li FQ, et al. Long-term high-frequency electro-acupuncture stimulation prevents neuronal degeneration and up-regulates BDNF mRNA in the substantia nigra and ventral tegmental area following medial forebrain bundle axotomy. Brain Res Mol Brain Res 2002; 108: 51–9.

64. Liang XB, Luo Y, Liu XY, et al. Electro-acupuncture improves behavior and upregulates GDNF mRNA in MFB transected rats. Neuroreport 2003; 14: 1177–81.

65. Qian ZN, Gu ZL, Pan JX. Effects of acupuncture analgesia on the monoamine transmitters levels in the striata and spinal cords in rats. [In Chinese]. Zhen Ci Yan Jiu 1985; 10: 199–201.

66. Kang JM, Park HJ, Choi YG, et al. Acupuncture inhibits microglial activation and inflammatory events in the MPTP-induced mouse model. Brain Res 2007; 1131: 211–19.

67. Lee MS, Shin BC, Kong JC, et al. Effectiveness of acupuncture for Parkinson's disease: a systematic review. Mov Disord 2008; 23: 1505–15.

68. Lam YC, Kum WF, Durairajan SS, et al. Efficacy and safety of acupuncture for idiopathic Parkinson's disease: a systematic review. J Altern Complement Med 2008; 14: 663–71.

69. Napadow V, Ahn A, Longhurst J, et al. The status and future of acupuncture mechanism research. J Altern Complement Med 2008; 14: 861–9.

70. Ding SQ. Clinical observation on treatment of 87 cases of Parkinson's disease with combined acupuncture and cupping therapies [in Chinese]. Liaoning J Tradit Chin Med 2006; 33: 737.

71. Paterson C, Allen JA, Browning M, et al. A pilot study of therapeutic massage for people with Parkinson's disease: the added value of user involvement. Complement Ther Clin Pract 2005; 11: 161–71.

72. Craig LH, Svircev A, Haber M, et al. Controlled pilot study of the effects of neuromuscular therapy in patients with Parkinson's disease. Mov Disord 2006; 21: 2127–33.

73. Elster EL. Upper cervical chiropractic management of a patient with Parkinson's disease: a case report. J Manipulative Physiol Ther 2000; 23: 573–7.

74. Burton RR. Parkinson's disease without tremor masquerading as mechanical back pain; a case report. J Can Chiropr Assoc 2008; 52: 185–92.

75. Reflexology association of Canada. Definition and Scope Standards of Practice for Reflexology/Reflexologist. Standards of Practice, Code of Ethics, Code of Conduct. 2005: 1–6.

76. Woodham A, Peters D, Parker C. Reflexology. In: Benson C, Beresford T, Weil C, Graville N, Chakraverty M, Martin A, eds. Encyclopedia of Natural Healing. London: A Dorling Kindersley Book, 2000: 66–9.

77. Ernst E, Posadzki P, Lee MS. Reflexology: an update of a systematic review of randomised clinical trials. Maturitas 2011; 68: 116–20.

78. Johns C, Blake D, Sinclair A. Can reflexology maintain or improve the well-being of people with Parkinson's disease? Complement Ther Clin Pract 2010; 16: 96–100.

79. Gedney JJ, Glover TL, Fillingim RB. Sensory and affective pain discrimination after inhalation of essential oils. Psychosom Med 2004; 66: 599–606.

80. Woodham A, Peters D, Parkes C. Reiki. In: Benson C, Beresford T, Weil C, Graville N, Chakraverty M, Martin A, eds. Encyclopedia of Natural Healing. London: A Dorling Kindersley Book, 2000: 107.

81. Lee MS, Pittler MH, Ernst E. Effects of reiki in clinical practice: a systematic review of randomised clinical trials. Int J Clin Pract 2008; 62: 947–54.

82. Woodham A, Peters D, Kelly K, et al. The Alexander technique. In: Benson C, Beresford T, Weil C, Graville N, Chakraverty M, Martin A, eds. Encyclopedia of Natural Healing. London: A Dorling Kindersley Book, 2000: 86–7.

83. Stallibrass C. An evaluation of the Alexander technique for the management of disability in Parkinson's disease–a preliminary study. Clin Rehabil 1997; 11: 8–12.
84. Stallibrass C, Sissons P, Chalmers C. Randomized controlled trial of the Alexander technique for idiopathic Parkinson's disease. Clin Rehabil 2002; 16: 695–708.
85. Woodham A, Peters D, Scholl B. Tragerwork. In: Benson C, Beresford T, Weil C, Graville N, Chakraverty M, Martin A, eds. Encyclopedia of Natural Healing. London: A Dorling Kindersley Book, 2000: 88.
86. Duval C, Lafontaine D, Hébert J, et al. The effect of Trager therapy on the level of evoked stretch responses in patients with Parkinson's disease and rigidity. J Manipulative Physiol Ther 2002; 25: 455–64.
87. Woodham A, Peters D, Bon JL. Osteopathy. In: Benson C, Beresford T, Weil C, Graville N, Chakraverty M, Martin A, eds. Encyclopedia of Natural Healing. London: A Dorling Kindersley Book, 2000: 76–81.
88. Wells MR, Giantinoto S, D'Agate D, et al. Standard osteopathic manipulative treatment acutely improves gait performance in patients with Parkinson's disease. J Am Osteopath Assoc 1999; 99: 92–8.
89. Sawabini KA, Watts RL. Treatment of depression in Parkinson's disease. Parkinsonism Relat Disord 2004; 10: S37–41.
90. Poewe W, Seppi K. Treatment options for depression and psychosis in Parkinson's disease. J Neurol 2001; 248: III12–21.
91. Gallagher DA, O'Sullivan SS, Evans AH, et al. Pathological gambling in Parkinson's disease: risk factors and differences from dopamine dysregulation. An analysis of published case series. Mov Disord 2007; 22: 1757–63.
92. Sproesser E, Viana MA, Quagliato EM, et al. The effect of psychotherapy in patients with PD: a controlled study. Parkinsonism Relat Disord 2010; 16: 298–300.
93. Dobkin RD, Menza M, Allen LA, et al. Cognitive-behavioral therapy for depression in Parkinson's disease: a randomized, controlled trial. Am J Psychiatry 2011; 168: 1066–74.
94. Pacchetti C, Mancini F, Aglieri R, et al. Active music therapy in Parkinson's disease: an integrative method for motor and emotional rehabilitation. Psychosom Med 2000; 62: 386–93.
95. Modugno N, Iaconelli S, Fiorlli M, et al. Active theater as a complementary therapy for Parkinson's disease rehabilitation: a pilot study. ScientificWorldJournal 2010; 10: 2301–13.
96. Bordet R, Devos D, Brique S, et al. Study of circadian melatonin secretion pattern at different stages of Parkinson's disease. Clin Neuropharmacol 2003; 26: 65–72.
97. Catala MD, Canete-Nicolas C, Iradi A, et al. Melatonin levels in Parkinson's disease: drug therapy versus electrical stimulation of the internal globus pallidus. Exp Gerontol 1997; 32: 553–8.
98. Zisapel N. Melatonin-dopamine interactions: from basic neurochemistry to a clinical setting. Cell Mol Neurobiol 2001; 21: 605–16.
99. Willis GL, Armstrong SM. A therapeutic role for melatonin antagonism in experimental models of Parkinson's disease. Physiol Behav 1999; 66: 785–95.
100. Willis GL, Robertson AD. Recovery of experimental Parkinson's disease with the melatonin analogues ML-23 and S-20928 in a chronic, bilateral 6-OHDA model: a new mechanism involving antagonism of the melatonin receptor. Pharmacol Biochem Behav 2004; 79: 413–29.
101. Paus S, Schmitz-Hübsch T, Wüllner U, et al. Bright light therapy in Parkinson's disease: a pilot study. Mov Disord 2007; 22: 1495–8.
102. Schlesinger I, Benyakov O, Erikh I, et al. Parkinson's disease tremor is diminished with relaxation guided imagery. Mov Disord 2009; 24: 2059–62.
103. Diederich NJ, Goetz CG. The placebo treatments in neurosciences: new insights from clinical and neuroimaging studies. Neurology 2008; 71: 677–84.

Index

AAAD. *See* Aromatic amino acid
    decarboxylase
Abalative surgery, 551
  speech and swallowing disorders,
    554–557
    collagen augmentation, 552
    cricopharyngeal myotomy, 552
    pallidotomy, 551
    thalamotomy and subthalamotomy, 551
    voice treatment, 554–560
Ablation, 158
Acoustic analyses, speech and voice
    disorders and, 540–541
Action Selection/Focused Attention theory,
    259, 260
Activities of daily living, 574
Actos®. *See* Pioglitazone
ADAGIO study, 438–439
Adenosine A_{2A} receptor antagonists,
    469–470
  istradefylline, 469
  preladenant, 469–470
Adjusting patient's home environment,
    532–533
ADL. *See* Activities of daily living
ADS-5102, dyskinesia treatment, 470
Advanced Parkinson's disease
  seligiline clinical trials and, 435–436
Adverse effects, rasagiline, 441
Advising and training caregivers, 528
ADX4862, dyskinesia treatment, 470
AFQ056, dyskinesia treatment, 470–471
Alexander technique, 581
Amantadine (Symmetrel®), 373–378
  clinical uses, 374–376
  history, 373
  mechanisms of action, 377–378
  pharmacokinetics and dosing, 373–374
  side effects, 376–377
American Academy of Neurology, 573
An Essay on the Shaking Palsy (Parkinson), 5

Animal models
  genetic models, 293
  invertebrate genetic models, 300
  methamphetamine (METH), 291–292
  multiple system atrophy (MSA), 301
  neurotoxin-induced models
    1-methyl-4-phenyl-1,2,3,
      6-tetrahydropyridine (MPTP),
      286–287
    6-hydroxydopamine, 283–286
    MPTP-lesioned mouse model, 287
    MPTP-lesioned nonhuman primate,
      287–290
    MPTP lesioning in other species,
      290–291
  paraquat (N, N'-dimethyl-4, 4'bipyridium
    dichloride), 292–293
  PD variants, models of, 300
  pharmacological/neurotoxin-induced
    models
    alpha-methyl-para-tyrosine (AMPT),
      282–283
    reserpine, 282
  progressive supranuclear palsy, 302
  rotenone, 292
  spontaneous rodent models, 294
  striatonigral degeneration (SND), 301
  tau-related disorders, 302
  transgenic mouse models, 294–300
    conditional knockout and vector
      targeting, 298–300
    DJ-1 gene (PARK7), 296
    leucine-rich repeat kinase 2 gene
      (LRRK2), 296
    multiple transgenic mouse models, 297
    Nurr1, 297
    other transgenic mice, 297–298
    parkin, 295–296
    phosphatase and tensin
      homolog-induced kinase-1
      (PINK1), 297

An environmentally friendly book printed and bound in England by www.printondemand-worldwide.com

PEFC Certified

This product is
from sustainably
managed forests
and controlled
sources

www.pefc.org

PEFC/16-33-415

®

MIX

Paper from
responsible sources

FSC

www.fsc.org

FSC® C004959

This book is made entirely of sustainable materials; FSC paper for the cover and PEFC paper for the text pages.

#0155 - 031013 - C4 - 234/156/33 [35] - CB